Visual
Nursing

A guide to diseases, skills, and treatments

2nd edition

Visual
Nursing

A guide to diseases, skills, and treatments

2nd edition

Wolters Kluwer | Lippincott Williams & Wilkins
Health

Philadelphia · Baltimore · New York · London
Buenos Aires · Hong Kong · Sydney · Tokyo

Staff

Publisher
J. Christopher Burghardt

Clinical Director
Joan M. Robinson, RN, MSN

Clinical Project Manager
Lorraine Hallowell, RN, BSN, RVS

Clinical Editor
Kate Stout, RN, MSN

Product Director
David Moreau

Product Manager
Rosanne Hallowell

Editor
Karen C. Comerford

Copy Editor
Linda Hager

Editorial Assistants
Karen J. Kirk, Jeri O'Shea,
Linda K. Ruhf

Art Director
Elaine Kasmer

Vendor Manager
Cynthia Rudy

Manufacturing Manager
Beth J. Welsh

Production and Indexing Services
Aptara, Inc.

Printed in China

VN011011-020513

Library of Congress Cataloging-in-Publication Data
Visual nursing : a guide to diseases, skills, and treatments. — 2nd ed.
    p. ; cm.
  Includes bibliographical references and index.
  ISBN 978-1-60913-650-5 (alk. paper)
  1. Nursing—Atlases. I. Lippincott Williams & Wilkins.
  [DNLM: 1. Nursing Care—Atlases. 2. Nursing Assessment—Atlases. WY 17]
  RT57.V57 2012
  610.73022′3—dc23
                                    2011022700

Contents

Contributors and consultants

Michael A. Carter,
DNSc, DNP, FAAN, FNP/GNP-BC
University Distinguished Professor
University of Tennessee Health
   Science Center
Memphis

Sharon Conner,
RN, MSN, CMSRN
Clinical Education Consultant
Integris Health
Oklahoma City

Anne W. Davis,
RN, PhD
Chair and Professor, Department
   of Nursing
East Central University
Ada, Okla.

Kathleen M. Lamaute,
EdD, FNP-BC, NEA-BC, CNE
Associate Professor
Molloy College
Rockville Centre, N.Y.

Anabel Quintanar,
RN, MSN, PHN
RN/Nursing Supervisor
Lompoc Valley Medical Center
Lompoc, Calif.

Donna Scemons,
PhD, FNP-BC, CNS, CWOCN
President
Healthcare Systems
Castaic, Calif.

Concha Carrillo Sitter,
MS, APN, FNP-BC, CGRN
Nurse Practitioner, Gastroenterology
Sterling Rock Falls Clinic
Sterling, Ill.

Kathy L. Stallcup,
RN, MSN, CCRN
Clinical Education Consultant
INTEGRIS Southwest Medical Center
Oklahoma City

Angela R. Starkweather,
PhD, ANP-C, CNRN
Assistant Professor
Virginia Commonwealth University
   School of Nursing
Richmond

Sharon Wing,
PhDc, RN-CNL
Associate Professor
Cleveland State University School of
   Nursing
Cleveland, Ohio

Foreword

Vivid images can be understood and recalled very quickly. Nurses and nursing students providing care for patients with complex diseases and treatments appreciate the value of excellent pictures and illustrations in supporting their continued learning.

Visual Nursing: A Guide to Diseases, Skills, and Treatments, 2nd edition, provides colorful images complemented by full descriptions. Informative photographs, artwork, and other visual aids are used frequently throughout the book to stimulate the reader's curiosity and enhance learning. The striking images in each section help focus attention to the topic; then, those images help simplify concepts and concisely organize text information in ways that promote retaining and recalling the information when it's needed at the bedside.

Chapter 1 brings attention to the assessment skills critical for effective nursing practice. Chapters that follow are organized by body system, with sections on diseases, tests, treatments, and procedures. For each disorder, the related pathophysiology, signs and symptoms, diagnostic tests, treatments and procedures, nursing considerations, and patient teaching points are described. This second edition includes new entries and images for peripheral arterial disease, venous thrombosis, and such interventions as abdominal pressure monitoring, vena cava filters, and aortic stent grafts.

Be sure to look for the "Picturing Patho" images, the "Hands On" procedure prompts, and the "Lesson Plans" summaries throughout the book. The "Picturing Patho" anatomical illustrations and flowcharts show the impact of complicated diseases on the body. The "Hands On" photographs illustrate how to perform nursing procedures and administer treatments using good technique. "Lesson Plans" summarize the most important information for nurses to teach patients and their caregivers.

As a reader, you can take advantage of the connections between images and words in this book to improve your comprehension and learning outcomes. Before you begin to read about a topic, skim through and preview the images in that section. Ask yourself what you should expect to learn and consider what else you might want to know about providing nursing care for patients in that situation.

After reading a section of the book, review the images again. Practice describing aloud what's happening in each anatomical illustration as though you were sharing that information with a colleague or a patient's family. Then, practice describing the procedures you see in the photographs as though you were explaining them to an anxious patient or to a colleague who has never seen the procedure.

Explaining what you see happening in the illustrations can help you clarify how your patients are affected by complicated disease processes. The ways that you and your nurse colleagues reflect to connect the vibrant images and descriptions in this book with your clinical experiences are powerful in promoting your lifelong learning and supporting your delivery of high-quality health care.

Debra Hagler, RN, PhD, ACNS-BC, CNE, ANEF
Clinical Professor & Coordinator
for Teaching Excellence
E3: Evaluation &
Educational Excellence
College of Nursing and
Health Innovation
Arizona State University
Phoenix

Chapter 1
Basic assessment skills

Health history

All assessments involve obtaining two kinds of data: objective and subjective. Objective data are obtained through hearing, touching, smelling, and seeing and are verifiable by someone other than the patient. For example, a red, swollen arm in a patient with arm pain is a kind of data that can be seen and verified by someone besides the patient. Subjective data can't be verified by anyone but the patient; they're gathered solely from the patient's own account—for example, "My stomach hurts" or "I have trouble getting up in the morning."

Here's a tip to help you remember the two types of data: you *observe* objective data, whereas only the *subject* provides subjective data.

Beginning the interview

To make the most of your patient interview, create an environment in which the patient feels comfortable, and use communication strategies to make the interaction most effective.

Asking questions

Questions can be characterized as open-ended or closed.

Open-ended questions

Open-ended questions require the patient to express feelings, opinions, and ideas. They also help gather more information than can be obtained through closed questions. Open-ended questions encourage a good nurse-patient rapport because they show that you're interested in what the patient has to say. Examples of such questions include:
▶ Why did you come to the hospital?
▶ How would you describe the problems you're having with your breathing?
▶ What lung problems, if any, do other members of your family have?

Closed questions

Closed questions elicit one- or two-word or yes-or-no responses. They limit the development of nurse-patient rapport. Closed questions can help "zoom in" on specific points, but they don't provide the patient with an opportunity to elaborate. Examples of closed questions include:
▶ Do you ever get short of breath?
▶ Are you the only one in your family with lung problems?

Interviewing tips

▶ Select a quiet, private setting.
▶ Choose terms carefully and avoid using medical jargon. Speak slowly and clearly.
▶ Use effective communication skills.
▶ Use appropriate body language.
▶ Confirm patient statements to avoid misunderstanding.
▶ Summarize and conclude with "Is there anything else?"

Components of a complete health history

Biographical data

Name _____
Address _____
Date of birth _____

Advance directive explained? ☐ Yes ☐ No
Living will on chart? ☐ Yes ☐ No

Name and phone numbers of two people to call if necessary:

NAME	RELATIONSHIP	PHONE #

Chief complaint

History of present illness
_____
_____

Current medications

DRUG AND DOSE	FREQUENCY	LAST DOSE

Medical history

Allergies
☐ Tape ☐ Iodine ☐ Latex ☐ No known allergies
☐ Drug:_____
☐ Food:_____
☐ Environmental:_____
☐ Blood reaction:_____
☐ Other:_____

Childhood illnesses   DATE
_____
_____

Previous hospitalizations
(Illness, accident or injury, surgery, blood transfusion)   DATE
_____
_____

Health problems   YES NO
Arthritis . . . . ☐ ☐
Blood problem (anemia, sickle cell, clotting, bleeding). ☐ ☐
Cancer . . . . ☐ ☐
Diabetes mellitus . . . . ☐ ☐
Eye problem (cataracts, glaucoma) . . . . ☐ ☐
Heart disease (heart failure, MI, valve disease) . . . . . ☐ ☐
Hiatal hernia. . . . . ☐ ☐
HIV/AIDS . . . . ☐ ☐
Hypertension . . . . ☐ ☐
Kidney problem . . . . ☐ ☐
Liver problem . . . . ☐ ☐
Lung problem (asthma, bronchitis, emphysema, pneumonia, TB, shortness of breath) . . . . ☐ ☐
Stroke . . . . ☐ ☐
Thyroid problem . . . . ☐ ☐
Ulcers (duodenal, peptic) . . . . ☐ ☐
Psychiatric disorder . . . . ☐ ☐

Obstetric history (females)
Last menstrual period
Gravida_____ Para_____
Menopause ☐ Yes ☐ No

Psychosocial history
Coping strategies
_____

Feelings of safety
_____

Social history
Smoke cigarettes? ☐ No ☐ Yes (# packs/day/# years)
Drink alcohol? ☐ No ☐ Yes (type, amount/day)
Use illicit drugs? ☐ No ☐ Yes (type)
Religious and cultural observances:
_____

Activities of daily living
Diet and exercise regimen_____
Elimination patterns_____
Sleep patterns_____
Work and leisure activities_____
Use of safety measures (seat belt, bike helmet, sunscreen)_____

Health maintenance history   DATE
Colonoscopy _____
Dental examination_____
Eye examination_____
Immunizations_____
Mammography_____

Family medical history

Health problems	YES	NO	Family member
Arthritis	☐	☐	
Cancer	☐	☐	
Diabetes mellitus	☐	☐	
Heart disease (heart failure, MI, valve disease)	☐	☐	
Hypertension	☐	☐	
Stroke	☐	☐	

Review of systems

The last part of the health history is a systematic review of each body system to make sure that important symptoms weren't missed. The order of the review of systems is head-to-toe. This helps ensure covering all areas.

Remember when questioning an elderly patient, he may have difficulty hearing or communicating. If the patient is confused or has trouble communicating, seek assistance from a family member for some or all of the health history.

If the patient is a child, direct as many questions as possible to him. Rely on the parents for information if the child is very young.

Here are some key questions to ask the patient about each system:

Head

Do you get headaches? If so, where are they and how painful are they? How often do they occur, and how long do they last? Does anything trigger them, and how do you relieve them? Have you ever had a head injury? Do you have lumps or bumps on your head?

Eyes

When was your last eye examination? Do you wear glasses? Do you have glaucoma, cataracts, or color blindness? Does light bother your eyes? Do you have excessive tearing; blurred vision; double vision; or dry, itchy, burning, inflamed, or swollen eyes? Have you ever had eye surgery? If so, why and when?

Ears

Do you have loss of balance, ringing in your ears, deafness, or poor hearing? Have you ever had ear surgery? If so, why and when? Do you wear a hearing aid? Are you having pain, swelling, or discharge from your ears? If so, has this problem occurred before, and how frequently?

Nose

Have you ever had nasal surgery? If so, why and when? Have you ever had sinusitis or nosebleeds? Do you have nasal problems that impair your ability to smell or that cause breathing difficulties, frequent sneezing, or discharge?

Mouth and throat

Do you have mouth sores, dry mouth, loss of taste, toothache, or bleeding gums? Do you wear dentures and, if so, do they fit? Do you have a sore throat, fever, or chills? How often do you get a sore throat, and have you seen a doctor for this?

Do you have difficulty swallowing? If so, is the problem with solids or liquids? Is it a constant problem or does it accompany a sore throat or another problem? What, if anything, makes it go away?

Neck

Do you have swelling, soreness, lack of movement, stiffness, or pain in your neck? If so, did something specific cause it to happen? How long have you had this symptom? Does anything relieve it or aggravate it?

Skin, hair, and nails

Do you presently have any skin disorders, such as psoriasis? Do you have any rashes, scars, sores, ulcers, or areas with abnormal skin color? Do you have skin growths, such as warts, moles, tumors, or masses? Do you experience skin reactions to hot or cold weather? Have you noticed changes to the amount, texture, or character of your hair? Have you noticed changes in your nails? Do you experience excessive nail splitting, cracking, or breaking?

Respiratory system

Do you ever have shortness of breath? Does anything relieve it or aggravate it? How many pillows do you use at night? Does breathing cause pain or wheezing? Do you have a productive cough? If so, describe the sputum. Do you have night sweats?

Have you ever been treated for pneumonia, asthma, emphysema, or frequent respiratory tract infections? Have you ever had a chest X-ray or tuberculin skin test? If so, when, and what were the results?

Cardiovascular system

Do you ever have chest pain, palpitations, irregular heartbeat, fast heartbeat, shortness of breath, or a persistent cough? If so, what aggravates it or relieves it? Have you ever had an electrocardiogram? If so, when, and what were the results?

Do you have high blood pressure, peripheral vascular disease, swelling of the ankles and hands, varicose veins, cold extremities, or intermittent pain in your legs? Have you experienced dizziness or fainting?

Breast and axilla

Ask women: Do you perform monthly breast self-examinations? Have you noticed a lump, a change in breast contour, breast pain, or discharge from your nipples? Have you ever had breast cancer? If not, has anyone else in your family had it? Have you ever had a mammogram? When, and what were the results?

Ask men: Do you have pain in your breasts? Have you ever noticed lumps or a change in contour?

Gastrointestinal system

Have you had nausea, vomiting, loss of appetite, heartburn, abdominal pain, frequent belching, or passing of gas? Have you lost or gained weight recently? If so, how much? How often do you have a bowel movement, and what color, odor, and consistency are your stools? Have you noticed a change in your regular elimination pattern? Do you use laxatives frequently?

Have you had hemorrhoids, rectal bleeding, hernias, gallbladder disease, or liver disease?

Genitourinary system

Do you have urinary problems, such as burning during urination, incontinence, urgency, retention, reduced urinary flow, or dribbling? Do you get up during the night to urinate? If so, how many times? What color is your urine? Have you ever noticed blood in it? Have you ever been treated for kidney stones?

Reproductive system

Ask women: How old were you when you started menstruating? How often do you get your period, and how long does it usually last? Do you have pain or pass clots? If you're past menopause, at what age did you stop menstruating? If you're in the transitional stage, what symptoms are you experiencing? Have you ever been pregnant? If so, how many times? How many pregnancies resulted in live births? What was the method of birth? How many resulted in miscarriages? Have you had an abortion?

What's your method of birth control? Are you involved in a long-term, monogamous relationship? Have you had vaginal infections or a sexually transmitted disease (STD)? When was your last gynecologic examination and Papanicolaou test? What were the results?

Ask men: Do you perform monthly testicular self-examinations? Have you ever had a prostate examination and if so, when? Have you noticed penile pain, discharge, lesions, or testicular lumps? Which form of birth control do you use? Have you had a vasectomy? Are you involved in a long-term, monogamous relationship? Have you ever had an STD?

Musculoskeletal system

Do you have difficulty walking, sitting, or standing? Are you steady on your feet or do you lose your balance easily? Do you have arthritis, gout, a back injury, muscle weakness, or paralysis? Have you ever had broken bones? If so, which bone and when did the injury occur?

Neurologic system

Have you ever had seizures? Do you ever experience tremors, twitching, numbness, tingling, or loss of sensation in a part of your body? Are you less able to get around than you think you should be?

Endocrine system

Have you been unusually tired lately? Do you feel hungry or thirsty more often than usual? Have you experienced an unexplained weight loss? How well do you tolerate heat or cold? Have you noticed changes in your hair color or texture? Have you been losing your hair? Do you take hormone medications?

Hematologic system

Have you ever been diagnosed with anemia or blood abnormalities? Have you ever had a blood transfusion? If so, did you have an adverse reaction? Do you bruise easily?

Psychological status

Do you ever experience mood swings or memory loss? Do you ever feel anxious, depressed, or unable to concentrate? Are you feeling unusually stressed? Do you ever feel unable to cope? Do you ever feel like hurting yourself? Do you feel safe in your home? Do you fear injury from anyone?

Evaluating a symptom

Your patient is vague in describing his chief complaint. Using interviewing skills, you discover his problem is related to abdominal distention. Now what? This flowchart will help you decide what to do next, using abdominal distention as the patient's chief complaint.

> Ask the patient to identify the symptom that's bothering him.
> He tells you, "My stomach gets bloated."

> Form a first impression. Does the patient's condition alert you to an emergency? For example, does he say the bloating developed suddenly? Does he mention that other signs or symptoms occur with it, such as sweating and light-headedness? (Both are indicators of hypovolemia.)

YES

> Take a brief history to gather more clues. For example, ask the patient if he has severe abdominal pain or difficulty breathing or if he ever had an abdominal injury.

NO

> Now, take a thorough history to get an overview of the patient's condition. Ask him about associated signs or symptoms. Especially note GI disorders that can lead to abdominal distention.

> Perform a focused physical examination to determine the severity of the patient's condition quickly. Check for bruising, lacerations, changes in bowel sounds, or abdominal rigidity.

> Now, thoroughly examine the patient to evaluate the chief sign or symptom and to detect additional signs and symptoms. Place the patient in a recumbent position, and observe for abdominal asymmetry. Inspect the skin, auscultate for bowel sounds, percuss and palpate the abdomen, and measure abdominal girth.

> Evaluate your findings. Are emergency signs or symptoms present, such as abdominal rigidity and abnormal bowel sounds?

YES

> Based on your findings, intervene appropriately to stabilize the patient. Notify the doctor immediately, place the patient in a comfortable position, administer oxygen, and start an I.V. line. GI or nasogastric tube insertion and emergency surgery may be needed.

NO

> Review your findings to consider possible causes, such as cancer, bladder distention, cirrhosis, heart failure, or gastric dilation.

> After the patient's condition is stabilized, review your findings to consider possible causes, such as cancer, bladder distention, cirrhosis, gastric dilation, heart failure, large-bowel obstruction, mesenteric artery occlusion, peritonitis, or trauma.

> Evaluate your findings, and devise an appropriate care plan. Position the patient comfortably, administer analgesics if appropriate, and prepare the patient for diagnostic tests.

Physical assessment

Before starting a physical assessment, assemble the necessary tools. Then perform a general survey to form an initial impression of the patient.

Obtain baseline data including height, weight, and vital signs. This information will direct the rest of the assessment.

Assessment tools

- Cotton balls
- Gloves
- Metric ruler
- Near vision and visual acuity charts
- Ophthalmoscope
- Otoscope
- Penlight
- Percussion hammer
- Safety pins
- Scale with height measurement
- Skin calipers
- Specula (nasal and vaginal)
- Sphygmomanometer
- Stethoscope
- Tape measure (cloth or paper)
- Thermometer
- Tuning fork
- Wooden tongue blade

HANDS ON

 Measuring blood pressure

- Position the patient with his upper arm at heart level and his palm turned up.
- Apply the cuff snugly, 1″ (2.5 cm) above the brachial pulse.
- Position the manometer at your eye level.
- Palpate the brachial or radial pulse with your fingertips while inflating the cuff.
- Inflate the cuff to 30 mm Hg above the point where the pulse disappears.
- Place the bell of your stethoscope over the point where you felt the pulse, as shown in the photo. (Using the bell will help you better hear Korotkoff's sounds, which indicate pulse.)

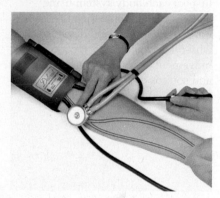

- Release the valve slowly, and note the point at which Korotkoff's sounds reappear. The start of the pulse sound indicates systolic pressure.
- The sounds will become muffled and then disappear. The last Korotkoff's sound you hear indicates the diastolic pressure.

Tips for interpreting vital signs

- Analyze all the patient's vital signs at the same time. Two or more abnormal values may provide clues to the patient's problem. For example, a rapid, thready pulse along with low blood pressure may signal shock.
- If you obtain an abnormal value, take the vital sign again to make sure it's accurate.

- Remember that normal readings vary with the patient's age. For example, temperature decreases with age, and respiratory rate can increase with age.
- Remember that an abnormal value for one patient may be a normal value for another, which is why baseline values are so important.

Physical assessment techniques

When you perform the physical assessment, you'll use four techniques: inspection, palpation, percussion, and auscultation.

Use these techniques in sequence except when you perform an abdominal assessment. Because palpation and percussion can alter bowel sounds, the sequence for assessing the abdomen is inspection, auscultation, percussion, and palpation.

Inspection

Inspect each body system using vision, smell, and hearing to assess normal conditions and deviations. Observe for color, size, location, movement, texture, symmetry, odors, and sounds as you assess each body system.

Palpation

Palpation requires you to touch the patient with different parts of your hands, using varying degrees of pressure. Keep your fingernails short and your hands warm. Wear gloves when palpating, especially for mucous membranes or areas in contact with body fluids. Palpate tender areas last.

Types of palpation

Light palpation

▸ Use this technique to feel for surface abnormalities.
▸ Depress the skin ½″ to ¾″ (1.5 to 2 cm) with your finger pads, using the lightest touch possible.
▸ Assess for texture, tenderness, temperature, moisture, elasticity, pulsations, superficial organs, and masses.

Deep palpation

▸ Use this technique to feel internal organs and masses for size, shape, tenderness, symmetry, and mobility.
▸ Depress the skin 1½″ to 2″ (4 to 5 cm) with firm, deep pressure.
▸ Use one hand on top of the other to exert firmer pressure if needed.

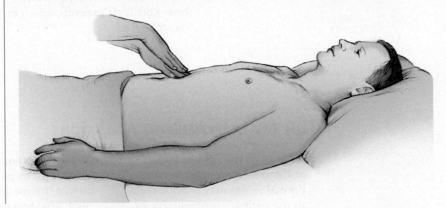

Percussion

Percussion involves tapping your fingers or hands quickly and sharply against parts of the patient's body to help you locate organ borders, identify organ shape and position, and determine if an organ is solid or filled with fluid or gas.

Auscultation

Auscultation, usually the last step, involves listening for various breath, heart, and bowel sounds with a stethoscope. Provide a quiet environment. Then make sure that the area to be auscultated is exposed. Auscultating over a gown or bed linens can interfere with sounds. Be sure to warm the stethoscope head in your hand to avoid startling the patient.

Types of percussion

Direct percussion

This technique reveals tenderness; it's commonly used to assess an adult patient's sinuses. Here's how to do it:

▸ Using one or two fingers, tap directly on the body part.
▸ Ask the patient to tell you which areas are painful, and watch his face for signs of discomfort.

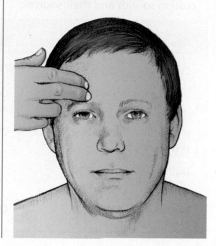

Indirect percussion

This technique elicits sounds that give clues to the makeup of the underlying tissue. Here's how to do it:

▸ Press the distal part of the middle finger of your nondominant hand firmly on the body part.
▸ Keep the rest of your hand off the body surface.
▸ Flex the wrist of your dominant hand.
▸ Using the middle finger of your dominant hand, tap quickly and directly over the point where your other middle finger touches the patient's skin.
▸ Listen to the sounds produced.

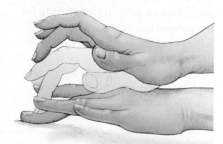

How to auscultate

▸ Use the diaphragm to pick up high-pitched sounds, such as first (S_1) and second (S_2) heart sounds. Hold the diaphragm firmly against the patient's skin, enough to leave a slight ring on the skin afterward.

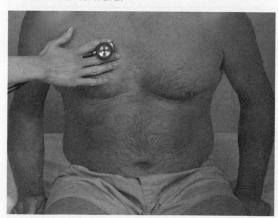

▸ Use the bell to pick up low-pitched sounds, such as third (S_3) and fourth (S_4) heart sounds. Hold the bell lightly against the patient's skin, just enough to form a seal. Holding the bell too firmly causes the skin to act as a diaphragm, obliterating low-pitched sounds.
▸ Listen and try to identify the characteristics of one sound at a time.

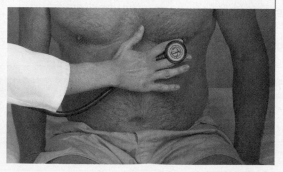

Documentation

Begin your documentation with general information, including the patient's age, race, sex, general appearance, height, weight, body mass, vital signs, communication skills, behavior, awareness, orientation, and level of cooperation. Next, precisely record all information you obtained using the four physical assessment techniques.

Just as you should follow an organized sequence in your examination, you should follow an organized pattern for recording your findings. Document all information about one body system, for example, before proceeding to another.

Locate landmarks

Use anatomic landmarks in your descriptions so other people caring for the patient can compare their findings with yours. For instance, you might describe a wound as 1½″ × 2½″ located 2½″ below the umbilicus at the midclavicular line."

With some structures, such as the tympanic membrane and breast, you can pinpoint a finding by its position on a clock. For instance, you might write "breast mass at 3 o'clock." If you use this method, however, make sure others recognize the same landmark for the 12 o'clock reference point.

Sounds and their sources

As you practice percussion, you'll recognize different sounds. Each sound is related to the structure underneath. This table offers a quick guide to percussion sounds and their sources.

Sound	Quality of sound	Where it's heard	Source
Tympany	Drumlike	Over enclosed air	Air in bowel
Resonance	Hollow	Over areas of part air and part solid	Normal lung
Hyper-resonance	Booming	Over air	Lung with emphysema
Dullness	Thudlike	Over solid tissue	Liver, spleen, heart
Flatness	Flat	Over dense tissue	Muscle, bone

Documenting your findings

Whether documenting an initial assessment of a patient admitted to your unit or writing a routine assessment note after a home visit, you'll need to use the appropriate form. Below is an example of part of an initial assessment form.

GENERAL INFORMATION

Age 55 Sex M Height 163 cm Weight 57 kg
T 37° C P 76 R 14 B/P(R) 150/90 sitting (L)

Room 328
Admission time 0800
Admission date 5/09/11
Doctor Manzel
Admitting diagnosis Pneumonia

Patient's stated reason for hospitalization To get rid of the pneumonia

Allergies penicillin, codeine
Current medications None

NAME	DOSAGE	LAST TAKEN

GENERAL SURVEY

In no acute distress, slender, appears younger than stated age. Is alert and well-groomed. Communicates well. Makes eye contact and expresses appropriate concern throughout exam.

— C. Smith, RN

Chapter 2
Cardiovascular care

DISEASES
Acute coronary syndrome

Acute myocardial infarction (MI), including ST-segment elevation MI, non-ST-segment elevation MI, and unstable angina are part of a group of diseases called *acute coronary syndrome* (ACS). Patients with ACS have some degree of coronary artery occlusion. Development begins with a rupture or erosion of plaque. The rupture results in platelet adhesions, fibrin clot formation, and activation of thrombin.

A thrombus progresses and occludes blood flow, although an early thrombus doesn't necessarily block blood flow. The effect is an imbalance in myocardial oxygen supply and demand. Depending on the degree of occlusion, ACS is defined as three types.

If the patient has unstable angina, a thrombus partially occludes a coronary vessel. This thrombus is full of platelets. The partially occluded vessel may have distal microthrombi that cause necrosis in some myocytes.

If smaller vessels infarct, the patient is at higher risk for MI, which may progress to a non-Q-wave MI. Usually, only the innermost layer of the heart is damaged.

A Q-wave MI results when reduced blood flow through one of the coronary arteries causes myocardial ischemia, injury, and necrosis. The damage extends through all myocardial layers. The destruction of healthy cardiac tissue from myocardial ischemia varies with the severity of the ACS involved and the promptness of effective diagnosis and treatment.

 ACS tissue destruction

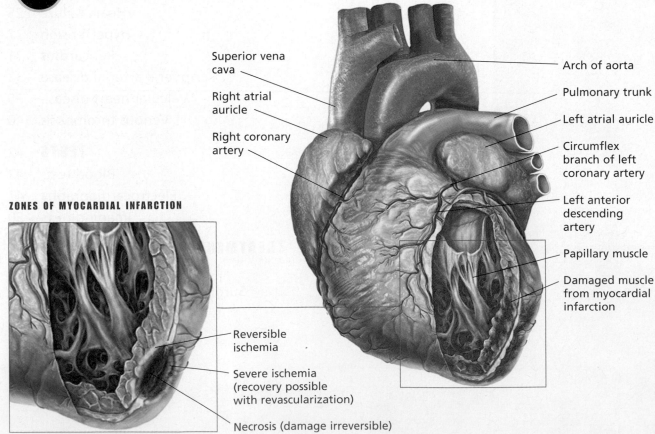

ZONES OF MYOCARDIAL INFARCTION

Superior vena cava

Right atrial auricle

Right coronary artery

Arch of aorta

Pulmonary trunk

Left atrial auricle

Circumflex branch of left coronary artery

Left anterior descending artery

Papillary muscle

Damaged muscle from myocardial infarction

Reversible ischemia

Severe ischemia (recovery possible with revascularization)

Necrosis (damage irreversible)

Comparing signs and symptoms of unstable angina and MI

	Unstable angina	Myocardial infarction
Character, location, and radiation	▸ Tightness, aching, crushing, burning, squeezing, substernal or retrosternal pain spreading across chest; may radiate to arm, neck, jaw, back, or shoulder.	▸ Severe, persistent substernal pain or pain over the pericardium; may spread widely throughout chest and be accompanied by pain in the shoulders, arms, jaw, belly, or back; may be described as crushing or squeezing
Duration of pain	▸ 5 to 30 minutes	▸ More than 20 minutes
Precipitating events	▸ Usually related to exertion, emotion, eating, and cold, but may occur without cause.	▸ Occurs spontaneously ▸ May be sequela to unstable angina
Relieving measures	▸ Rest, nitroglycerin, oxygen may be effective.	▸ Morphine sulfate, successful reperfusion of blocked coronary artery
Associated symptoms	▸ Shortness of breath ▸ Dizziness ▸ Nausea ▸ Palpitations ▸ Weakness	▸ Feeling of impending doom ▸ Fatigue ▸ Nausea and vomiting ▸ Shortness of breath ▸ Dizziness ▸ Palpitations ▸ Anxiety
Associated signs	▸ Hypotension or hypertension ▸ Tachycardia or bradycardia ▸ Diaphoresis	▸ Hypotension or hypertension ▸ Palpable precordial pulse ▸ Muffled heart sounds ▸ Arrhythmias ▸ Diaphoresis
Cardiac biomarkers	▸ Usually within normal range	▸ Elevated

The ABCs of ACS treatment

A—Antiplatelet therapy, anticoagulation, angiotensin-converting enzyme inhibitors, and angiotensin receptor blockade

B—Beta-adrenergic blockers and blood pressure control

C—Cholesterol-lowering treatment and cigarette smoking cessation

D—Diabetes management and diet

E—Exercise

Treatment
For angina
▸ Decrease in myocardial oxygen demand or increase in oxygen supply

For MI
▸ Pain relief
▸ Stabilization of heart rhythm
▸ Revascularization of the coronary artery
▸ Preservation of myocardial tissue
▸ Reduction of cardiac workload
▸ Thrombolytic therapy (unless contraindicated should be initiated within 30 to 60 minutes of arrival to emergency department)
▸ Percutaneous coronary interventions should be performed within 90 minutes of arrival

Nursing considerations
▸ Monitor and record the patient's electrocardiogram (ECG) readings, blood pressure, temperature, and heart and breath sounds.
▸ Assess pain and treat appropriately as ordered. Record the severity, location, type, duration, and relief of pain.
▸ Check the patient's blood pressure after giving nitroglycerin, especially the first dose.
▸ Continuously monitor ECG rhythm strips to detect rate changes and arrhythmias. Analyze rhythm strips, and place a representative strip in the patient's chart if any new arrhythmias are identified, if chest pain occurs, or at least every shift or according to facility protocol.
▸ During episodes of chest pain, obtain ECG readings and blood pressure and pulmonary artery catheter measurements, if applicable, to determine changes.

▶ Assess for crackles, cough, tachypnea, and edema, which may indicate impending left-sided heart failure. Carefully monitor daily weight, intake and output, respiratory rate, serum enzyme levels, ECG readings, and blood pressure. Auscultate for adventitious breath sounds periodically (patients on bed rest typically have atelectatic crackles, which may disappear after coughing) and for S_3 or S_4 gallops.

▶ Provide a stool softener to prevent straining during defecation, which causes vagal stimulation and may slow heart rate.

▶ Provide emotional support to help reduce stress and anxiety.

▶ After thrombolytic therapy, administer continuous heparin as ordered. Monitor the partial thromboplastin time every 6 hours, and monitor the patient for evidence of bleeding.

▶ Monitor ECG rhythm strips for reperfusion arrhythmias and treat according to facility protocol.

LESSON PLANS

Teaching about acute coronary syndrome

▶ Explain dosages and therapy to promote compliance with the prescribed medication regimen and other treatment measures.
▶ Review dietary restrictions.
▶ Encourage the patient to participate in a cardiac rehabilitation exercise program.
▶ Counsel the patient to resume sexual activity progressively.
▶ Advise the patient about appropriate responses to new or recurrent symptoms.
▶ Advise the patient to report typical or atypical chest pain.
▶ Stress the need to stop smoking. If necessary, refer the patient to a support group.

Aortic aneurysm

An aneurysm is a localized outpouching or abnormal dilation of a weakened arterial wall of the aorta. When developing, lateral pressure increases, causing the vessel lumen to widen and blood flow to slow. An aortic aneurysm may result in hemodynamic forces that can create pulsatile stresses on the weakened wall and press on the small vessels that supply nutrients to the arterial wall, causing the aorta to become bowed and torturous.

An aortic aneurysm may rupture or tear suddenly, possibly causing death. Rupture of an aortic aneurysm is a medical emergency requiring prompt treatment.

Aortic aneurysms are classified according to their anatomical location along the aorta, their shape, and how they are formed. Abdominal aneurysms are located along the portion of the aorta that passes through the abdomen. Ascending aneurysms are located in the ascending aorta and descending in the descending aorta.

Signs and symptoms
Abdominal
▶ Lumbar pain radiating to flank and groin
▶ Systolic bruit over aorta
▶ Tenderness on deep palpation
▶ Palpation of abdominal throbbing

Ascending
▶ Bradycardia
▶ Different blood pressures in right and left arms (more than 20 mm Hg)
▶ Jugular vein distention
▶ Murmur of aortic insufficiency
▶ Pain
▶ Pericardial friction rub
▶ Unequal carotid and radial pulses

Descending
▶ Dry cough
▶ Dysphagia
▶ Dyspnea and stridor
▶ Hoarseness
▶ Pain (sudden, between shoulder blades and chest)

Treatment
▶ Small, asymptomatic aneurysms (less than 4 cm in diameter): monitoring every 6 months with ultrasonography, X-ray, or computed tomography
▶ Large (5 cm or more) or symptomatic aneurysms: resection or repair to prevent rupture
▶ Monitoring of blood pressure and treatment with antihypertensives as needed.

Nursing considerations
▶ Allow the patient to express his fears and concerns. Help him identify effective coping strategies as he attempts to deal with his diagnosis.
▶ Before elective surgery, weigh the patient, insert an indwelling urinary catheter and an I.V. line, and assist with insertion of the arterial line and pulmonary artery catheter to monitor hemodynamic balance.

In an acute situation
▶ Insert multiple large-bore I.V. lines to facilitate blood replacement.
▶ Prepare the patient for impending surgery.
▶ As ordered, obtain blood samples for kidney function tests (such as blood urea nitrogen, creatinine, and electrolyte levels), a complete blood count with differential, blood typing and crossmatching, and arterial blood gas (ABG) levels.

Determining types of aortic aneurysms

Dissecting
A hemorrhagic separation in the aortic wall, usually within the medial layer

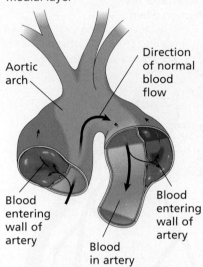

Aortic arch

Direction of normal blood flow

Blood entering wall of artery

Blood entering wall of artery

Blood in artery

Fusiform
A spindle-shaped enlargement encompassing the entire aortic circumference

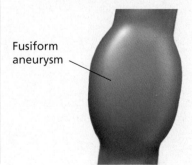

Fusiform aneurysm

Saccular
An outpouching of the arterial wall

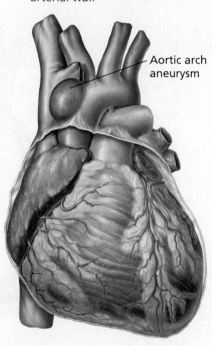

Aortic arch aneurysm

False
Caused by injury to entire arterial wall, resulting in a break in all layers of the wall; blood leaks out but is contained by the surrounding structures, creating a pulsatile hematoma

Pulsatile hematoma

▶ Monitor the patient's cardiac rhythm and vital signs. Assist with insertion of a pulmonary artery line to monitor for hemodynamic balance.

▶ Administer ordered medications, such as an antihypertensive and a beta-adrenergic blocker to control aneurysm progression and an analgesic to relieve pain.

▶ Be alert for signs of rupture, which may be fatal. Watch closely for any signs of acute blood loss (such as decreasing blood pressure, increasing pulse and respiratory rates, restlessness, decreased sensorium, and cool, clammy skin).

▶ If rupture occurs, transport the patient to surgery as soon as possible. Medical antishock trousers may be used while transporting him to surgery.

Teaching about aortic aneurysm

▶ Explain the surgical procedure and the expected postoperative care in the intensive care unit for patients undergoing open, complex abdominal surgery (I.V. lines, endotracheal and nasogastric intubation, and mechanical ventilation).

▶ Instruct the patient to take all medications as prescribed and to carry a list of medications at all times, in case of an emergency.

▶ Tell the patient not to push, pull, or lift heavy objects until the physician indicates that it's okay to do so.

Cardiac tamponade

Cardiac tamponade is a rapid, unchecked increase in pressure in the pericardial sac. It usually results from blood or fluid that accumulates in the sac and compresses the heart. This compression obstructs blood flow to the ventricles and reduces the amount of blood pumped out of the heart with each contraction. Possible causes include malignant disease, dissecting aorta, heart surgery, trauma or radiation to the chest, heart tumor, placement of a central line, myocardial infarction, pericarditis, or a reaction to certain drugs, such as procainamide or hydralazine.

Cardiac tamponade
With cardiac tamponade, blood or fluid fills the pericardial space, compressing the heart, decreasing cardiac output, and obstructing venous return.

PICTURING
PATHO

Understanding cardiac tamponade

Normal heart and pericardium
The pericardial space normally contains 10 to 30 ml of pericardial fluid, which lubricates the layers of the heart and reduces friction when the heart contracts.

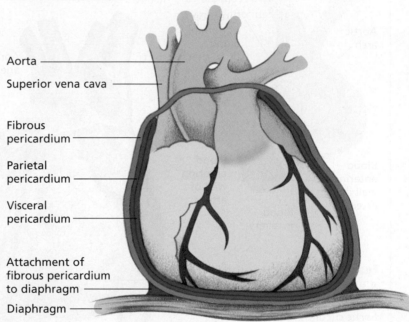

Aorta

Superior vena cava

Fibrous pericardium

Parietal pericardium

Visceral pericardium

Attachment of fibrous pericardium to diaphragm

Diaphragm

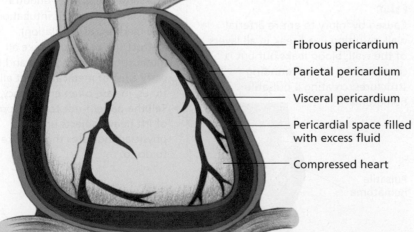

Fibrous pericardium

Parietal pericardium

Visceral pericardium

Pericardial space filled with excess fluid

Compressed heart

Signs and symptoms

Cardiac tamponade has three classic signs called *Beck's triad:*
▸ elevated central venous pressure (CVP) with jugular vein distention
▸ muffled heart sounds due to fluid accumulation
▸ pulsus paradoxus (inspiratory drop in systemic blood pressure greater than 15 mm Hg) due to arterial compression during inhalation.

Other symptoms include:
▸ Chest pain or discomfort sometimes relieved by sitting upright or leaning forward
▸ Pericardial friction rub
▸ dyspnea and cough due to compressed trachea and bronchi
▸ syncope, anxiety, and restlessness due to decreased oxygenation.

Treatment

▸ Supplemental oxygen
▸ Continuous electrocardiogram and hemodynamic monitoring
▸ Pericardiocentesis
▸ Surgical creation of pericardial window
▸ Pericardectomy
▸ Trial volume loading with crystalloids
▸ Inotropic drugs, such as dobutamine
▸ Posttraumatic injury: blood transfusion, thoracotomy to drain reaccumulating fluid, or repair of bleeding sites may be needed
▸ Heparin-induced tamponade: heparin antagonist protamine sulfate to stop bleeding
▸ Have emergency resuscitation equipment at the bedside
▸ Warfarin-induced tamponade: vitamin K to stop bleeding

Nursing considerations
After pericardiocentesis

▸ Reassure the patient to reduce his anxiety.
▸ Monitor blood pressure and CVP during and after pericardiocentesis. Infuse I.V. solutions, as ordered, to maintain blood pressure. Watch for a decrease in CVP and a concomitant increase in blood pressure, which indicate relief of cardiac compression.
▸ Administer oxygen therapy as needed.

After thoracotomy

▸ Give an antibiotic, protamine sulfate, or vitamin K as ordered.
▸ Postoperatively monitor critical parameters, such as vital signs and arterial blood gas levels, and assess heart and breath sounds. Give an analgesic as ordered. Maintain the chest drainage system and be alert for complications, such as hemorrhage and arrhythmias.

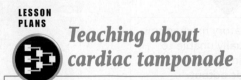

LESSON PLANS

Teaching about cardiac tamponade

Explain the procedure (pericardiocentesis or thoracotomy) to the patient. Tell him what to expect postoperatively (such as chest tubes, drains, and administration of oxygen). Teach him how to turn, deep breathe, and cough. If the patient isn't in an acute situation, teach these techniques preoperatively.

Cardiomyopathy

Cardiomyopathy is a disease of the heart where the heart muscle tissue can't work properly or as efficiently as it should. Cardiomyopathy can be classified as primary or secondary.

Primary cardiomyopathy refers to changes in the heart muscle without a specific cause. Secondary cardiomyopathy results from disorders that involve other organs as well as the heart.

There are four types of cardiomyopathy—dilated, restrictive, hypertrophic, and arrhythmogenic right ventricular dysplasia. Dilated or congestive cardiomyopathy (most common) and restrictive cardiomyopathy are discussed here.

CARDIOMYOPATHY, DILATED

Dilated cardiomyopathy results from extensively damaged myocardial muscle fibers. This disorder interferes with myocardial metabolism and grossly dilates all four chambers of the heart, giving the heart a globular appearance and shape. It usually isn't diagnosed until it has reached an advanced stage, and the prognosis is generally poor.

How dilated cardiomyopathy happens

Myocardial muscle fibers are extensively damaged.

↓

Contractility in the left ventricle decreases, lowering stroke volume.

↓

Early changes of heart failure (increased heart rate and left ventricular hypertrophy) help the heart to compensate functionally.

↓

The compensatory mechanisms are eventually unable to maintain adequate cardiac output.

↓

Severe left ventricular dilation occurs as venous return and systemic vascular resistance increase.

↓

Eventually, all chambers of the heart may dilate, causing generalized cardiomegaly with associated risk of arrhythmias and emboli.

PICTURING PATHO

Looking at dilated cardiomyopathy

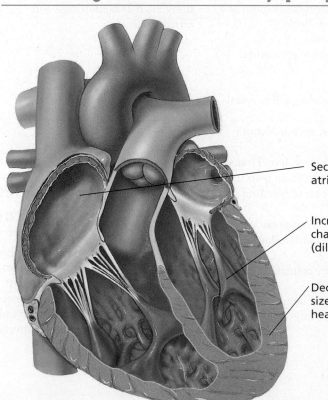

Secondary increased atrial chamber size

Increased ventricular chamber size (dilation)

Decreased muscle size but increased heart size

Signs and symptoms

▶ Shortness of breath, orthopnea, dyspnea on exertion, paroxysmal nocturnal dyspnea, fatigue, and a dry cough at night caused by left-sided heart failure
▶ Tachycardia with irregular pulse, if atrial fibrillation exists
▶ Pansystolic murmur associated with mitral and tricuspid insufficiency
▶ Peripheral cyanosis
▶ Peripheral edema, hepatomegaly, jugular vein distention, and weight gain caused by right-sided heart failure
▶ S_3 gallop

Treatment

▶ Management of underlying cause, if known
▶ Oxygen therapy
▶ Angiotensin-converting enzyme (ACE) inhibitors as first-line therapy
▶ Diuretics
▶ Digoxin (Lanoxin) for patients not responding to ACE inhibitors and diuretic therapy
▶ Vasodilators, such as hydralazine and isosorbide dinitrate (Isordil)
▶ Beta-adrenergic blockers for patients with mild or moderate heart failure
▶ Antiarrhythmics such as amiodarone (Cordarone)
▶ Cardioversion
▶ Automatic implanted cardioverter-defibrillator insertion
▶ Anticoagulants for patients with atrial fibrillation
▶ Revascularization, such as coronary artery bypass graft surgery, if dilated cardiomyopathy is due to ischemia
▶ Valvular repair or replacement if dilated cardiomyopathy is due to valve dysfunction
▶ Lifestyle modifications, such as smoking cessation; fluid restriction; low-fat, low-sodium diet; physical activity; and abstinence from alcohol
▶ Left ventricular assist device

Nursing considerations

▶ Alternate periods of rest with required activities of daily living and treatments. Provide personal care as needed to prevent fatigue.
▶ Provide active or passive range-of-motion exercises to prevent muscle atrophy.
▶ Consult a dietitian to provide a low-sodium diet.
▶ Monitor the patient for signs of progressive failure (decreased arterial pulses, increased jugular vein distention) and compromised renal perfusion (oliguria, increased blood urea nitrogen and serum creatinine levels, and electrolyte imbalances). Weigh the patient daily.
▶ Administer oxygen as needed.
▶ If the patient is receiving a vasodilator, check his blood pressure and heart rate frequently.
▶ If the patient is receiving a diuretic, monitor him for signs of resolving congestion (decreased crackles and dyspnea) or too-vigorous diuresis. Check his serum potassium level for hypokalemia, especially if therapy includes a cardiac glycoside.
▶ Allow the patient and his family to express their fears and concerns.
▶ Prevent constipation and stress ulcers to reduce cardiac workload.

LESSON PLANS

Teaching about dilated cardiomyopathy

▶ Before discharge, teach the patient about the illness and its treatment.
▶ Emphasize the need to restrict fluid and sodium intake, watch for weight gain, and take a cardiac glycoside if prescribed and watch for a toxic reaction to it (such as anorexia, nausea, and vomiting).
▶ Encourage family members to learn cardiopulmonary resuscitation because sudden cardiac arrest is possible.

CARDIOMYOPATHY, RESTRICTIVE

Restrictive cardiomyopathy is characterized by restricted ventricular filling (the result of left ventricular hypertrophy) and endocardial fibrosis and thickening. It's severe and irreversible, and the average survival after diagnosis is 9 years.

Signs and symptoms

▶ Fatigue
▶ Chest pain
▶ Dyspnea
▶ Edema
▶ High systemic and pulmonary venous pressure
▶ Liver engorgement
▶ Orthopnea
▶ Abdominal distention
▶ Palpitations

PICTURING PATHO

Looking at restrictive cardiomyopathy

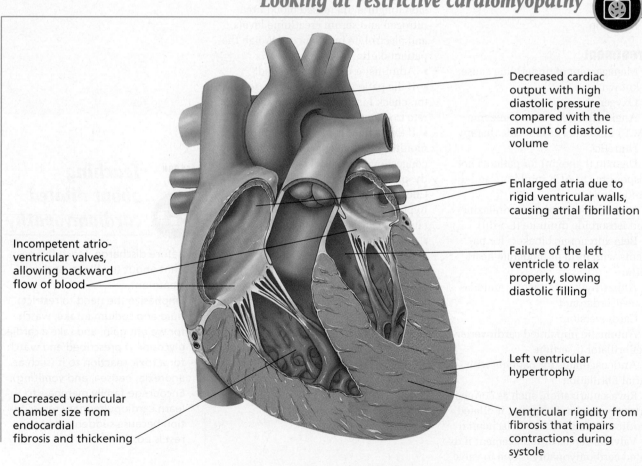

Decreased cardiac output with high diastolic pressure compared with the amount of diastolic volume

Enlarged atria due to rigid ventricular walls, causing atrial fibrillation

Failure of the left ventricle to relax properly, slowing diastolic filling

Left ventricular hypertrophy

Ventricular rigidity from fibrosis that impairs contractions during systole

Incompetent atrioventricular valves, allowing backward flow of blood

Decreased ventricular chamber size from endocardial fibrosis and thickening

Treatment

▶ Management of underlying cause (for example, administering deferoxamine to bind iron in restrictive cardiomyopathy due to hemochromatosis)
▶ Digoxin (Lanoxin), diuretics, and a restricted-sodium diet to ease the symptoms of heart failure (although no therapy exists for patients with restricted ventricular filling)
▶ Oral vasodilators
▶ Pacemaker
▶ Cardiac transplantation if intractable disease

Nursing considerations

▶ In the acute phase, monitor heart rate and rhythm, blood pressure, urine output, and pulmonary artery pressure readings to help guide treatment.
▶ Give psychological support. Provide appropriate diversionary activities for the patient restricted to prolonged bed rest. Because a poor prognosis may cause profound anxiety and depression, be especially supportive and understanding, and encourage the patient to express his fears. Refer him for psychosocial counseling, as necessary, for assistance in coping with his restricted lifestyle. Be flexible with visiting hours whenever possible.

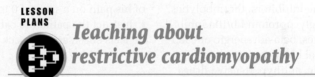

LESSON PLANS

Teaching about restrictive cardiomyopathy

Before discharge, teach the patient to watch for and report signs and symptoms of digoxin toxicity (anorexia, nausea, vomiting, and yellow vision); to record and report weight gain; and, if sodium restriction is ordered, to avoid canned foods, pickles, smoked meats, and use of table salt.

Coronary artery disease

Coronary artery disease (CAD) occurs when the arteries that supply blood to the heart muscle harden and narrow. The result is the loss of oxygen and nutrients to myocardial tissue because of diminished coronary blood flow. This reduction in blood flow can lead to coronary syndrome (angina or myocardial infarction).

Signs and symptoms
- Possibly none
- Abnormal stress test or echocardiogram findings
- Angina, typically with exertion or stress
- Uncontrolled hypertension and diabetes mellitus
- Major complications, such as acute coronary syndrome, heart failure, arrhythmias, or sudden death

Treatment
- Drug therapy: angiotensin-converting enzyme inhibitors, thrombolytics, diuretics, glycoprotein IIb/IIIa inhibitors, nitrates, beta-adrenergic or calcium channel blockers; antiplatelet, antilipemic, antihypertensive drugs
- Coronary artery bypass grafting (CABG)
- Minimally invasive surgery, an alternative to traditional CABG
- Angioplasty
- Arthrectomy
- Stent placement (especially drug-eluding) to maintain patency of reopened artery
- Lifestyle modifications to limit progression of CAD: smoking cessation, exercising regularly, maintaining ideal body weight, and eating a low-fat, low-sodium diet

Nursing considerations
- During anginal episodes, monitor blood pressure and heart rate. Take a 12-lead electrocardiogram before administering nitroglycerin or other nitrates. Record the duration of pain, the amount of medication required to relieve it, and accompanying symptoms.
- Ask the patient to grade the severity of his pain on a scale of 0 to 10.
- Instruct the patient to call whenever he feels chest, arm, or neck pain.
- After cardiac catheterization, review the expected course of treatment with the patient and family members. Monitor the catheter site for bleeding and check for distal pulses.
- After percutaneous transluminal coronary angioplasty (PTCA) and intravascular stenting, maintain heparinization, observe the patient for bleeding at the site, keep the affected leg immobile, and check for distal pulses. Precordial blood must be taken every 8 hours for 24 hours for cardiac enzyme levels. Complete blood count and electrolyte levels are monitored.
- After rotational ablation, monitor the patient for chest pain, hypotension, coronary artery spasm, and bleeding from the catheter site. Provide heparin and antibiotic therapy for 24 to 48 hours as ordered.
- After bypass surgery, monitor blood pressure, intake and output, breath sounds, chest tube drainage, and cardiac rhythm, watching for signs of ischemia and arrhythmias. Monitor capillary glucose, electrolyte levels, and arterial blood gases. Follow weaning parameters while patient is on a mechanical ventilator. I.V. epinephrine, nitroprusside, albumin, potassium, and blood products may be necessary. The patient may also need temporary epicardial pacing, especially if the surgery included replacement of the aortic valve.

PICTURING PATHO

Understanding atherosclerosis

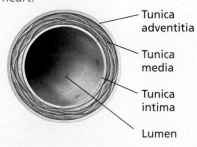

Coronary arteries are normally flexible and can adapt to the oxygen-carrying needs of the heart.

- Tunica adventitia
- Tunica media
- Tunica intima
- Lumen

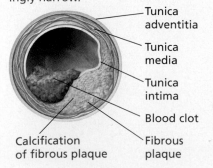

Atherosclerosis causes a buildup of fatty fibrous plaque in the vessel walls. Thrombi can also form if the plaque ruptures through the intimal layer. The lumen becomes increasingly narrow.

- Tunica adventitia
- Tunica media
- Tunica intima
- Blood clot
- Calcification of fibrous plaque
- Fibrous plaque

Stable angina

Angina is the classic sign of coronary artery disease. There are three forms of stable angina: chronic stable angina, microvascular (cardiac syndrome X) angina, and Prinzmetal's (variant) angina.

Chronic stable angina

▶ Characterized by exertional, rest-relieved discomfort, located anywhere between the umbilicus and the ears that may be associated with numbness of the arms or hands
▶ Doesn't increase in frequency or severity over time
▶ Generally caused by fixed obstructive atheromatous lesions
▶ Treated with rest and nitrates during attacks, and beta-adrenergic blockers for prevention

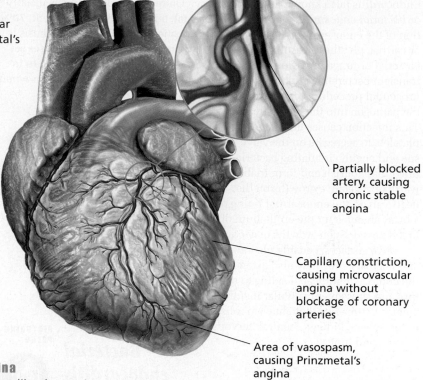

Partially blocked artery, causing chronic stable angina

Capillary constriction, causing microvascular angina without blockage of coronary arteries

Area of vasospasm, causing Prinzmetal's angina

Microvascular (cardiac syndrome X) angina

▶ Characterized by stable angina-like chest pain
▶ Caused by impairment of vasodilator reserve
▶ Poses no risk of cardiac ischemia because the capillaries are too small to block oxygenation of cardiac cells
▶ Treated with nitrates, beta-adrenergic blockers, or calcium channel blockers

Prinzmetal's (variant) angina

▶ Characterized by resting discomfort, which can cause the patient to awaken at night and persists for hours
▶ Caused by coronary artery vasospasm
▶ Causes reversible ST-segment elevation during event
▶ Treated with calcium channel blockers and nitrates, possibly beta-adrenergic blockers, or coronary stenting if intractable

LESSON PLANS

Teaching about CAD

▶ If the patient is scheduled for surgery, explain the procedure, provide a tour of the intensive care unit, introduce him to the staff, and discuss postoperative care.
▶ Help the patient determine which activities precipitate episodes of pain. Help him identify and select more effective coping mechanisms to deal with stress.

▶ Stress the need to follow the prescribed drug regimen.
▶ Encourage the patient to maintain the prescribed low-sodium diet and start a low-calorie diet as well.
▶ Explain that recurrent angina symptoms after PTCA or rotational ablation may signal reobstruction.
▶ Encourage regular, moderate exercise. Refer the patient to a cardiac

rehabilitation center or cardiovascular fitness program near his home or workplace.
▶ Reassure the patient that he can resume sexual activity and that modifications can allow for sexual fulfillment without fear of overexertion, pain, or reocclusion.
▶ Refer the patient to a smoking cessation program.

Endocarditis

Endocarditis (also known as *infective* or *bacterial endocarditis*) is an infection of the endocardium, heart valves, or cardiac prosthesis resulting from bacterial or fungal invasion. Even transient bacteremia after dental or urogenital procedures can introduce the pathogen into the bloodstream. This infection causes fibrin and platelets to aggregate on the valve tissue and engulf circulating bacteria or fungi that flourish and form friable, wartlike vegetative growths on the heart valves, the endocardial lining of a heart chamber, or the epithelium of a blood vessel. Such growths may cover the valve surfaces, causing ulceration and necrosis; they may also extend to the chordae tendineae, leading to rupture and subsequent valvular insufficiency. Ultimately, they may embolize to the spleen, kidneys, central nervous system, and lungs.

Untreated, endocarditis is usually fatal, but with proper treatment, 70% of patients recover. The prognosis is worst when endocarditis causes severe valvular damage, leading to insufficiency and heart failure, or when it involves a prosthetic valve.

Signs and symptoms

- Weakness and fatigue
- Anorexia
- Arthralgia
- Intermittent fever that may recur for weeks (in 90% of patients)
- Weight loss
- Loud, regurgitant murmur
- Petechiae
- Osler nodes
- Asymmetrical arthritis

Treatment

- Long-term antibiotic therapy: penicillin and aminoglycoside, usually gentamicin (Garamycin)
- Adequate rest periods
- Aspirin or acetaminophen for fever and aches
- Sufficient fluid intake
- Corrective surgery if refractory heart failure develops or heart structures are damaged
- Replacement of infected prosthetic valve
- Prophylactic treatment for high-risk individuals

Nursing considerations

- Stress the importance of adequate rest. Assist the patient with bathing if necessary. Provide a bedside commode because using a commode puts less stress on the heart than using a bedpan. Offer the patient diversionary, physically undemanding activities.
- To reduce anxiety, allow the patient to express his concerns about the effects of activity restrictions on his responsibilities and routines.
- Before giving an antibiotic, obtain a patient history of allergies. Administer the prescribed antibiotic on time to maintain a consistent drug level in the blood.
- Assess cardiovascular status frequently, and watch for signs and symptoms of left-sided heart failure, such as dyspnea, hypotension, tachycardia, tachypnea, crackles, and weight gain. Check for changes in cardiac rhythm or conduction.
- Administer oxygen and evaluate arterial blood gas levels, as needed, to ensure adequate oxygenation.
- Monitor the patient's renal status (including blood urea nitrogen levels, creatinine clearance, and urine output) to check for signs of renal emboli and drug toxicity.

Bacterial endocarditis

With bacterial endocarditis, the leaflets of the mitral valve erode and are eventually destroyed by bacterial invasion.

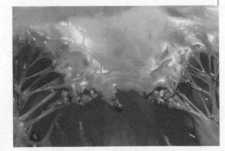

Libman-Sacks endocarditis

Found in patients with systemic lupus erythematosus, Libman-Sacks endocarditis is characterized by wartlike vegetations on the leaflets of the mitral valve.

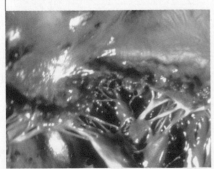

Teaching about endocarditis

▸ Teach the patient about the anti-infectives prescribed. Stress the importance of taking the medication and restricting activities for as long as the physician orders.
▸ Tell the patient to watch closely for fever, anorexia, and other signs and symptoms of relapse after treatment stops.

▸ Make sure the susceptible patient understands the need for a prophylactic antibiotic before, during, and after dental work, childbirth, and genitourinary, GI, or gynecologic procedures.
▸ Teach the patient to brush his teeth with a soft toothbrush and rinse his mouth thoroughly. Tell

him to avoid flossing his teeth and using irrigation devices.
▸ Teach the patient how to recognize symptoms of endocarditis, and tell him to notify the physician immediately if such symptoms occur.

Heart failure

Heart failure is a syndrome characterized by myocardial dysfunction that leads to impaired pump performance (diminished cardiac output) or to frank heart failure and abnormal circulatory congestion. Heart failure can be classified according to its pathophysiology. It may be right-sided or left-sided, systolic or diastolic, and acute or chronic.

Congestion of systemic or venous circulation may result in peripheral edema or hepatomegaly; congestion of pulmonary circulation may cause pulmonary edema, an acute life-threatening emergency. Pump failure usually occurs in a damaged left ventricle (left-sided heart failure) but may occur in the right ventricle (right-sided heart failure) either as a primary disorder or secondary to left-sided heart failure. Sometimes, left- and right-sided heart failure develop simultaneously.

LEFT-SIDED HEART FAILURE

Left-sided heart failure is the result of ineffective left ventricular contraction. It may lead to pulmonary congestion or pulmonary edema and decreased cardiac output. Left ventricular MI,

hypertension, and aortic or mitral valve stenosis or insufficiency are common causes. As the left ventricle's decreased pumping ability persists, fluid accumulates, backing into the left atrium, and then into the lungs. If this worsens, pulmonary edema and right-sided heart failure may also result.

PICTURING
PATHO

Left ventricular hypertrophy

Signs and symptoms
▸ Dyspnea, initially on exertion
▸ Confusion
▸ Dizziness
▸ Bibasilar crackles
▸ Cough
▸ Cyanosis or pallor
▸ Fatigue
▸ Muscle weakness
▸ Tachycardia

Hypertrophy of the left ventricle is one of the heart's first steps to compensate for increased pressures or increased blood volume.

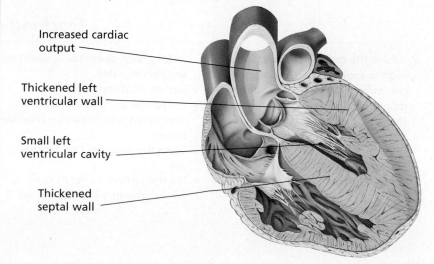

Increased cardiac output

Thickened left ventricular wall

Small left ventricular cavity

Thickened septal wall

RIGHT-SIDED HEART FAILURE

Right-sided heart failure is the result of ineffective right ventricular contraction. It may be caused by acute right ventricular infarction or pulmonary embolus. However, the most common cause is profound backward blood flow due to left-sided heart failure.

Signs and symptoms

▸ Edema, initially dependent
▸ Generalized weight gain
▸ Hepatomegaly
▸ Jugular vein distention
▸ Ascites

SYSTOLIC OR DIASTOLIC

With systolic heart failure, the left ventricle can't pump enough blood out to the systemic circulation during systole, and the ejection fraction fails. Consequently, blood backs up into the pulmonary circulation, pressure rises in the pulmonary venous system, and cardiac output fails.

With diastolic heart failure, the left ventricle can't relax and fill properly during diastole, and the stroke volume fails. Therefore, larger ventricular volumes are needed to maintain cardiac output.

ACUTE OR CHRONIC

The term *acute* refers to the timing of the onset of symptoms and whether compensatory mechanisms kick in. With acute heart failure, fluid status is typically normal or low, and sodium and water retention doesn't occur.

With chronic heart failure, signs and symptoms have been present for some time, compensatory mechanisms have taken effect, and fluid volume overload persists. Drugs, diet change, and activity restrictions usually control symptoms.

Treatment

Treatment of underlying disorders may improve heart failure. Lifestyle changes, such as smoking cessation and dietary adjustments, are important. Medications are prescribed according to the classification of signs and symptoms and recommendations of the New York Heart Association and the American College of Cardiology/American Heart Association.

Nursing interventions

▸ Place the patient in Fowler's position and give him supplemental oxygen to help him breathe more easily. Organize all activity to provide maximum rest periods.
▸ Weigh the patient daily (the best indicator of fluid retention), and check for peripheral edema. Also, monitor I.V. intake and urine output (especially if the patient is receiving a diuretic).
▸ Assess vital signs (for increased respiratory and heart rates and for narrowing pulse pressure) and mental status. Auscultate for abnormal heart and breath sounds. Report changes immediately.
▸ Frequently monitor blood urea nitrogen and serum creatinine, potassium, sodium, chloride, and magnesium levels.
▸ Provide continuous cardiac monitoring during acute and advanced stages to identify and treat arrhythmias promptly.
▸ To prevent deep vein thrombosis from vascular congestion, help the patient with range-of-motion exercises. Apply antiembolism stockings as needed. Check for calf pain and tenderness.

LESSON PLANS

Teaching about heart failure

▸ Advise the patient to avoid foods high in sodium, such as canned or commercially prepared foods and dairy products, to curb fluid overload.
▸ Stress the importance of taking digoxin (Lanoxin) exactly as prescribed. Tell the patient to watch for and immediately report signs of toxicity, such as anorexia, vomiting, and yellow vision.
▸ Explain fluid restrictions.
▸ Encourage the patient to participate in outpatient cardiac rehabilitation.
▸ Stress the need for regular check-ups.
▸ Tell the patient to notify the practitioner promptly if his pulse rate is unusually irregular or measures less than 60 beats/minute; if he experiences dizziness, blurred vision, shortness of breath, a persistent dry cough, palpitations, increased fatigue, paroxysmal nocturnal dyspnea, swollen ankles, or decreased urine output; or if he notices a rapid weight gain (3 to 5 lb [1.5 to 2.5 kg] in 1 week.
▸ Discuss the importance of smoking cessation.

Classifying signs and symptoms to determine treatment

Two sets of guidelines are available to help direct treatment of patients with heart failure. The New York Heart Association (NYHA) classification is based on functional capacity. The American College of Cardiology/American Heart Association (ACC/AHA) guidelines are based on objective assessment. These guidelines are compared below.

NYHA classification	ACC/AHA guidelines	Recommendations
	Stage A: Patient is at high risk for developing heart failure but has no structural heart disease or signs and symptoms of heart failure.	▹ Treatment of hypertension, lipid disorders, and diabetes ▹ Smoking cessation and regular exercise ▹ Discourage use of alcohol and illicit drugs ▹ Angiotensin-converting enzyme (ACE) inhibitor if indicated
Class I: Ordinary physical activity doesn't cause undue fatigue, palpitations, dyspnea, or angina.	**Stage B:** Patient has structural heart disease but no signs and symptoms of heart failure.	▹ All stage A therapies ▹ ACE inhibitor (unless contraindicated) ▹ Beta-adrenergic blocker (unless contraindicated)
Class II: Patient has slight limitation of physical activity but is asymptomatic at rest. Ordinary physical activity causes fatigue, palpitations, dyspnea, or anginal pain. **Class III:** Patient has marked limitation of physical activity but is typically asymptomatic at rest. Less than ordinary physical activity causes fatigue, palpitations, dyspnea, or angina.	**Stage C:** Patient has structural heart disease with prior or current signs and symptoms of heart failure.	▹ All stage A and B therapies ▹ Sodium-restricted diet ▹ Diuretics ▹ Digoxin ▹ Avoiding or withdrawing antiarrhythmics, most calcium channel blockers, and nonsteroidal anti-inflammatory drugs ▹ Drug therapy, including aldosterone antagonists, angiotensin receptor blockers, hydralazine, and nitrates
Class IV: Patient is unable to perform any physical activity without discomfort; symptoms may be present at rest. Discomfort increases with physical activity.	**Stage D:** Patient has end-stage disease requiring specialized treatment strategies, such as mechanical circulatory support, continuous inotropic infusion, or heart transplantation.	▹ All stage A, B, and C therapies ▹ Mechanical assist device, such as biventricular pacemaker or left ventricular assist device ▹ Continuous inotropic therapy ▹ Hospice care

Hypertension

Hypertension is an intermittent or sustained elevation in diastolic or systolic blood pressure. It may occur as essential (primary, idiopathic) where there is no identifiable cause, or secondary, resulting from an identifiable cause. Primary hypertension occurs in 90% to 95% of cases and tends to develop gradually over many years. Risk factors include obesity, stress, sedentary lifestyle, and smoking. Secondary hypertension tends to appear suddenly and causes higher blood pressure than does primary. Various conditions can lead to secondary hypertension, including renal disease, adrenal gland tumors, congenital coarctation, and obstructive sleep apnea. Medications that can cause secondary hypertension include hormonal contraceptives, cold remedies, certain pain relievers, and illegal drugs, such as cocaine and amphetamines. Malignant hypertension is a severe, fulminant form of hypertension common to both types. Hypertension is a major cause of stroke, cardiac disease, and renal failure. The prognosis is good if this disorder is detected early and treatment begins before complications develop. Severely elevated blood pressure (hypertensive crisis) may be fatal.

Signs and symptoms

- Possibly none
- Blurry vision
- Bruits over abdominal aorta or carotid, renal, and femoral arteries
- Confusion
- Dizziness or light-headedness
- Edema
- Elevated blood pressure from baseline
- Fatigue
- Nocturia
- Nose bleeds

The silent killer

Although patients may feel healthy, untreated or poorly controlled hypertension can damage their major organs. Organs at greatest risk are the brain, eyes, and kidneys.

Classification of blood pressure

The Seventh Report of the Joint National Committee on Prevention, Detection, Evaluation, and Treatment of High Blood Pressure recommends that a person's risk factors be considered in the treatment of his hypertension. The patient with more risk factors should be treated more aggressively.

Category	SBP mm Hg		DBP mm Hg
Normal	< 120	and	< 80
Prehypertension	120 to 139	or	80 to 89
Hypertension, stage 1	140 to 159	or	90 to 99
Hypertension, stage 2	≥ 160	or	≥ 100
KEY:	SBP = systolic blood pressure		DBP = diastolic blood pressure

BRAIN
Stroke

Stroke from blood clots occluding narrowed blood vessels or from hemorrhage of a weakened vessel wall (aneurysm) can be disabling or fatal.

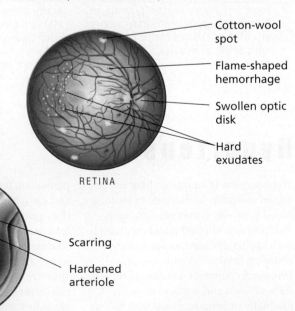

Infarct

Hemorrhage

Blood clot

EYE
Hypertensive retinopathy

Effects on the blood vessels within the retina can lead to hemorrhage, hard exudates, and swelling of the optic disk that may result in blindness.

Cotton-wool spot

Flame-shaped hemorrhage

Swollen optic disk

Hard exudates

RETINA

KIDNEY
Nephrosclerosis

Arterioles in the kidney harden and restrict oxygenation of the glomeruli, causing scarring and kidney failure.

Scarring

Hardened arteriole

GLOMERULUS

Treatment

The Seventh Report of the Joint National Commmittee on Prevention, Detection, Evaluation, and Treatment of High Blood Pressure has developed an innovative flowchart to guide the treatment of patients with hypertension.

Treating hypertension

Lifestyle modifications

Not at goal blood pressure (BP) (<140/90 mm Hg)
(<130/80 mm Hg for patients with diabetes or chronic kidney disease)

Initial drug choices

Without compelling indications

With compelling indications

Stage 1 hypertension

(systolic BP 140 to 159 mm Hg OR diastolic 90 to 99 mm Hg)

Thiazide-type diuretics for most; consider angiotensin-converting enzyme (ACE) inhibitors, angiotensin II receptor blockers (ARBs), beta-adrenergic blockers, calcium channel blockers, or combination

Stage 2 hypertension

(systolic BP ≥ 160 mm Hg OR diastolic BP ≥ 100 mm Hg)

Two-drug combination for most (usually thiazide-type diuretic and ACE inhibitor, ARB, beta-adrenergic blocker, or calcium channel blocker)

▸ Drug(s) for compelling indications (see prescriber)
▸ Other antihypertensive drugs (diuretics, ACE inhibitors, ARBs, beta-adrenergic blockers, calcium channel blockers) as needed

Not at goal BP

▸ Optimize dosages or add additional drugs until goal BP is achieved.
▸ Consider consultation with hypertension specialist.

Nursing considerations

▸ If a patient is hospitalized with hypertension, find out if he was taking his prescribed medications. If he wasn't, investigate the reasons. Refer him to the appropriate social service department for needed assistance, if appropriate.

▸ When routine blood pressure screening reveals elevated pressure, make sure the sphygmomanometer cuff size is appropriate for the patient's upper arm circumference. Take the pressure in both arms in lying, sitting, and standing positions. Ask the patient if he smoked, drank a beverage containing caffeine, or was emotionally upset before the reading. Advise him to return for blood pressure testing at frequent and regular intervals.

▸ To help identify hypertension and prevent untreated hypertension, participate in public education programs dealing with hypertension and ways to reduce risk factors. Encourage public participation in blood pressure screening programs. Routinely screen all patients, especially those at risk (blacks and those with family histories of hypertension, stroke, or heart attack).

LESSON
PLANS

 Teaching about hypertension

▸ Teach the patient to use a self-monitoring blood pressure cuff and to record the reading at least twice weekly in a journal for review by the physician at every office appointment.

▸ Tell the patient and family to keep a record of drugs used in the past, noting especially which ones are or aren't effective.

▸ To encourage compliance with antihypertensive therapy, suggest establishing a daily routine for taking medication. Tell him to report any adverse reactions to prescribed drugs. Advise him to avoid high-sodium antacids and over-the-counter cold and sinus medications containing harmful vasoconstrictors.

▸ Help the patient examine and modify his lifestyle. Suggest stress-reduction groups, dietary changes, and an exercise program, particularly aerobic walking, to improve cardiac status and reduce obesity and serum cholesterol levels.

▸ Encourage a change in dietary habits. Help the obese patient plan a reducing diet. Tell him to avoid high-sodium foods (such as pickles, potato chips, canned soups, and cold cuts), table salt, and foods high in cholesterol and saturated fat.

▸ Teach the patient and his family that this is a lifelong treatment. Warn the patient and family about complications that may occur from noncompliance and uncontrolled blood pressure, such as stroke and heart attack.

Pericarditis

Pericarditis is an inflammation of the pericardium, the fibroserous sac that envelops, supports, and protects the heart. It occurs in both acute and chronic forms. Acute pericarditis can be fibrinous or effusive with purulent, serous, or hemorrhagic exudate. Fluid buildup can cause pericardial effusion. If the effusion builds too rapidly, cardiac tamponade can occur.

Chronic constrictive pericarditis is characterized by dense fibrous pericardial thickening. This thickening causes constriction of normal heart size and movement, which can lead to permanently reduced stroke volume and cardiac output.

The prognosis depends on the underlying cause but is generally good in acute pericarditis, unless constriction occurs.

Signs and symptoms
Acute
▸ Pericardial friction rub at the left third intercostal space
▸ Sharp, sudden pain, usually starting over the sternum and radiating to the neck, shoulders, back, and arms
▸ Fever

Chronic
▸ Ascites and peripheral edema
▸ Chest pain with exertion
▸ Dyspnea
▸ Fatigue
▸ Inspiratory jugular vein distention (Kussmaul's sign)

Treatment
▸ Bed rest as long as fever and pain persist
▸ Treatment of underlying cause if it can be identified
▸ Nonsteroidal anti-inflammatory drugs, corticosteroids
▸ Antibacterial, antifungal, or antiviral therapy
▸ Partial or total pericardectomy
▸ Diuretics
▸ Pericardiocentesis

PICTURING PATHO

Pericarditis

Pericardial tissue damaged by bacteria or other substances releases chemical mediators of inflammation into the surrounding tissue.

Friction occurs as the inflamed pericardial layers rub against each other.

Histamines and other chemical mediators dilate vessels and increase vessel permeability.

Fluids and proteins (including fibrinogen) leak into the tissue causing extracellular edema.
Macrophages, neutrophils, and monocytes in the tissue begin to phagocytose the invading bacteria.

Gradually, the space fills with an exudate composed of necrotic tissue, dead neutrophils, and macrophages.
These products are eventually absorbed into healthy tissue.

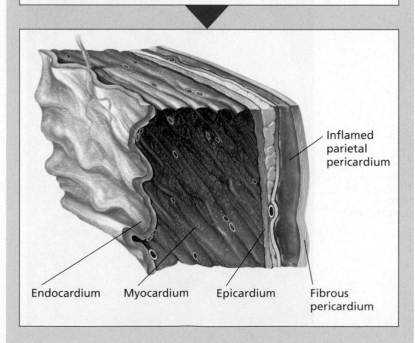

Endocardium   Myocardium   Epicardium   Fibrous pericardium

Inflamed parietal pericardium

Nursing considerations

▶ Stress the importance of bed rest.
▶ Assist the patient with bathing, if necessary.
▶ Place the patient in an upright position to relieve dyspnea and chest pain.
▶ Provide an analgesic to relieve pain and oxygen to prevent tissue hypoxia.
▶ Because cardiac tamponade requires immediate treatment, keep a pericardiocentesis tray handy if you suspect pericardial effusion.

▶ Assess cardiovascular status frequently, watching for signs of cardiac tamponade.
▶ To reduce anxiety, allow the patient to express his concerns about the effects of activity restrictions on his responsibilities and routines. Reassure him that the restrictions are temporary.
▶ Before giving an antibiotic, obtain a patient history of allergies. Administer the prescribed antibiotic on time to

maintain consistent drug levels in the blood.
▶ Observe the venipuncture site for signs of infiltration or inflammation, a possible complication of long-term I.V. administration. To reduce the risk of this complication, rotate venous access sites.

PICTURING PATHO

Chronic constrictive pericarditis

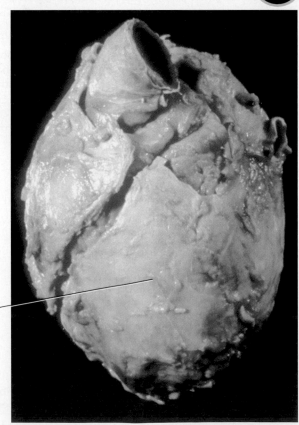

Thick, fibrous pericardium

LESSON PLANS

Teaching about pericarditis

▶ Explain to the patient all tests and treatments.
▶ If surgery is necessary, teach the patient how to perform coughing and deep-breathing exercises before he undergoes the procedure.
▶ Tell the patient to resume his daily activities slowly and to schedule rest periods into his daily routine, as instructed by the physician.

Peripheral arterial disease

Peripheral arterial disease (PAD) is a common complication of atherosclerosis. Obstruction or narrowing of the lumen of the aorta and its major branches causes an interruption of blood flow to the brain and extremities, most commonly the legs and feet. The obstruction may affect the arteries leading to the brain (carotid and vertebral), the arteries of the arm (subclavian, brachial, radial, and ulnar), and the arteries delivering blood to the legs and feet (iliac, femoral, popliteal, posterior tibial, anterior tibial, and peroneal).

PAD may be acute or chronic. An acute peripheral arterial occlusion requires emergent, aggressive treatment to revascularize the extremity and prevent limb loss. Chronic PAD may vary in severity from mild (with few symptoms) to severe ischemia (with tissue necrosis). Risk factors include smoking, aging, hypertension, hyperlipidemia, diabetes mellitus, and family history of vascular disorders, myocardial infarction, or stroke. Men suffer from PAD more often and at younger ages than women.

Pad sites

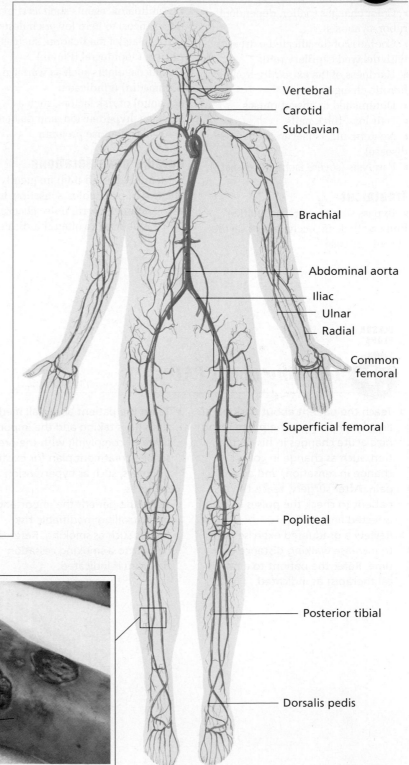

Vertebral

Carotid

Subclavian

Brachial

Abdominal aorta

Iliac

Ulnar

Radial

Common
femoral

Superficial femoral

Popliteal

Posterior tibial

Dorsalis pedis

Arterial ulcer

Hair loss

Thin, shiny
skin

Necrotic
tissue

Hardened
tissue

Rubor

Signs and symptoms

▶ Intermittent pain with exercise relieved with rest (chronic PAD)
▶ Abnormal sensation (pain at rest, tingling, numbness)
▶ Color changes (pallor, dependent rubor, cyanosis)
▶ Coolness of the affected extremity with delayed capillary refill
▶ Hardness of the extremity from fibrotic changes
▶ Diminished or absent pulses
▶ Hair loss, thick nails
▶ Necrotic ulcers (severe ischemic disease)
▶ Paralysis (severe ischemic disease)

Treatment

▶ Bypass surgery to revascularize limbs with acute occlusion or severe chronic disease
▶ Fibrinolytics to dissolve clot (acute arterial occlusion)
▶ Endovascular techniques, such as balloon angioplasty, atherectomy, or stenting
▶ Antilipemic agents such as simvastatin (Zocor) to help lower cholesterol
▶ Antiplatelet medication, such as aspirin or clopidogrel (Plavix)
▶ Anticoagulants such as warfarin (Coumadin) if indicated
▶ Control of risk factors, such as smoking, hypertension, and diabetes
▶ Regular exercise program

Nursing considerations

▶ Monitor affected limb frequently for changes in pain, color, sensation, and temperature. Perform pulse checks every shift or more often if indicated.
▶ Administer medications as ordered and analgesics to control pain. Monitor effects.
▶ Administer anticoagulants if indicated and monitor coagulation laboratory results.
▶ Monitor patient for increased bleeding.
▶ After surgery, monitor limb for circulation and wound healing. Encourage increasing activity as ordered and tolerated.
▶ Provide emotional support if acute occlusion results in amputation. Refer patient and caregivers to support groups as appropriate.

LESSON PLANS

 Teaching about PAD

▶ Teach the patient about peripheral arterial disease and help him recognize acute changes in his circulation, such as change in color, change in sensation, and acute pain. After surgery, teach the patient to check the pulses in his affected limb daily.
▶ Review a graduated exercise plan to increase walking distance over time. Refer the patient to a physical therapist as indicated.

▶ Teach the patient about all medications he is taking and the importance of complying with the prescribed treatment plan for existing disorders, such as hypertension and diabetes.
▶ Teach the patient the importance of controlling modifiable risk factors such as smoking. Refer the patient to a smoking cessation program if indicated.

▶ Teach the patient about atherosclerosis and how to help control it by following a low-fat diet, reducing weight, and maintaining a regular exercise program.

Valvular heart disease

AORTIC INSUFFICIENCY

Aortic insufficiency is the incomplete closure of the aortic semilunar valve. It's usually caused by scarring or retraction of valve leaflets. Aortic insufficiency can result from rheumatic fever, syphilis, hypertension, or endocarditis, or it may be idiopathic. It's also associated with Marfan syndrome and with ventricular septal defect, even after surgical closure.

Signs and symptoms

▸ Blowing diastolic murmur or S_3
▸ Cough
▸ Exertional dyspnea or chest pain
▸ Left-sided heart failure
▸ Pulsus bisferiens (rapidly rising and collapsing pulses)
▸ Fatigue, weakness
▸ Palpitations

Treatment

▸ Valve replacement
▸ Low-sodium diet
▸ Digoxin (Lanoxin), diuretics, vasodilators, and angiotensin-converting enzyme inhibitors

Nursing considerations

▸ Stress the importance of adequate rest. Assist with bathing if necessary. Provide a bedside commode because using a commode puts less stress on the heart than using a bedpan. Offer the patient diversionary, physically undemanding activities.
▸ Alternate periods of activity with periods of rest to prevent extreme fatigue and dyspnea.
▸ To reduce anxiety, allow the patient to express his concerns about the effects of activity restrictions on his responsibilities and routines. Reassure him that the restrictions are temporary.
▸ Keep the patient's legs elevated while he sits in a chair to improve venous return to the heart.
▸ Place the patient in an upright position to relieve dyspnea, if necessary, and administer oxygen to prevent tissue hypoxia.
▸ Keep the patient on a low-sodium diet. Consult a dietitian to make sure the patient receives foods that he likes while adhering to the diet restrictions.
▸ Monitor the patient for signs of heart failure, pulmonary edema, and adverse reactions to drug therapy.

PICTURING PATHO

Visualizing aortic insufficiency

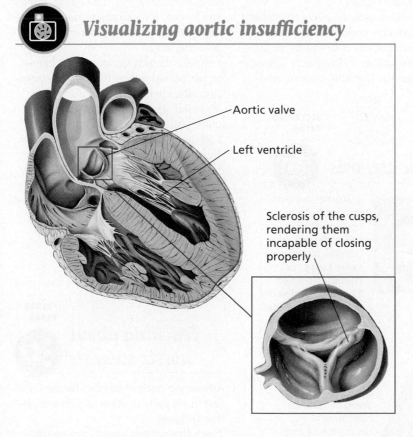

Aortic valve

Left ventricle

Sclerosis of the cusps, rendering them incapable of closing properly

LESSON PLANS

Teaching about aortic insufficiency

▸ Advise the patient to plan for periodic rest in his daily routine to prevent undue fatigue.
▸ Teach the patient about diet restrictions, medications, symptoms that should be reported, and the importance of consistent follow-up care.
▸ Tell the patient to elevate his legs whenever he sits.

AORTIC STENOSIS

With aortic stenosis, increased left ventricular pressure tries to overcome the resistance of the narrowed valvular opening. The added workload increases the demand for oxygen, and diminished cardiac output causes poor coronary artery perfusion, ischemia of the left ventricle, and left-sided heart failure.

Signs and symptoms

▶ Angina, palpitations, and cardiac arrhythmias
▶ Exertional dyspnea and paroxysmal nocturnal dyspnea
▶ Left-sided heart failure
▶ Syncope
▶ Systolic murmur at the base of the carotids

Treatment

▶ Commissurotomy (if patient is a child and if there are no calcifications)
▶ Valve replacement in symptomatic patients or those at risk for developing left-sided heart failure

▶ Percutaneous balloon aortic valvuloplasty in elderly patients with severe calcifications and in young children and adults with congenital aortic stenosis
▶ Antibiotic prophylaxis
▶ Digoxin (Lanoxin), diuretics, nitroglycerin or other drugs for symptoms
▶ Medication to control hypertension

Nursing considerations

▶ Stress the importance of adequate rest. Assist the patient with bathing if necessary; provide a bedside commode because using a commode puts less stress on the heart than using a bedpan. Offer the patient diversionary, physically undemanding activities.
▶ Alternate periods of activity with periods of rest to prevent extreme fatigue and dyspnea.
▶ To reduce anxiety, allow the patient to express his concerns about the effects of activity restrictions on his responsibilities and routines. Reassure him that the restrictions are temporary.

▶ Keep the patient's legs elevated while he sits in a chair to improve venous return to the heart.
▶ Place the patient in an upright position to relieve dyspnea, if needed. Administer oxygen to prevent tissue hypoxia, as needed.
▶ Keep the patient on a low-sodium diet. Consult with the dietitian to ensure that the patient receives foods that he likes while adhering to diet restrictions.
▶ Monitor the patient for signs of heart failure, pulmonary edema, and adverse reactions to drug therapy.
▶ Allow the patient to express his fears and concerns about the disorder, its impact on his life, and any upcoming surgery. Reassure him as needed.
▶ After cardiac catheterization, monitor the site for signs of bleeding. If the site bleeds, remove the pressure dressing and apply firm pressure until the bleeding stops.
▶ Notify the physician of any changes in peripheral pulses distal to the insertion site, changes in cardiac rhythm and vital signs, and complaints of chest pain.
▶ If the patient has surgery, watch for hypotension, arrhythmias, and thrombus formation. Monitor his vital signs, arterial blood gas levels, intake and output, daily weights, blood chemistry results, chest X-rays, and pulmonary artery catheter readings.

PICTURING PATHO

Looking at aortic stenosis

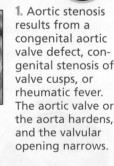

4. Diminished cardiac output causes poor coronary artery perfusion, ischemia of the left ventricle, and left-sided heart failure.

1. Aortic stenosis results from a congenital aortic valve defect, congenital stenosis of valve cusps, or rheumatic fever. The aortic valve or the aorta hardens, and the valvular opening narrows.

2. Left ventricular pressure rises to overcome the resistance of the narrowed valve.

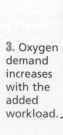

3. Oxygen demand increases with the added workload.

LESSON PLANS

Teaching about aortic stenosis

▶ Advise the patient to plan for periodic rest in his daily routine to prevent undue fatigue.
▶ Teach the patient about diet restrictions, medications, symptoms that should be reported, and the importance of consistent follow-up care.
▶ Tell the patient to elevate his legs whenever he sits.

What happens in mitral insufficiency

Blood flows from the left ventricle back into the left atrium during systole.
▼
Atrium enlarges to accommodate the backflow.
▼
Left ventricle dilates to accommodate the increased blood volume from the atrium and to compensate for diminished cardiac output.
▼
Ventricular hypertrophy and increased back pressure in the left atrium result in increased pulmonary artery pressure.
▼
Left- and right-sided heart failure result.

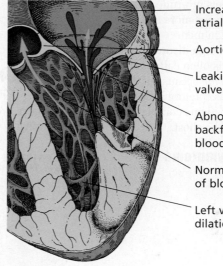

— Increased left atrial pressure

— Aortic valve

— Leaking mitral valve

— Abnormal backflow of blood

— Normal direction of blood flow

— Left ventricular dilation

MITRAL INSUFFICIENCY

An abnormality of the mitral leaflets, mitral annulus, chordae tendineae, papillary muscles, left atrium, or left ventricle can lead to mitral insufficiency. Acute mitral insufficiency can start suddenly, with the characteristic sign of dyspnea. Chronic mitral insufficiency is a slow process that's accompanied by such symptoms as fatigue and insomnia.

Signs and symptoms
▶ Angina and palpitations
▶ Fatigue
▶ New-onset atrial fibrillation
▶ Orthopnea or dyspnea
▶ Systolic murmur
▶ Light-headedness
▶ Cough, especially at night or when supine
▶ Pitting leg edema

Treatment
▶ Drugs to relieve symptoms
▶ Valvuloplasty or valve replacement

Nursing considerations
▶ Provide periods of rest between periods of activity to prevent excessive fatigue.
▶ To reduce anxiety, allow the patient to express his concerns about the effects of activity restrictions on his responsibilities and routines. Reassure him that the restrictions are temporary.
▶ Keep the patient on a low-sodium diet; consult with the dietitian to ensure that the patient receives as many favorite foods as possible during the restriction.
▶ Monitor the patient for left-sided heart failure, pulmonary edema, and adverse reactions to drug therapy. Provide oxygen to prevent tissue hypoxia as needed.
▶ If the patient has surgery, monitor him postoperatively for hypotension, arrhythmias, and thrombus formation.
▶ Monitor the patient's vital signs, arterial blood gas levels, intake and output, daily weights, blood chemistry results, chest X-rays, and pulmonary artery catheter readings.

Teaching about mitral insufficiency

▶ Teach the patient about diet restrictions, medications, signs and symptoms that should be reported, and the importance of consistent follow-up care.
▶ Explain all tests and treatments.
▶ Make sure the patient and his family understand the need to comply with prolonged antibiotic therapy and follow-up care, and the need for an additional antibiotic during dental procedures.
▶ Tell the patient to stop the drug and call the physician immediately if he develops a rash, fever, chills, or other signs or symptoms of allergy at any time during penicillin therapy.
▶ Instruct the patient and his family to watch for and report early signs and symptoms of heart failure, such as dyspnea and a hacking, nonproductive cough.

MITRAL VALVE PROLAPSE

With mitral valve prolapse, one or both valve leaflets protrude into the left atrium. It occurs more commonly in women than in men.

Typically a benign disorder, mitral valve prolapse is often called *click-murmur syndrome* because of the auscultatory sounds commonly associated with it. Some patients complain of palpitations of the chest.

Signs and symptoms
▶ Possibly none
▶ Chest pain
▶ Dizziness
▶ Heart murmur
▶ Palpitations
▶ Syncope
▶ Fatigue
▶ Dyspnea

Treatment
▶ None unless symptomatic
▶ Beta blockers, aspirin, or other anticoagulants
▶ Valve repair or replacement

Nursing considerations
▶ Provide periods of rest between periods of activity to prevent excessive fatigue.
▶ To reduce anxiety, allow the patient to express her concerns about the effects of activity restrictions on her responsibilities and routines. Reassure her that the restrictions are temporary.
▶ Keep the patient on a low-sodium diet; consult with the dietitian to ensure that the patient receives as many favorite foods as possible during the restriction.
▶ If the patient has surgery, monitor postoperatively for hypotension, arrhythmias, and thrombus formation.
▶ Monitor the patient's vital signs, arterial blood gas levels, intake and output, daily weights, blood chemistry results, chest X-rays, and pulmonary artery catheter readings.

PICTURING PATHO

Understanding mitral valve prolapse

Mitral valve prolapse is a billowing and subsequent improper closing of the mitral valve.

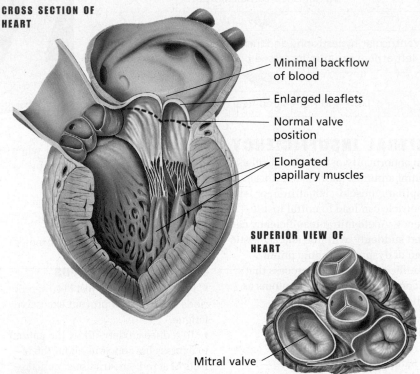

CROSS SECTION OF HEART

- Minimal backflow of blood
- Enlarged leaflets
- Normal valve position
- Elongated papillary muscles

SUPERIOR VIEW OF HEART

Mitral valve

LESSON PLANS

Teaching about mitral valve prolapse

▶ Explain all tests and treatments to the patient.
▶ Advise the patient to plan for periodic rest in her daily routine to prevent undue fatigue.
▶ Teach the patient about diet restrictions, medications, symptoms that should be reported, and the importance of consistent follow-up care.

▶ Make sure the patient and her family understand the need to comply with prolonged antibiotic therapy and follow-up care, and the need for an additional antibiotic during dental or other surgical procedures.

Understanding mitral valve stenosis

**PULMONARY
HYPERTENSION DEVELOPS**

**LUNG CONGESTION AND
PRESSURE**

**RIGHT-SIDED HEART
FAILURE**

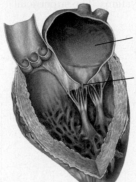

Left atrium
dilation

Narrowed
mitral valve

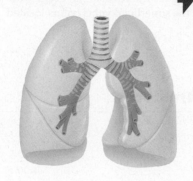

MITRAL VALVE STENOSIS

Mitral stenosis involves narrowing of the valve by valvular abnormalities, fibrosis, or calcification that obstructs blood flow from the left atrium to the left ventricle. Consequently, left atrial volume and pressure rise, and the chamber dilates. Greater resistance to blood flow causes pulmonary hypertension, right ventricular hypertrophy, and right-sided heart failure. Also, inadequate filling of the left ventricle produces low cardiac output.

Signs and symptoms

▶ A holosystolic murmur at apex, a possible split S_2, and an S_3
▶ Angina
▶ Crackles
▶ Dyspnea
▶ Fatigue
▶ Hepatomegaly (right-sided heart failure)
▶ Jugular vein distention
▶ Orthopnea
▶ Palpitations
▶ Peripheral edema
▶ Pulmonary edema
▶ Tachycardia

Treatment

▶ Anticoagulants
▶ Drugs for heart failure
▶ Synchronized cardioversion for atrial fibrillation
▶ Valvuloplasty or valve replacement

Nursing considerations

▶ Before giving penicillin, ask the patient if he has ever had a hypersensitivity reaction to it. Even if he hasn't, warn him that such a reaction is possible.
▶ Stress the importance of adequate rest. Assist with bathing, as necessary. Provide a bedside commode because using a commode puts less stress on the heart than using a bedpan. Offer the patient diversionary, physically undemanding activities.
▶ To reduce anxiety, allow the patient to express concerns over his inability to meet his responsibilities because of activity restrictions. Give reassurance that activity limitations are temporary.
▶ Watch closely for signs of heart failure, pulmonary edema, and adverse reactions to drug therapy.
▶ Place the patient in an upright position to relieve dyspnea if needed. Administer oxygen to prevent tissue hypoxia as needed.

▶ If the patient has had surgery, watch for hypotension, arrhythmias, and thrombus formation. Monitor vital signs, arterial blood gas levels, intake and output, daily weights, blood chemistry results, chest X-rays, and pulmonary artery catheter readings.
▶ Keep the patient on a low-sodium diet; provide as many favorite foods as possible.

Teaching about mitral stenosis

▶ Explain all tests and treatments.
▶ Advise the patient to plan for periodic rest in his daily routine to prevent undue fatigue.
▶ Teach the patient about diet restrictions, medications, symptoms that should be reported, and the importance of consistent follow-up care.
▶ Make sure the patient and his family understand the need to comply with prolonged antibiotic therapy and follow-up care, and the need for an additional antibiotic during dental or other surgical procedures.

Venous thrombosis

Venous thrombosis is an acute condition characterized by inflammation and the formation of thrombus within a vein. In venous thrombosis, damage to the epithelial lining of the vein wall causes platelets to aggregate and releases clotting factors that cause fibrin in the blood to form a clot.

Venous thrombosis can occur within the superficial veins (veins located above the aponeurotic fascia and closer to the skin), the deep veins (veins located below the aponeurotic fascia and typically accompanying arteries), or within both systems. The superficial

Looking at venous thrombosis

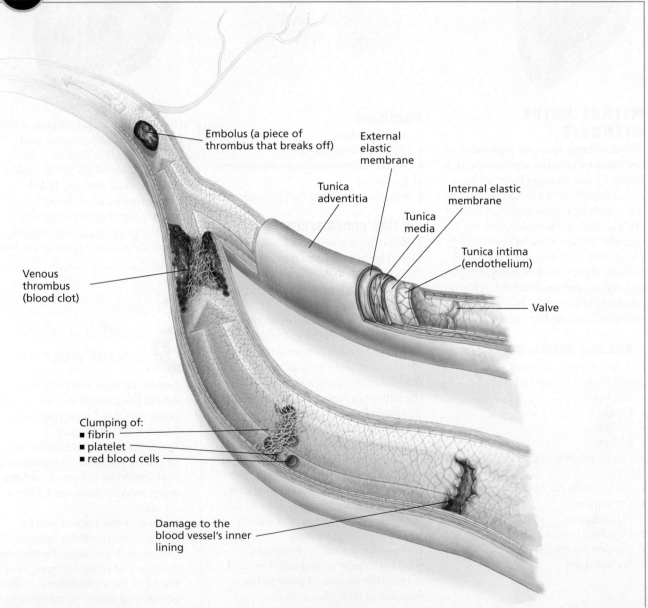

Embolus (a piece of thrombus that breaks off)

External elastic membrane

Tunica adventitia

Internal elastic membrane

Tunica media

Tunica intima (endothelium)

Venous thrombus (blood clot)

Valve

Clumping of:
- fibrin
- platelet
- red blood cells

Damage to the blood vessel's inner lining

veins drain blood into the deep veins and the deep veins return deoxygenated blood to the heart and lungs. Thrombus that forms within the superficial venous system is known as *superficial thrombophlebitis*. Thrombus that forms within the deep veins is known as *deep vein thrombosis* (DVT). Superficial thrombophlebitis is usually self-limiting and rarely embolizes. DVT impairs venous blood flow, and chronic vein changes may persist even with aggressive treatment. Chronic DVT is a significant cause of venous insufficiency, edema, and ulcers.

A venous *thromboembolus* occurs when a portion of a clot breaks off (generally from a deep vein) and travels to a distant site. A *pulmonary embolus* (PE) occurs when a thrombus dislodges (most commonly from the leg) and travels through the venous system and through the heart, where it lodges in a branch of the pulmonary artery. Once there, the thrombus obstructs blood flow to the lung. A large PE may cause respiratory failure, right-sided heart failure, and death.

Risk factors for venous thrombosis include obesity; history of cancer, coagulation disorders, or a prior thrombosis; age of 75 or older; an existing acute infectious process; pregnancy; immobility for more than 3 days; varicose veins or venous valvular disease; an in-place central venous catheter; oral contraceptive, estrogen, or I.V. drug use; and recent surgery.

Signs and symptoms
Superficial thrombophlebitis
▶ Palpable induration of the affected vein
▶ Heat and redness along the vein
▶ Pain and tenderness along the vein

DVT
▶ Fever, chills, and malaise
▶ Severe pain in the affected extremity
▶ Sudden nonpitting edema of the affected extremity
▶ Prominent superficial veins
▶ Erythema of the affected extremity
▶ Cool, pale, edematous extremity (in advanced DVT)

Treatment
▶ Anticoagulants, such as heparin, warfarin (Coumadin), or low-molecular-weight heparin (enoxaparin [Lovenox]) for DVT or PE
▶ Thrombolytics (alteplase) to dissolve the clot (in extensive PE)
▶ Venal caval filter to prevent PE
▶ Bed rest and elevation of the extremity
▶ Warm, moist soaks to the area
▶ Analgesics as needed
▶ Thrombectomy

Nursing considerations
▶ Perform a risk assessment for DVT on admission and at each shift to direct treatment. Patients at higher risk will receive prophylactic medication such as enoxaparin; patients with a lower risk may need antiembolism or compression stockings.
▶ Administer anticoagulants and oxygen therapy as ordered.
▶ Measure the girth of the affected extremity daily to detect worsening venous outflow obstruction and possible clot extension.
▶ Monitor patients with a diagnosed DVT for signs and symptoms of PE (shortness of breath, chest pain, respiratory distress).
▶ Encourage ambulation when appropriate, or limb exercises for immobile patients.
▶ Elevate affected limb and administer analgesics, if needed. Assess for effects of treatment.
▶ Monitor coagulation studies for effectiveness of treatment; observe for signs and symptoms of bleeding.

LESSON PLANS

Teaching about venous thrombosis

▶ Teach the patient about all medications he is taking, the signs and symptoms that should be reported, and the importance of regular coagulation laboratory tests if he is taking warfarin.
▶ Explain all tests and treatments.
▶ Teach the patient to apply compression hose, elevate the affected limb as ordered, and report worsening edema, pain, or dyspnea.
▶ Teach the patient to exercise his limbs and minimize immobility.

TESTS
Blood tests

TESTS TO IDENTIFY MYOCARDIAL INFARCTION

After a myocardial infarction (MI), damaged cardiac tissue releases significant amounts of enzymes and proteins into the blood. Specific blood test results help reveal the extent of cardiac damage and help monitor healing progress.

Myoglobin

▶ Elevated
▶ First marker of cardiac injury after acute MI

CK-MB

▶ Returns to normal quickly
▶ Most reliable when reported as a percentage of total creatine kinase (CK) (relative index)

Troponin I

▶ Isotypes of troponin found only in myocardium
▶ Elevated
▶ Specific to myocardial damage

Troponin T

▶ Isotype of troponin that's less specific to myocardial damage (can indicate renal failure)
▶ Elevated
▶ Determined quickly at bedside

Release of cardiac enzymes and proteins

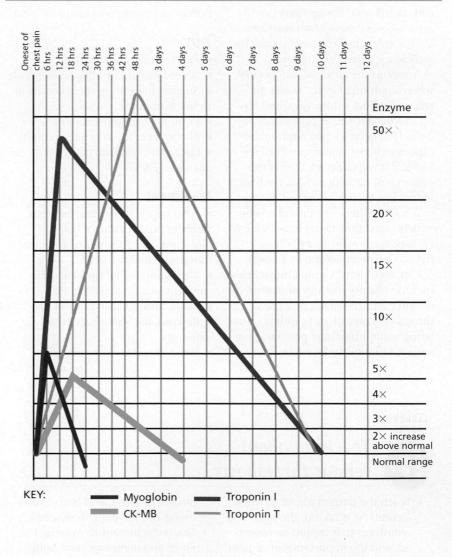

KEY:
— Myoglobin   — Troponin I
— CK-MB   — Troponin T

TESTS TO IDENTIFY THE RISK OF HEART DISEASE

Homocysteine (tHcy)
▶ Normal level: ≤13 µmol/L
▶ Excess levels
– Irritate blood vessels, leading to atherosclerosis
– Raise low-density lipoprotein (LDL) levels
– Make blood clot more easily

High-sensitivity C-reactive protein (hs-CRP)
▶ Normal level: 0.2 to 0.8 mg/dl
▶ Excess levels: May indicate increased risk of coronary artery disease (CAD)

Triglycerides
▶ Normal level: < 150 mg/dl
▶ Excess levels: Identification of hyperlipidemia in patients at risk for CAD

Total cholesterol
▶ Normal level: < 200 mg/dl for adults and less than 170 mg/dl for children and adolescents; borderline high up to 240 mg/dl; high if > 240 mg/dl
▶ Excess levels: May indicate hereditary lipid disorders, CAD

Lipoprotein fractionation
▶ Isolates and measures high-density lipoproteins (HDLs), LDLs, and very-low-density lipoproteins (VLDLs)
▶ Each of these particles composed of protein, cholesterol, and triglyceride in varying amounts

HDL
▶ Primarily protein
▶ Test measures the actual amount in the blood
▶ The *higher* the level, the *lower* the risk of CAD
▶ Normal values for males: 37 to 70 mg/dl; for females, 40 to 85 mg/dl

LDL
▶ Mainly cholesterol
▶ Equal to total cholesterol—HDL cholesterol minus VLDL cholesterol (when triglyceride level is < 400 mg/dl)
▶ The *higher* the LDL level, the *higher* the incidence of CAD
▶ Normal levels for individuals without CAD, < 130 mg/dl; borderline high, 130 to 159 mg/dl; high >160 mg/dl
▶ Optimal levels for individuals who have CAD, < 100 mg/dl

VLDL
▶ Mainly triglycerides
▶ Calculated as the triglyceride level divided by five
▶ The *higher* the VLDL level, the *higher* the incidence of CAD
▶ Can be measured with LDLs in blood with a more sensitive test when high-risk patients and those with triglycerides of 400 mg/dl or more require complex medical management

Evaluating lipid test results

Use this chart to determine an adult patient's risk for coronary artery disease (CAD).

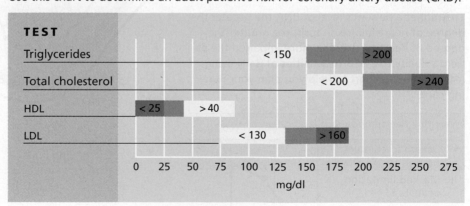

TEST		
Triglycerides	< 150	> 200
Total cholesterol	< 200	> 240
HDL	< 25	> 40
LDL	< 130	> 160

0   25   50   75   100   125   150   175   200   225   250   275
mg/dl

KEY:
Desirable level — No treatment
Borderline level — May need conservative treatment
High risk of CAD — Requires careful medical management

TESTS TO IDENTIFY THE RISK OF HEART FAILURE

Cardiac cells produce and store two neurohormones—A-type natriuretic peptide (ANP) and B-type natriuretic peptide (BNP)—that help ensure cardiac equilibrium. Disruptions in fluid balance within the circulatory system trigger release of these hormones, which act as natural diuretics and antihypertensives.

ANP
▶ Found in atrial tissue
▶ Normal value: 20 to 77 pg/ml

BNP
▶ Found in ventricular tissues
▶ Helps accurately diagnose and grade the severity of heart failure
▶ Normal value: < 100 pg/ml

Correlating the degree of heart failure with BNP level

The higher a patient's level of BNP, the greater the degree of heart failure. In turn, the greater the degree of heart failure, the more impaired the patient's ability to perform activities of daily living (ADLs). Use this chart to help you plan your nursing care.

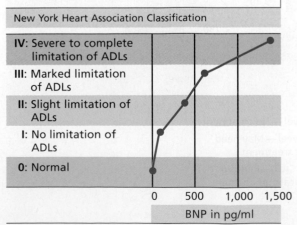

New York Heart Association Classification

IV: Severe to complete limitation of ADLs				
III: Marked limitation of ADLs				
II: Slight limitation of ADLs				
I: No limitation of ADLs				
0: Normal				

0   500   1,000   1,500

BNP in pg/ml

Understanding ANP and BNP

ANP is released by the atria in response to acute increased fluid volume and pressure.

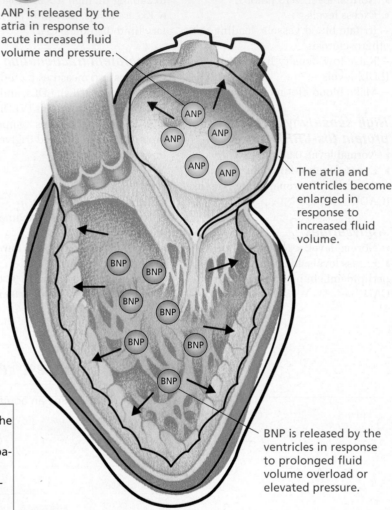

The atria and ventricles become enlarged in response to increased fluid volume.

BNP is released by the ventricles in response to prolonged fluid volume overload or elevated pressure.

ELECTROLYTE TESTS

Electrolytes—which occur in the fluids both inside and outside cells—are crucial for nearly all cellular reactions and functions.

Potassium level

▶ Normal levels: 3.5 to 5 mEq/L
▶ Most critical value
▶ Has narrow therapeutic range
▶ Imbalances causing life-threatening arrhythmias
▶ Affected by diuretics, penicillin G, and low insulin levels

Calcium level

▶ Normal levels: 8.2 to 10.3 mg/dl
▶ High levels causing cardiac toxicity and arrhythmias
▶ Elevations commonly indicate cancer or hyperparathyroidism

Magnesium level

▶ Normal levels: 1.3 to 2.1 mg/dl
▶ Low levels causing electrocardiogram (ECG) changes, ventricular tachycardia, and ventricular fibrillation
▶ High levels causing ECG changes, bradycardia, and hypotension

Sodium level

▶ Normal levels: 135 to 145 mEq/L
▶ Maintains osmotic pressure, acid-base balance, and nerve impulse transmission
▶ Low levels indicating severe heart failure
▶ Decreased levels caused by diuretics, high triglycerides, and low blood protein

Chloride level

▶ Normal levels: 100 to 108 mEq/L
▶ Partners with sodium to maintain fluid and acid-base balance
▶ Low levels indicating heart failure and metabolic acidosis

Carbon dioxide level

▶ Normal levels: 23 to 30 mEq/L
▶ Primarily made up of bicarbonate
▶ Regulated by the kidneys
▶ Reduced by thiazide diuretics

COAGULATION TESTS

Partial thromboplastin time, prothrombin time (PT), and activated clotting time are tests that measure clotting time. They're used to measure response to treatment as well as to screen for clotting disorders.

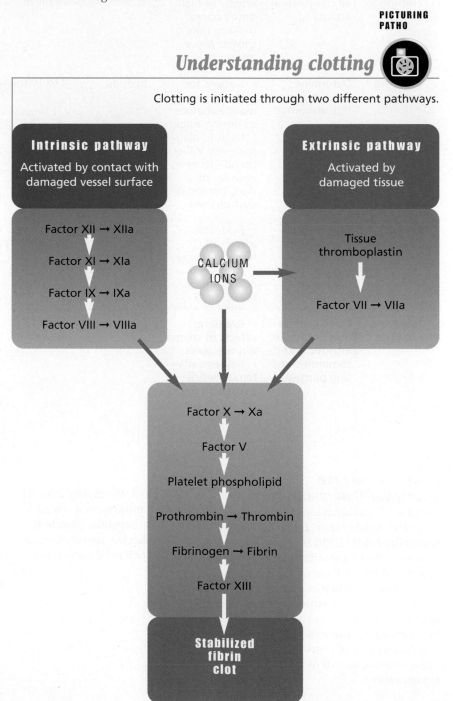

PICTURING PATHO

Understanding clotting

Clotting is initiated through two different pathways.

Intrinsic pathway
Activated by contact with damaged vessel surface

Factor XII → XIIa
Factor XI → XIa
Factor IX → IXa
Factor VIII → VIIIa

CALCIUM IONS

Extrinsic pathway
Activated by damaged tissue

Tissue thromboplastin

Factor VII → VIIa

Factor X → Xa
Factor V
Platelet phospholipid
Prothrombin → Thrombin
Fibrinogen → Fibrin
Factor XIII

Stabilized fibrin clot

Common tests for clotting

Test	Action	Clinical uses	Where performed	Normal range	Therapeutic range	Panic value
Activated clotting time	Measures overall coagulation activity	▸ Evaluates effects of high-dose heparin therapy during cardiac procedures	Bedside	70 to 120 seconds	2 times normal range	Unknown
Bleeding time	Determines platelet function abnormalities	▸ Screens for platelet abnormalities before or during surgery ▸ Used to diagnose von Willebrand's disease, vascular disorders, hemostatic dysfunctions	Bedside	3 to 10 minutes	Unknown	> 15 minutes
Partial thromboplastin time	Measures defects in intrinsic and common clotting pathways	▸ Evaluates effects of heparin therapy ▸ Assesses overall coagulation system	Laboratory	21 to 35 seconds	2 to 2.5 times normal range	> 70 seconds
Prothrombin time	Directly measures defects in intrinsic and common clotting pathways	▸ Evaluates effects of coumadin therapies ▸ Assesses vitamin K deficiency ▸ Used to diagnose liver failure	Laboratory	11 to 13 seconds	2 to 2.5 times normal range	> 30 seconds

Understanding the International Normalized Ratio

Because PT measurements vary from laboratory to laboratory, International Normalized Ratio (INR) is generally viewed as the best standarized measurement of PT. Both are used for monitoring warfarin (Coumadin) treatment. Guidelines for patients receiving warfarin recommend an INR of 2.9 to 3.0 except for patients with mechanical prosthetic heart valves. For those patients, an INR of 2.5 to 3.5 is recommended.

Increased INR values may indicate disseminated intravascular coagulation, cirrhosis, hepatitis, vitamin K deficiency, salicylate intoxication, or uncontrolled oral anticoagulation.

Electrocardiography

12-LEAD ECG

A commonly used diagnostic tool, the standard 12-lead electrocardiogram (ECG) can help identify myocardial ischemia, myocardial infarction, rhythm and conduction disturbances, chamber enlargement, electrolyte imbalances, and drug toxicity. It measures electrical potential from 12 different views (leads).

Understanding ECG leads

ECG waveforms vary depending on the leads being viewed and the rhythm of the heart. To make an accurate assessment of the heart's electrical activity, a 12-lead ECG evaluates the heart from 12 different views to determine malfunctions.

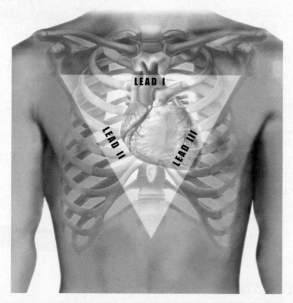

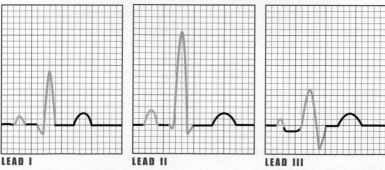

LEAD I   LEAD II   LEAD III

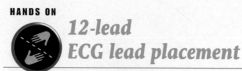

12-lead ECG lead placement

Six unipolar precordial leads (V_1 to V_6) show the heart from the horizontal plane.

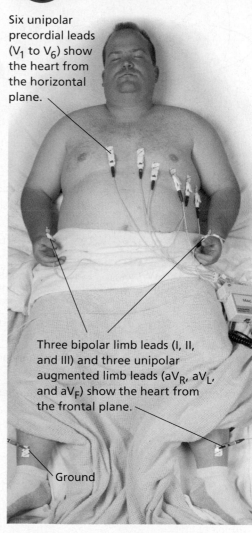

Three bipolar limb leads (I, II, and III) and three unipolar augmented limb leads (aV_R, aV_L, and aV_F) show the heart from the frontal plane.

Ground

A right-sided ECG may be used to diagnose a right ventricular infarct. Leads V_1 and V_2 are placed in the same position as for a left-sided ECG. Leads V_3 to V_6 are placed along the right chest wall in a mirror position to the left-sided ECG.

Locating myocardial damage with a 12-lead ECG

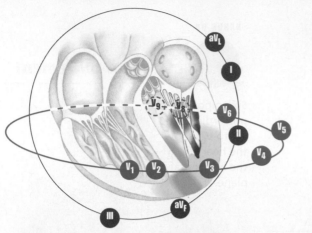

KEY:

Anteroseptal wall

Anterior wall

Lateral wall

Inferior wall

Posterior wall

Wall affected	Leads	Artery involved	Reciprocal changes
Antero-septal	V_1, V_2, V_3, V_4	Left anterior descending (LAD)	None
Anterior	V_2, V_3, V_4	Left coronary artery (LCA)	II, III, aV_F
Antero-lateral	I, aV_L, V_3, V_4, V_5, V_6	LAD and diagonal branches, circumflex, and marginal branches	II, III, aV_F
Lateral	I, aV_L, V_5, V_6	Circumflex branch of LCA	II, III, aV_F
Inferior	II, III, aV_F	Right coronary artery (RCA)	I, aV_L
Posterior	V_8, V_9	RCA or circumflex	V_1, V_2, V_3, V_4 (R greater than S in V_1 and V_2, ST-segment depression, elevated T waves)

EXERCISE ECG

Exercise ECG, or stress testing, is a noninvasive procedure that helps assess the heart's response to an increased workload. If the patient experiences chest pain, fatigue, severe dyspnea, claudication, weakness or dizziness, hypotension, pallor or vaso-constriction, disorientation, ataxia, ischemic ECG changes (with or without pain), rhythm disturbances or heart block, or ventricular conduction abnormalities, the test is stopped.

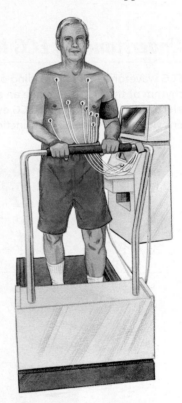

Drug-induced stress tests

If a patient can't tolerate physical activity, a drug such as regadenoson (Lexiscan), adenosine (Adenoscan), or dobutamine can be administered to cause the heart to react as if the person were exercising. The drug is given I.V. along with thallium (a radioactive substance known as a *tracer*). The areas of the heart that lack adequate blood supply pick up the tracer very slowly, if at all.

A nuclear scanner records an initial set of images and then a second set of images taken 3 to 4 hours later. A cardiologist uses these images to determine areas of heart muscle with diminished blood supply or permanent damage from a myocardial infarction.

HOLTER MONITORING

Also called *ambulatory ECG,* Holter monitoring records the heart's activity as the patient follows his normal routine. The patient wears a small electronic recorder connected to electrodes placed on his chest and keeps a diary of his activities and associated symptoms. Used to identify intermittent arrhythmias, this test usually lasts about 24 hours (about 100,000 cardiac cycles).

A look at a Holter monitor

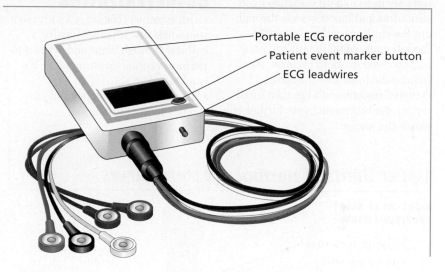

- Portable ECG recorder
- Patient event marker button
- ECG leadwires

Normal conduction intervals in adults

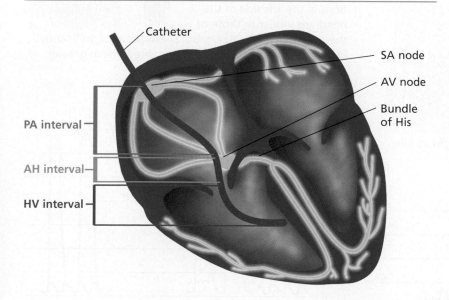

- Catheter
- SA node
- AV node
- Bundle of His

PA interval

AH interval

HV interval

PA interval = conduction from sinatrial (SA) node to atrioventricular (AV) node
= 20 to 40 msec

AH interval = conduction from AV node to bundle of His
= 4 to 150 msec

HV interval = conduction from bundle of His to ventricles
= 35 to 55 msec

ELECTROPHYSIOLOGY STUDIES

Electrophysiology studies are used to help determine the cause of an arrhythmia and the best treatment for it. A bipolar or tripolar electrode catheter is threaded into a vein, through the right atrium, and across the septal leaflet of the tricuspid valve. The femoral vein is the most common choice for the catheter insertion. However, the subclavian, internal jugular, or brachial vein may also be used. The heart's usual conduction is recorded first. The catheter sends electrical signals to the heart to change the heart rate and initiate an arrhythmia. Various drugs are then tried to terminate the arrhythmia.

Also, sometimes the cardiologist can induce an arrhythmia and then immediately treat it using radiofrequency ablation, a pacemaker, or an implantable cardioverter-defibrillator.

Imaging tests

Various imaging and radiographic tests are used to help visualize heart structures and blood vessels throughout the cardiovascular system. Although many of these tests are noninvasive and quick to perform, some require the insertion of a cardiac catheter, injection of a contrast medium, or nuclear medicine to further enhance the image.

CARDIAC CATHETERIZATION

Cardiac catheterization is an invasive procedure that involves passing a catheter through veins and arteries to perform various measurements. It's used to:

▶ measure heart chamber and pulmonary artery pressures

▶ check blood flow between the heart chambers
▶ determine valve competence
▶ monitor cardiac wall contractility
▶ detect intracardiac status
▶ visualize the coronary arteries.

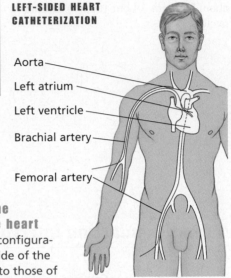

LEFT-SIDED HEART CATHETERIZATION

Aorta
Left atrium
Left ventricle
Brachial artery
Femoral artery

Upper limits of normal pressure curves

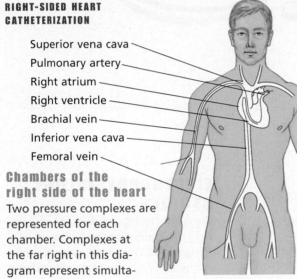

RIGHT-SIDED HEART CATHETERIZATION

Superior vena cava
Pulmonary artery
Right atrium
Right ventricle
Brachial vein
Inferior vena cava
Femoral vein

Chambers of the right side of the heart

Two pressure complexes are represented for each chamber. Complexes at the far right in this diagram represent simultaneous recordings of pressures from the right atrium, right ventricle, and pulmonary artery.

Pressure
(mm Hg)
100
80
60
40
20
0

a v a   1   3 4
             2   5
RA   RV   PA   RA RV PA

KEY:
RA = Right atrium
RV = Right ventricle
PA = Pulmonary artery
a wave = Contraction
v wave = Passive filling

1 = RV peak systolic pressure
2 = RV end-diastolic pressure
3 = PA peak systolic pressure
4 = PA dicrotic notch
5 = PA diastolic pressure

Chambers of the left side of the heart

Overall pressure configurations in the left side of the heart are similar to those of the right side of the heart, but pressures are significantly higher because systemic flow resistance is much greater than pulmonary resistance.

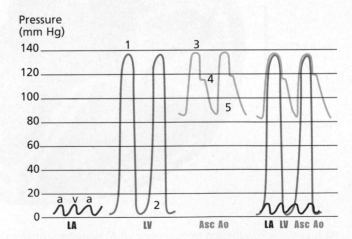

Pressure
(mm Hg)
140
120
100
80
60
40
20
0

a v a   1   3
                     4
                     5
        2
LA   LV   Asc Ao   LA LV Asc Ao

KEY:
LA = Left atrium
LV = Left ventricle
Asc Ao = Ascending aorta
a wave = Contraction
v wave = Passive filling

1 = LV peak systolic pressure
2 = LV end-diastolic pressure
3 = PA peak systolic pressure
4 = PA dicrotic notch
5 = PA diastolic pressure

ECHOCARDIOGRAPHY

An echocardiograph uses ultra-high-frequency sound waves to help examine the size, shape, and motion of the heart's structures. A special transducer is placed over the patient's chest over an area where bone and tissues are absent. It directs sound waves to the heart structures and converts them to electrical impulses. These electrical impulses are sent to the echocardiograph and displayed on a screen. The image is then recorded on a strip chart or videotaped.

A look at echocardiography

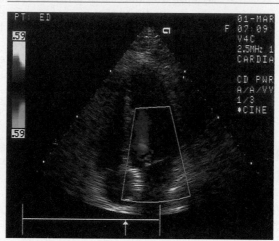

This computer graphic depicts an image of the heart's chambers and valves that's more detailed than an X-ray film. The ultrasound waves that rebound (or echo) off the heart can show the size, shape, and movement of cardiac structures as well as the flow of blood through the heart, which helps analyze valvular function and heart pressures.

Two types of echocardiography

The most commonly used echocardiographic techniques are motion mode (M-mode) and two-dimensional (2-D). In many cases, the techniques are performed together to complement each other. Echocardiography may be used to detect mitral stenosis, mitral valve prolapse, aortic insufficiency, wall motion abnormalities, and pericardial effusion.

In M-mode echocardiography, a single, pencil-like ultrasound beam strikes the heart, producing a vertical, or "ice pick," view of cardiac structures. The echo tracings are plotted against time. This mode is especially useful for precisely viewing cardiac structures.

In 2-D echocardiography, the ultrasound beam rapidly sweeps through a 30-degree arc, producing a cross-sectioned, or fan-shaped, view of cardiac structures. Appearing as a real-time video display, this technique is useful for recording lateral motion and providing the correct spatial relationship between cardiac structures.

The shaded areas beneath the transducer identify cardiac structures that intercept and reflect the transducer's ultrasonic waves.

Transducer

Anterolateral chest wall

Right ventricular anterior wall

Right ventricle

Intraventricular septum

Aortic valve

Left ventricle

Left atrium

Left ventricular posterior wall

Transesophageal echocardiography

In transesophageal echocardiography (TEE), ultrasonography is combined with endoscopy to provide a better view of the heart's structures.

TEE is used to evaluate valvular disease or repairs. It's also used to diagnose:

▶ thoracic and aortic disorders
▶ endocarditis
▶ congenital heart disease
▶ intracardiac thrombi
▶ tumors.

CARDIAC MAGNETIC RESONANCE IMAGING

Also known as *nuclear magnetic resonance,* cardiac magnetic resonance imaging (MRI) yields high-resolution, tomographic, three-dimensional images of the heart. Cardiac MRI permits visualization of valve leaflets and structures, pericardial abnormalities and processes, ventricular hypertrophy, cardiac neoplasm, infarcted tissue, anatomic malformations, and structural deformities. It can be used to monitor the progression of ischemic heart disease and the effectiveness of treatment.

How TEE is performed

A small transducer is attached to the end of a gastroscope and inserted into the esophagus so that images of the heart's structure can be taken from the posterior of the heart. This test causes less tissue penetration and interference from chest wall structures and produces high-quality images of the thoracic aorta (except for the superior ascending aorta, which is shadowed by the trachea).

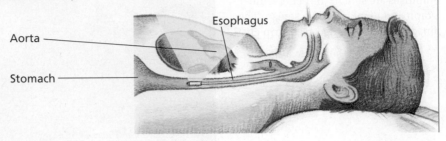

Picturing MRI

The magnetic resonance imaging (MRI) scanner records the electromagnetic signals the nuclei emit. The scanner then translates the signals into detailed pictures. The resulting images show tissue characteristics without lung or bone interference, as shown here.

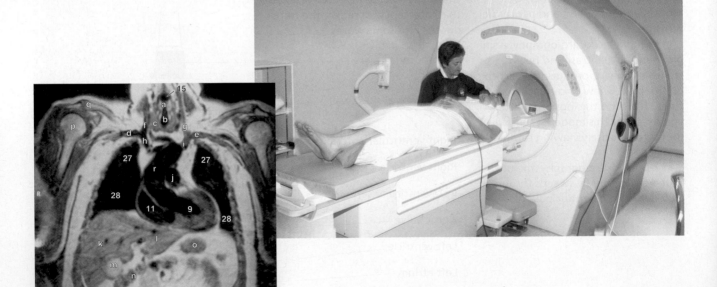

CARDIAC POSITRON EMISSION TOMOGRAPHY

Cardiac positron emission tomography (PET) scanning combines elements of computed tomography scanning and conventional radionuclide imaging. Radioisotopes are administered to the patient by injection, inhalation, or I.V. infusion. One isotope targets blood; one targets glucose. These isotopes emit particles called *positrons*. The PET scanner detects and reconstructs the positrons to form an image.

A PET scan can show the following:
▶ Normal blood flow and glucose metabolism indicates good coronary perfusion.
▶ Decreased blood flow with increased glucose metabolism indicates ischemia.
▶ Decreased blood flow with decreased glucose metabolism shows necrotic or scarred heart tissue.

CARDIAC BLOOD POOL IMAGING

Cardiac blood pool imaging (also called *multiple-gated acquisition [MUGA] scanning*) is used to evaluate regional and global ventricular performance.

Many variations of the MUGA scan are available:
▶ In the *stress MUGA* test, the same test is performed at rest and after exercise to detect changes in ejection fraction and cardiac output.
▶ In the *nitroglycerin MUGA* test, the scintillation camera records points in the cardiac cycle after the sublingual administration of nitroglycerin to assess the drug's effect on ventricular function.

Picturing MUGA scanning

During a multiple-gated acquisition (MUGA) scan, the camera records 14 to 64 points of a single cardiac cycle, yielding sequential images that can be studied like a motion picture film. This allows physicians to evaluate regional motion and determine ejection fraction and other indices of cardiac function.

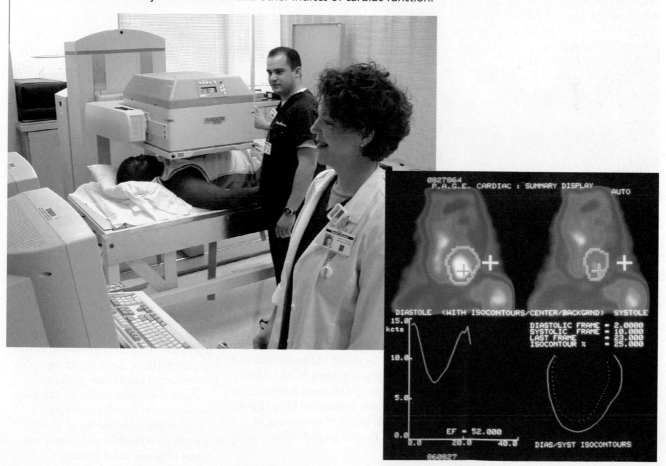

HOT AND COLD SPOT IMAGING

Technetium-99m (^{99m}Tc) pyrophosphate scanning, also known as hot spot imaging or PYP scanning, helps diagnose acute myocardial injury by showing the location and size of newly damaged myocardial tissue. In this test, the patient receives an injection of ^{99m}Tc pyrophosphate, a radioactive material absorbed by damaged cells. Damaged areas show as orange to bright red spots on the image. A spot's size usually corresponds to the injury size. The scan reveals transmural infarction, right ventricular, and posterior infarctions. It also helps assess ventricular aneurysms and heart tumors.

Also known as *cold spot imaging,* thallium-201 (^{201}TI) scanning evaluates myocardial blood flow and myocardial cell status. This test helps determine areas of ischemic myocardium and infarcted tissue. It can also help evaluate ventricular function and pericardial effusion.

^{201}TI is a radioactive isotope that emits gamma rays. When injected I.V. the isotope is absorbed quickly by healthy myocardial tissue. However, unhealthy tissue absorbs the isotope slowly. Damaged areas show as dark blue to purple spots on the image.

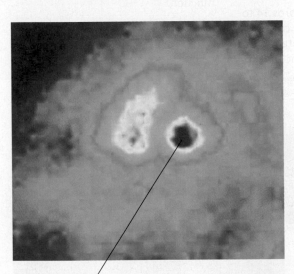

Damaged area

DOPPLER ULTRASONOGRAPHY

Duplex Doppler ultrasonography involves the use of high-frequency sound waves to image vessels and evaluate blood flow in the major vessels of the trunk (heart and intra-abdominal organs) and extremities (arms and legs) and in the extracranial cerebrovascular system (neck). This noninvasive test shows the speed, direction, and patterns of blood flow and is used to detect narrowing or blockages in arteries and veins.

A handheld transducer directs high-frequency sound waves to the artery or vein being tested. The sound waves strike moving red blood cells and are reflected back to the transducer at frequencies that correspond to blood flow velocity through the vessel. The transducer then amplifies the sound waves to permit direct listening and graphic recording of blood flow patterns.

Pulse volume recorder testing may be performed along with duplex Doppler ultrasonography to yield a quantitative recording of changes in blood pressure in an extremity.

Measuring the ankle-brachial index

A hand-held Doppler ultrasound device can also be used to measure the ankle-brachial index to help identify peripheral vascular disease of the lower extremities. To perform this test, follow these steps.

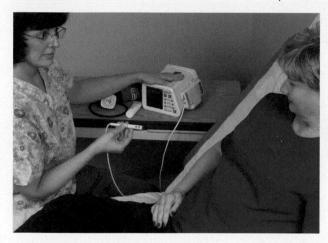

1. Confirm the patient's identity using two patient identifiers according to facility policy.

2. Gather your materials and wash your hands.

3. Explain the procedure to the patient.

4. Apply an appropriate-sized blood pressure cuff to the upper arm.

5. Apply warm conductive gel to the patient's arm where the brachial pulse has been palpated and then obtain the systolic reading of both arms.

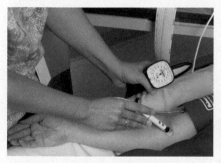

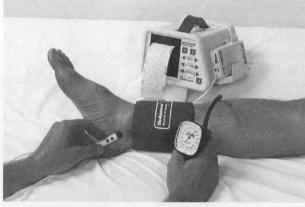

6. Apply an appropriate-sized blood pressure cuff just above the right ankle. Locate the posterior tibial pulse and record the systolic pressure. Then, locate the dorsalis pedis pulse and repeat the procedure.

7. Repeat the procedure on the left ankle.

Normally, venous blood flow fluctuates with respiration, so observing changes in sound wave frequency during respiration helps detect venous occlusive disease. Compression maneuvers can help detect occlusion of the veins as well. Abnormal images and Doppler signals may indicate plaque, stenosis, occlusion, dissection, aneurysm, carotid body tumor, arteritis, and venous thrombosis.

Doppler of popliteal artery
The image at right shows a color flow duplex image of a popliteal artery with normal triphasic Doppler signal.

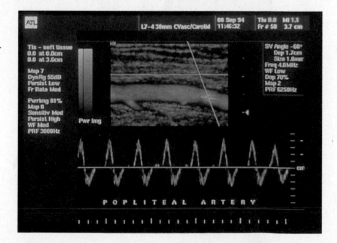

Calculating ABI

To calculate the ankle-brachial index (ABI), divide the higher systolic pressure obtained from each leg (dorsalis pedis or posterior tibial) by the higher brachial systolic pressure.

Systolic readings (mm Hg)	Left	Right
Posterior tibial	128	96
Dorsalis pedis	130	90
Brachial	132	130
Calculations	130 ÷ 132 = 0.98	96 ÷ 132 = 0.73

and interpreting the results

Greater than 1.3: Unreliable and inconclusive; false-high readings possibly produced by calcified vessels (such as occurs in diabetes)

1.01 to 1.3: Correlates with patient history (especially in diabetes)

0.97 to 1: Normal

0.8 to 0.96: Mild ischemia

0.4 to 0.79: Moderate to severe ischemia

0.39 or less: Severe ischemia, danger of limb loss

Venography

Also known as *ascending contrast phlebograpy,* venography is radiographic examination of veins in a lower extremity and is used less frequently than other methods. During this test, a catheter is inserted into a vein (usually through the foot) and a contrast medium is injected. X-rays are then used to determine the patency of the vein by viewing the flow of the contrast medium through the vessel.

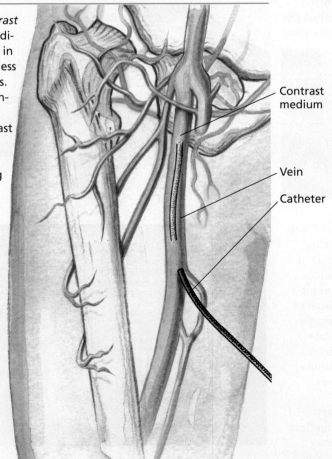

Contrast medium

Vein

Catheter

PERIPHERAL ARTERIOGRAPHY

Peripheral arteriography, or *angiography*, is the injection of a contrast medium into the peripheral arteries accompanied by cineangiograms (rapidly changing movies on an intensified fluoroscopic screen), which record the passage of the contrast medium through the vascular system. Arteriography can also be done using a magnetic resonance scanner and contrast medium.

Arteriography demonstrates the location and degree of obstruction and collateral circulation. This procedure is particularly useful in chronic disease or for evaluating candidates for reconstructive surgery.

Angiograph of the femoral artery and its branches

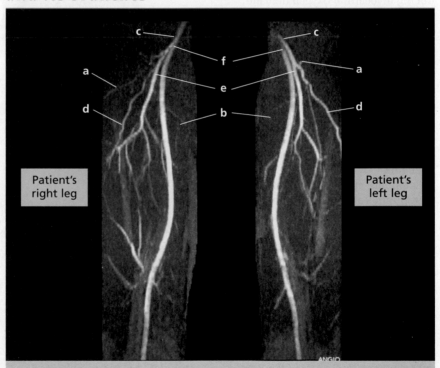

Patient's right leg

Patient's left leg

KEY:
a = Lateral circumflex femoral artery
b = Medial circumflex femoral artery
c = Femoral artery
d = Descending branch of the profunda femoris artery
e = Profunda femoris artery
f = Femoral artery

TREATMENTS AND PROCEDURES
Drug therapy

Several types of drugs are critical to the treatment of cardiovascular disorders. These drugs include:

▶ antianginals
▶ antiarrhythmics
▶ anticoagulants
▶ antihypertensives
▶ antilipemics
▶ inotropics
▶ thrombolytics.

ANTIANGINALS

Antianginals relieve chest pain by reducing myocardial oxygen demand, increasing the supply of oxygen to the heart, or both. The three main types are:

Beta-adrenergic blockers

▶ Reduce myocardial oxygen demands by slowing the heart rate and increasing the force of myocardial contractions
▶ Prescribed for long-term prevention of angina
▶ Examples: atenolol (Tenormin), metoprolol (Lopressor), nadolol (Corgard), propranolol (Inderal)

Calcium channel blockers

▶ Dilate coronary and peripheral arteries and prevent coronary vasospasm
▶ Used when other drugs fail to prevent angina
▶ Examples: amlodipine (Norvase), diltiazem (Cardizem), nicardipine (Cardene), verapamil (Calan)

Nitrates

▶ Produce vasodilation, decrease preload and afterload, and reduce myocardial oxygen consumption
▶ Used primarily to treat angina
▶ Examples: nitroglycerin (Nitro-Bid, Nitrostat, Nitrolingual), isosorbide dinitrate (Isordil)

How antianginal drugs work

When the coronary arteries can't supply enough oxygen to the myocardium, angina occurs. This forces the heart to work harder, increasing heart rate, preload, afterload, and the force of myocardial contractility. Antianginal drugs relieve angina by decreasing one or more of these four factors.

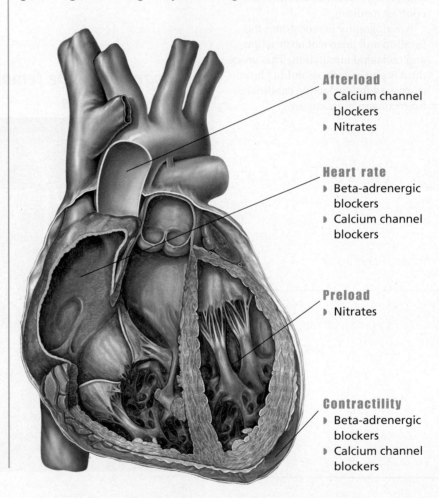

Afterload
▶ Calcium channel blockers
▶ Nitrates

Heart rate
▶ Beta-adrenergic blockers
▶ Calcium channel blockers

Preload
▶ Nitrates

Contractility
▶ Beta-adrenergic blockers
▶ Calcium channel blockers

Classes of antiarrhythmics

Antiarrhythmics are used to treat disturbances in normal heart rhythm and are grouped in one of four classes.

Class	Features	Rhythms treated	Examples
I Sodium channel blockers	▸ Largest class ▸ Three subdivisions plus adenosine ▸ Decrease automaticity, conduction velocity, and membrane responsiveness	▸ IA: atrial and ventricular arrhythmias ▸ IB: acute ventricular arrhythmias ▸ IC: severe refractory ventricular arrhythmias ▸ Adenosine: paroxysmal supraventricular tachycardia	▸ IA: disopyramide (Norpace) ▸ IB: lidocaine (Xylocaine) ▸ IC: flecainide (Tambocor)
II Beta-adrenergic blockers	▸ Slow automaticity of sinoatrial node ▸ Reduce conduction of atrioventricular node and pacer cells ▸ Decrease strength of contraction	▸ Atrial flutter and fibrillation ▸ Paroxysmal atrial tachycardia	▸ Atenolol (Tenormin) ▸ Metoprolol (Lopressor) ▸ Propranolol (Inderal)
III Potassium channel blockers	▸ Act on tissues in all chambers of the heart ▸ May slow repolarization ▸ May prolong refractory period	▸ Ventricular arrhythmias	▸ Amiodarone (Cordarone) ▸ Dofetilide (Tikosyn) ▸ Sotalol (Betapace)
IV Calcium channel blockers	▸ Decrease cardiac contractility and oxygen demand ▸ Dilate coronary arteries and arterioles	▸ Supraventricular arrhythmias with rapid ventricular response	▸ Diltiazem (Cardizem) ▸ Amlodipine (Norvasc) ▸ Verapamil (Calan)

ANTIARRHYTHMICS

Antiarrhythmics are used to treat disturbances in the normal heart rhythm, and are grouped in one of four classes: I (sodium channel blockers), II (beta-adrenergic blockers), III (potassium channel blockers), and IV (calcium channel blockers).

ANTICOAGULANTS

Anticoagulants reduce the blood's ability to clot. They're prescribed for mitral insufficiency and atrial fibrillation, or to prevent clots in an artery or vein.

Types of anticoagulants

Anticoagulants reduce the blood's ability to clot. They're prescribed for mitral insufficiency or atrial fibrillation or to reduce the amount of clots that block an artery.

Category	Features	Examples
Heparins	‣ Used in patients with unstable angina, myocardial infarction, and deep vein thrombosis (DVT) ‣ Act immediately when given I.V. ‣ Available in regular and low-molecular-weight forms	‣ Heparin ‣ Low-molecular-weight anticoagulant (dalteparin [Fragmin], enoxaparin [Lovenox])
Coumarin derivatives	‣ Antagonize production of vitamin K–dependent clotting factors ‣ Prevent DVT and thrombus formation ‣ Used in patients who have undergone prosthetic heart valve surgery, or revascularization with prosthetic bypass grafts, those with diseased valves, and those with chronic atrial fibrillation ‣ Take days to reach effect ‣ Available only in oral form	‣ Warfarin (Coumadin)
Antiplatelet drugs	‣ Prevent thromboembolism ‣ Prevent cardiac and cerebral episodes in paients with coronary artery disease risk factors ‣ Prevent thrombosis after revascularization surgery	‣ Aspirin ‣ Clopidogrel (Plavix) ‣ Dipyridamole (Persantine) ‣ Sulfinpyrazone (Anturane) ‣ Ticlopidine (Ticlid)
Direct thrombin inhibitors	‣ Treat heparin-induced thrombocytopenia ‣ Used when heparin can't be ‣ Prophylactically used before angioplasty and stent placement ‣ Available I.V.	‣ Argatroban ‣ Bivalirudin (Angiomax) ‣ Lepirudin (Refludan)
Activated factor X inhibitors	‣ Prevent DVT after total hip or knee replacement surgery or postoperatively with hip fractures	‣ Fondaparinux (Arixtra)

ANTIHYPERTENSIVES

Treatment for hypertension begins with modifying diet, encouraging exercise and, if indicated, counseling about weight loss. If these measures aren't enough, drugs can help control blood pressure.

Angiotensin-converting enzyme (ACE) inhibitors

‣ Decrease vasoconstriction and re-uptake of fluids by preventing angiotensin I from converting to angiotensin II
‣ Examples: captopril (Capoten), enalapril (Vasotec)

Angiotensin II receptor blockers (ARBs)

‣ Inhibit vasoconstriction
‣ Protect against renal failure in patients with type 2 diabetes
‣ Examples: losartan (Cozaar), olmesartan (Benicar)

Beta-adrenergic blockers

‣ Block catecholamine-induced increase in blood pressure
‣ Examples: metoprolol (Lopressor), nadolol (Corgard)

Calcium channel blockers

‣ Dilate the arteries to lower blood pressure
‣ Decrease cardiac contractility
‣ Examples: amlodipine (Norvasc), diltiazem (Cardizem)

Diuretics

‣ Help kidneys excrete water and electrolytes, which lowers blood pressure
‣ Thiazide example: hydrochlorothiazide (HydroDIURIL)
‣ Loop example: furosemide (Lasix)
‣ Potassium-sparing example: spironolactone (Aldactone)

PICTURING
PATHO

Antihypertensives and the renin-angiotensin-aldosterone system

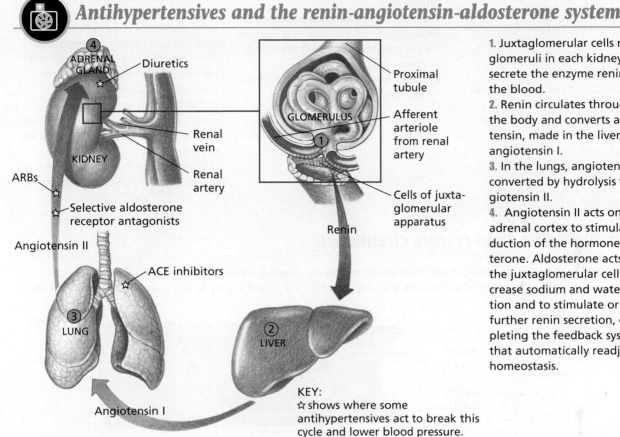

1. Juxtaglomerular cells near the glomeruli in each kidney secrete the enzyme renin into the blood.
2. Renin circulates throughout the body and converts angiotensin, made in the liver, to angiotensin I.
3. In the lungs, angiotensin I is converted by hydrolysis to angiotensin II.
4. Angiotensin II acts on the adrenal cortex to stimulate production of the hormone aldosterone. Aldosterone acts on the juxtaglomerular cells to increase sodium and water retention and to stimulate or depress further renin secretion, completing the feedback system that automatically readjusts homeostasis.

KEY:
☆ shows where some antihypertensives act to break this cycle and lower blood pressure.

Selective aldosterone receptor antagonists
- Used as a second-line treatment when other drugs fail
- Only example: eplerenone (Inspra)

Sympatholytics
- Decrease peripheral vascular resistance by inhibiting the sympathetic nervous system
- Examples: clonidine (Catapres), doxazosin (Cardura), carvedilol (Coreg)

Vasodilators
- Relax arteries, veins, or both
- Examples: hydralazine (Apresoline), I.V. nitroprusside (Nitropress), diazoxide (Hyperstat I.V.)

ANTILIPEMICS
Antilipemics lower cholesterol, triglyceride, and phospholipid levels. They're used in combination with lifestyle changes to decrease the risk of coronary artery disease.

Bile-sequestering drugs
- Remove excess bile acids from fat deposits
- Lower low-density lipoprotein (LDL) levels
- Example: cholestyramine (Questran)

Cholesterol absorption inhibitors
- Lower total cholesterol levels
- Example: ezetimibe (Zetia)

Fibric-acid derivatives
- Lower triglyceride levels
- Minimally increase high-density lipoprotein (HDL) levels
- Examples: fenofibrate (Tricor), gemfibrozil (Lopid)

HMG-CoA reductase inhibitors
- Also known as *statins*
- Lower total cholesterol and LDL levels
- Minimally increase HDL levels
- Examples: atorvastatin (Lipitor), simvastatin (Zocor)

Nicotinic acid (niacin)
- Water-soluble vitamin
- Lowers triglyceride levels
- Increases HDL levels

INOTROPICS

Inotropics increase the force of the heart's contractions. The two types are cardiac glycoside and phosphodiesterase inhibitors.

Cardiac glycoside

▶ Slows the heart rate and electrical impulse conduction through the sinoatrial and the atrioventricular nodes
▶ Example: digoxin (Lanoxin)

Phosphodiesterase (PDE) inhibitors

▶ Provide short-term management of heart failure or long-term management for patients awaiting heart transplant surgery
▶ Examples: inamrinone (Amrinone), milrinone (Primacor)

FIBRINOLYTICS

Fibrinolytics can dissolve a clot or thrombus that has caused acute MI, ischemic stroke or peripheral artery occlusion, or pulmonary embolus. They can also dissolve thrombi and reestablish blood flow in arteriovenous cannulas, grafts, and I.V. catheters. In an acute or emergency situation, they must be administered within 3 to 6 hours after the onset of symptoms. Fibrinolytics include alteplase (Activase), reteplase (Retavase), and urokinase (Abbokinase).

How fibrinolytics help restore circulation

When a thrombus forms in an artery, it obstructs the blood supply, causing ischemia and necrosis. Fibrinolytics can dissolve thrombi in the coronary and pulmonary arteries, restoring the blood supply to the area beyond the blockage.

Obstructed artery
A thrombus blocks blood flow through the artery, causing distal ischemia.

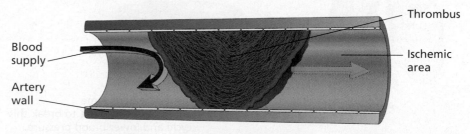

Inside the thrombus
The fibrinolytic enters the thrombus and binds to the fibrin-plasminogen complex, converting inactive plasminogen into active plasmin. Active plasmin digests fibrin, dissolving the thrombus. As the thrombus dissolves, blood flow resumes.

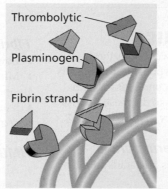
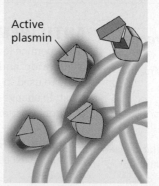
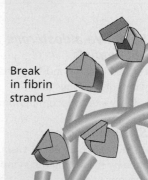

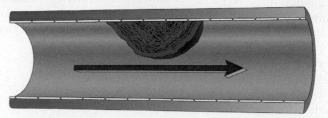

Surgical and other procedures

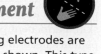
HANDS ON

CARDIAC PACING

When the electrical conduction of the heart is disrupted, cardiac output is diminished and perfusion of blood and oxygen to all body tissues is affected. Treatment to restore the heart's conduction needs to begin quickly. Some treatments include pacemaker insertion (temporary and permanent) and an implantable cardioverter-defibrillator (ICD).

Temporary pacing

Temporary pacing is used in arrhythmic emergencies, such as bradycardia and tachyarrhythmias, or other conduction system disturbances. Temporary pacemakers contain external, battery-powered pulse generators and a lead or electrode system and can be transcutaneous or transvenous.

Temporary transvenous pacemaker

Transvenous pacing provides a more reliable pacing beat. This type of pacing is more comfortable for the patient because the pacing wire is inserted in the heart via a major vein.

Transcutaneous electrode placement

For a noninvasive temporary pacemaker, the two pacing electrodes are placed at heart level on the patient's chest and back, as shown. This type of pacemaker can be quickly applied in an emergency but is uncomfortable for the patient.

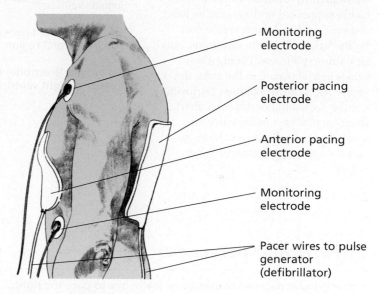

- Monitoring electrode
- Posterior pacing electrode
- Anterior pacing electrode
- Monitoring electrode
- Pacer wires to pulse generator (defibrillator)

Transvenous pulse generator

Sense meter registers every time the patient's heart beats.

Pace meter registers every pacing stimulus delivered to the heart.

Rate control sets the minimum heart rate at which point the pacemaker takes over.

Sensitivity control adjusts pacemaker sensitivity to the patient's heart rate. When the dial is set on ASYNC the pacemaker delivers a set rate regardless of the patient's intrinsic rate.

Output control determines the number of milliamps of electricity sent to the heart.

Connector attaches the pacing wires to the pulse generator.

Battery compartment

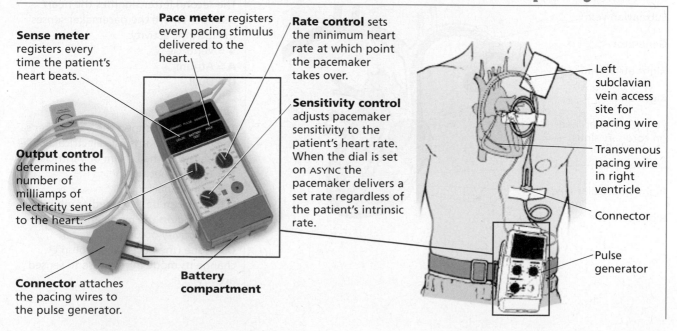

- Left subclavian vein access site for pacing wire
- Transvenous pacing wire in right ventricle
- Connector
- Pulse generator

Permanent pacing

A permanent pacemaker is a self-contained device that's surgically implanted in a pocket under the patient's skin. Permanent pacemakers allow the patient's heart to beat on its own but keep the heartbeat from falling below a preset rate. Pacemakers treat persistent bradyarrhythmias, complete heart block, congenital or degenerative heart diseases, Stokes-Adams syndrome, Wolff-Parkinson-White syndrome, and sick sinus syndrome. Pacing electrodes can be placed in the atria, the ventricles, or both chambers (atrioventricular sequential or dual chamber). Biventricular pacemakers also are available for cardiac resynchronization therapy in patients with heart failure.

Permanent pacemaker

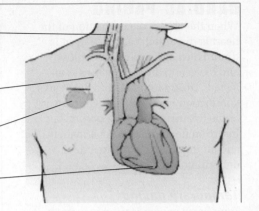

Pacemaker lead in external jugular vein

Pacemaker lead tunneled subcutaneously between pacemaker and external jugular vein

Generator placed beneath skin in pectoral region

Tip of wire (electrode) lodged in apex of right ventricle

Biventricular pacemaker

A biventricular pacemaker uses three leads: one to pace the right atrium, one to pace the right ventricle, and one to pace the left ventricle. The left ventricular lead is placed in the coronary sinus. Both ventricles are paced at the same time, causing them to contract simultaneously, improving cardiac output.

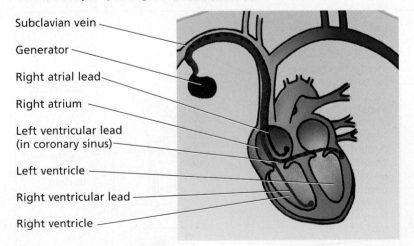

Subclavian vein

Generator

Right atrial lead

Right atrium

Left ventricular lead (in coronary sinus)

Left ventricle

Right ventricular lead

Right ventricle

Understanding pacemaker codes

First letter
The first letter of a pacemaker code identifies the heart chambers that are paced:
V = Ventricle
A = Atrium
D = Dual (ventricle and atrium)

Second letter
The second letter signifies the heart chamber where the pacemaker senses the intrinsic activity:
V = Ventricle
A = Atrium
D = Dual

Third letter
The third letter shows the pacemaker's response to the intrinsic electrical activity it senses in the atrium or ventricle.
T = Triggers pacing
I = Inhibits pacing
D = Dual (can be triggered or inhibited depending on the mode and where intrinsic activity occurs)
O = None (the pacemaker doesn't change its mode in response to sensed activity)

Fourth letter

The fourth letter signifies the rate modulation ability of the pacemaker (attempt to replicate the ability of a normal heart to increase heart rate in response to metabolic demand).
R = Rate modulated
O = Not programmable

Fifth letter

The fifth letter designates the location of multisite pacing.
V = Ventricle
A = Atrium
D = Dual
O = None

Implantable cardioverter-defibrillators

ICDs are used for arrhythmia pacing, cardioversion, and defibrillation. Some defibrillators have the ability to pace the atrium and the ventricle, and some can perform biventricular pacing. A lead or leads are placed transvenously in the endocardium of the appropriate chambers. The lead connects to a generator box implanted in the right or left upper chest near the clavicle. If a lethal rhythm is detected, such as ventricular tachycardia, a shock is delivered to convert the rhythm.

A look at an ICD

An ICD typically consists of a programmable pulse generator and an electrode. It detects ventricular bradyarrhythmias and tachyarrhythmias and responds with appropriate therapies.

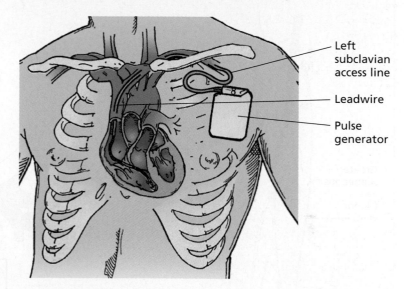

Left subclavian access line

Leadwire

Pulse generator

Types of ICD therapies

Implantable cardioverter-defibrillators (ICDs) can deliver a range of therapies, depending on the arrhythmia that's detected and how the device is programmed. These include antitachycardia pacing, cardioversion, defibrillation, and bradycardia pacing. Some newer ICDs can also provide biventricular pacing or treatment for atrial fibrillation.

Therapy	What it does
Antitachycardia pacing	A series of small, rapid, electrical pacing pulses are used to terminate ventricular tachycardia (VT) and return the heart to its normal rhythm.
Cardioversion	A low- or high-energy shock (up to 35 joules) is timed to the R wave to terminate VT and return the heart to its normal rhythm.
Defibrillation	A high-energy shock (up to 35 joules) is used to terminate ventricular fibrillation and return the heart to its normal rhythm.
Bradycardia pacing	Electrical pacing pulses are used when the heart's natural electrical signals are too slow. Most ICD systems can pace one chamber (VVI pacing) of the heart at a preset rate. Some systems sense and pace both chambers (DDD pacing).

CORONARY ARTERY BYPASS GRAFT SURGERY

Coronary artery bypass graft (CABG) surgery relieves the symptoms of coronary artery disease and decreases risk of future heart attack or heart failure.

The surgery is performed either "on pump" (the traditional method) or "off pump" (also called the "beating heart method" or OPCAB).

Bypass surgery may involve multiple vessels and may be termed according to how many vessels are bypassed; for example, "triple bypass" refers to three vessels, "quadruple bypass" refers to four vessels.

Patients who have had CABG surgery are monitored for such complications as severe hypotension, decreased cardiac output, and cardiogenic shock.

How CABG is performed

Coronary artery bypass graft (CABG) surgery circumvents an occluded coronary artery by using a segment of the saphenous vein, radial artery, or internal mammary artery to restore blood flow to the heart.

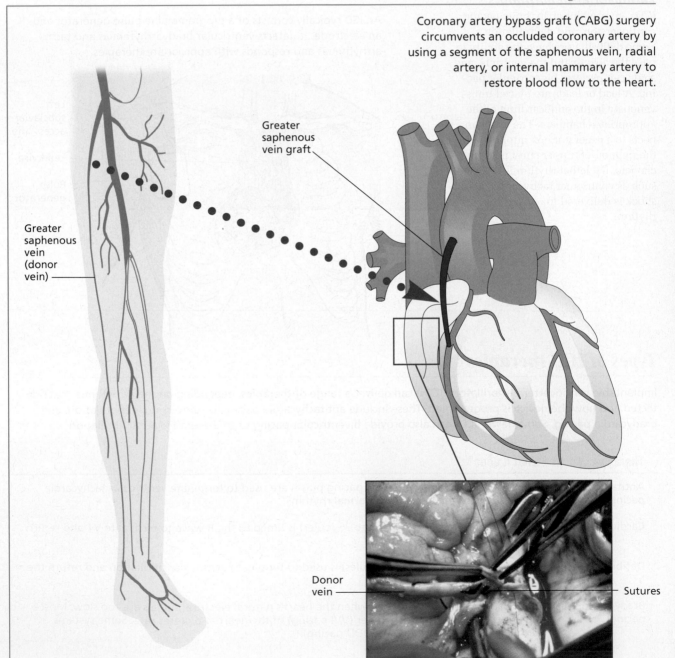

Greater saphenous vein graft

Greater saphenous vein (donor vein)

Donor vein

Sutures

Minimally invasive direct coronary artery bypass

Minimally invasive direct coronary artery bypass (MIDCAB) is performed on a beating heart through a small thoracotomy incision. The patient receives only right lung ventilation and drugs to slow the heart rate and reduce heart movement during surgery. Because the procedure is minimally invasive, it results in shorter hospital stays, fewer postoperative complications, earlier extubation, reduced cost, smaller incisions, and an earlier return to work. Patients eligible for MIDCAB include those with proximal left anterior descending lesions and some lesions of the right coronary and circumflex arteries.

The MIDCAB procedure

The MIDCAB procedure is performed through a short incision in the left chest cavity. The internal mammary artery is sewn to the left anterior descending artery in the front of the heart, as shown here.

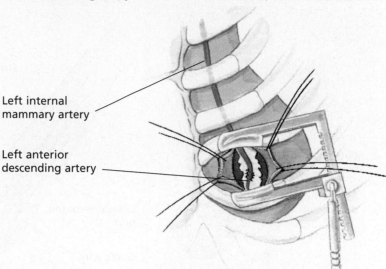

Left internal mammary artery

Left anterior descending artery

Comparing types of CABG

Features	On-pump CABG	OPCAB	MIDCAB
Access site	▸ Breastbone severed for heart access	▸ Breastbone severed for heart access	▸ Incision made between ribs for anterior heart access, no bones cut
Indications	▸ Suitable for multivessel disease, any coronary artery	▸ Suitable for multivessel disease, any coronary artery	▸ Only used for one-vessel diseases in anterior portions of heart, such as left anterior descending artery, or some portions of the right coronary and circumflex arteries
Graft types	▸ Combination of artery and vein grafts	▸ Combination of artery and vein grafts	▸ Arterial grafts (better long-term results)
Complications	▸ Highest risk of postoperative complications	▸ Reduced blood usage, fewer rhythm problems, less kidney dysfunction than on-pump CABG	▸ Reduced blood usage, fewest complications, fastest recovery
Intubation	▸ Up to 24 hours	▸ Up to 24 hours	▸ Usually for 2 to 4 hours
Incisions	▸ Leg incisions for vein grafting, possibly arm incision for radial artery grafting	▸ Leg incisions for vein grafting, possibly arm incision for radial artery grafting	▸ No leg incisions, possibly arm incision for radial artery grafting
Heart and lung function	▸ Heart and lung circulation bypassed mechanically, affecting blood cells	▸ Drugs and special equipment used to slow heart and immobilize it; cardiopulmonary and systemic circulation still function	▸ Drugs used to slow heart; cardiopulmonary and systemic circulation still function

Atherectomy

Atherectomy is the use of a small, rotating knife to remove fatty deposits from blocked coronary arteries. The catheter is advanced to the arterial obstruction, the knife is positioned precisely on the fatty deposit, and then the fatty deposit is shaved off the artery wall.

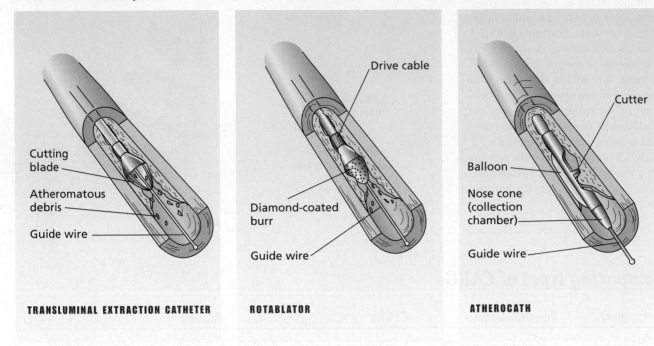

TRANSLUMINAL EXTRACTION CATHETER

Cutting blade
Atheromatous debris
Guide wire

ROTABLATOR

Drive cable
Diamond-coated burr
Guide wire

ATHEROCATH

Cutter
Balloon
Nose cone (collection chamber)
Guide wire

Intravascular stents

An intravascular stent may be used to hold the walls of a vessel open. Some stents are coated with a drug that's slowly released to inhibit further aggregation of fibrin or clots.

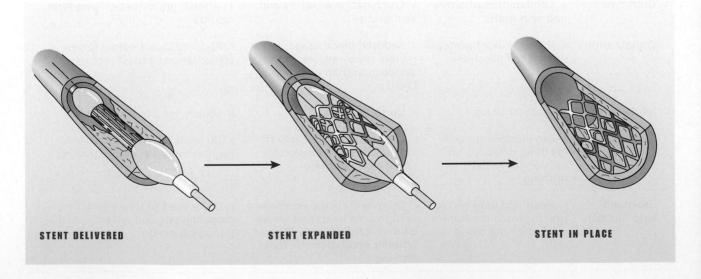

STENT DELIVERED   **STENT EXPANDED**   **STENT IN PLACE**

Heart transplantation surgery

The illustrations below outline the process of removing the donor heart and transplanting it into the recipient.

The donor's heart
The donor's heart is removed after the surgeon cuts along these dissection lines.

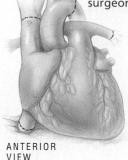

ANTERIOR VIEW

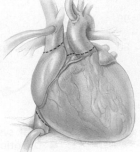

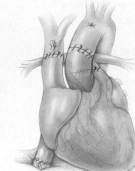

The recipient's heart
Before it can be removed, the recipient's heart is resected along these lines.

The transplanted heart
The transplanted heart is sutured in place within the recipient.

HEART TRANSPLANTATION

With heart transplantation, a patient's failing heart is replaced with a donor heart. Used to treat end-stage cardiac disease in patients who have poor quality of life and aren't expected to survive for more than 6 to 12 months, heart transplantation doesn't provide a cure.

Patients who receive donor hearts must be treated for rejection with monoclonal antibodies and potent immunosuppressants that can increase the risk of life-threatening infection.

INTRA-AORTIC BALLOON PUMP COUNTERPULSATION

Intra-aortic balloon pump (IABP) counterpulsation temporarily reduces left ventricular workload and improves coronary perfusion. It's used to treat cardiogenic shock caused by acute MI, septic shock, intractable angina before surgery, intractable ventricular arrhythmias, ventricular septal or papillary muscle ruptures, and pump failure.

Understanding an IABP

An IABP consists of a polyurethane balloon attached to an external pump console by means of a large-lumen catheter. It's inserted percutaneously through the femoral artery and positioned in the descending aorta, just distal to the left subclavian artery and above the renal arteries.

This external pump works in precise counterpoint to the left ventricle, inflating the balloon with helium early in diastole and deflating it just before systole. As the balloon inflates, it forces blood toward the aortic valve, thereby raising pressure in the aortic root and augmenting diastolic pressure to improve coronary perfusion. It also improves peripheral circulation by forcing blood through the brachiocephalic, common carotid, and subclavian arteries arising from the aortic trunk.

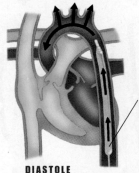

DIASTOLE

Balloon inflated during early diastole

The balloon deflates rapidly at the end of diastole, creating a vacuum in the aorta. This reduces aortic volume and pressure, thereby decreasing the resistance to left ventricular ejection (afterload). This decreased workload, in turn, reduces the heart's oxygen requirements and, combined with the improved myocardial perfusion, helps prevent or diminish myocardial ischemia.

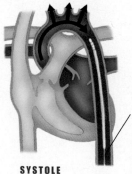

SYSTOLE

Balloon deflated just before systole

Timing IABP counterpulsation

IABP counterpulsation is synchronized with either the electrocardiogram or the arterial waveform. Ideally, balloon inflation should begin when the aortic valve closes—at the dicrotic notch on the arterial waveform. Deflation should occur just before diastole.

Timing of the counterpulsation is crucial. Early inflation can damage the aortic valve by forcing it closed, whereas late inflation permits most of the blood emerging from the ventricle to flow past the balloon, reducing the pump's effectiveness.

Late deflation may cause cardiac arrest because it increases the resistance to left ventricle pumping. IABP counterpulsation boosts peak diastolic pressure and lowers peak systolic and end-diastolic pressures.

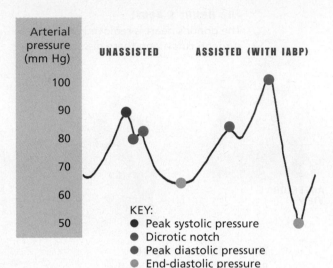

Arterial pressure (mm Hg)

UNASSISTED ASSISTED (WITH IABP)

100
90
80
70
60
50

KEY:
● Peak systolic pressure
● Dicrotic notch
● Peak diastolic pressure
● End-diastolic pressure

ENHANCED EXTERNAL COUNTERPULSATION

Enhanced eternal counterpulsation (EECP) provides pain relief for patients who suffer from recurrent stable angina when standard treatments fail. It's a noninvasive technique that increases oxygen-rich blood flow to the heart and reduces the heart's workload. EECP can reduce angina pain, improve exercise tolerance, and stimulate collateral circulation.

EECP treatment

With enhanced external counterpulsation (EECP), three pneumatic cuffs are wrapped around the patient's calf, lower thigh, and upper thigh. These cuffs sequentially inflate and gently compress blood vessels in the legs, forcing blood back to the heart.

1. The cuffs inflate on the calf, initiating a retrograde pulse wave.

2. The cuffs inflate on the lower thigh.

3. The cuffs inflate on the upper thigh.

4. All three cuffs simultaneously deflate.

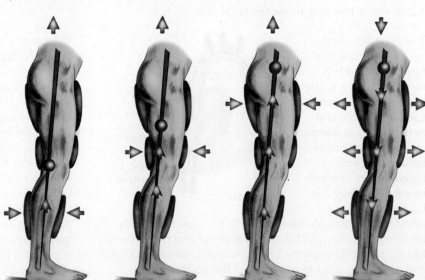

PERCUTANEOUS TRANSLUMINAL CORONARY ANGIOPLASTY

Percutaneous transluminal coronary angioplasty (PTCA), also called *angioplasty*, is a nonsurgical alternative to CABG. Performed in the cardiac catheterization laboratory under local anesthesia, it involves the use of a balloon-tipped catheter to dilate the blocked coronary artery. In most cases, the patients recuperate quickly, usually walking the same day and returning to work in 2 weeks.

PTCA works best when lesions are readily accessible, noncalcified, less than 10 mm, concentric, discrete, and smoothly tapered. Possible complications include vessel closure and late atherosclerosis.

RADIOFREQUENCY ABLATION

Radiofrequency ablation is used to treat arrhythmias in patients who don't respond to antiarrhythmic drugs or cardioversion. During the procedure, a special catheter is inserted in a vein and advanced to the heart. After the source of the arrhythmia is identified, radiofrequency energy destroys the abnormal electrical impulses or conduction pathway. The tissue that's destroyed can no longer conduct electrical impulses.

Understanding PTCA

In PTCA, a guide catheter is threaded into the coronary artery by way of the femoral artery. Then, a balloon-tipped catheter is inserted through the occlusion and inflated to flatten the plaque until the vessel is opened.

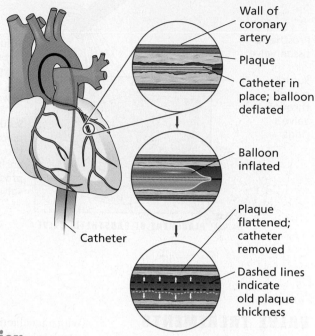

Catheter

Wall of coronary artery

Plaque

Catheter in place; balloon deflated

Balloon inflated

Plaque flattened; catheter removed

Dashed lines indicate old plaque thickness

Types of ablation

AV node ablation

If a rapid arrhythmia originates above the atrioventricular (AV) node, the AV node may be destroyed to block impulses from reaching the ventricles.

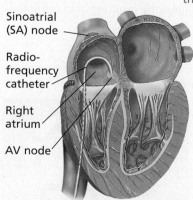

Sinoatrial (SA) node

Radiofrequency catheter

Right atrium

AV node

The radiofrequency ablation catheter is directed to the base of the pulmonary vein.

Pulmonary vein ablation

If the pulmonary vein is the source of the arrhythmia, such as in atrial fibrillation, radiofrequency energy is used to destroy the tissue in the area of the atrium that connects to the pulmonary vein. The scar that forms blocks impulses from firing within the pulmonary vein, preventing arrhythmias.

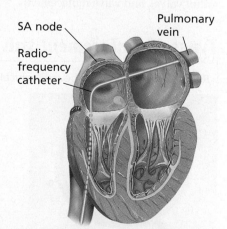

SA node

Radiofrequency catheter

Pulmonary vein

Radiofrequency energy is used to destroy the tissue where the atrium connects to the pulmonary vein.

Valve replacement

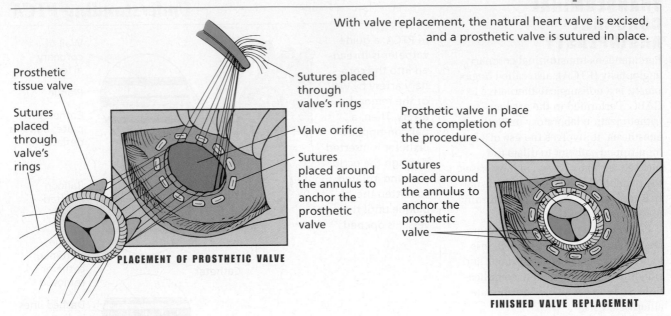

With valve replacement, the natural heart valve is excised, and a prosthetic valve is sutured in place.

Prosthetic tissue valve

Sutures placed through valve's rings

Sutures placed through valve's rings

Sutures placed through valve's rings

Valve orifice

Sutures placed around the annulus to anchor the prosthetic valve

Prosthetic valve in place at the completion of the procedure

Sutures placed around the annulus to anchor the prosthetic valve

PLACEMENT OF PROSTHETIC VALVE

FINISHED VALVE REPLACEMENT

VALVE TREATMENTS

Valve treatments are used to prevent heart failure in patients with valvular stenosis or insufficiency accompanied by severe, unmanageable symptoms. Depending on the patient's condition, he may undergo one of three types of valve surgery. Types of valve surgery include valvuloplasty (valvular repair), commissurotomy (separation of the adherent, thickened leaflets of the mitral valve), and valve replacement (with a mechanical or prosthetic valve). When valve surgery isn't an option, percutaneous balloon valvuloplasty is used to enlarge the orifice of a stenotic heart valve, improving valvular function.

Although valve surgery carries a low risk of mortality, it can cause serious complications. Hemorrhage, for instance, may result from unligated vessels, anticoagulant therapy, or coagulopathy resulting from cardiopulmonary bypass during surgery. Stroke may result from thrombus formation caused by turbulent blood flow through the prosthetic valve or from poor cerebral perfusion during cardiopulmonary bypass. With valve replacement, bacterial endocarditis can develop within days of implantation or months later. Valve dysfunction or failure may occur as the prosthetic device wears out.

Types of replacement valves

Replacement valves can be mechanical or tissue.

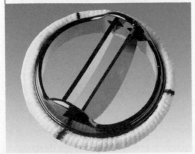

BILEAFLET VALVE
(St. Jude, mechanical)

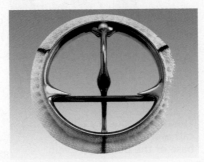

TILTING-DISK VALVE
(Medtronic-Hall, mechanical)

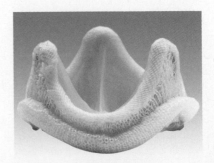

PORCINE HETEROGRAFT VALVE
(Carpentier-Edwards, tissue)

Valve leaflet resection and repair

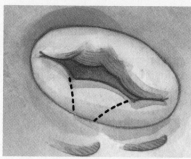

The section between the dashed line is excised.

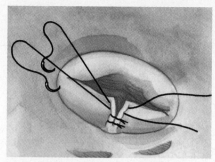

The edges are approximated and sutured.)

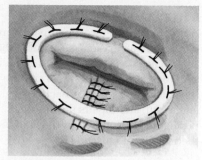

The repair is finished off with an annuloplasty ring.

Commissurotomy of mitral valve

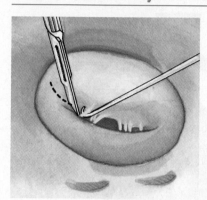

In commissurotomy, the thickened valve leaflets are surgically separated.

Percutaneous balloon valvuloplasty

During valvuloplasty, a surgeon inserts a small balloon catheter through the skin at the femoral vein and advances it until it reaches the affected valve. The balloon is then inflated, forcing the valve opening to widen.

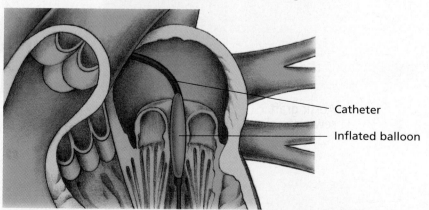

Catheter

Inflated balloon

Vascular interventions

Aortic aneurysm resection

Aortic aneurysm resection involves removing an aneurysmal segment of the aorta. The surgeon first makes an incision to expose the aneurysm site. He then clamps the aorta, resects the aneurysm, and repairs the damaged portion of the aorta by sewing a prosthetic graft into place.

Aortic endovascular stent graft

Endovascular stent grafting is a minimally invasive procedure used to repair abdominal aortic aneurysm and other aneurysmal arteries by reinforcing the vessel walls. The surgeon uses fluoroscopic guidance to insert a delivery catheter with an attached compressed graft through a small incision into the iliac or femoral artery. The catheter is advanced into the aorta and positioned across the aneurysm below the renal arteries. The stent graft prevents blood from entering the aneurysmal area of the artery but maintains blood flow distally. This helps prevent the aneurysm from enlarging and possibly rupturing.

Aortic aneurysm resection

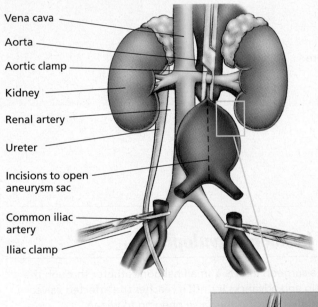

Vena cava

Aorta

Aortic clamp

Kidney

Renal artery

Ureter

Incisions to open aneurysm sac

Common iliac artery

Iliac clamp

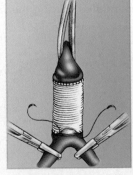

Aortic graft sewn into place

Aortic endovascular stent graft

AORTO-ILIAC STENT GRAFT

Right renal artery

Left renal artery

Stent graft

Aortic aneurysm

Right iliac artery

Left iliac artery aneurysm

Arterial bypass graft

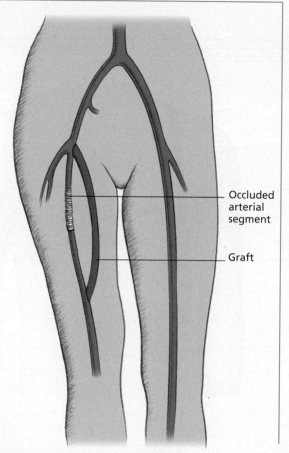

Occluded
arterial
segment

Graft

Embolectomy

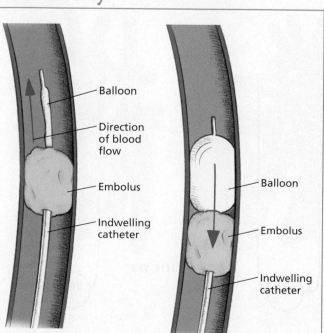

Balloon

Direction
of blood
flow

Embolus

Indwelling
catheter

Balloon

Embolus

Indwelling
catheter

Arterial bypass graft
Bypass grafting serves to bypass an arterial obstruction resulting from arteriosclerosis. After exposing the affected artery, the surgeon anastomoses a synthetic or autogenous graft to divert blood flow around the occluded arterial segment.

Embolectomy
To remove an embolism from an artery, a surgeon may perform an embolectomy by inserting a balloon-tipped indwelling catheter in the artery and passing it through the embolus. He then inflates the balloon and withdraws the catheter to remove the occlusion.

Vena caval filter
A vena caval filter, or umbrella, traps emboli originating from the pelvis or lower extremities in the vena cava, preventing them from reaching the pulmonary vessels but allowing venous blood flow.

Vena caval filter

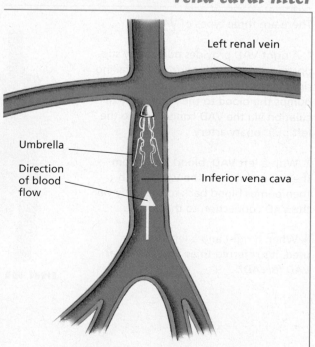

Left renal vein

Umbrella

Direction
of blood
flow

Inferior vena cava

VENTRICULAR ASSIST DEVICE

A ventricular assist device (VAD) is an implantable device that consists of a blood pump, cannulas, and a pneumatic or electrical drive console. The pump is synchronized to the patient's electrocardiogram and functions as the heart's ventricle. It decreases the heart's workload while increasing cardiac output.

Pump options

VADs are available as continuous flow or pulsatile pumps. A continuous flow pump fills continuously and returns blood to the aorta at a constant rate. A pulsatile pump may work in one of two ways:

▸ It may fill during systole and pump blood into the aorta during diastole.
▸ It may pump regardless of the patient's cardiac cycle.

Left VAD

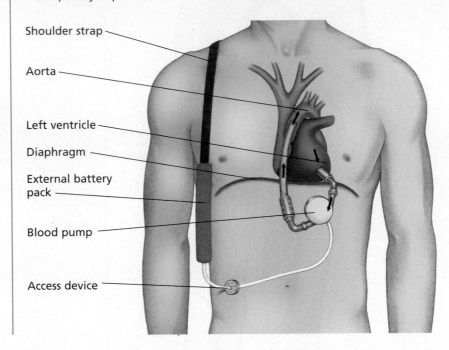

A completely implanted left VAD is shown here.

Shoulder strap
Aorta
Left ventricle
Diaphragm
External battery pack
Blood pump
Access device

A closer look at VADs

There are three types of VADs.

1. A right VAD provides pulmonary support by diverting blood from the failing right ventricle to the VAD, which then pumps the blood to the pulmonary circulation via the VAD connection to the left pulmonary artery.

2. With a left VAD, blood flows from the left ventricle to the VAD, which then pumps blood back to the body via the VAD connection to the aorta.

3. When a right and a left VAD are used, it's referred to as a *biventricular VAD (BiVAD).*

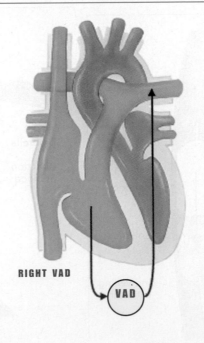

RIGHT VAD

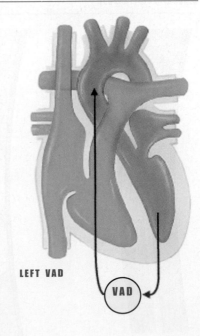

LEFT VAD

Chapter 3

Respiratory care

DISEASES
Acute respiratory distress syndrome

Acute respiratory distress syndrome (ARDS), also called *shock lung* or *adult respiratory distress syndrome*, results from increased permeability of the alveolocapillary membrane. Fluid accumulates in the lung interstitium, alveolar spaces, and small airways, causing the lung to stiffen. Effective ventilation is thus impaired, prohibiting adequate oxygenation of pulmonary capillary blood. Severe ARDS can cause intractable and fatal hypoxemia. However, patients who recover may have little or no permanent lung damage.

ARDS results from a variety of respiratory and nonrespiratory insults, such as:

◗ aspiration of gastric contents
◗ massive blood transfusions
◗ drug overdose (barbiturates, glutethimide, or opioids)
◗ gestational hypertension
◗ hydrocarbon and paraquat ingestion
◗ increased intracranial pressure
◗ microemboli (fat or air emboli or disseminated intravascular coagulation)
◗ near drowning
◗ oxygen toxicity
◗ pancreatitis, uremia, or miliary tuberculosis (rare)
◗ prolonged heart bypass surgery
◗ radiation therapy
◗ sepsis (primarily gram-negative)
◗ shock
◗ smoke or chemical inhalation (nitrous oxide, chlorine, or ammonia)
◗ trauma
◗ viral, bacterial, or fungal pneumonia
◗ leukemia
◗ thrombotic thrombocytopenic purpura.

 What happens in ARDS

Shock, sepsis, and trauma are the most common causes of acute respiratory distress syndrome (ARDS). Trauma-related factors, such as fat emboli, pulmonary contusions, and multiple transfusions, may increase the likelihood that microemboli will develop.

Phase 1
In *phase 1,* injury reduces normal blood flow to the lungs. Platelets aggregate and release histamine (H), serotonin (S), and bradykinin (B).

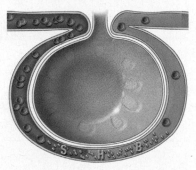

Phase 2
In *phase 2,* those substances—especially histamine—inflame and damage the alveolocapillary membrane, increasing capillary permeability. Fluids then shift into the interstitial space.

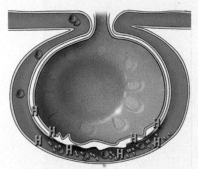

Phase 3
In *phase 3,* as capillary permeability increases, proteins and fluids leak out, increasing interstitial osmotic pressure and causing pulmonary edema.

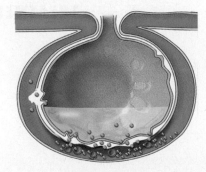

Phase 4
In *phase 4,* decreased blood flow and fluids in the alveoli damage surfactant and impair the cell's ability to produce more. As a result, alveoli collapse, impeding gas exchange and decreasing lung compliance.

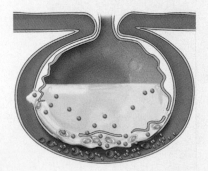

Signs and symptoms

▶ Apprehension
▶ Crackles
▶ Dyspnea
▶ Hypoxemia
▶ Intercostal and suprasternal retractions
▶ Cough
▶ Confusion
▶ Hypotension
▶ Mental sluggishness
▶ Motor dysfunction
▶ Rapid, shallow breathing
▶ Restlessness
▶ Rhonchi
▶ Tachycardia

Treatment

▶ Correction of the underlying cause
▶ Prevention of progression and the potentially fatal complications of hypoxemia and respiratory acidosis
▶ Administration of humidified oxygen with continuous positive airway pressure
▶ Possibly ventilatory support with intubation, volume ventilation, and positive end-expiratory pressure (PEEP)
▶ Fluid restriction
▶ Diuretics
▶ Correction of electrolyte and acid-base abnormalities
▶ Treatment to reverse severe metabolic acidosis with sodium bicarbonate may be necessary, although in severe cases, this may worsen the acidosis if carbon dioxide can't be cleared adequately
▶ Administration of fluids and vasopressors to maintain blood pressure
▶ Antibiotic administration
▶ Administration of prostaglandins

Nursing considerations

▶ Frequently assess the patient's respiratory status.
▶ Check for clear, frothy sputum, which may indicate pulmonary edema.
▶ Maintain a patent airway.
▶ Closely monitor heart rate and blood pressure. Watch for arrhythmias that may result from hypoxemia, acid-base disturbances, or electrolyte imbalance.
▶ Monitor serum electrolytes and correct imbalances.
▶ Measure intake and output; weigh the patient daily.
▶ Check ventilator settings frequently.
▶ Monitor arterial blood gas studies and pulse oximetry.
▶ Give sedatives, as needed, to reduce restlessness.
▶ If the patient is receiving PEEP, check for hypotension, tachycardia, and decreased urine output.
▶ Give tube feedings and parenteral nutrition, as ordered.
▶ Perform passive range-of-motion exercises or help the patient perform active exercises, if possible, to help maintain joint mobility.
▶ Provide meticulous skin care to prevent skin breakdown.
▶ Plan patient care to allow periods of adequate rest.
▶ Provide emotional support.
▶ Place in prone position to improve chest wall compliance and drainage of bronchial secretions.

Phase 5

In *phase 5,* sufficient oxygen (O_2) can't cross the alveolocapillary membrane, but carbon dioxide (CO_2) can and is lost with every exhalation. O_2 and CO_2 levels decrease in the blood.

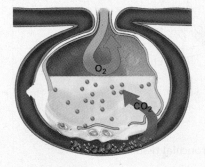

Phase 6

In *phase 6,* pulmonary edema worsens, inflammation leads to fibrosis, and gas exchange is further impeded.

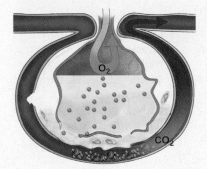

LESSON PLANS

Teaching about ARDS

▶ Explain the disorder to the patient and his family. Tell them which signs and symptoms may occur, and review necessary treatment.
▶ Orient the patient and his family to the unit and health care facility surroundings. Explain equipment needed to provide adequate oxygenation.
▶ Tell a recuperating patient that recovery takes time and that he'll feel weak for a while. Urge him to share his concerns with the staff.

Asthma

Asthma is a reversible lung disease characterized by obstruction or narrowing of the airways, which are typically inflamed and hyperresponsive to a variety of stimuli. It may resolve spontaneously or with treatment. Its symptoms range from mild wheezing and dyspnea to life-threatening respiratory failure. Symptoms of bronchial airway obstruction may persist between acute episodes.

Signs and symptoms

▸ Chest tightness
▸ Coughing with thick, clear, or yellow mucus
▸ Cyanosis (late sign)
▸ Diaphoresis
▸ Nasal flaring
▸ Pursed-lip breathing
▸ Sudden dyspnea
▸ Tachycardia
▸ Tachypnea
▸ Use of accessory muscles for breathing
▸ Wheezing accompanied by coarse rhonchi

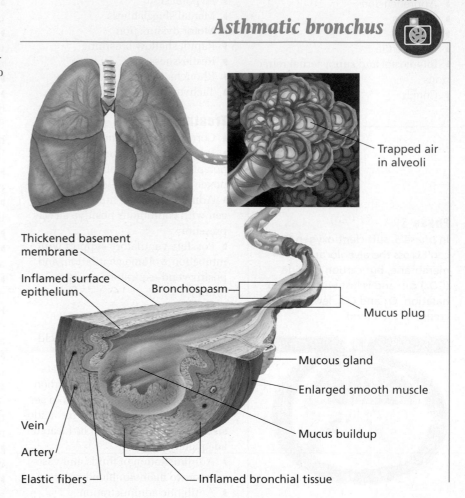

PICTURING PATHO

Asthmatic bronchus

Trapped air in alveoli

Thickened basement membrane
Inflamed surface epithelium
Bronchospasm
Mucus plug
Mucous gland
Enlarged smooth muscle
Mucus buildup
Vein
Artery
Elastic fibers
Inflamed bronchial tissue

Determining asthma's severity

Current guidelines for classifying asthma severity for patients age 12 and older are listed here.

Intermittent	Mild persistent	Moderate persistent	Severe persistent
▸ Attacks no more than twice per week ▸ Nighttime attacks no more than twice per month ▸ Rescue inhaler used no more than twice per week ▸ Asthma doesn't interfere with daily activities ▸ Normal FEV_1 (forced expiratory volume in 1 second)	▸ Attacks more than twice per week but not every day ▸ Nighttime attacks three to four nights per month ▸ Rescue inhaler used more than 2 days per week ▸ Asthma minorly interferes with daily activities ▸ FEV_1 greater than 80% of normal lung function most of the time	▸ Daily attacks ▸ Nighttime attacks more than once per week ▸ Rescue inhaler used daily ▸ Asthma moderately interferes with daily activities ▸ FEV_1 greater than 60% but less than 80%	▸ Continual, severe daily attacks ▸ Nighttime attacks daily ▸ Rescue inhaler used multiple times per day ▸ Asthma severely interferes with daily activities ▸ FEV_1 less than 60%

Treatment

‣ Identification and avoidance of precipitating factors
‣ Desensitization to specific antigens
‣ Low-flow humidified oxygen
‣ Inhaled steroids such as triamcinolone acetonide (Azmacort)
‣ Leukotriene inhibitors such as montelukast (Singulair)
‣ Long-acting bronchodilators such as formoterol (Foradil Aerolizer)
‣ Mast cell stabilizers, such as cromolyn sodium (Intal) or nedocromil (Alocril)
‣ Aminophyllin (Truphylline) or theophylline (Slo-bid)
‣ Short-acting bronchodilators, such as albuterol (Proventil) or levalbuterol (Xopenex)
‣ Oral or I.V. corticosteroids
‣ Mechanical ventilation
‣ Nebulized atropine
‣ Omalizumab (Xolair)
‣ Bronchial thermoplasty

Nursing considerations

‣ Administer the prescribed treatments and assess the patient's response.
‣ Place the patient in high Fowler's position.
‣ Monitor the patient's vital signs, especially respiratory status.
‣ Administer prescribed humidified oxygen.
‣ Anticipate intubation and mechanical ventilation if the patient fails to maintain adequate oxygenation.
‣ Monitor serum theophylline levels.
‣ Observe for signs and symptoms of theophylline toxicity (vomiting, diarrhea, and headache).
‣ Perform postural drainage and chest percussion.
‣ Provide emotional support.
‣ Anticipate the need for bronchoscopy or bronchial lavage when a lobe or larger area collapses.
‣ Review arterial blood gas levels, pulmonary function test results, and SaO_2 readings.

How status asthmaticus progresses

A potentially fatal complication, status asthmaticus arises when impaired gas exchange and heightened airway resistance increase the work of breathing. This flowchart shows the stages of status asthmaticus.

> Obstructed airways hamper gas exchange and increase airway resistance, leading to labored breathing.

> The patient hyperventilates, lowering partial pressure of arterial carbon dioxide ($PaCO_2$).

> Respiratory alkalosis and hypoxemia develop.

> Hypoxia and labored breathing tire the patient. His respiratory rate drops to normal.

> $PaCO_2$ rises to a higher-than-baseline level (an asthmatic patient's $PaCO_2$ is usually low).

> The patient hypoventilates from exhaustion.

> Respiratory acidosis begins as partial pressure of oxygen in arterial blood drops and $PaCO_2$ continues to rise.

> Without treatment, the patient experiences acute respiratory failure.

> Hypoxia and cellular death from lack of oxygen and accumulation of carbon dioxide can result.

LESSON PLANS

Teaching about asthma

‣ Teach the patient to avoid known allergens and irritants.
‣ Describe prescribed drugs, including their names, dosages, actions, adverse effects, and special instructions.
‣ Teach the patient how to use a metered-dose inhaler.
‣ If the patient has moderate to severe asthma, explain how to use a peak flowmeter and to keep a record of peak flow readings.
‣ Tell the patient to seek immediate medical attention if he develops a fever above 100° F (37.8° C), chest pain, shortness of breath without coughing or exercising, or uncontrollable coughing.
‣ Teach diaphragmatic and pursed-lip breathing and effective coughing techniques.
‣ Urge the patient to drink at least 3 qt (3 L) of fluids daily to help loosen secretions and maintain hydration.
‣ Explain the importance of seeking immediate medical attention if the peak flow drops suddenly.

Cystic fibrosis

Cystic fibrosis is a generalized dysfunction of the exocrine glands that affects multiple organ systems. Transmitted as an autosomal recessive trait, it's the most common fatal genetic disease in white children. Affecting about 30,000 U.S. children and adults, cystic fibrosis is most common in Whites (1 in 3,300 births) and less common in Blacks (1 in 15,300 births), Native Americans, and Asians. It occurs equally in both sexes.

Most cases of cystic fibrosis arise from a mutation that affects the genetic coding for a single amino acid, resulting in a protein that doesn't function properly. The abnormal protein resembles other transmembrane transport proteins. It lacks phenylalanine (an essential amino acid) that's usually produced by normal genes. This abnormal protein may interfere with chloride transport by preventing adenosine triphosphate from binding to the protein and interfering with activation by protein kinase. The lack of essential amino acids leads to dehydration and mucosal thickening in the respiratory and intestinal tracts.

Signs and symptoms
- Excessive salty taste to skin
- Barrel chest
- Clubbing of fingers and toes
- Crackles and wheezing
- Cyanosis
- Dyspnea
- Failure to thrive, poor weight gain, distended abdomen
- Frequent bouts of pneumonia
- Frequent bulky and foul-smelling stools (steatorrhea)
- Frequent upper respiratory tract infections
- Intestinal obstruction (meconium ileus in infants)
- Persistent cough
- Thick secretions

Treatment
- Diet with increased fat and sodium
- Salt supplements
- Pancreatic enzyme replacement
- Breathing exercises, chest percussion, and postural drainage
- Inhaled beta-adrenergics
- Broad-spectrum antimicrobials
- Sodium channel blockers
- Heart or lung transplant
- Dornase alfa (Pulmozyme)
- High-frequency chest compression vest
- Oxygen therapy as needed
- Bronchodilators
- Mucolytic aerosols
- Corticosteroids

Nursing considerations
- Give medications as ordered. Administer pancreatic enzymes with meals and snacks.
- Perform chest physiotherapy, including postural drainage and chest percussion several times per day.
- Administer oxygen therapy as ordered. Check levels of arterial oxygen saturation using pulse oximetry.
- Provide a well-balanced, high-calorie, high-protein diet. Include plenty of fats.
- Administer vitamin A, D, E, and K supplements, if laboratory analysis indicates deficiencies.
- Make sure the patient receives plenty of liquids to prevent dehydration, especially in warm weather.
- Provide exercise and activity periods.
- Encourage deep-breathing exercises.
- Provide the young child with play periods and enlist the help of physical and play therapists.
- Provide emotional support to the patient and parents. Encourage them to discuss their fears and concerns and answer questions as honestly as possible.
- Include the family in all phases of patient care.

LESSON PLANS

 Teaching about cystic fibrosis

- Tell the patient and his family about the disease and thoroughly explain all treatments. Make sure they know about tests to determine whether family members carry the cystic fibrosis gene.
- Explain aerosol therapy, including intermittent nebulizer treatments before postural drainage. Tell the patient and his family that these treatments help loosen secretions and dilate bronchi.
- Instruct family members in proper methods of chest physiotherapy.
- Teach the patient and his family signs of infection and sudden changes they should report to the physician, including increased coughing, decreased appetite, sputum that thickens or contains blood, shortness of breath, and chest pain.

Emphysema

Emphysema is a form of chronic obstructive pulmonary disease characterized by the abnormal, permanent enlargement of the acini accompanied by destruction of alveolar walls without fibrosis. Obstruction results from tissue changes rather than mucus production, which occurs in asthma and chronic bronchitis. The distinguishing characteristic of emphysema is airflow limitation caused by thick elastic recoil in the lungs.

Senile emphysema results from degenerative changes that cause stretching without destruction of the smooth muscle. Connective tissue usually isn't affected.

Signs and symptoms
▶ Accessory muscle use for breathing
▶ Anorexia with resultant weight loss
▶ Barrel chest
▶ Chronic cough with or without sputum production
▶ Clubbed fingers and toes
▶ Crackles and wheezing on inspiration
▶ Decreased breath sounds
▶ Decreased chest expansion
▶ Decreased tactile fremitus
▶ Dyspnea on exertion
▶ Hyperresonance
▶ Malaise
▶ Mental status changes, if carbon dioxide retention worsens
▶ Prolonged expiration and grunting
▶ Tachypnea

PICTURING PATHO

Lung changes in emphysema

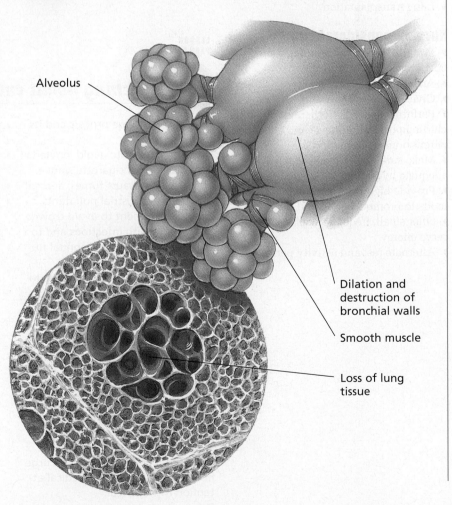

Alveolus

Dilation and destruction of bronchial walls

Smooth muscle

Loss of lung tissue

Treatment

◗ Avoidance of tobacco smoke and air pollution
◗ Bronchodilators, such as beta-adrenergic blockers and albuterol (Proventil), aminophylline
◗ Antibiotics
◗ Flu vaccine to prevent influenza
◗ Pneumovax to prevent pneumococcal pneumonia
◗ Adequate hydration
◗ Chest physiotherapy
◗ Oxygen therapy
◗ Mucolytics
◗ Aerosolized or systemic corticosteroids
◗ Lung volume reduction surgery
◗ Lung transplantation

Nursing considerations

◗ Provide incentive spirometry and encourage deep breathing.
◗ Administer oxygen.
◗ Give antibiotics as ordered.
◗ Perform chest physiotherapy including postural drainage and chest percussion as ordered.
◗ Make sure that the patient receives adequate hydration.
◗ Provide high-calorie, protein-rich foods to promote health and healing.
◗ Offer small, frequent meals to conserve energy.
◗ Alternate rest and activity periods.

LESSON PLANS

Teaching about emphysema

◗ Explain the disease process and its treatments.
◗ Urge the patient to avoid inhaled irritants, such as cigarette smoke, automobile exhaust fumes, aerosol sprays, and industrial pollutants.
◗ Advise the patient to avoid crowds and people with infections and to obtain pneumonia and annual flu vaccines.
◗ Warn the patient that exposure to blasts of cold air may trigger bronchospasm; suggest that he avoid cold, windy weather and that he cover his mouth and nose with a scarf or mask if he must go outside in such conditions.
◗ Explain all drugs, including their indications, dosages, adverse effects, and special considerations.
◗ Inform the patient about signs and symptoms that suggest ruptured alveolar blebs and bullae, and urge him to seek immediate medical attention if they occur.
◗ Demonstrate how to use a metered-dose inhaler.

◗ Teach the safe use of home oxygen therapy.
◗ Teach the patient and his family how to perform postural drainage and chest physiotherapy.
◗ Discuss the importance of drinking plenty of fluids to liquefy secretions.
◗ For family members of a patient with familial emphysema, recommend a blood test for alpha$_1$-antitrypsin. If a deficiency is found, stress the importance of not smoking and avoiding areas (if possible) where smoking is permitted.
◗ Promote smoking cessation, if appropriate.

Lung cancer

Even though it's largely preventable, lung cancer has long been the most common cause of cancer death in men and is an increasing cause of cancer death in women. Lung cancer usually develops within the wall or epithelium of the bronchial tree. The most common type is non-small-cell cancer, which includes epidermoid (squamous cell) carcinoma, adenocarcinoma, and large cell (anaplastic) carcinoma. Less common is small-cell lung cancer. Prognosis varies with the extent of metastasis at the time of diagnosis and the cell type growth rate.

Signs and symptoms

▶ Cough, hoarseness, wheezing, dyspnea, hemoptysis, and chest pain
▶ Bone and joint pain
▶ Clubbing of fingers
▶ Cushing's syndrome
▶ Fever, weight loss, weakness, and anorexia
▶ Hemoptysis, atelectasis, pneumonitis, and dyspnea
▶ Hypercalcemia
▶ Jugular vein distention and facial, neck, and chest edema
▶ Piercing chest pain, increasing dyspnea, and severe arm pain
▶ Pleural friction rub
▶ Rust-colored or purulent sputum
▶ Shoulder pain and unilateral paralysis of diaphragm
▶ Wheezing

Treatment

▶ Lobectomy, wedge resection, or pneumonectomy
▶ Video-assisted chest surgery
▶ Laser surgery
▶ Radiation
▶ Chemotherapy
▶ Cisplastin and p53 gene therapy

PICTURING PATHO

Tumor infiltration in lung cancer

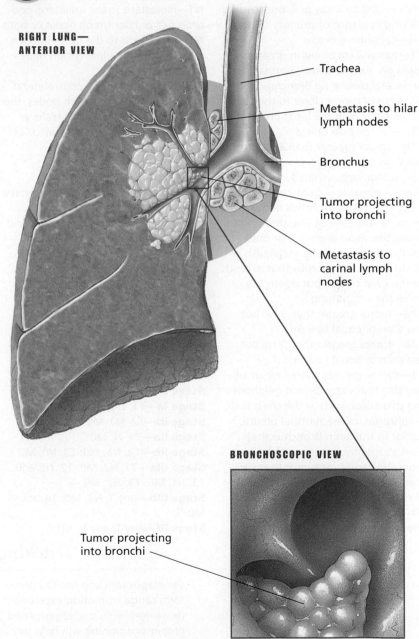

RIGHT LUNG—
ANTERIOR VIEW

Trachea

Metastasis to hilar lymph nodes

Bronchus

Tumor projecting into bronchi

Metastasis to carinal lymph nodes

BRONCHOSCOPIC VIEW

Tumor projecting into bronchi

Staging lung cancer

Using the TNM (tumor, node, metastasis) classification system, the American Joint Committee on Cancer stages lung cancer as follows.

Primary tumor

TX—primary tumor can't be assessed, or malignant tumor cells are detected in sputum or bronchial washings but undetected by X-ray or bronchoscopy

T0—no evidence of primary tumor

Tis—carcinoma in situ

T1—tumor 3 cm or less in greatest dimension, surrounded by normal lung or visceral pleura; no bronchoscopic evidence of cancer closer to the center of the body than the lobar bronchus

T1a—tumor 2 cm or less

T1b—tumor greater than 2 cm but less than or equal to 3 cm

T2—tumor larger than 3 cm but less than or equal to 7 cm; one that involves the main bronchus and is 2 cm or more from the carina; one that invades the visceral pleura; or one that's accompanied by atelectasis or obstructive pneumonitis that extends to the hilar region but doesn't involve the entire lung

T2a—tumor greater than 3 cm but less than or equal to 5 cm

T2b—tumor greater than 5 cm but less than or equal to 7 cm

T3—tumor greater than 7 cm or of any size that extends into neighboring structures, such as the chest wall, diaphragm, or mediastinal pleura; tumor in the main bronchus that doesn't involve but is less than 2 cm from the carina; or tumor that's accompanied by atelectasis or obstructive pneumonitis of the entire lung

T4—tumor of any size that invades the mediastinum, heart, great vessels, trachea, esophagus, vertebral body, or carina; or tumor with malignant pleural effusion

Regional lymph nodes

NX—regional lymph nodes can't be assessed

N0—no detectable metastasis to lymph nodes

N1—metastasis to the ipsilateral peribronchial or hilar lymph nodes or both

N2—metastasis to the ipsilateral mediastinal or subcarinal lymph nodes or both

N3—metastasis to the contralateral mediastinal or hilar lymph nodes, the ipsilateral or contralateral scalene lymph nodes, or the supraclavicular lymph nodes

Distant metastasis

M0—no evidence of distant metastasis

M1—distant metastasis

M1a—tumor with malignant pleural or pericardial effusion or pleural nodules; separate tumor nodules in contralateral lobe

M1b—metastasis in extrathoracic organs

Staging categories

Lung cancer progresses from mild to severe as follows:

Occult carcinoma—TX, N0, M0

Stage 0—Tis, N0, M0

Stage Ia—T1, N0, M0

Stage Ib—T2, N0, M0

Stage IIa—T1, N, M0

Stage IIb—T2, N1, M0; T3, N0, M0

Stage IIIa—T1, N2, M0; T2, N2, M0; T3, N1, M0; T3, N2, M0

Stage IIIb—any T, N3, M0; T4, any N, M0

Stage IV—any T, any N, M1

Nursing considerations

▶ Give comprehensive, supportive care and provide patient teaching to minimize complications and speed the patient's recovery from surgery, radiation, and chemotherapy.

▶ Urge the patient to voice his concerns and schedule time to answer his questions. Be sure to explain procedures before performing them.

After thoracic surgery

▶ Maintain a patent airway and monitor chest tubes.

▶ Check vital signs and watch for and report abnormal respirations and other changes.

▶ Suction the patient as needed and encourage him to begin deep breathing and coughing as soon as possible. Check secretions often. Initially sputum will appear thick and dark with blood, but it should become thinner and grayish-yellow within 1 day.

▶ Monitor and document amount and color of closed chest drainage. Keep chest tubes patent and draining effectively. Watch for fluctuation in the water seal chamber on inspiration and expiration, indicating that the chest tube remains patent. Watch for air leaks and report them immediately. Position the patient on the surgical side to promote drainage and lung reexpansion.

▶ Monitor intake and output and maintain hydration.

▶ Encourage early ambulation.

LESSON PLANS

Teaching about lung cancer

▶ Preoperatively, teach the patient about postoperative procedures and equipment. Teach him how to cough and breathe deeply from the diaphragm and how to perform range-of-motion exercises. Reassure him that analgesics and proper positioning will help to control postoperative pain.

▶ If the patient will have chemotherapy or radiation therapy, make sure he understands the adverse effects that occur and measures to prevent or reduce their severity.

▶ To help prevent lung cancer, teach high-risk patients to stop smoking.

Refer smokers who want to quit to the local branch of the American Cancer Society or American Lung Association. Explain that nicotine

gum or a nicotine patch and an antidepressant may be prescribed in combination with educational and support groups.

Pneumonia

Pneumonia is an acute infection of the lung parenchyma that commonly impairs gas exchange. The prognosis is generally good for people who have normal lungs and adequate host defenses before the onset of pneumonia; however, pneumonia is the sixth leading cause of death in the United States.

Pneumonia can be classified by microbiologic etiology, location, or type.

▶ *Microbiologic etiology*—Pneumonia can be viral, bacterial, fungal, protozoan, mycobacterial, mycoplasmal, or rickettsial in origin.

▶ *Location*—Bronchopneumonia involves distal airways and alveoli; lobular pneumonia, part of a lobe; and lobar pneumonia, an entire lobe.

▶ *Type*—Pneumonia may be described by the setting in which it was acquired. Community-acquired pneumonia is the most common type and occurs outside the health care setting. Hospital-acquired pneumonia (HAC) occurs in the health care setting. Ventilator-associated pneumonia is a type of HAC occurring in ventilator patients. Health care–associated pneumonia occurs in other health care settings, such as nursing homes. Aspiration pneumonia refers to pneumonia that results from a foreign substance, such as emesis, entering the lungs.

Predisposing factors for bacterial and viral pneumonia include:

▶ abdominal and thoracic surgery
▶ aspiration
▶ atelectasis
▶ cancer (particularly lung cancer)
▶ chronic illness and debilitation
▶ common colds or other viral respiratory infections
▶ exposure to noxious gases
▶ immunosuppressive therapy
▶ influenza

▶ malnutrition
▶ smoking
▶ tracheostomy.

Predisposing factors for aspiration pneumonia include:

▶ artificial airway use
▶ debilitation
▶ decreased level of consciousness
▶ impaired gag reflex
▶ nasogastric (NG) tube feedings
▶ advanced age
▶ poor oral hygiene
▶ positioning during and after eating or feeding.

Signs and symptoms

▶ Coughing
▶ Crackles and decreased breath sounds
▶ Dyspnea
▶ Fatigue
▶ Fever
▶ Headache
▶ Pleuritic chest pain
▶ Rapid, shallow breathing
▶ Shaking chills
▶ Shortness of breath
▶ Sputum production
▶ Sweating
▶ Decreased pulse oximetry reading

PICTURING PATHO

Locations of pneumonia

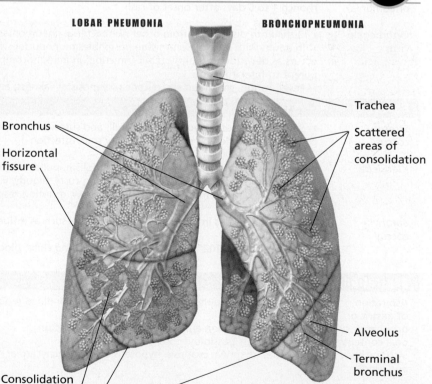

LOBAR PNEUMONIA   BRONCHOPNEUMONIA

Trachea

Scattered areas of consolidation

Bronchus

Horizontal fissure

Alveolus

Terminal bronchus

Consolidation in one lobe

Oblique fissure

Distinguishing sources of pneumonia

The characteristics and prognosis of different types of pneumonia vary.

Type	Characteristics
Viral	
Influenza	▶ Prognosis poor even with treatment ▶ 50% mortality from cardiopulmonary collapse ▶ Cough (initially nonproductive; later, purulent sputum), marked cyanosis, dyspnea, high fever, chills, substernal pain and discomfort, moist crackles, frontal headache, and myalgia
Adenovirus	▶ Insidious onset ▶ Typically affects young adults ▶ Good prognosis; usually clears with no residual effects ▶ Sore throat, fever, cough, chills, malaise, small amounts of mucoid sputum, retrosternal chest pain, anorexia, rhinitis, adenopathy, scattered crackles, and rhonchi
Respiratory syncytial virus	▶ Most common in infants and children ▶ Complete recovery in 1 to 3 weeks; may cause death in premature infants younger than age 6 months ▶ Listlessness, irritability, tachypnea with retraction of intercostal muscles, slight sputum production, fever, severe malaise, possible cough or croup, and fine, moist crackles
Measles (rubeola)	▶ Typically more severe in adults than in children ▶ Fever, dyspnea, cough, small amounts of sputum, rash, cervical adenopathy, and profusely runny nose
Chickenpox (varicella pneumonia)	▶ Uncommon in children but present in 30% of adults with varicella ▶ Characteristic rash, cough, dyspnea, cyanosis, tachypnea, pleuritic chest pain, and hemoptysis and rhonch 1 to 6 days after onset of rash
Cytomegalo-virus	▶ Difficult to distinguish from other nonbacterial pneumonias ▶ In adults with healthy lung tissue, resembles mononucleosis and typically is benign; in neonates, occurs as devastating multisystemic infection; in immunocompromised hosts, varies from clinically inapparent to fatal infection ▶ Fever, cough, shaking chills, dyspnea, cyanosis, weakness, and diffuse crackles
Bacterial	
Streptococcus	▶ Sudden onset of a single, shaking chill, and sustained temperature of 102° to 104° F (38.9° to 40° C); commonly preceded by upper respiratory tract infection
Klebsiella	▶ More likely in patients with chronic alcoholism, pulmonary disease, and diabetes ▶ Fever and recurrent chills; cough producing rusty, bloody, viscous sputum (currant jelly); cyanosis of lips and nail beds from hypoxemia; and shallow, grunting respirations
Staphylococcus	▶ Commonly occurs in patients with viral illness, such as influenza or measles, and in those with cystic fibrosis ▶ Temperature of 102° to 104° F, recurrent shaking chills, bloody sputum, dyspnea, tachypnea, and hypoxemia
Aspiration	
Aspiration of gastric or oropharyngeal contents into trachea and lungs	▶ Noncardiogenic pulmonary edema possible with damage to respiratory epithelium from contact with gastric acid ▶ Subacute pneumonia possible with cavity formation ▶ Lung abscess possible if foreign body present ▶ Crackles, dyspnea, cyanosis, hypotension, and tachycardia

Treatment

▶ Antimicrobial therapy that varies with the causative agent (should be reevaluated early in the course of treatment)
▶ Humidified oxygen therapy for hypoxemia
▶ Mechanical ventilation for respiratory failure
▶ High-calorie diet and adequate fluid intake
▶ Bed rest
▶ Analgesics to relieve pleuritic chest pain
▶ Positive end-expiratory pressure to facilitate adequate oxygenation for patients with severe pneumonia who are on mechanical ventilation
▶ Administration of bronchodilators
▶ Administration of corticosteroids

Nursing considerations

▶ Maintain a patent airway and adequate oxygenation. Monitor pulse oximetry. Measure arterial blood gas levels and administer supplemental oxygen as indicated.
▶ Teach the patient how to cough and perform deep-breathing exercises.
▶ If the patient requires endotracheal intubation or tracheostomy, provide thorough respiratory care. Suction the patient as needed, using sterile technique.
▶ Obtain sputum specimens as ordered.
▶ Administer antibiotics as ordered and pain medication as needed; record the patient's response to medications.
▶ Administer I.V. fluids and electrolyte replacement therapy as ordered.
▶ Maintain adequate nutrition and ask the dietary department to provide a high-calorie, high-protein diet consisting of soft, easy-to-eat foods.
▶ Provide a quiet, calm environment for the patient, with frequent rest periods.
▶ Provide emotional support, especially if respiratory failure occurs.

LESSON PLANS

 Teaching about pneumonia

▶ Explain the disease process and the treatment plan.
▶ Teach the patient how to cough and perform deep-breathing exercises to clear secretions; encourage him to do so often.
▶ Give emotional support by explaining all procedures (especially intubation and suctioning) to the patient and his family.
▶ To control the spread of infection, tell the patient to sneeze and cough into a disposable tissue; tape a lined bag to the side of the bed for used tissues.

▶ Teach the patient strategies to prevent pneumonia:
– Advise against using antibiotics indiscriminately during minor viral infections because doing so may encourage upper airway colonization by antibiotic-resistant bacteria.
– Encourage pneumonia and annual flu vaccination for high-risk patients, such as those with chronic obstructive pulmonary disease, chronic heart disease, or sickle cell disease.
– Urge all bedridden and postoperative patients to perform deep-breathing and coughing exercises often. Tell caregivers to reposition such patients frequently to promote full aeration and drainage of secretions. Encourage early ambulation in postoperative patients.
– Urge patients to avoid irritants that stimulate secretions, such as cigarette smoke, dust, and environmental pollution.

Pulmonary edema

Pulmonary edema is the accumulation of fluid in the extravascular spaces of the lung. With cardiogenic pulmonary edema, fluid accumulation results from elevations in pulmonary venous and capillary hydrostatic pressures. A common complication of cardiac disorders, pulmonary edema can occur as a chronic condition or it can develop quickly and cause death.

Pulmonary edema usually results from left-sided heart failure due to arteriosclerotic, hypertensive, cardiomyopathic, or valvular heart disease. With such disorders, the compromised left ventricle can't maintain adequate cardiac output; increased pressures are transmitted to the left atrium, pulmonary veins, and pulmonary capillary bed. This increased pulmonary capillary hydrostatic force promotes transudation of intravascular fluids into the pulmonary interstitium, decreasing lung compliance and interfering with gas exchange.

Signs and symptoms

▶ Cold, clammy, and sweaty skin
▶ Cough
▶ Decreased level of consciousness
▶ Dependent crackles or wheezing
▶ Diastolic (S_3) gallop
▶ Dyspnea on exertion
▶ Frothy, bloody sputum
▶ Hypoxemia
▶ Jugular vein distention
▶ Orthopnea
▶ Paroxysmal nocturnal dyspnea
▶ Restlessness and anxiety
▶ Tachycardia
▶ Tachypnea
▶ Thready pulse

How pulmonary edema develops

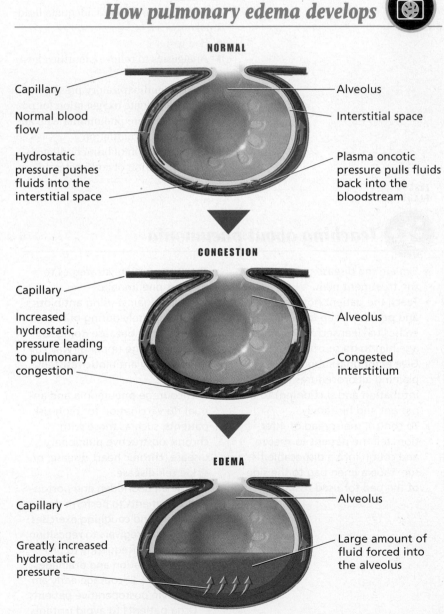

NORMAL

Capillary

Normal blood flow

Hydrostatic pressure pushes fluids into the interstitial space

Alveolus

Interstitial space

Plasma oncotic pressure pulls fluids back into the bloodstream

CONGESTION

Capillary

Increased hydrostatic pressure leading to pulmonary congestion

Alveolus

Congested interstitium

EDEMA

Capillary

Greatly increased hydrostatic pressure

Alveolus

Large amount of fluid forced into the alveolus

Treatment

▶ High concentrations of oxygen by cannula, face mask and, if necessary, assisted ventilation
▶ Angiotensin-converting enzyme inhibitors, diuretics, inotropic drugs such as digoxin (Lanoxin), antiarrhythmic agents, beta-adrenergic blockers, and human B-type natriuretic peptide to treat heart failure
▶ Vasodilator drugs, such as nitroprusside (Nipride) to reduce preload and afterload in acute episodes of pulmonary edema
▶ Morphine to reduce anxiety and dyspnea as well as to dilate the systemic venous bed, promoting blood flow from pulmonary circulation to the periphery

Nursing considerations

▶ Administer oxygen, as ordered, and monitor pulse oximetry.
▶ Monitor vital signs every 15 to 30 minutes while giving nitroprusside in dextrose 5% in water by I.V. drip.
▶ Watch for arrhythmias in patients receiving cardiac glycosides and diuretics and for marked respiratory depression in those receiving morphine.
▶ Assess the patient's condition frequently, and record response to treatment. Monitor arterial blood gas levels, electrolytes, oral and I.V. fluid intake, urine output and, in the patient with a pulmonary artery catheter, pulmonary end-diastolic and wedge pressures. Check cardiac monitor often. Report changes immediately.
▶ Reassure the patient, who will have anxiety due to hypoxia and respiratory distress. Explain all procedures. Provide emotional support to his family as well.
▶ Place the patient in high Fowler's position to enhance lung expansion.

LESSON PLANS

Teaching about pulmonary edema

▶ Explain all procedures to the patient and his family.
▶ Review all prescribed drugs with the patient. If he takes digoxin (Lanoxin), show him how to monitor his own pulse rate and warn him to report signs of toxicity.
▶ Encourage the patient to eat potassium-rich foods to lower the risk of cardiac arrhythmias.
▶ If the patient takes a vasodilator, teach him the signs of hypotension and emphasize the need to avoid alcohol.

▶ Urge the patient to comply with the prescribed drug regimen to avoid future episodes of pulmonary edema.
▶ Emphasize the need to report early signs of fluid overload.
▶ Discuss ways to conserve physical energy.

Pulmonary embolism

Pulmonary embolism is an obstruction of the pulmonary arterial bed that occurs when a mass—such as a dislodged thrombus—lodges in a pulmonary artery branch, partially or completely obstructing it. This causes a ventilation-perfusion mismatch, resulting in hypoxemia, as well as intrapulmonary shunting.

The prognosis varies. Although the pulmonary infarction that results from embolism may be so mild that the patient is asymptomatic, massive embolism (more than 50% obstruction of pulmonary arterial circulation) and infarction can cause rapid death.

In most patients, pulmonary embolism results from a dislodged thrombus (blood clot) that originates in the leg veins. More than one-half of such thrombi arise in the deep veins of the legs; usually multiple thrombi arise. Other, less common sources of thrombi include the pelvic, renal, and hepatic veins, the right side of the heart, and the upper extremities.

Signs and symptoms
▶ Cyanosis
▶ Dyspnea or unexplained shortness of breath
▶ Hypotension
▶ Jugular vein distention
▶ Low-grade fever
▶ Pleuritic pain or chest pain
▶ Productive cough (sputum may be blood tinged)
▶ Tachycardia or arrhythmia

Treatment
▶ Oxygen therapy
▶ Fibrinolytic therapy
▶ Anticoagulation with heparin
▶ Embolectomy
▶ Vasopressors and antibiotics
▶ Vena caval ligation, plication, or insertion of a device to filter blood returning to the heart and lungs to prevent future pulmonary emboli

Understanding thrombus formation

Thrombus formation results from vascular wall damage, venous stasis, and hypercoagulability of the blood. Trauma, clot dissolution, intravascular pressure changes, or a change in peripheral blood flow can cause the thrombus to loosen or become fragmented. Then, the thrombus—now called an *embolus*—floats to the heart's right side and enters the lung through the pulmonary artery.

There, the embolus may dissolve, become more fragmented, or grow.

By occluding the pulmonary artery, the embolus prevents alveoli from producing enough surfactant to maintain alveolar integrity. As a result, alveoli collapse and atelectasis develops. If the embolus enlarges, it may clog most or all pulmonary vessels and cause right-sided heart failure and death.

Who's at risk for pulmonary embolism?

Many disorders and treatments increase the risk of pulmonary embolism. Risk is particularly high for patients who have had recent surgery. The anesthetic used during surgery can injure lung vessels, and surgery or prolonged immobility can promote venous stasis, further compounding the risk.

Predisposing disorders
▶ Lung disorders, especially chronic types
▶ Cardiac disorders
▶ Infection
▶ Cancer
▶ History of thromboembolism, thrombophlebitis, or venous insufficiency
▶ Sickle cell disease
▶ Autoimmune hemolytic anemia
▶ Polycythemia
▶ Osteomyelitis
▶ Long-bone fracture
▶ Manipulation or disconnection of central lines
▶ Coagulation disorders

Venous stasis
▶ Prolonged immobilization
▶ Obesity
▶ Age older than 40
▶ Burns
▶ Pregnancy or recent childbirth
▶ Orthopedic casts

Venous injury
▶ Surgery, particularly of the legs, pelvis, abdomen, or thorax
▶ Leg or pelvic fractures or injuries
▶ I.V. drug abuse
▶ I.V. therapy

Increased blood coagulability
▶ Use of high-estrogen hormonal contraceptives
▶ Dehydration
▶ Family history

Nursing considerations

▶ As ordered, give oxygen by nasal cannula or mask. If the patient has worsening dyspnea, check his arterial blood gas levels. If breathing is severely compromised, assist with endotracheal intubation and provide assisted ventilation as ordered.

▶ Administer heparin as ordered by I.V. push or continuous drip. Monitor coagulation studies frequently.

▶ During heparin therapy, watch closely for epistaxis, petechiae, and other signs of abnormal bleeding. Also check the patient's stools for occult blood. Don't administer I.M. injections.

▶ After the patient stabilizes, encourage him to ambulate, and assist with isometric and range-of-motion exercises. Check his temperature and the color of his feet to detect venous stasis. Never vigorously massage his legs; that could cause thrombi to dislodge.

▶ Apply antiembolism stockings to promote venous return.

▶ If the patient needs surgery, make sure he ambulates as soon as possible afterward to promote circulation.

▶ Provide the patient with adequate nutrition and fluids to promote healing.

▶ If the patient has pleuritic chest pain, administer the ordered analgesic.

▶ Provide incentive spirometry to help the patient with deep breathing. Provide tissues and a bag for easy disposal of tissues.

▶ Provide adequate rest periods.

PICTURING PATHO

A *closer look at pulmonary emboli*

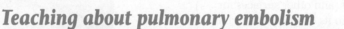

Multiple emboli in small branches of left pulmonary artery

Infarcted area

Embolus in branch of right pulmonary artery

LESSON PLANS

Teaching about pulmonary embolism

▶ Explain all procedures and treatments to the patient and family.

▶ Teach about the signs and symptoms of thrombophlebitis and pulmonary embolism.

▶ Teach the patient receiving anticoagulant therapy the signs of bleeding to watch for (bloody stools, blood in urine, large bruises).

▶ Tell the patient that he can help prevent bleeding by shaving with an electric razor and by brushing his teeth with a soft toothbrush.

▶ Make sure that the patient understands the importance of taking drugs exactly as prescribed. Tell him not to take other drugs, especially aspirin, without asking the physician.

▶ Stress the importance of follow-up laboratory tests, such as prothrombin time, to monitor anticoagulant therapy.

▶ Tell the patient that he must inform all of his health care providers—including dentists—that he's receiving anticoagulant therapy.

▶ To prevent pulmonary emboli in a high-risk patient, encourage him to walk and exercise his legs and to wear support or antiembolism stockings. Tell him not to cross or massage his legs and to report leg pain or edema.

Severe acute respiratory syndrome

Severe acute respiratory syndrome (SARS) is a viral respiratory infection that can progress to pneumonia and, eventually, death. The disease was first recognized in 2003 with outbreaks in China, Canada, Singapore, Taiwan, and Vietnam, with other countries—including the United States—reporting smaller numbers of cases.

SARS is caused by the SARS-associated coronavirus (SARS-CoV). Coronaviruses are a common cause of mild respiratory illnesses in humans, but researchers believe that a virus may have mutated, allowing it to cause this potentially life-threatening disease.

Close contact with a person who's infected with SARS, including contact with infectious aerosolized droplets or body secretions, is the transmission mode. Most people who contracted the disease during the 2003 outbreak contracted it during travel to endemic areas. However, the virus has been found to live on human hands, disposable tissues, and other surfaces for up to 6 hours in its droplet form. It has also been found to live in the stools of people with SARS for up to 4 days. The virus may be able to live for months or years in below-freezing temperatures.

Signs and symptoms

▶ Chills
▶ Diarrhea
▶ Dry cough
▶ Fever (greater than 100.4° F [38° C])
▶ General discomfort
▶ Headache
▶ Myalgia
▶ Rhinorrhea
▶ Rigors
▶ Shortness of breath
▶ Sore throat

PICTURING PATHO

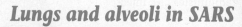

Lungs and alveoli in SARS

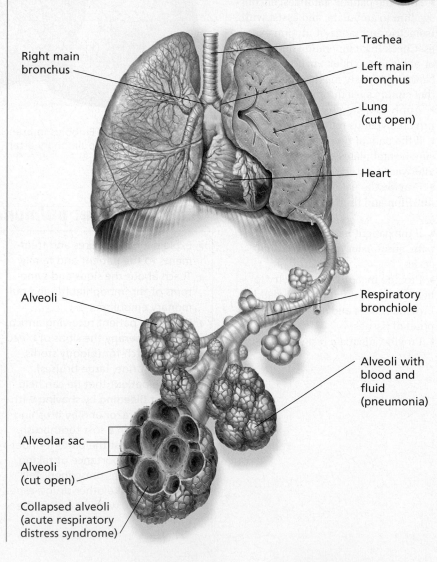

Trachea

Right main bronchus

Left main bronchus

Lung (cut open)

Heart

Alveoli

Respiratory bronchiole

Alveoli with blood and fluid (pneumonia)

Alveolar sac

Alveoli (cut open)

Collapsed alveoli (acute respiratory distress syndrome)

Treatment
▸ Patent airway maintenance
▸ Adequate nutrition
▸ Supplemental oxygen as needed
▸ Chest physiotherapy
▸ Mechanical ventilation
▸ Contact precautions requiring gowns and gloves for all hospitalized patients and their contacts, and airborne precautions utilizing a negative pressure isolation room and properly fitted N-95 respirators
▸ Quarantine to prevent the spread of infection
▸ Antibiotics to treat bacterial causes of atypical pneumonia
▸ Antiviral medications
▸ High doses of corticosteroids to reduce lung inflammation
▸ In some serious cases, serum from individuals who have already recovered from SARS (convalescent serum); general benefit of these treatments not conclusive

Nursing considerations
▸ Report suspected cases of SARS to local and national health organizations.
▸ Frequently monitor the patient's vital signs and respiratory status.
▸ Maintain isolation as recommended. Provide emotional support to deal with anxiety and fear related to the diagnosis of SARS and as a result of isolation.
▸ Administer medications, as ordered, and evaluate response.
▸ Provide oxygen as needed and monitor pulse oximetry.

LESSON PLANS

Teaching about SARS

▸ Teach the patient about the need for isolation. Provide emotional support to help him deal with anxiety and fear related to his diagnosis and as a result of isolation.
▸ Emphasize the importance of frequent hand washing, covering the mouth and nose when coughing or sneezing, and avoiding close personal contact while infected or potentially infected.

▸ Instruct the patient and family that such items as eating utensils, towels, and bedding shouldn't be shared until they've been washed with soap and hot water, and that disposable gloves and household disinfectant should be used to clean any surface that may have been exposed to the patient's body fluids.
▸ Emphasize the importance of not going to work, school, or other public places until recommended by the health care provider.

Tuberculosis

An acute or chronic infection caused by *Mycobacterium tuberculosis,* tuberculosis (TB) is characterized by pulmonary infiltrates, formation of granulomas with caseation, fibrosis, and cavitation. People who live in crowded, poorly ventilated conditions and those who are immunocompromised are most likely to become infected. In patients with strains that are sensitive to the usual antitubercular agents, the prognosis is excellent with correct treatment. However, in those with strains that are resistant to two or more of the major antitubercular agents, mortality is 50%.

After exposure to *M. tuberculosis,* about 5% of infected people develop active TB within 1 year; in the remainder, microorganisms cause a latent infection. The host's immune system usually controls the tubercle bacillus by enclosing it in a tiny nodule (tubercle). The bacillus may lie dormant within the tubercle for years and later reactivate and spread.

Although the primary infection site is the lung, mycobacteria commonly exist in other parts of the body. A number of factors increase the risk of infection reactivation: gastrectomy, uncontrolled diabetes mellitus, Hodgkin's disease, leukemia, silicosis, acquired immunodeficiency syndrome, treatment with corticosteroids or immunosuppressants, and advanced age.

PICTURING PATHO

Appearance of tuberculosis in the lungs

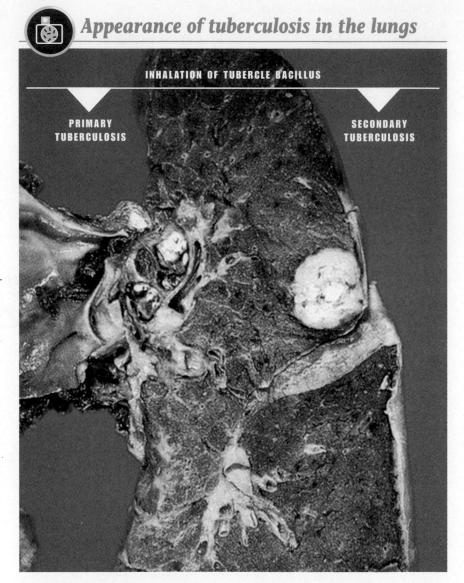

INHALATION OF TUBERCLE BACILLUS

PRIMARY TUBERCULOSIS

SECONDARY TUBERCULOSIS

Signs and symptoms

In primary infection, after an incubation period of 4 to 8 weeks, TB usually produces no symptoms; however, it may initially produce nonspecific symptoms, such as:
- anorexia
- fatigue
- low-grade fever
- night sweats
- weakness
- weight loss.

In reactivation, symptoms may include:
- chest pains
- cough that produces mucopurulent sputum
- occasional hemoptysis.

Treatment

▶ Isoniazid, rifampin, ethambutol, and pyrazinamide
▶ Daily INH for 9 months to treat latent TB; RIF daily for 4 months for people with latent TB whose contacts are INH resistant
▶ For most adults with active TB, administration of all four drugs daily for 2 months, followed by 4 to 7 months of INH and RIF recommended; drug therapy selected according to patient condition and organism susceptibility
▶ First-line drug such as rifapentine (Priftin) and second-line drugs, such as cycloserine, ethionamide, amino-salicylic acid (Paser), streptomycin, and capreomycin (reserved for special circumstances or drug-resistant strains)
▶ Interruption of drug therapy requiring initiation of therapy from the beginning of the regimen

Nursing considerations

▶ Initiate acid-fast bacillus (AFB) isolation precautions immediately for all patients suspected or confirmed to have TB.
▶ Continue AFB isolation until there's clinical evidence of reduced infectiousness (substantially decreased cough, fewer organisms on sequential sputum smears).
▶ Teach the infectious patient to cough and sneeze into tissues and to dispose of all secretions properly. Place a covered trash can nearby or tape a lined bag to the side of the bed to dispose of used tissues.
▶ Instruct the patient to wear a mask when outside of his room.
▶ Visitors and staff members should wear N-95 respirators that fit properly when they're in the patient's room.
▶ Provide adequate rest periods. Provide balanced meals to promote recovery. If the patient is anorectic, urge him to eat small meals frequently. Record weight weekly.
▶ Be alert for adverse effects of medications. Because INH sometimes leads to hepatitis or peripheral neuritis, monitor aspartate aminotransferase and alanine aminotransferase levels. To prevent or treat peripheral neuritis, give pyridoxine (vitamin B_6), as ordered. If the patient receives EMB, watch for optic neuritis; if it develops, discontinue the drug. If he receives RIF, watch for hepatitis and purpura. Observe the patient for other complications such as hemoptysis.
▶ Advise staff members and other persons who have been exposed to infected patients to receive tuberculin tests; chest X-rays and prophylactic INH may also be ordered.

LESSON PLANS

Teaching about tuberculosis

▶ Teach the infectious patient to cough and sneeze into tissues and to dispose of all secretions properly. Place a covered trash can nearby or tape a lined bag to the side of the bed to dispose of used tissues.
▶ Instruct the patient to wear a mask when out of his room.
▶ Remind the patient to get plenty of rest. Stress the importance of eating balanced meals to promote recovery. If the patient is anorectic, urge him to eat small, frequent meals.

▶ Before discharge, advise the patient to watch for adverse drug effects and to report them immediately. Emphasize the importance of regular follow-up examinations. Teach the patient and his family about signs and symptoms of recurring tuberculosis. Stress the need to follow long-term treatment faithfully.
▶ Emphasize the importance of taking the drugs daily as prescribed. To avoid the development of drug-resistant organisms, the patient may participate in a supervised administration program.

TESTS
Blood tests

Blood tests used to help diagnose respiratory disorders include arterial blood gas (ABG) analysis, arterial-to-alveolar oxygen ratio, white blood cell (WBC) count, and WBC differential.

ARTERIAL BLOOD GAS ANALYSIS

ABG analysis is one of the first tests ordered to assess respiratory status because it helps evaluate gas exchange in the lungs by measuring:

▶ pH: indicates the blood's hydrogen ion concentration, which shows the blood's acidity or alkalinity

▶ partial pressure of arterial carbon dioxide ($Paco_2$): reflects the adequacy of the lungs' ventilation and carbon dioxide elimination; known as the *respiratory parameter*

▶ partial pressure of arterial oxygen (Pao_2): reflects the body's ability to pick up oxygen from the lungs

▶ bicarbonate level (HCO_3^-): reflects the kidneys' ability to retain and excrete bicarbonate; known as the *metabolic parameter*

The respiratory and metabolic systems work together to keep the body's acid-base balance within normal limits. If respiratory acidosis develops, for example, the kidneys attempt to compensate by conserving HCO_3^-. Therefore, if respiratory acidosis is present, expect to see the HCO_3^- value rise above normal. Similarly, if metabolic acidosis develops, the lungs try to compensate by increasing the respiratory rate and depth to eliminate carbon dioxide. Therefore, expect to see the $Paco_2$ level fall below normal. These compensatory measures attempt to balance the pH of the blood.

Balancing pH

To measure the acidity or alkalinity of a solution, chemists use a pH scale of 1 to 15 that measures hydrogen ion concentrations. As hydrogen ions and acidity increase, pH falls below 7.0, which is neutral. Conversely, when hydrogen ions decrease, pH and alkalinity increase. Acid-base balance, or homeostasis of hydrogen ions, is necessary if the body's enzyme systems are to work properly.

The slightest change in ionic hydrogen concentration alters the rate of cellular chemical reactions; a sufficiently severe change can be fatal. To maintain a normal blood pH—generally between 7.35 and 7.45—the body relies on three mechanisms: buffers, respiration, and urinary excretion.

Buffers

Chemically composed of two substances, buffers prevent radical pH changes by replacing strong acids added to a solution (such as blood) with weaker ones. For example, strong acids capable of yielding many hydrogen ions are replaced by weaker ones that yield fewer hydrogen ions. Because of the principal buffer coupling of bicarbonate and carbonic acid—normally in a ratio of 20:1—the plasma acid-base level rarely fluctuates. Increased bicarbonate, however, indicates alkalosis, whereas decreased bicarbonate points to acidosis. Increased carbonic acid indicates acidosis, and decreased carbonic acid indicates alkalosis.

Respiration

Respiration is important in maintaining blood pH. The lungs convert carbonic acid to carbon dioxide and water. With every expiration, carbon dioxide and water leave the body, decreasing the carbonic acid content of the blood. Consequently, fewer hydrogen ions are formed, and blood pH increases. When the blood's hydrogen ion or carbonic acid content increases, neurons in the respiratory center stimulate respiration.

Hyperventilation eliminates carbon dioxide and hence carbonic acid from the body, reduces hydrogen ion formation, and increases pH.

Conversely, increased blood pH from alkalosis—decreased hydrogen ion concentration—causes hypoventilation, which restores blood pH to its normal level by retaining carbon dioxide and thus increasing hydrogen ion formation.

Urinary excretion

The third factor in acid-base balance is urine excretion. Because the kidneys excrete varying amounts of acids and bases, they control urine pH, which in turn affects blood pH. For example, when blood pH is decreased, the distal and collecting tubules remove excessive hydrogen ions (carbonic acid forms in the tubular cells and dissociates into hydrogen and bicarbonate) and displaces them in urine, thereby eliminating hydrogen from the body. In exchange, basic ions in the urine—usually sodium—diffuse into the tubular cells, where they combine with bicarbonate. This sodium bicarbonate is then reabsorbed in the blood, resulting in decreased urine pH and, more importantly, increased blood pH.

Understanding acid-base disorders

Disorders and ABG findings	Possible causes	Signs and symptoms
Respiratory acidosis (excess CO_2 retention)		
▶ pH < 7.35 (SI, < 7.35) ▶ HCO_3^- > 26 mEq/L (SI, > 26 mmol/L) (if compensating) ▶ $Paco_2$ > 45 mm Hg (SI, > 5.3 kPa)	▶ Central nervous system depression from drugs, injury, or disease ▶ Asphyxia ▶ Hypoventilation due to pulmonary, cardiac, musculoskeletal, or neuromuscular disease ▶ Obesity ▶ Postoperative pain ▶ Abdominal distention	Diaphoresis, headache, tachycardia, confusion, restlessness, apprehension, drowsiness, tremor, myoclonic jerks, asterixis, stupor (carbon dioxide narcosis), hypoxia
Respiratory alkalosis (excess CO_2 excretion)		
▶ pH > 7.45 (SI, > 7.45) ▶ HCO_3^- < 22 mEq/L (SI, < 22 mmol/L) (if compensating) ▶ $Paco_2$ < 35 mm Hg (SI, < 4.7 kPa)	▶ Hyperventilation due to anxiety, pain, or improper ventilator settings ▶ Respiratory stimulation caused by drugs, disease, hypoxia, fever, or high room temperature ▶ Gram-negative bacteremia ▶ Compensation for metabolic acidosis (chronic renal failure)	Rapid, deep breathing; paresthesia; light-headedness; twitching; anxiety; fear; confusion; cramps; syncope; hyperpnea; tachypnea; carpopedal spasm; peripheral and circumoral paresthesia
Metabolic acidosis (HCO_3^- loss, acid retention)		
▶ pH < 7.35 (SI, < 7.35) ▶ HCO_3^- < 22 mEq/L (SI, < 22 mmol/L) ▶ $Paco_2$ < 35 mm Hg (SI, < 4.7 kPa) (if compensating)	▶ HCO_3^- depletion due to renal disease, diarrhea, or small-bowel fistulas ▶ Excessive production of organic acids due to hepatic disease; endocrine disorders, including diabetes mellitus, hypoxia, shock, and drug intoxication ▶ Inadequate excretion of acids due to renal disease	Rapid, deep breathing; fruity breath; fatigue; headache; lethargy; drowsiness; nausea; vomiting; coma (if severe)
Metabolic alkalosis (HCO_3^- retention, acid loss)		
▶ pH > 7.45 (SI, > 7.45) ▶ HCO_3^- > 26 mEq/L (SI, > 26 mmol/L) ▶ $Paco_2$ > 45 mm Hg (SI, > 5.3 kPa)	▶ Loss of hydrochloric acid from prolonged vomiting or gastric suctioning ▶ Loss of potassium due to increased renal excretion (as in diuretic therapy) or steroid overdose ▶ Excessive alkali ingestion ▶ Compensation for chronic respiratory acidosis	Slow, shallow breathing; hypertonic muscles; restlessness; twitching; confusion; irritability; apathy; tetany; seizures; coma (if severe); headache; lethargy

ARTERIAL-TO-ALVEOLAR OXYGEN RATIO

Using calculations based on the patient's laboratory values, the arterial-to-alveolar oxygen ratio (also known as *a/A ratio*) can help identify the cause of hypoxemia and intrapulmonary shunting by providing an approximation of the partial pressure of oxygenation of the alveoli and arteries. It may help differentiate the cause as ventilated alveoli but no perfusion, unventilated alveoli with perfusion, or collapse of the alveoli and capillaries.

WHITE BLOOD CELL COUNT

The WBC, or *leukocyte*, count measures the number of WBCs in a microliter of whole blood. This is done through the use of electronic devices. A WBC count can be useful in diagnosing infection and inflammation as well as in monitoring a patient's response to chemotherapy or radiation therapy. WBC counts can also help determine whether further tests are needed. An elevated WBC count (leukocytosis) commonly signals infection, such as an abscess, meningitis, appendicitis, or tonsillitis. A high count may also indicate leukemia or tissue necrosis caused by burns, myocardial infarction, or gangrene.

WHITE BLOOD CELL DIFFERENTIAL

A WBC differential can provide more specific information about a patient's immune system. In a WBC differential, the laboratory classifies 100 or more WBCs in a stained film of blood according to five major types of leukocytes—neutrophils, eosinophils, basophils, lymphocytes, and monocytes—and determines the percentage of each type. Abnormally high levels of WBCs are associated with allergic reactions and parasitic infections. After the normal values for the patient have been determined, an assessment can be made.

Sputum and pleural fluid tests

Sputum tests include sputum analysis, nasopharyngeal culture, and throat culture. Pleural fluid tests include thoracentesis.

SPUTUM ANALYSIS

Analysis of a sputum specimen (the material expectorated from a patient's lungs and bronchi during deep coughing) helps diagnose respiratory disease, determine the cause of respiratory infection (including viral and bacterial causes), identify abnormal lung cells, and manage lung disease.

Culture and sensitivity testing identifies a specific microorganism and its antibiotic sensitivities. A negative culture may suggest a viral infection.

Flora commonly found in the respiratory tract include alpha-hemolytic streptococci, *Neisseria* species, diphtheroids, some *Haemophilus* species, pneumococci, staphylococci, and yeasts such as *Candida*. However, the presence of normal flora doesn't rule out infection. A culture isolate must be interpreted in light of the patient's overall clinical condition.

Pathogenic organisms most commonly found in sputum include

HANDS ON

Using an in-line trap

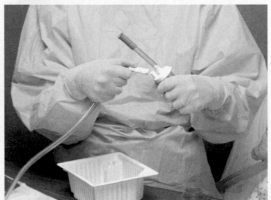

Push the suction tubing onto the male adapter of the in-line trap.

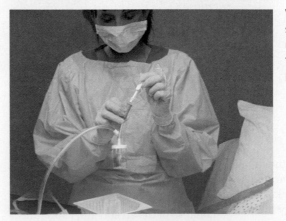

With one hand, insert the suction catheter into the rubber tubing of the trap. Then suction the patient.

Streptococcus pneumoniae, Mycobacterium tuberculosis, Klebsiella pneumoniae (and other Enterobacteriaceae), *H. influenzae, Staphylococcus aureus,* and *Pseudomonas aeruginosa.* Other pathogens, such as P*neumocystis carinii,* Legionella species, *Mycoplasma pneumoniae,* and respiratory viruses, may exist in the sputum and can cause lung disease, but they usually require serologic or histologic diagnosis rather than diagnosis by sputum culture.

NASOPHARYNGEAL CULTURE

Direct microscopic inspection of a Gram-stained smear of a nasopharyngeal specimen provides preliminary identification of organisms, which may guide clinical management and determine the need for additional testing. Streaking a culture plate with the swab—allowing any organisms present to grow—permits isolation and identification of pathogens. Cultured pathogens may require susceptibility testing to determine the appropriate antimicrobial agent.

Flora commonly found in the nasopharynx include nonhemolytic streptococci, alpha-hemolytic streptococci, *Neisseria* species (except *N. meningitidis* and *N. gonorrhoeae*), *Staphylococcus epidermidis* and, methicillin-resistant *S. aureus.*

THROAT CULTURE

A throat culture requires swabbing the throat, streaking a culture plate, and allowing the organisms to grow for isolation and identification of pathogens. A Gram-stained smear may provide preliminary identification, which may guide clinical management and determine the need for further tests. Culture results must be interpreted in light of clinical status, recent antimicrobial therapy, and the amount of normal flora.

Possible pathogens cultured include group A beta-hemolytic streptococci (*Streptococcus pyogenes*), which can cause scarlet fever or pharyngitis; *Candida albicans*, which can cause thrush; *Corynebacterium diphtheriae*, which can cause diphtheria; and *Bordetella pertussis*, which can cause whooping cough. Other cultured bacteria include *Legionella* species, *Mycoplasma pneumoniae, Staphylococcus aureus, Streptococcus pneumoniae,* and *H. influenzae.* Cultured bacteria are also used to screen for carriers of *N. meningitidis.* Fungi include *Histoplasma capsulatum, Coccidioides immitis,* and *Blastomyces dermatitidis.* Viruses include adenovirus, enterovirus, herpesvirus, rhinovirus, influenza virus, and parainfluenza virus.

HANDS ON *Obtaining a nasopharyngeal specimen*

When the swab passes into the nasopharynx, gently but quickly rotate it to collect a specimen. Then remove the swab, taking care not to injure the nasal mucous membrane.

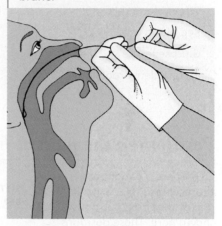

THORACENTESIS

Thoracentesis, also known as *pleural fluid aspiration,* is used to obtain a sample of pleural fluid for analysis, relieve lung compression through fluid removal and, occasionally, obtain a lung tissue biopsy specimen.

The pleural cavity should contain less than 20 ml of serous fluid. Pleural effusion results from the abnormal formation or reabsorption of pleural fluid. Certain characteristics classify pleural fluid as either a transudate or an exudate.

Pleural fluid may contain blood, chyle, or pus and necrotic tissue. A high percentage of neutrophils suggests septic inflammation. Pleural fluid glucose levels that are 30 to 40 mg/dl (SI, 1.5 to 2 mmol/L) lower than blood glucose levels may indicate cancer, bacterial infection, nonseptic inflammation, or metastasis. Increased amylase levels occur with pleural effusions associated with pancreatitis.

After suctioning, disconnect the in-line trap from the suction tubing and catheter. To seal the container, connect the rubber tubing to the female adapter of the trap.

Characteristics of pulmonary transudate and exudate

These characteristics help classify pleural fluid as either a transudate or an exudate.

Characteristic	Transudate	Exudate
Appearance	Clear	Cloudy, turbid
Specific gravity	< 1.016	> 1.016
Clot (fibrinogen)	Absent	Present
Protein	< 3 g/dl (SI, < 30 g/L)	> 3 g/dl (SI, > 30 g/L)
White blood cells	Few lymphocytes	Many lymphocytes; may be purulent
Red blood cells	Few	Variable
Glucose level	Equal to serum level	May be less than serum level
Lactate dehydrogenase	Low	High

Positioning the patient for thoracentesis

To prepare a patient for thoracentesis, place him in one of the three positions shown here. These positions serve to widen the intercostal spaces and permit easy access to the pleural cavity. Using pillows (as shown) will make the patient more comfortable.

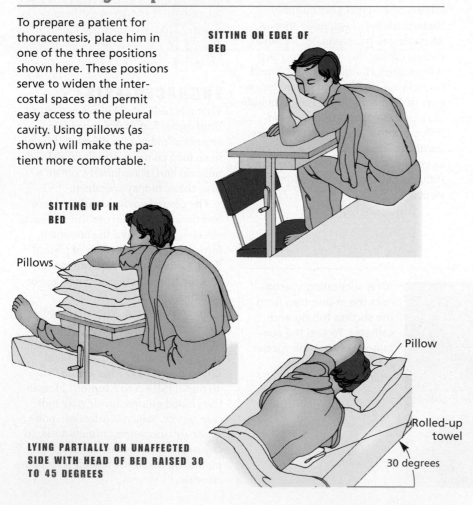

SITTING ON EDGE OF BED

SITTING UP IN BED

Pillows

LYING PARTIALLY ON UNAFFECTED SIDE WITH HEAD OF BED RAISED 30 TO 45 DEGREES

Pillow

Rolled-up towel

30 degrees

Recognizing complications of thoracentesis

You can identify complications of thoracentesis by watching for characteristic signs and symptoms:

▶ *pneumothorax*—apprehension, increased restlessness, cyanosis, sudden breathlessness, tachycardia, chest pain
▶ *tension pneumothorax*—dyspnea, chest pain, tachycardia, hypotension, absent or diminished breath sounds on the affected side
▶ *subcutaneous emphysema*—local tissue swelling, crackling on palpation of site
▶ *infection*—fever, rapid pulse rate, pain
▶ *mediastinal shift*—labored breathing, cardiac arrhythmias, pulmonary edema
▶ *bleeding*—bruising, pain, dyspnea, hypotension, altered mental status.

Endoscopic and imaging tests

Endoscopic and imaging tests include bronchoscopy, chest X-ray, indirect laryngoscopy, direct laryngoscopy, magnetic resonance imaging (MRI), mediastinoscopy, pulmonary angiography, thoracic computed tomography (CT) scan, thoracoscopy, and ventilation-perfusion ($\dot{V}/\dot{Q}$) scan.

BRONCHOSCOPY

Bronchoscopy is direct inspection of the larynx, trachea, and bronchi through a flexible fiber-optic or rigid metal bronchoscope. A more recent approach is the use of virtual bronchoscopy. Although a flexible fiber-optic bronchoscope allows a wider view and is used more commonly, the rigid metal bronchoscope is required to remove foreign objects, excise endobronchial lesions, and control massive hemoptysis. A brush biopsy, forceps, or catheter may be passed through the bronchoscope to obtain specimens for cytologic examination.

CHEST X-RAY

Because normal pulmonary tissue is radiolucent, foreign bodies, infiltrates, fluids, tumors, and other abnormalities appear as densities (white areas) on a chest X-ray. It's most useful when compared with the patient's previous films, which allow the radiologist to detect changes.

By itself, a chest X-ray film may not provide information for a definitive diagnosis. For example, it may not reveal mild to moderate obstructive pulmonary disease. Even so, it can show the location and size of lesions and identify structural abnormalities that influence ventilation and diffusion. Examples of abnormalities visible on X-ray include pneumothorax, fibrosis, atelectasis, and infiltrates.

Virtual bronchoscopy

Using a computer and data from a spiral computed tomography (CT) scan, physicians can now examine the respiratory tract noninvasively with virtual bronchoscopy. Although still in its early stages, researchers believe that this test can enhance screening, diagnosis, preoperative planning, surgical technique, and postoperative follow-up.

Advantages

Unlike its counterpart—conventional bronchoscopy—virtual bronchoscopy is noninvasive, doesn't require sedation, and provides images for examination beyond the segmental bronchi, thus allowing for possible diagnosis of areas that may be stenosed, obstructed, or compressed from an external source. The images obtained from the CT scan include views of the airways and lung parenchyma. Anatomic structures and abnormalities can be precisely identified and, therefore, can be helpful in locating potential biopsy sites to be obtained with conventional bronchoscopy and provide simulation for planning the optimal surgical approach.

Disadvantages

Virtual bronchoscopy does have disadvantages. This technique doesn't allow for biopsy specimens to be obtained from tissue sources. It also can't demonstrate details of the mucosal surface, such as color or texture. Moreover, if an area contains viscous secretions, such as mucus, blood, or a foreign object, visualization becomes difficult and removal isn't possible.

More research on this technique is needed. However, researchers believe that virtual bronchoscopy may play a major role in the screening and early detection of certain cancers, thus allowing for treatment at an earlier, possibly curable stage.

Selected clinical implications of chest X-ray films

Normal anatomic location and appearance	Possible abnormality
Trachea Visible midline in the anterior mediastinal cavity; translucent tubelike appearance	▸ Deviation from midline ▸ Narrowing with hourglass appearance and deviation to one side
Heart Visible in the anterior left mediastinal cavity; solid appearance due to blood contents; edges may be clear in contrast with surrounding air density of the lung	▸ Shift ▸ Hypertrophy ▸ Cardiac borders obscured by stringy densities ("shaggy heart")
Aortic knob Visible as water density; formed by the arch of the aorta	▸ Solid densities, possibly indicating calcifications ▸ Tortuous shape
Mediastinum (mediastinal shadow) Visible as the space between the lungs; shadowy appearance that widens at the hilum of the lungs	▸ Deviation to nondiseased side; deviation to diseased side by traction ▸ Gross widening
Ribs Visible as thoracic cage	▸ Break or misalignment ▸ Widening of intercostal spaces
Spine Visible midline in the posterior chest; straight bony structure	▸ Spinal curvature ▸ Break or misalignment
Clavicles Visible in upper thorax; intact and equidistant in properly centered X-ray films	▸ Break or misalignment
Hila (lung roots) Visible above the heart, where pulmonary vessels, bronchi, and lymph nodes join the lungs; appear as small, white, bilateral densities	▸ Shift to one side ▸ Accentuated shadows
Mainstem bronchus Visible; part of the hila with translucent tubelike appearance	▸ Spherical or oval density
Bronchi Usually not visible	▸ Visible
Lung fields Usually not visible throughout, except for the blood vessels	▸ Visible ▸ Irregular
Hemidiaphragm Rounded, visible; right side ⅜" to ¾" (1 to 2 cm)	▸ Elevation of diaphragm (difference in elevation can be measured on inspiration and expiration to detect movement) ▸ Flattening of diaphragm ▸ Unilateral elevation of either side ▸ Unilateral elevation of left side only

Implications

- Tension pneumothorax, atelectasis, pleural effusion, consolidation, mediastinal nodes or, in children, enlarged thymus
- Substernal thyroid or stenosis secondary to trauma

- Atelectasis, pneumothorax
- Cor pulmonale, heart failure
- Cystic fibrosis

- Atherosclerosis
- Atherosclerosis

- Pleural effusion or tumor, fibrosis or collapsed lung

- Neoplasms of esophagus, bronchi, lungs, thyroid, thymus, peripheral nerves, lymphoid tissue; aortic aneurysm; mediastinitis; cor pulmonale

- Fractured sternum or ribs
- Emphysema

- Scoliosis, kyphosis
- Fracture

- Fractures

- Atelectasis
- Pneumothorax, emphysema, pulmonary abscess, tumor, enlarged lymph nodes

- Bronchogenic cyst

- Bronchial pneumonia

- Atelectasis
- Resolving pneumonia, infiltrates, silicosis, fibrosis, neoplasm

- Active tuberculosis, pneumonia, pleurisy, acute bronchitis, active disease of the abdominal viscera, bilateral phrenic nerve involvement, atelectasis
- Asthma, emphysema
- Possible unilateral phrenic nerve paresis
- Perforated ulcer (rare), gas distention of stomach or splenic flexure of colon, free air in abdomen

INDIRECT LARYNGOSCOPY

Indirect laryngoscopy allows inspection of the nasopharynx and posterior soft palate using a small mirror or an instrument that resembles a telescope. While the mirror is inserted, slight pressure is applied to the tongue, and the patient is instructed to say, "a" and then "e," which elevates the soft palate. The instrument shouldn't touch the tongue to prevent stimulation of the gag reflex. The nasopharynx is then inspected for drainage, bleeding, ulceration, or masses.

DIRECT LARYNGOSCOPY

Direct laryngoscopy allows visualization of the larynx by the use of a fiber-optic endoscope or laryngoscope passed through the mouth or nose and pharynx to the larynx. It's indicated for any condition requiring direct visualization or specimen samples for diagnosis, such as in patients with strong gag reflexes due to anatomic abnormalities, and those who have had no response to short-term therapy for symptoms of pharyngeal or laryngeal disease, such as stridor and hemoptysis. Secretions or tissue may be removed during this procedure for further study. The test is usually contraindicated in patients with epiglottiditis but may be performed on them in an operating room with resuscitative equipment available.

MAGNETIC RESONANCE IMAGING

MRI is a noninvasive test that uses a powerful magnet, radio waves, and a computer to help diagnose respiratory disorders. It provides high-resolution, cross-sectional images of lung structures and traces blood flow. The greatest advantage of an MRI is its ability to "see through" bone and to delineate fluid-filled soft tissue in great detail, without using ionizing radiation or contrast media.

MEDIASTINOSCOPY

Mediastinoscopy is performed under general anesthesia and involves insertion of a mirrored-lens instrument that's similar to a bronchoscope but is inserted through an incision at the base of the anterior neck. A biopsy of mediastinal lymph nodes is obtained. Because mediastinal lymph nodes drain lymphatic drainage from the lungs, specimens can identify carcinoma, granulomatous infection, sarcoidosis, coccidioidomycosis, or histoplasmosis. It can also be used to stage lung cancer or determine the extent of lung tumor metastasis.

PULMONARY ANGIOGRAPHY

Pulmonary angiography, also called *pulmonary arteriography,* allows radiographic examination of the pulmonary circulation. After injecting a radioactive contrast dye through a catheter inserted into the pulmonary artery or one of its branches, a series of X-rays is taken to detect blood flow abnormalities, possibly caused by emboli or pulmonary infarction. This test provides more reliable results than a V̇/Q̇ scan but carries higher risks, including cardiac arrhythmias.

THORACIC CT SCANNING

A thoracic CT scan provides cross-sectional views of the chest by passing an X-ray beam from a computerized scanner through the body at different angles and depths. The CT scan provides a three-dimensional image of the lung, allowing the physician to assess abnormalities in the configuration of the trachea or major bronchi and evaluate masses or lesions, such as tumors and abscesses, and abnormal lung shadows. A contrast agent is sometimes used to highlight blood vessels and to allow greater visual discrimination. Pulmonary emboli may also be identified.

THORACOSCOPY

A thoracoscopy is an invasive diagnostic procedure that uses a fiber-optic endoscope to examine the thoracic cavity. Thoracoscopy allows visualization of the visceral and parietal pleura, pleural spaces, mediastinum, thoracic walls, and pericardium. It can also be used to perform laser procedures, to assess pleural effusion, tumor growth, emphysema, inflammatory disease, and conditions that would predispose the patient to pneumothorax. Biopsies of the pleura, mediastinal lymph nodes, and lungs can also be obtained during thoracoscopy.

Video-assisted thorascopic surgery is a minimally invasive procedure used to diagnose and treat lung disorders. A thoracoscope is inserted in the chest through small incisions and transmits images onto a video monitor. This procedure is used for many purposes, such as biopsy or tumor removal.

V̇/Q̇ SCAN

Although less reliable than pulmonary angiography, a V̇/Q̇ scan carries fewer risks. This test indicates lung perfusion and ventilation. It's used to evaluate V̇/Q̇ mismatch, to detect pulmonary emboli, atelectasis, obstructing tumors, and chronic obstructive pulmonary disease and to evaluate pulmonary function, particularly in preoperative patients with marginal lung reserves.

Usually, in a V̇/Q̇ scan two radionuclides are administered. One is technetium-99. Injected I.V., it's used for the perfusion part of the study. Areas of decreased uptake of radioactivity correspond to decreased blood flow in the area of the embolization.

For the ventilation portion of the test, the other radionuclide commonly used is xenon-133 gas. This test, as the name implies, requires the patient to "ventilate" or breathe the radioactive particles into his lungs. Decreased areas of radioactivity correspond to irregular lung function.

Comparing normal and abnormal ventilation scans

The normal lung ventilation scan on the left, taken 30 minutes to 1 hour after the start of the wash-out phase, shows equal gas distribution. The abnormal lung ventilation scan on the right, taken 1¼ to 2 hours after the start of the wash-out phase, shows unequal gas distribution, represented by the area of poor wash-out on both the left and right sides.

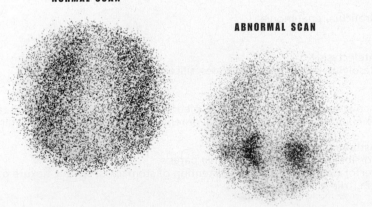

NORMAL SCAN

ABNORMAL SCAN

Biopsies

Biopsies include lung and pleural biopsies.

LUNG BIOPSY

In a lung biopsy, a specimen of pulmonary tissue is excised for examination, using the closed or the open technique. The closed technique, performed under local anesthesia, includes needle and transbronchial biopsies. The open technique, performed under general anesthesia in the operating room, includes limited and standard thoracotomies.

Needle biopsy is appropriate when the lesion is readily accessible. This procedure provides a much smaller specimen than the open technique. Transbronchial biopsy, the removal of multiple tissue specimens through a fiber-optic bronchoscope, is appropriate for some lung abnormalities or when the patient's condition won't tolerate an open biopsy.

Examination of lung tissue specimens can reveal squamous cell or oat cell carcinoma and adenocarcinoma.

PLEURAL BIOPSY

Pleural biopsy is the removal of pleural tissue, by needle biopsy or open biopsy, for examination. A pleural biopsy is usually ordered when pleural fluid obtained during a thoracentesis suggests infection, cancer, or tuberculosis. Performed under local anesthesia, pleural biopsy usually follows thoracentesis—aspiration of pleural fluid—which is performed when the cause of the effusion is unknown. However, it can be performed separately.

Open pleural biopsy, performed in the absence of pleural effusion, permits direct visualization of the pleura and the underlying lung. It's performed in the operating room.

Microscopic examination of the tissue specimen can reveal malignant disease, tuberculosis, or viral, fungal, parasitic, or collagen vascular disease.

Other diagnostic tests

Other diagnostic tests include pulmonary function tests (PFTs), pulse oximetry, and sweat testing.

PULMONARY FUNCTION TESTS

There are two types of PFTs: volume and capacity. These tests aid diagnosis in patients with suspected respiratory dysfunction. The physician orders these tests to:

▶ evaluate ventilatory function through spirometric measurements
▶ determine the cause of dyspnea
▶ assess the effectiveness of medications, such as bronchodilators and steroids
▶ determine whether a respiratory abnormality stems from an obstructive or restrictive disease process
▶ evaluate the extent of dysfunction.

Of the five pulmonary volume tests, tidal volume and expiratory reserve volume are measured through direct spirography. Minute volume, inspiratory reserve volume, and residual volume are calculated from the results of other PFTs.

Of the pulmonary capacity tests, functional residual capacity, total lung capacity, and maximal midexpiratory flow must be calculated. Vital capacity and inspiratory capacity may be measured directly or calculated indirectly. Direct spirographic measurements include forced vital capacity, forced expiratory volume, and maximal voluntary ventilation. The amount of carbon monoxide exhaled permits calculation of the diffusing capacity for carbon monoxide.

Interpreting pulmonary function tests

Pulmonary function test	Method of calculation	Implications
Tidal volume (V_T)		
Amount of air inhaled or exhaled during normal breathing	Determining the spirographic measurement for 10 breaths and then dividing by 10	Decreased V_T may indicate restrictive lung disease and requires further testing, such as full pulmonary function studies or chest X-rays.
Minute volume (MV)		
Total amount of air expired per minute	Multiplying V_T by the respiratory rate	Normal MV can occur in emphysema; decreased MV may indicate other diseases such as pulmonary edema. Increased MV can occur with acidosis, increased carbon dioxide (CO_2), decreased partial pressure of arterial oxygen, exercise, and low compliance states.
Carbon dioxide response		
Increase or decrease in MV after breathing various CO_2 concentrations	Plotting changes in MV against increasing inspired CO_2 concentrations	Reduced CO_2 response may occur in emphysema, myxedema, obesity, hypoventilation syndrome, and sleep apnea.
Inspiratory reserve volume (IRV)		
Amount of air inspired over above-normal inspiration	Subtracting V_T from inspiratory capacity (IC)	Abnormal IRV alone doesn't indicate respiratory dysfunction; IRV decreases during normal exercise.
Expiratory reserve volume (ERV)		
Amount of air exhaled after normal expiration	Direct spirographic measurement	ERV varies, even in healthy people, but usually decreases in obese people.
Residual volume (RV)		
Amount of air remaining in the lungs after forced expiration	Subtracting ERV from functional residual capacity (FRC)	RV > 35% of total lung capacity (TLC) after maximal expiratory effort may indicate obstructive lung disease.
Vital capacity (VC)		
Total volume of air that can be exhaled after maximum inspiration	Direct spirographic measurement or adding V_T, IRV, and ERV	Normal or increased VC with decreased flow rates may indicate any condition that causes a reduction in functional pulmonary tissue such as pulmonary edema. Decreased VC with normal or increased flow rates may indicate decreased respiratory effort resulting from neuromuscular disease, drug overdose, or head injury; decreased thoracic expansion; or limited diaphragm movement.
Inspiratory capacity (IC)		
Amount of air that can be inhaled after normal expiration	Direct spirographic measurement or adding IRV and V_T	Decreased IC indicates restrictive lung disease.
Thoracic gas volume (TGV)		
Total volume of gas in the lungs from ventilated and nonventilated airways	Body plethysmography	Increased TGV indicates air trapping, which may result from obstructive lung disease.
Functional residual capacity (FRC)		
Amount of air remaining in the lungs after normal expiration	Nitrogen washout, helium dilution technique, or adding ERV and RV	Increased FRC indicates overdistention of the lungs, which may result from obstructive lung disease.

Interpreting pulmonary function tests (continued)

Pulmonary function test	Method of calculation	Implications
Total lung capacity (TLC)		
Total volume of the lungs when maximally inflated	Adding V_T, IRV, ERV, and RV; FRC and IC; or VC and RV	Low TLC indicates restrictive lung disease; high TLC indicates overdistended lungs caused by obstructive lung disease.
Forced vital capacity (FVC)		
Amount of air exhaled forcefully and quickly after maximum inspiration	Direct spirographic measurement; expressed as a percentage of the total volume of gas exhaled	Decreased FVC indicates flow resistance in the respiratory system from obstructive lung disease such as chronic bronchitis or from restrictive lung disease such as pulmonary fibrosis.
Flow-volume curve (also called *flow-volume loop*)		
Greatest rate of flow (V_{max}) during FVC maneuvers versus lung volume change	Direct spirographic measurement at 1-second intervals; calculated from flow rates (expressed in L/second) and lung volume changes (expressed in liters) during maximal inspiratory and expiratory maneuvers	Decreased flow rates at all volumes during expiration indicate obstructive lung disease of the small airways such as emphysema. A plateau of expiratory flow near TLC, a plateau of inspiratory flow at mid-VC, and a square wave pattern through most of VC indicate obstructive lung disease of large airways. Normal or increased peak expiratory flow rate (PEFR), decreased flow with decreasing lung volumes, and markedly decreased VC indicate restrictive lung disease.
Forced expiratory volume (FEV)		
Volume of air expired in the first, second, or third second of an FVC maneuver	Direct spirographic measurement; expressed as a percentage of FVC	Decreased FEV_1 and increased FEV_2 and FEV_3 may indicate obstructive lung disease; decreased or normal FEV_1 may indicate restrictive lung disease.
Forced expiratory flow (FEF)		
Average rate of flow during the middle half of FVC	Calculated from the flow rate and the time needed for expiration of the middle 50% of FVC	Low FEF (25% to 75%) indicates obstructive lung disease of the small and medium-sized airways.
Peak expiratory flow rate (PEFR)		
V_{max} during forced expiration	Calculated from the flow-volume curve or by direct spirographic measurement using a pneumotachometer or electronic tachometer with a transducer to convert flow to electrical output display	Decreased PEFR may indicate a mechanical problem, such as upper airway obstruction, or obstructive lung disease. PEFR is usually normal in restrictive lung disease but decreases in severe cases. Because PEFR is effort dependent, it's also low in a person who has poor expiratory effort or doesn't understand the procedure.
Maximal voluntary ventilation (MVV) (also called *maximum breathing capacity*)		
The greatest volume of air breathed per unit of time	Direct spirographic measurement	Decreased MVV may indicate obstructive lung disease; normal or decreased MVV may indicate restrictive lung disease such as myasthenia gravis.
Diffusing capacity for carbon monoxide (DL_{CO})		
Milliliters of CO diffused per minute across the alveolocapillary membrane	Calculated from analysis of the amount of CO exhaled compared with the amount inhaled	Decreased DL_{CO} due to a thickened alveolocapillary membrane occurs in interstitial lung diseases, such as pulmonary fibrosis, asbestosis, and sarcoidosis; DL_{CO} is reduced in emphysema because of alveolocapillary membrane loss.

PULSE OXIMETRY

Pulse oximetry is a continuous noninvasive study of arterial blood oxygen saturation using a clip or probe attached to a sensor site (usually an earlobe or a fingertip). The percentage expressed is the ratio of oxygen to hemoglobin. Readings are generally accurate for saturated oxygen ranges between 70% and 100%. Readings can be affected by decreased perfusion, movement, abnormal hemoglobin, or fingernail polish.

SWEAT TEST

The sweat test is a quantitative measurement of electrolyte concentrations (primarily sodium and chloride) in sweat, usually performed using pilocarpine iontophoresis (pilocarpine is a sweat inducer). This test is considered the "gold standard" to confirm cystic fibrosis (CF) in children. It's also performed in adults to determine if they're homozygous or heterozygous for CF. Genetic testing for CF has also become available.

It's recommended that the sweat test be performed at Cystic Fibrosis Foundation–accredited facilities to ensure accurate results.

HANDS ON

Performing pulse oximetry

Follow these instructions to perform pulse oximetry:
- Select a finger for the test. Although the index finger is commonly used, a smaller finger may be selected.
- Clean the selected area and allow it to dry.

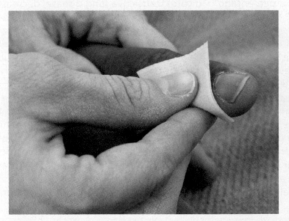

- Remove nail polish and artificial nails according to the manufacturer's instructions for the pulse oximeter.
- Apply the probe securely to the finger, making sure that the light-emitting sensor and the light-receiving sensors are directly opposite each other on the finger.

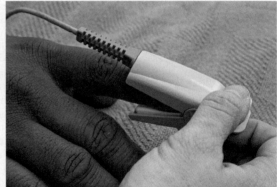

- Set the alarm limits for high and low readings according to the manufacturer's instruction or the practitioner's order.
- Check the patient's oxygen saturation levels at regular intervals or as ordered by the practitioner.

TREATMENTS AND PROCEDURES

HANDS ON

Diagnosing pulse oximeter problems

To maintain a continuous display of arterial oxygen saturation (SpO_2) levels, you'll need to keep the monitoring site clean and dry. Make sure that the skin doesn't become irritated from adhesives used to keep disposable probes in place. You may need to change the site if this happens. Disposable probes that irritate the skin can also be replaced by nondisposable models that don't need tape.

Another common problem with pulse oximeters is the failure of the devices to obtain a signal. Your first reaction if this happens should be to check the patient's vital signs. If they're sufficient to produce a signal, check for the following problems.

Venous pulsations

Erroneous readings may be obtained if the pulse oximeter detects venous pulsations. This may occur in patients with tricuspid insufficiency or pulmonary hypertension or if a finger probe is taped too tightly to the finger.

Poor concentration

See if the sensors are properly aligned. Make sure that the wires are intact and securely fastened and that the pulse oximeter is plugged into a power source.

Inadequate or intermittent blood flow to the site

Check the patient's pulse rate and capillary refill time and take corrective action if blood flow to the site is decreased. This may mean loosening restraints, removing tight-fitting clothes, taking off a blood pressure cuff, or checking arterial and I.V. lines. If none of these interventions work, you may need to find an alternate site. Finding a site with proper circulation may also prove challenging when a patient is receiving vasoconstrictive drugs.

Equipment malfunction

If you think the equipment might be malfunctioning, remove the pulse oximeter from the patient, set the alarm limits at 85% and 100%, and try the instrument on yourself or another healthy person. This will tell you if it's working correctly.

Penumbra effect

The penumbra effect may occur when an adult oximetry probe is placed on an infant's or a small child's finger. Because of a different path length of tissue for each of the wavelengths, the oximeter can underread or overread the SpO_2 level. To avoid the penumbra effect, use probes specifically designed for infants and children.

Tag-It Cystic Fibrosis Kit

The U.S. Food and Drug Administration approved the use of a deoxyribonucleic acid test for diagnosing cystic fibrosis (CF). The test, called the Tag-It Cystic Fibrosis Kit, is a blood test that screens for genetic mutations and variations in the cystic fibrosis transmembrane conductance regulator (CFTR) gene. This test identifies 23 genetic mutations and 4 variations in the CFTR gene. It also screens for 16 additional mutations in the gene that are involved in many cases of CF.

The test is recommended for use in detecting and identifying these mutations and variations in the gene as a means for determining carrier status in adults, screening neonates, and for confirming diagnostic testing in neonates and children. There are over 1,300 genetic variations in the CFTR gene responsible for causing CF. Therefore, the test isn't recommended as the only means for diagnosing CF. Test results need to be viewed along with the patient's condition, ethnic background, and family history. Genetic counseling is suggested to help patients understand the results and their implications.

TREATMENTS AND PROCEDURES

Respiratory disorders interfere with airway clearance, breathing patterns, and gas exchange. If not corrected, they can adversely affect many other body systems and can be life-threatening. Treatments for respiratory disorders include drug therapy, inhalation therapy, surgical procedures, and other treatments and procedures.

Drug therapy

Certain drugs are used for airway management in patients with such disorders as acute respiratory failure, acute respiratory distress syndrome, asthma, emphysema, and chronic bronchitis. They're used to improve respiratory function and include aerosol anti-infectives, antitussives, beta$_2$-adrenergic agonists, corticosteroids, decongestants, expectorants, leukotriene modifiers, mast cell stabilizers, methylxanthines, and mucus-controlling agents (mucolytics).

AEROSOL ANTI-INFECTIVES
‣ Provide direct, targeted local airway delivery of anti-infectives with minimal systemic blood levels

‣ Examples: pentamidine (NebuPent), ribavirin (Virazole), tobramycin (TOBI), and zanamivir (Relenza)

ANTITUSSIVES
‣ Suppress or inhibit coughing
‣ Administered orally as a liquid and typically used to treat dry, nonproductive coughs
‣ Examples: benzonatate, codeine, dextromethorphan hydrobromide, and hydrocodone bitartrate

BETA$_2$-ADRENERGIC AGONISTS
‣ Treat symptoms associated with asthma and chronic obstructive pulmonary disease
‣ Increase levels of cyclic adenosine monophosphate through the stimulation of the beta$_2$-adrenergic receptors in the smooth muscle, resulting in bronchodilation
‣ May be short- or long-acting
‣ Examples:
− Short-acting inhaled beta$_2$-adrenergic agonists: albuterol and pirbuterol (Maxair)
− Long-acting agent combined with an anti-inflammatory: salmeterol (Serevent)

CORTICOSTEROIDS
‣ Inhaled or systemic anti-inflammatories for short- and long-term control of asthma symptoms
‣ Suppress immune responses, reduce inflammation, and prevent asthma exacerbations

Understanding corticosteroids

Use this table to learn about the indications, adverse reactions, and nursing considerations associated with corticosteroids.

Drug	Indications	Adverse reactions	Nursing considerations
Systemic corticosteroids ‣ Dexamethasone ‣ Methylprednisolone ‣ Prednisone	‣ Anti-inflammatory in acute respiratory failure, acute respiratory distress syndrome, and chronic obstructive pulmonary disease ‣ Anti-inflammatory and immunosuppressant in asthma	‣ Heart failure, cardiac arrhythmias, edema, circulatory collapse, thromboembolism, pancreatitis, peptic ulcer	‣ Use cautiously in patients with recent myocardial infarction, hypertension, renal disease, and GI ulcer. ‣ Monitor blood pressure and blood glucose levels.
Inhaled corticosteroids ‣ Beclomethasone ‣ Budesonide ‣ Flunisolide ‣ Fluticasone ‣ Triamcinolone	‣ Long-term asthma control	‣ Hoarseness, dry mouth, wheezing, bronchospasm, oral candidiasis	‣ Do *not* use to treat an acute asthma attack. ‣ Use a spacer to reduce adverse effects. ‣ Instruct patient to rinse mouth after use to prevent oral fungal infection.

▶ Examples of systemic form: dexamethasone, methylprednisolone (Medrol), and prednisone
▶ Examples of inhaled form: beclomethasone (QVAR), budesonide (Pulmicort Turbuhaler), flunisolide (AeroBid), and fluticasone (Flovent)

DECONGESTANTS

▶ Classified as systemic decongestants or topical decongestants
▶ Systemic decongestants reduce swelling of the respiratory tract's vascular network
▶ Topical decongestants act as powerful vasoconstrictors and provide immediate relief from nasal congestion and swollen mucous membranes when applied directly to nasal mucosa
▶ Examples of systemic form: pseudoephedrine hydrochloride (Sudafed) and pseudoephedrine sulfate
▶ Example of topical form: oxymetazoline (Afrin)

EXPECTORANTS

▶ Thin mucus so that it's cleared more easily out of airways
▶ Soothe mucous membranes in the respiratory tract
▶ Example: guaifenesin (Mucinex)

LEUKOTRIENE MODIFIERS

▶ Released from mast cells, eosinophils, and basophils
▶ Result in smooth-muscle contraction of the airways, increased permeability of the vasculature, increased secretions, and activation of other inflammatory mediators
▶ Examples: zafirlukast (Accolate) and montelukast (Singulair)

MAST CELL STABILIZERS

▶ Inhibit the release of inflammatory mediators by stabilizing the mast cell membrane, possibly through the inhibition of chloride channels
▶ Administered by inhalation
▶ Examples: cromolyn sodium (Intal)

MUCOLYTICS

▶ Act directly on mucus, breaking down sticky, thick secretions so they're more easily eliminated
▶ Administered by inhalation
▶ Examples: acetylcysteine (Mucomyst) and dornase alfa (Pulmozyme)

XANTHINES

▶ Xanthines, also called *methylxanthines* (theophylline and derivatives), and adrenergics; used to dilate bronchial passages and reduce airway resistance
▶ Administered orally or by inhalation
▶ Decrease airway reactivity and relieve bronchospasm by relaxing bronchial smooth muscle
▶ Theophylline inhibiting phosphodiesterase resulting in smooth-muscle relaxation in addition to decreased inflammatory mediators, such as mast cells, T-cells, and eosinophils
▶ Example: theophylline

Inhalation therapy

Inhalation therapy employs carefully controlled ventilation techniques to help the patient maintain optimal ventilation in the event of respiratory distress. Techniques include aerosol treatments, continuous positive airway pressure (CPAP), endotracheal (ET) intubation, end-tidal carbon dioxide (ETCO$_2$) monitoring, mixed venous oxygen saturation (S$\bar{v}$O$_2$) monitoring, incentive spirometry, mechanical ventilation, and oxygen therapy.

AEROSOL TREATMENTS

Aerosol therapy is a means of administering medication into the airways. The administration method can be used through small-volume nebulizers or oropharyngeal inhalers. These devices deliver topical medications to the respiratory tract, producing local and systemic effects. The mucosal lining of the respiratory tract absorbs the inhalant almost immediately.

Common inhalants are bronchodilators, used to improve airway patency and facilitate mucus drainage; mucolytics, which attain a high local concentration to liquify tenacious bronchial secretions; and corticosteroids, used to decrease inflammation.

Small-volume nebulizers

A small-volume nebulizer is a type of inhaler that sprays a fine, liquid mist of medication. The medication is instilled into the nebulizer chamber, as shown below.

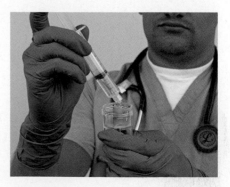

The nebulizer is then attached to either an oxygen source or a compressor (for home use). A facial mask or mouthpiece is connected to a machine via plastic tubing to deliver the medication, as shown below.

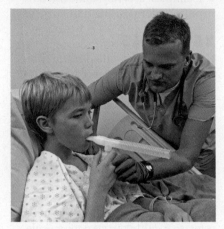

Oropharyngeal inhalers

Handheld oropharyngeal inhalers include the metered-dose inhaler, the turbo-inhaler, and the diskus. These devices deliver topical medications to the respiratory tract, producing local and systemic effects. The mucosal lining of the respiratory tract absorbs the inhalant almost immediately.

Types of handheld inhalers

Handheld inhalers use air under pressure to produce a mist containing tiny droplets of medication.

Metered-dose inhalers

Metered-dose inhalers (MDI) are handheld inhalers that use air under pressure to produce a mist containing medication. Drugs delivered in this form (such as bronchodilators and mucolytics) can travel deep into the lungs. They're portable, compact, and relatively easy to use.

The pressurized canisters contain a micronized powder form of the medication that's either dissolved or suspended in one or more liquid propellants along with oily, viscous substances called surfactants that are used to keep the drug suspended in the propellants. The surfactant also lubricates the valve mechanism of the MDI. They do require hand-breath coordination to successfully deliver the aerosol during the patient's inhalation.

METERED-DOSE INHALER

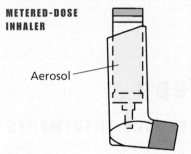

Aerosol

Spacers

Inhalers with a special attachment called a spacer provide greater therapeutic benefits for children and patients with poor coordination. The spacer attachment, an extension to the inhaler's mouthpiece, provides more dead-air space for mixing medication.

INHALER WITH BUILT-IN SPACER

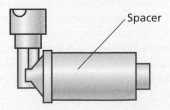

Spacer

Turbo-inhalers

Turbo-inhalers administer dry powder medication without the use of propellants and don't require hand-breath coordination. Used to dispense terbutaline (Brethine) or budesonide (Pulmicort), the inhaler is stocked with 200 doses of medication.

The patient holds the device in the upright position and twists the lower ring to load the medication. He then exhales and places his mouth over the dispenser and inhales the medication. The dispenser has a dose counter so that the patient knows when he has 20 doses remaining.

TURBO-INHALER

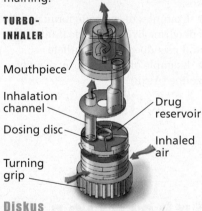

Mouthpiece

Inhalation channel

Dosing disc

Turning grip

Drug reservoir

Inhaled air

Diskus

A diskus incorporates a disk that contains 60 sealed pockets on an aluminum foil strip within the disk. A lever that the patient activates advances the strip. As the drug pocket reaches the mouthpiece, the cover is peeled away and the medication is dispensed and ready for inhalation.

DISKUS DRY POWDER INHALER

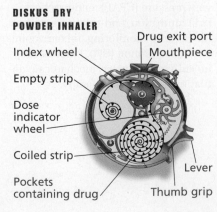

Index wheel

Empty strip

Dose indicator wheel

Coiled strip

Pockets containing drug

Drug exit port

Mouthpiece

Lever

Thumb grip

CONTINUOUS POSITIVE AIRWAY PRESSURE

As its name suggests, CPAP ventilation maintains positive pressure in the airways throughout the patient's respiratory cycle. Originally delivered only with a ventilator, CPAP may now be delivered to intubated or nonintubated patients through an artificial airway, a mask, or nasal prongs by means of a ventilator or a separate high-flow generating system.

Nasal CPAP has proved successful for long-term treatment of obstructive sleep apnea. With this type of CPAP, high-flow compressed air is directed into a mask that covers only the patient's nose. The pressure supplied through the mask serves as a backpressure splint, preventing the unstable upper airway from collapsing during inspiration.

ENDOTRACHEAL INTUBATION

ET intubation involves insertion of a tube into the lungs through the mouth or nose to establish a patent airway and provide ventilation. It protects the patient from aspiration by sealing off the trachea from the digestive tract and permits removal of tracheobronchial secretions in the patient who can't cough effectively.

With orotracheal intubation, the oral cavity is used as the route of insertion. It's preferred in emergency situations because it's easier and faster. However, maintaining proper tube placement is more difficult because of mouth movement and oral secretions. The tube must be well secured to avoid kinking and prevent bronchial obstruction or accidental extubation. It's also uncomfortable for the conscious patient because it stimulates salivation, coughing, and retching.

With nasal intubation, the nasal passage is used as the route of insertion. Nasal intubation is preferred for elective insertion when the patient is capable of spontaneous ventilation for a short period.

Using nasal CPAP

This illustration shows the continuous positive-airway pressure (CPAP) apparatus used to apply positive pressure to the airway to prevent obstruction during inspiration in patients with obstructive sleep apnea.

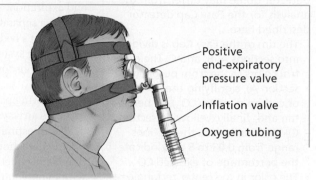

- Positive end-expiratory pressure valve
- Inflation valve
- Oxygen tubing

HANDS ON

Endotracheal tube care

- Wash your hands and put on personal protective equipment.
- Support the endotracheal (ET) tube and tubing as needed. Preferably, two people should help change the ties.
- Perform oral hygiene using a pediatric or soft toothbrush at least twice per day.
- Use oral swabs with a 1.5% hydrogen peroxide solution to clean the mouth every 2 to 4 hours.
- Suction the oral cavity as needed to remove secretions.
- Remove the old tape or securing device, making sure that the ET tube is stabilized. Note tube position by looking at the markings on the tube.

- Remove the bite block or oral airway if present.
- Move the ET tube to the opposite side of the mouth.
- Ensure proper cuff inflation and tube position.

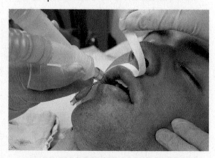

- Secure the ET tube by using tape or a securing device.

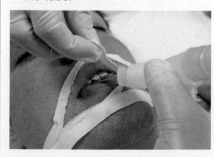

Analyzing CO₂ levels

Depending on the end-tidal carbon dioxide (ETCO_2) detector you use, the meaning of color changes within the detector dome may differ from the analysis for the Easy Cap detector described here.

▸ The rim of the Easy Cap is divided into sections A, B, and C. Their control colors range from purple (in section A), signifying the absence of carbon dioxide (CO_2), to beige, tan and, finally, yellow (in section C). The numbers in the sections range from 0.03 to 5 and indicate the percentage of exhaled CO_2.

▸ The color in the center rectangle reflects the patient's CO_2 level. It should fluctuate during ventilation from purple (matching section A) during inspiration to yellow (matching section C) at the end of expiration. This indicates that the ETCO_2 levels are adequate—above 2%.

▸ An end-expiratory color change from the C range to the B range may be the first sign of hemodynamic instability.

▸ During cardiopulmonary resuscitation (CPR), an end-expiratory color change from the A or B range to the C range may mean the return of spontaneous ventilation.

▸ During prolonged cardiac arrest, inadequate pulmonary perfusion leads to inadequate gas exchange. The patient exhales little or no CO_2, so the color stays in the purple range even with proper intubation. Ineffective CPR also leads to inadequate pulmonary perfusion.

COLOR INDICATORS ON ETCO_2 DETECTOR

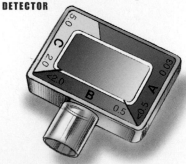

END-TIDAL CARBON DIOXIDE MONITORING

ETCO_2 monitoring is used to measure the carbon dioxide concentration at end expiration. An ETCO_2 monitor may be a separate monitor or part of the patient's bedside hemodynamic monitoring system.

Indications for ETCO_2 monitoring include:

▸ monitoring patency of the airway (in acute airway obstruction and apnea) and respiratory function

▸ early detection of changes in carbon dioxide production and elimination with hyperventilation therapy, or hypercapnia or hyperthermia states

▸ assessing effectiveness of interventions, such as mechanical ventilation or neuromuscular blockade used with mechanical ventilation, and prone positioning.

With ETCO_2 monitoring, a photodetector measures the amount of infrared light absorbed by the airway during inspiration and expiration. (Light absorption increases along with the carbon dioxide concentration.) The monitor converts these data to a carbon dioxide value and a corresponding waveform or capnogram, if capnography is used.

Values are obtained by monitoring samples of expired gas from an ET tube or an oral or nasopharyngeal airway. Although the values are similar, the ETCO_2 values are usually 2 to 5 mm Hg lower than the partial pressure of arterial carbon dioxide value. Capnograms and ETCO_2 monitoring reduce the need for frequent arterial blood gas sampling.

Comparing normal and S̄vo₂ waveforms

This tracing represents a stable, normal mixed venous oxygen saturation (S̄vo₂) level: higher than 60% and lower than 80%. Note the relatively constant line.

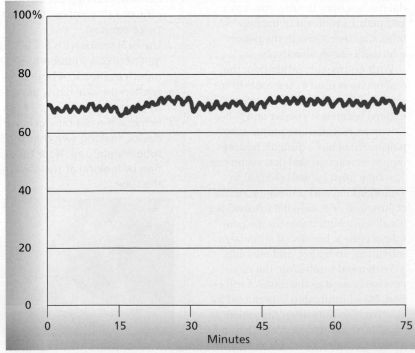

MIXED VENOUS OXYGEN SATURATION MONITORING

$S\bar{v}O_2$ reflects the oxygen saturation level of venous blood. It's determined by measuring the amount of oxygen extracted and used or consumed by the body's tissues.

$S\bar{v}O_2$ monitoring uses a fiber-optic thermodilution pulmonary artery catheter to continuously monitor oxygen delivery to tissues and oxygen consumption by tissues. Monitoring of $S\bar{v}O_2$ allows rapid detection of impaired oxygen delivery, as from decreased cardiac output, hemoglobin level, or arterial oxygen saturation. It also helps evaluate a patient's response to drug therapy, ET tube suctioning, ventilator setting changes, positive-end-expiratory pressure, and fraction of inspired oxygen (FIO_2).

Using incentive spirometry

Volume incentive spirometer

The volume incentive spirometer is activated when the patient inhales a certain volume of air. By estimating the volume of air inhaled, it measures lung inflation. It's used with patients at high risk for atelectasis.

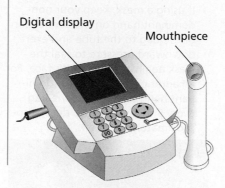

Digital display

Mouthpiece

Flow incentive spirometer

The flow incentive spirometer contains floats, which rise according to how much air the patient pulls through the device during inhalation. It's used with patients at low risk for atelectasis.

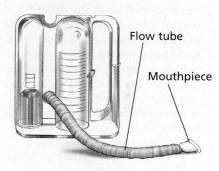

Flow tube

Mouthpiece

This waveform shows typical changes in the $S\bar{v}O_2$ level as a result of various activities.

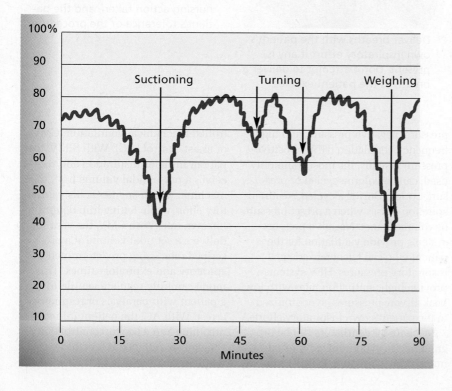

INCENTIVE SPIROMETRY

Incentive spirometry involves using a breathing device to help the patient achieve maximal ventilation. The device measures respiratory flow or respiratory volume and induces the patient to take a deep breath and hold it for several seconds. This deep breath:
▸ increases lung volume
▸ boosts alveolar inflation
▸ promotes venous return.

This exercise also establishes alveolar hyperinflation for a longer time than is possible with a normal deep breath, thus preventing and reversing the alveolar collapse that causes atelectasis and pneumonitis.

Devices used for incentive spirometry provide a visual incentive to breathe deeply. Some are activated when the patient inhales a certain volume of air; the device then estimates the amount of air inhaled. Others contain plastic floats, which rise according to the amount of air the patient pulls through the device when he inhales.

Understanding manual ventilation

A handheld resuscitation bag is an inflatable device that can be attached to a face mask or directly to a tracheostomy or an endotracheal (ET) tube to allow manual delivery of oxygen or room air to the lungs of a patient who can't breathe by himself.

Although usually used in an emergency, manual ventilation can also be performed while the patient is temporarily disconnected from a mechanical ventilator, such as during a tubing change, during transport, or before suctioning. In such instances, the use of the handheld resuscitation bag maintains ventilation. Oxygen administration with a resuscitation bag can help improve a compromised cardiorespiratory system.

Ventilation guidelines

To manually ventilate a patient with a mask or an ET or tracheostomy tube, follow these guidelines:

▶ If oxygen is readily available, connect the handheld resuscitation bag to the oxygen. Attach one end of the tubing to the bottom of the bag and the other end to the nipple adapter on the flowmeter of the oxygen source.

▶ Turn on the oxygen and adjust the flow rate to 15 L.

▶ Before attaching the handheld resuscitation bag, suction the ET or tracheostomy tube to remove any secretions that may obstruct the airway.

▶ Remove the mask from the ventilation bag and attach the handheld resuscitation bag directly to the tube.

▶ If using a mask, keep your nondominant hand on the connection of the bag to the tube and exert downward pressure to seal the mask against the patient's face. For an adult patient, use your dominant hand to compress the bag every 5 to 8 seconds to deliver approximately 1 L of air.

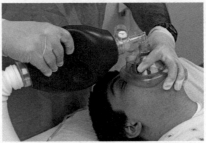

▶ Deliver breaths with the patient's own inspiratory effort if any is present. Don't attempt to deliver a breath as the patient exhales.

▶ Observe the patient's chest to ensure that it rises and falls with each compression. If ventilation fails to occur, check the connection and patency of the patient's airway; if necessary, suction.

▶ Be alert for possible underventilation. The volume of air delivered to the patient varies with the type of bag used and the hand size of the person compressing the bag. An adult with a small- or medium-sized hand may not consistently deliver 1 L of air. For these reasons, have someone assist with the procedure if possible.

▶ Keep in mind that air is forced into the patient's stomach with manual ventilation using a mask, placing the patient at risk for aspiration of vomitus (possibly resulting in pneumonia) and gastric distention.

▶ Record the date and time of the procedure, the reason and length of time the patient was disconnected from mechanical ventilation and received manual ventilation, complications and the nursing action taken, and the patient's tolerance of the procedure.

MECHANICAL VENTILATION

Mechanical ventilation corrects profoundly impaired ventilation, evidenced by hypercapnia and symptoms of respiratory distress (such as nostril flaring, intercostal retractions, decreased blood pressure, and diaphoresis). It's also used for respiratory depression or respiratory arrest. Requiring an ET or tracheostomy tube, it delivers up to 100% room air under positive pressure or oxygen-enriched air in concentrations up to 100%.

Major types of mechanical ventilation systems include positive-pressure, negative-pressure, and high-frequency ventilation (HFV). Positive-pressure systems, the most commonly used, can be volume-cycled or pressure-cycled. During a cycled breath, inspiration ceases when a preset pressure or volume is met. Negative-pressure systems provide ventilation for the patient who can't generate adequate inspiratory pressures. HFV systems provide high ventilation rates with low peak airway pressures, synchronized to the patient's own inspiratory efforts.

Mechanical ventilators can be programmed to synchronized intermittent mandatory ventilation (SIMV), controlled mechanical ventilation (CMV), or assist control (AC). With SIMV, the patient initiates inspiration and receives a preset tidal volume from the machine, which augments his ventilatory effort while letting him determine his own rate. With CMV, the ventilator delivers a set tidal volume at a prescribed rate, using predetermined inspiratory and expiratory times. This mode can fully regulate ventilation in a patient with paralysis or respiratory arrest. With AC, the patient initiates breathing and a backup control delivers a preset number of breaths at a set volume.

OXYGEN THERAPY

Oxygen therapy is delivered by mask, nasal prongs, nasal catheter, or transtracheal catheter to prevent or reverse hypoxemia and reduce the work of breathing. The equipment used depends on the patient's age, condition, and the required FIO_2.

Oxygen delivery systems

Patients may receive oxygen through one of several administration systems, including a nasal cannula, simple mask, nonrebreather mask, Venturi mask, and tracheostomy collar.

Nasal cannula

Oxygen is delivered at 1 to 6 L/minute in concentrations of less than 40% through a plastic cannula in the patient's nostrils.

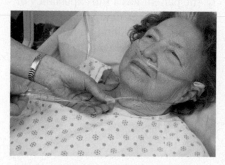

Nonrebreather mask

On inhalation, the one-way inspiratory valve opens, directing oxygen from a reservoir bag into the mask. On exhalation, gas exits the mask through the one-way expiratory valves and enters the atmosphere. The patient breathes air only from the bag. It delivers the highest possible oxygen concentration (60% to 90%), short of intubation and mechanical ventilation.

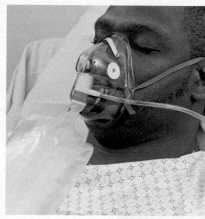

Venturi mask

The mask is connected to a Venturi device, which mixes a specific volume of air and oxygen. It delivers highly accurate oxygen concentration (24% to 55%) despite the patient's respiratory pattern.

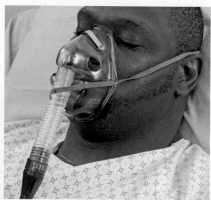

Simple mask

Oxygen flows through an entry port at the bottom of the mask and exits through large holes on the sides of the mask. It delivers oxygen in concentrations of 40% to 60%.

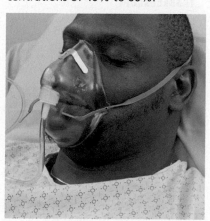

Tracheostomy collar

A tracheostomy collar is connected to wide-bore tubing that delivers high-humidity oxygen.

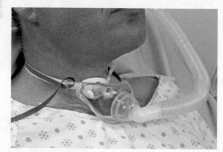

Surgical procedures

If drugs or other therapeutic approaches fail to maintain airway patency and protect healthy tissues from respiratory disease, surgical intervention may be necessary. Respiratory surgeries include chest tube insertion, lung volume reduction surgery, lung transplantation, and tracheotomy.

CHEST TUBE INSERTION

A chest tube may be required to help treat pneumothorax, hemothorax, empyema, pleural effusion, or chylothorax. Inserted into the pleural space, the tube allows blood, fluid, pus, or air to drain and allows the lung to reinflate. With pneumothorax, the tube restores negative pressure to the pleural space through an underwater-seal drainage system. The water in the system prevents air from being sucked back into the pleural space during inspiration. If a leak occurs through the bronchi and can't be sealed, suction applied to the underwater-seal system removes air from the pleural space faster than it can collect.

LUNG VOLUME REDUCTION SURGERY

Lung volume reduction surgery is removal of the diseased portion of the lung to increase chest cavity space. The procedure can alter the flattened diaphragm to assume a normal shape, making it function better, and result in diminished shortness of breath, greater exercise tolerance, and better quality of life.

It can be performed through a unilateral or bilateral thoracoscopy, which is a minimally invasive technique. Three small incisions are made between the ribs. A videoscope is placed through one of the incisions. A stapler and grasper are placed in the other incisions and the diseased portions of the lungs are removed

It can also be performed using a bilateral sternotomy approach, where an incision is made through the breastbone to expose both lungs. Both lungs are then reduced at the same time. This is the most invasive technique and is only used when thoracoscopy isn't appropriate.

LUNG TRANSPLANTATION

Lung transplantation involves the replacement of one or both lungs with those of a donor. Cystic fibrosis is the most common underlying disease that necessitates lung transplantation; others include bronchopulmonary dysplasia, pulmonary hypertension, and pulmonary fibrosis.

In some cases, only one lobe may be involved in transplantation. Single lung transplantation is considered for patients with end-stage chronic obstructive pulmonary disease. Typically, the patient has a life expectancy of less than 2 years. One-year survival rates after transplantation range from 75% to 85%, decreasing to 50% after 5 years.

Lung volume reduction surgery

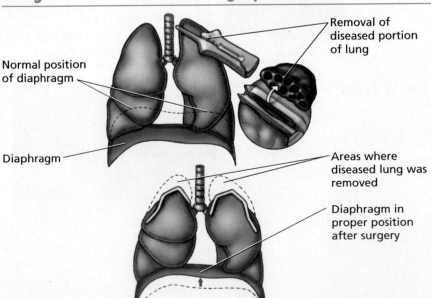

Removal of diseased portion of lung

Normal position of diaphragm

Diaphragm

Areas where diseased lung was removed

Diaphragm in proper position after surgery

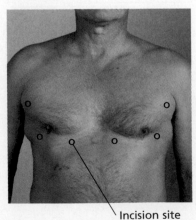

THORACOSCOPY

Incision site

To be a candidate for lung transplantation, a patient must:

▸ have forced vital capacity less than 40%

▸ have forced expiratory volume less than 30% of predicted value

▸ have partial pressure of arterial oxygen less than 60 mm Hg on room air at rest

▸ exhibit evidence of major pulmonary complications

▸ demonstrate increased antibiotic resistance.

The major complication after lung transplantation is organ rejection, which occurs because the recipient's body responds to the implanted tissue as a foreign body and triggers an immune response. This leads to fibrosis and scar formation.

Another major complication after lung transplantation is infection due to immunosuppressive therapy. Other possible complications include hemorrhage and reperfusion edema. Long-term complications (typically occurring after 3 years) include obliterative bronchiolitis and posttransplant lymphoproliferative disorder. Either may be fatal.

TRACHEOTOMY

A tracheotomy provides a stable airway for an intubated patient who needs prolonged mechanical ventilation and allows removal of lower tracheobronchial secretions from a patient who can't clear them. It's also performed in emergencies when endotracheal intubation isn't possible, to prevent an unconscious or paralyzed patient from aspirating food or secretions, and to bypass upper airway obstruction due to trauma, burns, epiglottiditis, or a tumor.

After the physician creates the surgical opening, he inserts a tracheostomy tube to permit access to the airway. He may select from several tube styles, depending on the patient's condition.

Comparing tracheostomy tubes

Tracheostomy tubes are made of plastic or metal and come in uncuffed, cuffed, or fenestrated varieties. Tube selection depends on the patient's condition and the physician's preference. Make sure you're familiar with the advantages and disadvantages of these commonly used tracheostomy tubes.

Uncuffed
(plastic or metal)

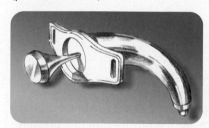

Advantages
▸ Free flow of air around tube and through larynx
▸ Reduced risk of tracheal damage
▸ Mechanical ventilation possible in patient with neuromuscular disease

Disadvantages
▸ Increased risk of aspiration in adults due to lack of cuff
▸ Adapter possibly needed for ventilation

Plastic cuffed
(low pressure and high volume)

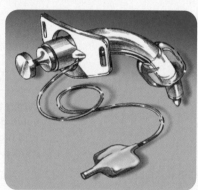

Advantages
▸ Disposable
▸ Cuff bonded to tube (won't detach accidentally inside trachea)
▸ Low cuff pressure that's evenly distributed against tracheal wall (no need to deflate periodically to lower pressure)
▸ Reduced risk of tracheal damage

Disadvantages
▸ Possibly more expensive than other tubes

Fenestrated

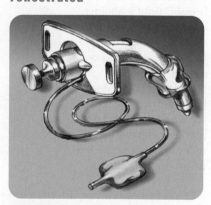

Advantages
▸ Speech possible through upper airway when external opening is capped and cuff is deflated
▸ Breathing by mechanical ventilation possible with inner cannula in place and cuff inflated
▸ Easy removal of inner cannula for cleaning

Disadvantages
▸ Possible occlusion of fenestration
▸ Possible dislodgment of inner cannula
▸ Cap removal necessary before inflating cuff

Other treatments and procedures

Other respiratory treatments and procedures include chest physiotherapy, mucus-clearance device, and suctioning.

CHEST PHYSIOTHERAPY

Chest physiotherapy is usually performed with other treatments, such as suctioning, incentive spirometry, and administration of such medications as small-volume nebulizer aerosol treatments and expectorants. Recent studies indicate that percussional vibration isn't an effective treatment of most diseases; exceptions include cystic fibrosis and bronchiectasis. Improved breath sounds, increased partial pressure of arterial oxygen, sputum production, and improved airflow suggest successful treatment.

MUCUS-CLEARANCE DEVICE

The patient with a chronic respiratory disorder, such as cystic fibrosis, bronchitis, or bronchiectasis, requires therapy to mobilize and remove mucus secretions from the lungs. A handheld mucus-clearance device, also known as the *flutter valve device,* can help these patients cough up secretions more easily. This device is basically a ball valve that vibrates as the patient exhales vigorously through it. The vibrations propagate throughout the airways during expiration, thereby loosening the mucus. As the patient repeats this process, the mucus progressively moves up the airways until it can be coughed out easily. The frequency and duration with which this device can be used should be determined by a licensed practitioner.

HANDS ON

Performing percussion and vibration

To perform percussion, instruct the patient to breathe slowly and deeply, using the diaphragm, to promote relaxation. Hold your hands in a cupped shape, with fingers flexed and thumbs pressed tightly against your index fingers. Percuss each segment for 1 to 2 minutes by alternating your hands against the patient in a rhythmic manner. Listen for a hollow sound on percussion to verify correct performance of the technique.

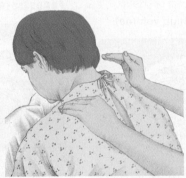

To perform vibration, ask the patient to inhale deeply and then exhale slowly through pursed lips. During exhalation, firmly press your fingers and the palms of your hands against the chest wall. Tense the muscles of your arms and shoulders in an isometric contraction to send fine vibrations through the chest wall. Vibrate during five exhalations over each chest segment.

Flutter valve device

When the patient exhales through the flutter valve device, both positive expiratory pressure and high-frequency oscillations help move mucus.

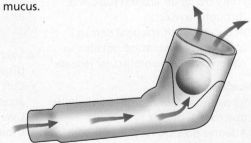

SUCTIONING

Oronasopharyngeal suction

Oronasopharyngeal suction removes secretions from the pharynx by a suction catheter inserted through the mouth or nostril. Performed to maintain a patent airway, this procedure helps the patient who can't clear his airway effectively with coughing and expectoration, such as the unconscious or severely debilitated patient. The procedure should be done as often as necessary, depending on the patient's condition.

Oronasopharyngeal suction is an aseptic procedure that requires sterile equipment. However, clean technique may be used for a tonsil tip suction device. In fact, an alert patient can use a tonsil tip suction device himself to remove secretions. This type of suctioning should be used with caution in patients who have nasopharyngeal bleeding or spinal fluid leakage into the nasopharyngeal area, in trauma patients, in patients receiving anticoagulant therapy, and in those who have blood diseases because these conditions increase the risk of bleeding.

Tracheal suctioning

Tracheal suctioning involves the removal of secretions from the trachea or bronchi by means of a catheter inserted through the mouth or nose, a tracheal stoma, a tracheostomy tube, or an endotracheal tube.

Assess the patient's vital signs, breath sounds, and general appearance to establish a baseline for comparison after suctioning. Review the patient's arterial blood gas values and oxygen saturation levels if they're available. If you'll be performing nasotracheal suctioning, check the patient's history for a deviated septum, nasal polyps, nasal obstruction, nasal trauma, epistaxis, or mucosal swelling.

Performing nasopharyngeal and oropharyngeal suctioning

HANDS ON

- Assess the patient's vital signs.
- Place the patient in semi-Fowler's position if he's conscious and in a lateral position facing you if he's unconscious.
- Put on protective equipment and gloves.
- Without applying suction, insert the sterile suction catheter into the patient's nostril, as shown.

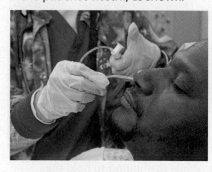

- Apply suction intermittently by occluding the port of the catheter with your thumb as shown, and gently rotating the catheter as it's being withdrawn from the nostril.

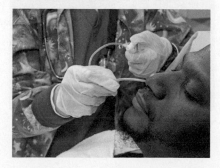

- Flush the catheter with saline and repeat the suctioning as needed to clear the airway.
- To suction the oropharynx; put on a clean pair of gloves and use a new suction catheter.
- Without applying suction, insert the sterile suction catheter into the patient's oral cavity, as shown.

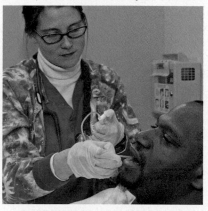

- Repeat the procedures as necessary to remove secretions.
- Auscultate the patient's chest for breath sounds to assess the effectiveness of the suctioning.

Closed tracheal suctioning

The closed tracheal suction system can ease removal of secretions and reduce patient complications. Consisting of a sterile suction catheter in a clear plastic sleeve, the system lets the patient remain connected to the ventilator during suctioning. As a result, the patient can maintain the tidal volume, oxygen concentration, and positive end-expiratory pressure delivered by the ventilator while being suc-

tioned. In turn, this reduces the occurrence of suction-induced hypoxemia.

Another advantage of this system is a reduced risk of infection, even when the same catheter is used many times. Because the catheter remains in a protective sleeve, gloves aren't required but are still recommended. The caregiver doesn't need to touch the catheter and the ventilator circuit remains closed.

HANDS ON

Performing closed tracheal suctioning

To perform closed tracheal suctioning, gather a closed suction control valve, a T-piece to connect the artificial airway to the ventilator breathing circuit, and a catheter sleeve that encloses the catheter and has connections at each end for the control valve and the T-piece. Put on personal protective equipment, if you haven't already done so. Then follow these steps:

▸ Remove the closed suction system from its wrapping. Attach the control valve to the connecting tubing.
▸ Depress the thumb suction control valve, and keep it depressed while setting the suction pressure to the desired level.
▸ Connect the T-piece to the ventilator breathing circuit, making sure that the irrigation port is closed; then connect the T-piece to the patient's endotracheal or tracheostomy tube.

▸ With one hand keeping the T-piece parallel to the patient's chin, use the thumb and index finger of the other hand to advance the catheter through the tube and into the patient's tracheobronchial tree (as shown below). It may be necessary to gently retract the catheter sleeve as you advance the catheter.

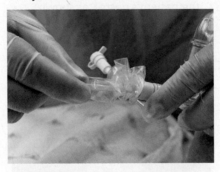

▸ While continuing to hold the T-piece and control valve, apply intermittent suction (as shown below).

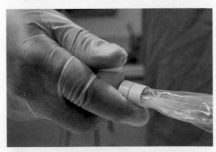

▸ Withdraw the catheter until it reaches its fully extended length in the sleeve (as shown below). Repeat the procedure as necessary.

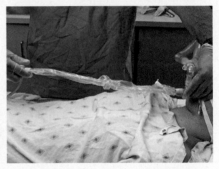

▸ After you've finished suctioning, flush the catheter by maintaining suction while slowly introducing normal saline solution or sterile water into the irrigation port.
▸ Place the thumb control valve in the off position.
▸ Dispose of and replace the suction equipment and supplies according to your facility's policy.
▸ Change the closed suction system every 24 hours to minimize the risk of infection.

Chapter 4

Neurologic care

DISEASES
Alzheimer's disease

Alzheimer's disease, also called *primary degenerative dementia,* accounts for more than half of all dementias. It results in memory loss, confusion, impaired judgment, personality changes, disorientation, and loss of language skills; it essentially steals away the patient's mind. Because this is a primary progressive dementia, the prognosis for a patient with this disease is poor.

The cause of Alzheimer's disease is unknown; however, several factors are thought to be implicated in this disease. These include *neurochemical factors,* such as deficiencies in the neurotransmitter acetylcholine, somatostatin, substance P, and norepinephrine; *environmental factors;* and *genetic immunologic factors.* Genetic studies show that an autosomal dominant form of Alzheimer's disease is associated with early onset and early death, accounting for about 100,000 deaths per year. A family history of Alzheimer's disease and the presence of Down syndrome are two established risk factors. Alzheimer's disease isn't exclusive to the elder population; its onset begins in middle age in 1% to 10% of cases.

The brain tissue of patients with Alzheimer's disease has three hallmark features: neurofibrillary tangles, neuritic plaques, and granulovascular degeneration.

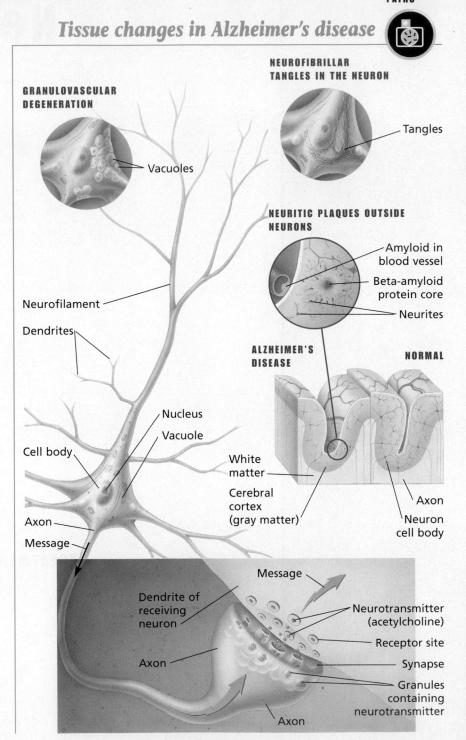

PICTURING PATHO

Tissue changes in Alzheimer's disease

GRANULOVASCULAR DEGENERATION

Vacuoles

NEUROFIBRILLAR TANGLES IN THE NEURON

Tangles

NEURITIC PLAQUES OUTSIDE NEURONS

Amyloid in blood vessel

Beta-amyloid protein core

Neurites

ALZHEIMER'S DISEASE

NORMAL

Neurofilament

Dendrites

Nucleus

Vacuole

Cell body

White matter

Cerebral cortex (gray matter)

Axon

Axon

Message

Neuron cell body

Message

Dendrite of receiving neuron

Neurotransmitter (acetylcholine)

Receptor site

Axon

Synapse

Granules containing neurotransmitter

Axon

Signs and symptoms
▶ Forgetfulness
▶ Progressive memory loss
▶ Difficulty learning and remembering new information
▶ Deterioration in personal hygiene and appearance
▶ Inability to concentrate
▶ Progressive difficulty in communication
▶ Severe deterioration in memory, language, and motor function
▶ Loss of coordination
▶ Inability to write or speak
▶ Personality changes (restlessness, irritability)
▶ Nocturnal awakenings
▶ Loss of eye contact
▶ Anxiety

Treatment
▶ Cholinesterase inhibitors such as tacrine (Cognex), donepezil (Aricept), rivastigmine (Exelon), and galantamine (Razadyne)
▶ *N*-methyl-D-aspartate antagonist: nemantine (Namenda)
▶ Antidepressants
▶ Routine physical activity and exercise
▶ Behavioral therapy

Nursing considerations
Overall care is focused on supporting the patient's remaining abilities and compensating for those he has lost.
▶ Establish an effective communication system with the patient and his family to help them adjust to the patient's altered cognitive abilities.
▶ Offer emotional support to the patient and his family.
▶ Monitor the patient for periods of anxiety. Provide reassurance and note which methods are successful in calming the patient.

▶ Provide the patient with a safe environment. Encourage him to exercise, as ordered, to help maintain mobility.

LESSON PLANS

Teaching about Alzheimer's disease

▶ Teach the patient, his family, and caregiver about the disease and its treatments, and refer them to social services and community resources for support.
▶ Explain the need for activity and exercise to maintain mobility and help prevent complications.
▶ Discuss dietary adjustments for patients with restlessness, dysphagia, or coordination problems.

▶ Emphasize the importance of establishing a daily routine, providing a safe environment, and avoiding overstimulation.
▶ Instruct the patient, his family, and caregiver about self-care, including the importance of adequate rest, good nutrition, and private time.

Amyotrophic lateral sclerosis

Amyotrophic lateral sclerosis (ALS), also called *Lou Gehrig disease,* is the most common of the motor neuron diseases that cause muscle atrophy. Symptoms don't develop until age 50. ALS is a chronic, progressively debilitating disease; ALS patients survive an average of 3 years.

ALS affects about 2 out of 100,000 people per year. The exact cause of ALS is unknown, but about 10% of cases have a genetic component. In these patients, it's an autosomal dominant trait and affects men and women equally.

Other than a family member affected with the hereditary form, there are no known risk factors.

Classically, ALS affects two or more levels of motor neurons. Affected lower motor neurons lead to progressive musle weakness and atrophy. Stiffness, spasticity, and abnormally active reflexes occur when upper motor neurons are affected.

PICTURING
PATHO

Motor neuron changes in ALS

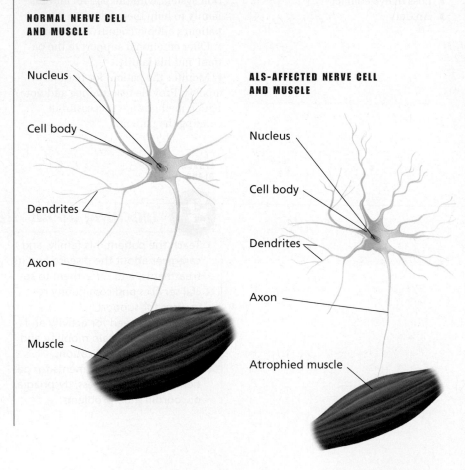

NORMAL NERVE CELL
AND MUSCLE

Nucleus

Cell body

Dendrites

Axon

Muscle

ALS-AFFECTED NERVE CELL
AND MUSCLE

Nucleus

Cell body

Dendrites

Axon

Atrophied muscle

Signs and symptoms

▶ Progressive loss of muscle strength and coordination
▶ Fasciculations
▶ Atrophy and weakness, especially in the muscles of the feet and the hands
▶ Impaired speech
▶ Difficulty chewing, swallowing, and breathing
▶ Choking
▶ Excessive drooling
▶ Muscle cramps
▶ Loss of dexterity
▶ Uncontrolled laughing or crying

Treatment

▶ Aims to control symptoms and provide emotional, psychological, and physical support
▶ Riluzole (Rilutek): may increase quality of life and survival but doesn't reverse or stop disease progression
▶ Baclofen (Lioresal) or tizanidine (Zanaflex): helps control spasticity that interferes with activities of daily living
▶ Sympathomimetics, anticholinergics, botulinum toxin type B or salivary gland irradiation: may be needed to control saliva
▶ Mucolytics: to thin secretions
▶ Percutaneous endoscopic gastrostomy: may be needed early to prevent aspiration
▶ Physical therapy, rehabilitation, and use of appliances or orthopedic intervention: may be required to maximize function
▶ Noninvasive ventilatory support initially; mechanical ventilation may eventually be needed

Nursing considerations

▶ Implement a rehabilitation program designed to maintain independence as long as possible.
▶ Help the patient obtain assistive equipment, such as a walker and a wheelchair.
▶ Arrange for a visiting nurse to oversee the patient's status, to provide support, and to teach the patient's family about the illness.
▶ Depending on the patient's muscular capacity, assist with bathing, personal hygiene, and transfers from wheelchair to bed.
▶ Help establish a regular bowel and bladder routine.
▶ Provide good skin care if the patient is bedridden. Turn him often, keep his skin clean and dry, and use pressure-reducing devices such as an alternating air mattress.
▶ If the patient has trouble swallowing, give him soft, solid foods and position him upright during meals. Gastrostomy and nasogastric tube feedings may be necessary to prevent aspiration.
▶ Provide emotional support.
▶ Discuss end-of-life care with the patient and family. Assist with advance directives, as appropriate.
▶ Provide information about hospice programs and local ALS support groups.

**LESSON
PLANS**

 Teaching about ALS

▶ Teach the patient, his family, and caregiver how motor neuron degeneration affects muscles and their motor function.
▶ Urge the patient to exercise to maintain strength in unaffected muscles.
▶ Describe dietary changes that ease swallowing.
▶ Demonstrate how to operate a wheelchair safely.
▶ Explain how to prevent and manage complications such as pressure ulcers.
▶ Help the patient develop alternative communication techniques.

▶ Teach the patient to suction himself if he's unable to handle an increased accumulation of secretions.
▶ If the patient has a gastrostomy tube, show the patient's family and caregiver how to administer tube feedings.
▶ Discuss advance directives regarding health care decisions.
▶ Teach the patient about his medications, including indication, dosage, administration, and possible adverse effects.

Guillain-Barré syndrome

Guillain-Barré syndrome is an acute, rapidly progressive, and potentially fatal form of polyneuritis that causes muscle weakness and mild distal sensory loss most often in an ascending pattern. Recovery is spontaneous and complete in about 85% of patients within 6 to 12 months, although mild motor or reflex deficits in the feet and legs may persist. The prognosis is best when symptoms clear between 15 and 20 days after onset.

Precisely what causes Guillain-Barré syndrome is unknown, but it may be a cell-mediated immunologic attack on peripheral nerves in response to a virus. The major pathologic effect is segmental demyelination of the peripheral nerves. Because this syndrome causes inflammation and degenerative changes in both the posterior (sensory) and anterior (motor) nerve roots, signs of sensory and motor losses occur simultaneously.

The clinical course of Guillain-Barré syndrome is divided into three phases:

Initial phase
▶ Begins when the first definitive symptom appears
▶ Ends 1 to 3 weeks later, when no further deterioration occurs

Plateau phase
▶ Lasts several days to 2 weeks
▶ Followed by the recovery phase, which is believed to coincide with remyelination and axonal process regrowth

Recovery phase
▶ Extends over a period of 4 to 6 months
▶ Patients with severe disease may take up to 2 years to recover, and recovery may not be complete

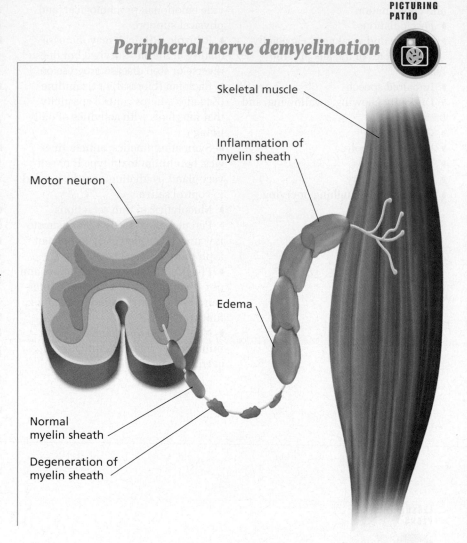

PICTURING PATHO

Peripheral nerve demyelination

Skeletal muscle

Inflammation of myelin sheath

Motor neuron

Edema

Normal myelin sheath

Degeneration of myelin sheath

Signs and symptoms
▶ A history of minor febrile illness (10 to 14 days before onset)
▶ Symmetrical muscle weakness
▶ Muscle weakness develops in the arms first (descending type) or in the arms and legs simultaneously
▶ In milder forms, muscle weakness nonexistent or affecting only the cranial nerves
▶ Paresthesia
▶ Facial diplegia (possibly with ophthalmoplegia)
▶ Dysphagia or dysarthria

Treatment
▶ Endotracheal (ET) intubation or tracheotomy if the patient has difficulty clearing secretions or maintaining adequate ventilation
▶ Plasmapheresis—useful in decreasing severity of symptoms, thereby facilitating a more rapid recovery
▶ I.V. immune globulin—equally effective in reducing the severity and duration of symptoms

Nursing considerations

▸ Monitor the patient for ascending sensory loss, which precedes motor loss.

▸ Monitor vital signs and level of consciousness.

▸ Assess and treat respiratory dysfunction. If respiratory muscles are weak, take serial vital capacity recordings.

▸ Obtain arterial blood gas measurements.

▸ Be alert for signs of rising partial pressure of carbon dioxide (such as confusion and tachypnea).

▸ Auscultate breath sounds, turn and position the patient, and encourage coughing and deep breathing. Provide respiratory support at the first sign of dyspnea or with decreasing partial pressure of arterial oxygen.

▸ If respiratory failure becomes imminent, assist with insertion of an ET tube.

▸ Give meticulous skin care to prevent skin breakdown. Establish a strict turning schedule; inspect the skin (especially sacrum, heels, and ankles) for breakdown, and reposition the patient every 2 hours.

▸ Perform passive range-of-motion exercises within the patient's pain limits. When the patient's condition stabilizes, change to gentle stretching and active assistance exercises.

▸ To prevent aspiration, test the gag reflex, and elevate the head of the bed before giving the patient anything to eat or drink. If the gag reflex is absent, give nasogastric feedings until this reflex returns.

▸ As the patient regains strength and can tolerate a vertical position, be alert for postural hypotension. Monitor blood pressure and pulse during tilting periods.

▸ Inspect the patient's legs regularly for signs of thrombophlebitis (localized pain, tenderness, erythema, edema, and positive Homans' sign), a common complication of Guillain-Barré syndrome. To prevent thrombophlebitis, apply antiembolism or compression stockings and give prophylactic anticoagulants, as ordered.

▸ If the patient has facial paralysis, give eye and mouth care every 4 hours.

▸ Measure and record intake and output every 8 hours, and watch for urine retention.

▸ Encourage adequate fluid intake of 2 qt (2 L) per day, unless contraindicated. If urine retention develops, begin intermittent catheterization as ordered.

▸ To prevent or relieve constipation, offer plenty of water, prune juice, and a high-bulk diet. If necessary, give daily or alternate-day suppositories (glycerin or bisacodyl) or enemas, as ordered.

▸ Refer the patient's family to the Guillain-Barré Syndrome Foundation International.

LESSON PLANS

Teaching about Guillain-Barré syndrome

▸ Explain the disease and its signs and symptoms to the patient and his family. Explain the diagnostic tests that will be performed.

▸ If the patient loses his gag reflex, tell him tube feeding will be needed to maintain nutritional status.

▸ Advise family members to help the patient maintain mental alertness, fight boredom, and avoid depression. Suggest that they plan frequent visits to help distract the patient as much as possible.

▸ Before discharge, teach the patient how to transfer from bed to wheelchair and from wheelchair to toilet or tub and how to walk short distances with a walker or a cane.

▸ Instruct the patient's family on how to help the patient eat and drink compensating for facial weakness, and how to help him avoid skin breakdown.

▸ Emphasize the importance of establishing a regular bowel and bladder elimination routine.

▸ Refer the patient for physical therapy, occupational therapy, and speech therapy, as needed.

Herniated disk

A herniated disk (also known as a *herniated nucleus pulposus* or a *slipped disk*) occurs when all or part of the nucleus pulposus—an intervertebral disk's gelatinous center—extrudes through the disk's weakened or torn outer ring (anulus fibrosus). The resultant pressure on spinal nerve roots or on the spinal cord itself causes back pain and other symptoms of nerve root irritation.

About 90% of herniations affect the lumbar (L) and lumbosacral spine; 8% occur in the cervical (C) spine and 1% to 2% in the thoracic spine. The most common site for herniation is the L4-L5 disk space. Other sites include L5-S1, L2-L3, L3-L4, C6-C7, and C5-C6.

Lumbar herniation usually develops in people ages 20 to 45 and cervical herniation in those ages 45 or older. Herniated disks affect more men than women.

Herniated disks may result from severe trauma or strain, or they may be related to intervertebral joint degeneration. In an elderly person with degenerative disk changes, minor trauma may cause herniation. A person with a congenitally small lumbar spinal canal or with osteophytes along the vertebrae may be more susceptible to nerve root compression with a herniated disk. This person is also more likely to exhibit neurologic symptoms.

Signs and symptoms

Vary according to location and extent of herniation.
▶ Severe lower back pain to the buttocks, legs, and feet, usually unilaterally
▶ Sudden pain after trauma, subsiding in a few days and then recurring at shorter intervals and with progressive intensity
▶ Sciatic pain beginning as a dull pain in the buttocks

How a herniated disk develops

A spinal disk has two parts: the soft center called the *nucleus pulposus* and the tough, fibrous, surrounding ring called the *anulus fibrosus*. The nucleus pulposus acts as a shock absorber, distributing the mechanical stress applied to the spine when the body moves.

NORMAL VERTEBRA AND INTERVERTEBRAL DISK

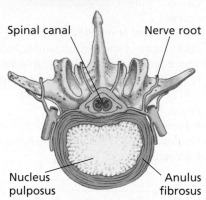

Spinal canal   Nerve root

Nucleus pulposus   Anulus fibrosus

Physical stress—usually a twisting motion—can cause the anulus fibrosus to tear or rupture, allowing the nucleus pulposus to push through (herniate) into the spinal canal. This process allows the vertebrae to move closer together as the disk compresses. This, in turn, causes pressure on the nerve roots as they exit between the vertebrae. Pain and, possibly, sensory and motor loss follow.

A herniated disk can also occur with intervertebral joint degeneration. If the disk has begun to degenerate, minor trauma may cause herniation.

Herniation occurs in three stages: protrusion, extrusion, and sequestration.

Protrusion
The nucleus pulposus presses against the anulus fibrosus.

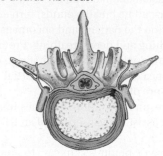

Extrusion and sequestration
The nucleus pulposus bulges forcefully through the anulus fibrosus, pushing against the nerve root. Then the anulus fibrosus gives way as the core of the disk bursts through to press against the nerve root.

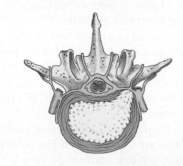

- Sensory and motor loss in the area innervated by the compressed spinal nerve root and in later stages, weakness and atrophy of the leg muscles

Treatment

- Unless neurologic impairment progresses rapidly, conservative initial treatment, consisting of bed rest (possibly with pelvic traction) for several days, supportive devices (such as a brace), heat or ice applications, and exercise or physical therapy
- Nonsteroidal anti-inflammatory drugs, steroidal drugs such as dexamethasone (Decadron), or muscle relaxants such as diazepam (Valium) or methocarbamol (Robaxin), to reduce inflammation and edema at the injury site
- Laminectomy and spinal fusion
- Chemonucleolysis—injection of the enzyme chymopapain into the herniated disk to dissolve the nucleus pulposus: possible alternative to a laminectomy

- Microdiscectomy to remove fragments of the nucleus pulposus
- Analgesics
- Weight reduction

Nursing considerations

- Assess the patient's pain. Give pain medications as ordered, and assess the patient's response.
- Offer supportive care, patient teaching, and encouragement to help the patient cope with the discomfort and frustration of back pain and impaired mobility. Include the patient and family members in all phases of his care.
- Encourage the patient to verbalize his concerns about his disorder. Answer all of the patient's questions.
- Encourage the patient to perform as much self-care as his immobility and pain allow.
- Help the patient identify and perform activities that promote rest and relaxation.

- If the patient will undergo myelography, ask him about allergies to iodides, iodine-containing substances, or seafood because such allergies may indicate sensitivity to a radiopaque contrast agent used in the test. Monitor intake and output. Watch for seizures and an allergic reaction.
- If the patient is in traction, make sure that the pelvic straps are properly positioned and that the weights are suspended. Periodically remove the traction to inspect the skin. Also remember to monitor the patient for deep vein thrombosis.
- After laminectomy, microdiskectomy, or spinal fusion, enforce bed rest as ordered. If the patient has a blood drainage system (Hemovac) in place, check the tubing frequently for patency and a secure vacuum seal. Report colorless moisture on dressings (possible cerebrospinal fluid leakage) or excessive drainage immediately. Check the neurovascular status of the patient's legs (color, motion, temperature, and sensation).
- Monitor vital signs, and check for bowel sounds and abdominal distention. Use the logrolling technique to turn the patient. Administer analgesics as ordered, especially about 30 minutes before attempts to sit or walk.
- Encourage participation in physical therapy.

LESSON PLANS

Teaching about herniated disk

- Teach the patient about treatments, which may include bed rest and pelvic traction; heat application to the area to decrease pain; an exercise program; medications to decrease pain, inflammation, and muscle spasms; and surgery.
- If weight reduction is indicated, teach the patient about appropriate dietary changes and refer him to a dietitian.

- Before myelography, reinforce previous explanations of the need for this test, and tell the patient to expect some pain. Assure him that he'll receive a sedative before the test, if needed, to keep him as calm and comfortable as possible. After the test, urge the patient to remain in bed with his head elevated (especially if metrizamide was used) and to drink plenty of fluids.
- If surgery is required, explain all preoperative and postoperative procedures and treatments to the patient and his family.
- Prepare the patient for discharge and encourage participation in prescribed physical therapy.

Meningitis

With meningitis, the brain and the spinal cord meninges become inflamed, usually as a result of a viral or a bacterial infection. Such inflammation may involve all three meningeal membranes—the dura mater, the arachnoid, and the pia mater. If the disease is recognized early and the infecting organism responds to antibiotics, the prognosis is good and complications are rare; however, mortality in untreated meningitis is 70% to 100%. The prognosis is worse for infants and the elderly, particularly if antibiotic therapy isn't started within hours of symptom onset.

Meningitis is almost always a complication of another bacterial infection—bacteremia (especially from pneumonia, empyema, osteomyelitis, or endocarditis), sinusitis, otitis media, encephalitis, myelitis, or brain abscess—usually caused by *Neisseria meningitidis*, *Haemophilus influenzae* (in children and young adults), or *Streptococcus pneumoniae* (in adults). In some cases, a virus is suspected. Meningitis may also follow skull fracture, a penetrating head wound, lumbar puncture, or ventricular shunting procedure. Aseptic meningitis may result from a virus or other organism. Sometimes, no causative organism can be found. Meningitis commonly begins as an inflammation of the pia-arachnoid, which may progress to congestion of adjacent tissues and destruction of some nerve cells.

PICTURING PATHO

Inflammation in meningitis

NORMAL MENINGES

Dura mater
Arachnoid
Pia mater

INFLAMMATION IN MENINGITIS

Swelling of the meninges interfering with normal brain functioning

Understanding aseptic viral meningitis

A benign syndrome, aseptic viral meningitis results from infection with enterovirus (most common), arbovirus, herpes simplex virus, mumps virus, or lymphocytic choriomeningitis virus.

Signs and symptoms usually begin suddenly with a temperature up to 104° F (40° C), drowsiness, confusion, stupor, and slight neck or spine stiffness when the patient bends forward. The patient history may reveal a recent illness.

Other signs and symptoms include headache, nausea, vomiting, abdominal pain, poorly defined chest pain, and sore throat.

A complete patient history and knowledge of seasonal epidemics are key to differentiating among the many forms of aseptic viral meningitis. Negative bacteriologic cultures and cerebrospinal fluid (CSF) analysis showing pleocytosis (increased number of cells in the CSF) and increased protein suggest the diagnosis. Isolation of the virus from CSF confirms it.

Treatment for aseptic viral meningitis includes bed rest, maintenance of fluid and electrolyte balance, analgesics for pain, and exercises to combat residual weakness. Careful handling of excretions and good hand-washing technique prevent the spread of the disease.

Signs and symptoms
◗ Fever
◗ Chills
◗ Malaise
◗ Headache
◗ Vomiting
◗ Nuchal rigidity
◗ Seizures
◗ Positive Brudzinski's and Kernig's signs
◗ Exaggerated and symmetrical deep tendon reflexes
◗ Opisthotonos
◗ Irritability, confusion
◗ Sinus arrhythmias
◗ Photophobia
◗ Diplopia (and other visual problems)
◗ Delirium
◗ Deep stupor
◗ Coma

Treatment
◗ I.V. antibiotics (if bacterial)—for at least 2 weeks—followed by oral antibiotics
◗ I.V. fluids
◗ Mannitol to decrease cerebral edema
◗ Anticonvulsants (usually given I.V.)
◗ Sedative to reduce restlessness
◗ Aspirin or acetaminophen (Tylenol) to relieve headache and fever
◗ Bed rest
◗ Isolation (if nasal cultures are positive)

Nursing considerations
◗ Assess neurologic function often. Observe level of consciousness (LOC) and signs of increased intracranial pressure (plucking at the bedcovers, vomiting, seizures, and a change in motor function and vital signs). Watch for signs of cranial nerve involvement (ptosis, strabismus, and diplopia).
◗ Be especially alert for a temperature increase up to 102° F (38.9° C), deteriorating LOC, onset of seizures, and altered respirations, all of which may signal an impending crisis.
◗ Monitor fluid balance. Maintain adequate fluid intake to avoid dehydration, but avoid fluid overload because of the danger of cerebral edema. Measure central venous pressure and intake and output accurately.
◗ Watch for adverse effects of I.V. antibiotics and other drugs.
◗ Position the patient carefully to prevent joint stiffness and neck pain. Turn him often, according to a planned positioning schedule. Assist with range-of-motion exercises.
◗ Maintain adequate nutrition and elimination.
◗ Ensure the patient's comfort. Provide mouth care regularly. Maintain a quiet environment.
◗ Provide reassurance and support.

HANDS ON

Important signs of meningitis

A positive response to the following tests helps diagnose meningitis.

Brudzinski's sign
Place the patient in a dorsal recumbent position; then put your hands behind his neck and bend it forward. Pain and resistance may indicate neck injury or arthritis. But if the patient also involuntarily flexes the hips and knees, chances are he has meningeal irritation and inflammation, a sign of meningitis.

Kernig's sign
Place the patient in a supine position. Flex his leg at the hip and knee; then straighten the knee. Pain or resistance suggests meningitis.

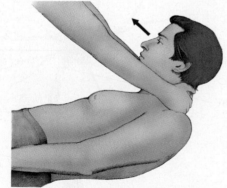
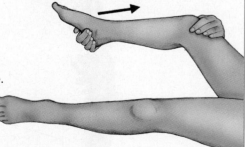

LESSON PLANS

Teaching about meningitis

◗ Teach the patient and his family about meningitis and its signs and symptoms, including its effects on behavior. Reassure the family that the delirium and behavior changes caused by meningitis usually disappear.
◗ Urge the patient to take drugs exactly as prescribed.
◗ To help prevent meningitis, teach patients with chronic sinusitis or other chronic infections—as well as those exposed to people with meningitis—the importance of quick and proper medical treatment.
◗ Encourage those in close contact with patient to receive prophylactic treatment.

Multiple sclerosis

Multiple sclerosis (MS) is a progressive disease caused by demyelination of the white matter of the brain and spinal cord. With this disease, sporadic patches of demyelination throughout the central nervous system induce widely disseminated and varied neurologic dysfunction. Characterized by exacerbations and remissions, MS is a major cause of chronic disability in young adults.

Prognosis varies; MS may progress rapidly, disabling some patients by early adulthood or causing death within months of onset. However, 70% of patients lead active, productive lives with prolonged remissions.

The exact cause of MS is unknown, but current theories suggest a slow-acting or latent viral infection and an autoimmune response. Other theories suggest that environmental and genetic factors may also be linked to MS. Emotional stress, overwork, fatigue, pregnancy, and acute respiratory tract infections have been known to precede the onset of this illness.

Signs and symptoms

▶ Vary with the extent and site of myelin destruction, the extent of remyelination, and the adequacy of subsequent restored synaptic transmission
▶ May be transient or may last for hours or weeks; may wax and wane with no predictable pattern, vary from day to day, and be difficult for the patient to describe; may be so mild that the patient is unaware of them or so bizarre that he appears hysterical
▶ Visual problems
▶ Numbness
▶ Tingling sensations (paresthesia)

▶ Optic neuritis, diplopia, ophthalmoplegia, blurred vision, and nystagmus
▶ Weakness, paralysis ranging from monoplegia to quadriplegia, spasticity, hyperreflexia, intention tremor, and gait ataxia
▶ Incontinence, frequency, urgency, and frequent infections
▶ Mood swings, irritability, euphoria, and depression
▶ Poorly articulated or scanning speech and dysphagia

PICTURING PATHO

Demyelination in multiple sclerosis

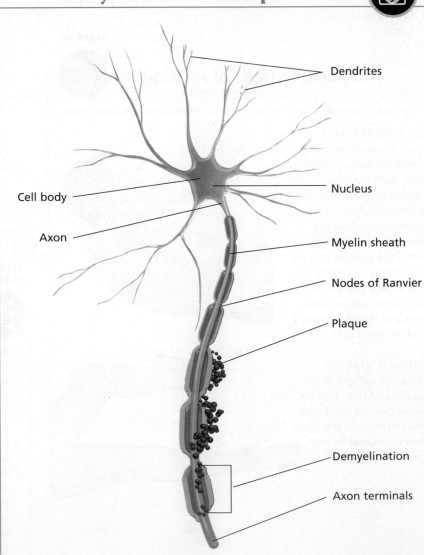

Dendrites

Nucleus

Cell body

Axon

Myelin sheath

Nodes of Ranvier

Plaque

Demyelination

Axon terminals

Treatment

‣ Immune-modulating therapy, with interferon or glatiramer acetate (Copaxone)
‣ Steroids—used to reduce the associated edema of the myelin sheath during exacerbations
‣ Baclofen (Lioresal), tizanidine (Zanaflex), or diazepam (Valium) to relieve spasticity
‣ Cholinergic agents to relieve urine retention and minimize frequency and urgency
‣ Amantadine (Symmetrel) or modafinil (Provigil) to relieve fatigue
‣ Antidepressants
‣ Comfort measures such as massages
‣ Fatigue prevention
‣ Pressure ulcer prevention
‣ Bowel and bladder training (if necessary)
‣ Antibiotics for bladder infections
‣ Physical therapy
‣ Counseling
‣ Speech therapy
‣ Occupational therapy
‣ Planned exercise programs—help with maintaining muscle tone
‣ Avoidance of extreme heat

Nursing considerations

‣ Assist with physical therapy.
‣ Assist with active, resistive, and stretching exercises to maintain muscle tone and joint mobility, decrease spasticity, improve coordination, and boost morale.
‣ Evaluate the need for bowel and bladder training during hospitalization. Encourage adequate fluid intake and regular urination.
‣ Promote emotional stability. Help the patient establish a daily routine to maintain optimal functioning. Encourage daily physical exercise and regular rest periods to prevent fatigue.
‣ For more information, refer the patient to the National Multiple Sclerosis Society.

‣ Provide adequate nutrition and refer the patient to a nutritionist if appropriate.

LESSON
PLANS

Teaching about multiple sclerosis

‣ Teach the patient and his family about the disease process, including its symptoms, complications, and treatments.
‣ Teach about prescribed drugs, including their names, indications, dosages, adverse effects, and special considerations.
‣ Discuss the chronic course of multiple sclerosis (MS), including that exacerbations are unpredictable and demand physical and emotional adjustments.
‣ Emphasize the need to avoid temperature extremes, stress, fatigue, and infections and other illnesses, all of which can trigger an MS attack.
‣ Advise the patient to maintain independence by developing new ways of performing daily activities.

‣ Stress the importance of eating a nutritious, well-balanced diet that contains sufficient roughage and adequate fluids to prevent constipation.
‣ Teach correct use of suppositories to help attain a regular bowel schedule.
‣ Discuss methods to relieve urinary incontinence and urine retention, including Credé's maneuver and self-catheterization.
‣ Encourage daily physical exercise and regular rest periods to prevent fatigue.
‣ Discuss sexual dysfunction and childbearing concerns.
‣ Supply the patient and family with information regarding support services.

Myasthenia gravis

Myasthenia gravis produces sporadic but progressive weakness and abnormal fatigability of striated (skeletal) muscles, exacerbated by exercise and repeated movement, but improved by anticholinesterase drugs. Usually, this disorder affects muscles innervated by the cranial nerves (face, lips, tongue, neck, and throat), but it can affect any muscle group. Myasthenia gravis follows an unpredictable course of recurring exacerbations and periodic remissions. There's no known cure. Drug treatment has improved prognosis and allows patients to lead relatively normal lives except during exacerbations. When the disease involves the respiratory system, it may be life-threatening.

Myasthenia gravis causes a failure in transmission of nerve impulses at the neuromuscular junction. Theoretically, such impairment may result from an autoimmune response, ineffective acetylcholine release, or inadequate muscle fiber response to acetylcholine.

Signs and symptoms

◗ Skeletal muscle weakness and fatigability
◗ Weak eye closure
◗ Ptosis
◗ Blank, expressionless face
◗ Nasal vocal tone
◗ Frequent nasal regurgitation of fluids
◗ Difficulty chewing and swallowing
◗ Neck muscles becoming too weak to support the head without bobbing
◗ Weak respiratory muscles and decreased tidal volume and vital capacity, making breathing difficult

Treatment

◗ Anticholinesterase inhibitors, such as neostigmine (Prostigmin) and pyridostigmine (Mestinon)
◗ Corticosteroids
◗ Immunomodulatory therapy
◗ Thymectomy
◗ Tracheotomy
◗ Positive-pressure ventilation
◗ Plasmapheresis

PICTURING PATHO

Understanding myasthenia gravis

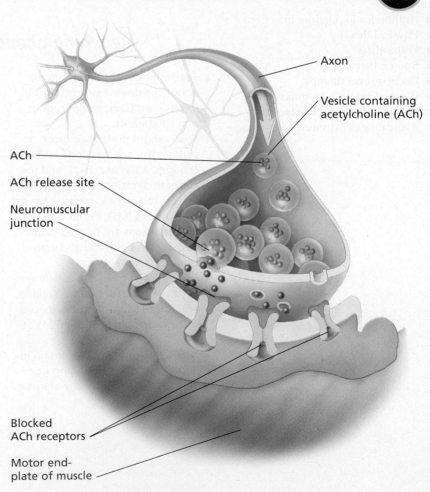

Axon

Vesicle containing acetylcholine (ACh)

ACh

ACh release site

Neuromuscular junction

Blocked ACh receptors

Motor end-plate of muscle

Nursing considerations

▶ Establish an accurate neurologic and respiratory baseline. Thereafter, monitor tidal volume and vital capacity regularly. Suction as needed to remove accumulating secretions.

▶ Be alert for signs of an impending crisis (increased muscle weakness, respiratory distress, and difficulty in talking or chewing).

▶ Plan exercise, meals, patient care, and activities to make the most of energy peaks and avoid fatigue.

▶ Monitor swallowing ability. Give soft, solid foods instead of liquids to lessen the risk of choking.

▶ Warn the patient to avoid strenuous exercise, stress, infection, and needless exposure to the sun or cold. All of these may worsen signs and symptoms.

▶ For more information and support, refer the patient to the Myasthenia Gravis Foundation.

LESSON PLANS

Teaching about myasthenia gravis

▶ Teach the patient and his family about the disease process, including its symptoms, complications, and treatments.

▶ Teach about prescribed drugs, including their names, indications, dosages, adverse effects, and special considerations.

▶ Help the patient plan daily activities to coincide with energy peaks.

▶ Stress the need for frequent rest periods throughout the day.

▶ Explain that remissions, exacerbations, and daily fluctuations are common.

▶ Teach the patient how to recognize adverse effects and evidence of toxicity from anticholinesterase drugs (headaches, weakness, sweating, abdominal cramps, nausea, vomiting, diarrhea, excessive salivation, and bronchospasm) and corticosteroids (euphoria, insomnia, edema, and increased appetite).

▶ Warn the patient to avoid strenuous exercise, stress, infection, and needless exposure to the sun or cold, which can worsen signs and symptoms.

▶ Teach the patient about thymectomy if indicated.

▶ Encourage regular follow-up visits with the primary physician.

Parkinson's disease

Parkinson's disease is a neurodegenerative disorder that characteristically produces progressive muscle rigidity, akinesia, involuntary tremor, and dementia. Death may result from aspiration pneumonia or an infection.

Although the cause of Parkinson's disease is unknown, study of the extrapyramidal brain nuclei (corpus striatum, globus pallidus, and substantia nigra) has established that a dopamine deficiency prevents affected brain cells from performing their normal inhibitory function within the central nervous system. Parkinson's disease occurs in families in some cases; in others, it may be secondary to external factors such as medications used to treat schizophrenia.

Signs and symptoms

▶ Early signs: decreased sense of smell, REM behavior disorder
▶ Muscle rigidity: causes resistance to passive muscle stretching, which may be uniform (lead-pipe rigidity) or jerky (cogwheel rigidity)
▶ Insidious resting tremor that begins in the fingers (unilateral pill-roll tremor), increases during stress or anxiety, and decreases with purposeful movement and sleep
▶ Difficulty walking (gait lacks parallel motion and may be retropulsive or propulsive)
▶ Rigidity
▶ Bradykinesia
▶ Drooling and excessive sweating
▶ Masklike facial expression
▶ Dysarthria, dysphagia, or both
▶ Orthostatic hypotension
▶ Dementia

Treatment

▶ Levodopa and carbidopa (combination [Sinemet]) to halt peripheral dopamine synthesis)
▶ Anticholinergics such as trihexyphenidyl (Artane)
▶ Amantadine (Symmetrel)

Neurotransmitter action in Parkinson's disease

PICTURING PATHO

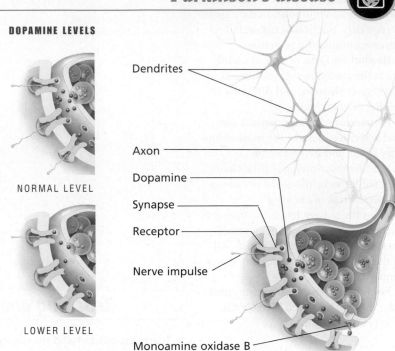

DOPAMINE LEVELS

NORMAL LEVEL

LOWER LEVEL

Dendrites
Axon
Dopamine
Synapse
Receptor
Nerve impulse
Monoamine oxidase B

▶ Dopamine agonist rotigotine (Neupro) transdermal patch
▶ Neuroprotective therapy, such as selegiline (Eldepryl) and rasagiline (Azilect)
▶ Stereotactic neurosurgery, such as subthalamotomy and pallidotomy
▶ Brain stimulator implantation
▶ Active and passive range-of-motion exercises, routine daily activities, walking, and baths and massage to help relax muscles

Nursing considerations

▶ Monitor drug treatment and observe for adverse effects.
▶ If the patient has surgery, watch for signs of hemorrhage and increased intracranial pressure by frequently checking level of consciousness and vital signs.

▶ Encourage independence and participation in physical and occupational therapy.
▶ Advise the patient to change position slowly and dangle his legs before getting out of bed.
▶ Help establish a regular bowel routine by encouraging him to drink at least 2 qt (2 L) of liquids daily and eat high-fiber foods.
▶ Provide emotional support.
▶ Refer the patient and his family to the National Parkinson Foundation or the United Parkinson Foundation for more information.

Teaching about Parkinson's disease

▶ Teach the patient and his family about the disorder, including its progressive symptoms, complications, and treatments.
▶ Discuss warning signs of complications that require immediate attention.
▶ Teach the patient about prescribed drugs, including their names, indications, dosages, adverse effects, and special considerations (such as dietary restrictions and the need to stand up slowly if the patient takes Sinemet).
▶ Reinforce the importance of range-of-motion exercises, routine daily activities, walking, and baths and massage to help relax muscles.

▶ Explain to the patient and his family how to prevent pressure ulcers and contractures by proper positioning.
▶ Explain household safety measures to prevent accidents.
▶ Reinforce a swallowing therapy regimen to prevent aspiration.
▶ Provide information regarding support services as needed.

Seizure disorder

Seizure disorder, or *epilepsy*, is a condition of the brain characterized by recurrent seizures (paroxysmal events associated with abnormal electrical discharges of neurons in the brain). The prognosis is good if the patient adheres strictly to the prescribed treatment.

Primary seizure disorder or epilepsy is idiopathic without apparent structural changes in the brain.

Secondary epilepsy, characterized by structural changes or metabolic alterations of the neuronal membranes, causes increased automaticity.

In about one-half of seizure disorder cases, the cause is unknown. Some possible causes are:
▶ birth trauma (such as inadequate oxygen supply to the brain, blood incompatibility, or hemorrhage)
▶ perinatal infection
▶ anoxia
▶ infectious diseases (meningitis, encephalitis, or brain abscess)
▶ head injury or trauma.

Some neurons in the brain may depolarize easily or be hyperexcitable, firing more readily than normal when

stimulated. On stimulation, the electrical current spreads to surrounding cells, which fire in turn. The impulse thus cascades to:
▶ one side of the brain (a partial seizure)
▶ both sides of the brain (a generalized seizure)
▶ cortical, subcortical, and brain stem areas.

The brain's metabolic demand for oxygen increases dramatically during a seizure. If this demand isn't met, hypoxia and brain damage result.

Firing of inhibitory neurons causes the excited neurons to slow their firing and eventually stop. Without this inhibitory action, the result is status epilepticus (seizures occurring one right after another). Without treatment, resulting anoxia is fatal.

Understanding status epilepticus

Status epilepticus is a continuous seizure state that must be interrupted by emergency measures. It can occur during all types of seizures. For example, generalized tonic-clonic status epilepticus is a continuous generalized tonic-clonic seizure without an intervening return of consciousness.

Status epilepticus can result from withdrawal of antiepileptic drugs, hypoxic or metabolic encephalopathy, acute head trauma, or septicemia caused by encephalitis or meningitis.

Emergency treatment usually includes lorazepam (Ativan), phenytoin (Dilantin), or phenobarbital (Luminal); I.V. dextrose 50% when seizures are caused by hypoglycemia; and I.V. thiamine in patients with chronic alcoholism or who are undergoing withdrawal.

Understanding types of seizures

Use these guidelines to understand different seizure types. Remember that patients may be affected by more than one type of seizure.

Partial seizures

Partial seizures start in a localized area in the brain and may spread to the entire brain (generalized seizure). Partial seizures include simple (jacksonian and sensory), complex, and secondarily generalized.

Simple partial seizure

Simple partial seizures are localized motor or sensory seizures that spread to adjacent areas of the brain. Symptoms include twitching and jerky, unilateral movement of an extremity, the face, or eye. The patient seldom loses consciousness, but the seizure may generalize to tonic-clonic.

Sensory seizure

Symptoms of sensory seizures include hallucinations, flashing lights, tingling, vertigo, déjà vu, and smelling a foul odor.

Complex partial seizure

Signs and symptoms of a complex partial seizure vary but may start with an aura and usually include purposeless behavior, including a glassy stare, picking at clothes, aimless wandering, lip-smacking or chewing motions, and unintelligible speech. The seizure may last a few seconds to 20 minutes. After, confusion may last several minutes and make the person look intoxicated or psychotic. The patient has no memory of his actions during the seizure.

Secondarily generalized seizure

A secondarily generalized seizure is a seizure that can be simple or complex and can generalize. An aura may occur first, with loss of consciousness immediately or 1 to 2 minutes later.

Generalized seizures

Generalized seizures cause a generalized electrical abnormality in the brain.

Absence seizure

Most common in children, absence seizure usually causes a mild change in consciousness (blinking or rolling the eyes, blank stare, slight mouth movements) and lasts 1 to 10 seconds. Untreated, these seizures can recur up to 100 times per day and become generalized tonic-clonic seizures.

Myoclonic seizure

Also called *bilateral massive epileptic myoclonus,* a myoclonic seizure is marked by brief, involuntary, possibly rhythmic muscular jerks of the body or limbs and a brief loss of consciousness.

Generalized tonic-clonic seizure

A generalized tonic-clonic seizure usually starts with a loud cry. The person loses consciousness and falls to the ground, first stiff (tonic) and then alternating spasm and relaxation (clonic). He may have tongue biting, incontinence, labored breathing, apnea, and cyanosis. After 2 to 5 minutes, abnormal electrical discharge stops and the person regains consciousness but is confused, drowsy, fatigued, sore, or weak. He may have a headache and fall asleep.

Akinetic seizure

Akinetic seizure affects young children and may be called a drop attack. It causes a loss of postural tone and temporary loss of consciousness.

Signs and symptoms

▶ Recurring partial or generalized seizures, or a combination

Treatment

▶ For generalized tonic-clonic seizures and complex partial seizures, phenytoin (Dilantin), fosphenytoin (Cerebyx), carbamazepine (Tegretol), valproic acid (Depakote), gabapentin (Neurontin), and primidone (Mysoline)
▶ For absence seizures only, ethosuximide (Zarontin)
▶ For status epilepticus, I.V. diazepam (Valium), lorazepam (Ativan), phenytoin (Dilantin), or phenobarbital
▶ Administration of dextrose (when seizures are secondary to hypoglycemia) or thiamine (in chronic alcoholism or withdrawal)
▶ Surgery to remove a demonstrated focal lesion if drug therapy is ineffective or to remove an underlying cause, such as a tumor, abscess, or vascular problem
▶ Vagus nerve stimulator implant

Nursing considerations

▶ Monitor a patient taking anticonvulsants for signs of toxicity, such as nystagmus, ataxia, lethargy, dizziness, drowsiness, slurred speech, irritability, nausea, and vomiting.
▶ When administering phenytoin or fosphenytoin I.V., use a large vein, administer according to guidelines, and monitor vital signs often.
▶ Initiate seizure precautions to maintain the patient's safety.
▶ Encourage the patient and his family to express their feelings about the patient's condition.
▶ Stress the need for compliance with the prescribed drug schedule.
▶ Emphasize the importance of having blood levels of anticonvulsants checked at regular intervals.

Tonic-clonic interventions

Generalized tonic-clonic seizures may necessitate the following interventions:

◗ Avoid restraining the patient during a seizure.

◗ Help the patient to a lying position, loosen any tight clothing, and place something flat and soft, such as a pillow, under his head.

◗ Clear the area of hard objects.

◗ Don't force anything into the patient's mouth if his teeth are clenched.

◗ Turn the patient's head or turn him on his side to provide an open airway.

◗ After the seizure, reassure the patient that he's all right, orient him to time and place, and tell him that he had a seizure.

LESSON
PLANS

 ### Teaching about seizure disorder

◗ Teach the patient and his family about the disease process, including its signs and symptoms, complications, and treatments.

◗ Teach about prescribed drugs, including their names, indications, dosages, frequencies, and special considerations.

◗ Stress the need to comply with the prescribed drug schedule.

◗ Warn against possible adverse effects that should be reported immediately—drowsiness, lethargy, hyperactivity, confusion, and vision and sleep disturbances—all of which indicate the need for dosage adjustment.

◗ Emphasize the importance of having anticonvulsant blood levels checked at regular intervals, even if the seizures are under control.

◗ Warn the patient against drinking alcoholic beverages.

◗ Discuss warning signs and symptoms of complications that require immediate medical attention.

◗ Review any activity restrictions, such as driving, if applicable.

◗ Discuss safety procedures to be used when a seizure is imminent.

◗ Teach the patient's family members how to protect the patient from injury and aspiration during a seizure and to observe and report the seizure activity.

◗ Stress the importance of wearing or carrying medical identification.

Stroke, acute ischemic

A stroke, also called *brain attack,* is a sudden impairment of cerebral circulation in one or more of the blood vessels supplying the brain. A stroke interrupts or diminishes oxygen supply and commonly causes serious damage or necrosis in brain tissues. The sooner circulation returns to normal after a stroke, the better chances are for complete recovery. However, about half of those who survive a stroke remain permanently disabled and experience a recurrence within weeks, months, or years.

The major causes of stroke are thrombosis and embolism. Factors that increase the risk of stroke include history of transient ischemic attacks (TIAs), atherosclerosis, hypertension, kidney disease, arrhythmias (specifically atrial fibrillation), electrocardiogram changes, rheumatic heart disease, carotid artery disease, diabetes mellitus, postural hypotension, cardiac or myocardial enlargement, high serum triglyceride levels, lack of exercise, use of hormonal contraceptives, cigarette smoking, and family history of stroke.

Understanding transient ischemic attack

A transient ischemic attack (TIA) is a neurologic deficit that lasts seconds to hours. It's usually considered a warning sign of an impending thrombotic stroke; 50% to 80% of patients who have had a cerebral infarction from thrombosis have also had a TIA. The age of onset varies after age 50 and is highest among blacks and men.

In a TIA, microemboli released from a thrombus temporarily interrupt blood flow, especially in the small distal branches of the brain's arterial tree. Small spasms in those arterioles may precede TIA and also impact blood flow. The most distinctive characteristics of TIAs are the transient nature of the neurologic deficits and the complete return of normal function. Signs and symptoms correlate with the location of the affected artery. They include double vision, unilateral blindness, staggering or uncoordinated gait, unilateral weakness or numbness, falling because of weakness in the legs, dizziness, and speech deficits, such as slurring or thickness.

During a TIA, treatment aims to prevent a completed stroke and consists of aspirin or anticoagulants to minimize the risk of thrombosis. After or between attacks, preventive treatment includes carotid endarterectomy or cerebral microvascular bypass.

Ischemic stroke

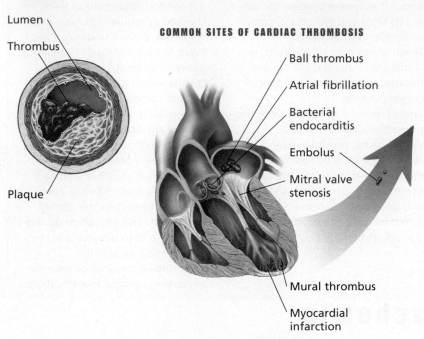

Lumen

Thrombus

Plaque

COMMON SITES OF CARDIAC THROMBOSIS

Ball thrombus

Atrial fibrillation

Bacterial endocarditis

Embolus

Mitral valve stenosis

Mural thrombus

Myocardial infarction

COMMON SITES OF PLAQUE FORMATION, EMBOLISM, AND INFARCTION

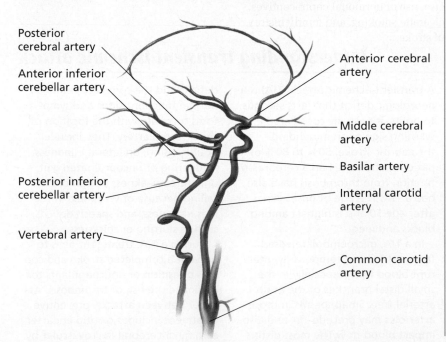

Posterior cerebral artery

Anterior inferior cerebellar artery

Posterior inferior cerebellar artery

Vertebral artery

Anterior cerebral artery

Middle cerebral artery

Basilar artery

Internal carotid artery

Common carotid artery

Strokes are classified according to their course of progression. The least severe is the TIA, or "little stroke," which results from a temporary interruption of blood flow, most commonly in the carotid and vertebrobasilar arteries. A progressive stroke, or stroke-in-evolution (thrombus-in-evolution), begins with slight neurologic deficit and worsens in 1or 2 days. In a completed stroke, neurologic deficits are maximal at onset.

Signs and symptoms

◗ Vary with the artery affected and the region of the brain it supplies, the severity of damage, and the extent of collateral circulation that develops (a stroke in one hemisphere causes signs and symptoms on the opposite side of the body; a stroke that damages cranial nerves affects structures on the same side)

Treatment
General
◗ Intracranial pressure (ICP) management with monitoring, hyperventilation, and osmotic diuretics
◗ Anticonvulsants (if patient has seizures)
◗ Antihypertensives
◗ Surgery for large cerebellar infarction
◗ Percutaneous transluminal angioplasty or stent insertion
◗ Stool softeners
◗ Rehabilitation with physical and occupational therapy

Ischemic stroke
◗ Thrombolytic therapy within 3 hours after onset of symptoms
◗ Microvascular bypass
◗ Anticoagulant therapy
◗ Antiplatelet agents
◗ Carotid enterectomy

Neurologic deficits in stroke

With stroke, functional loss reflects damage to the brain area normally perfused by the occluded or ruptured artery. Whereas one patient may experience only mild hand weakness, another may develop unilateral paralysis. Hypoxia and ischemia may produce edema that affects distal parts of the brain, causing further neurologic deficits. The signs and symptoms that accompany stroke at different sites are described below.

Site	Signs and symptoms
Anterior cerebral artery	▶ Confusion ▶ Impaired motor and sensory functions ▶ Incontinence ▶ Numbness on the affected side (especially in the arm) ▶ Paralysis of the contralateral foot and leg with accompanying footdrop ▶ Personality changes, such as flat affect and distractibility ▶ Poor coordination ▶ Weakness
Internal carotid artery	▶ Altered level of consciousness ▶ Aphasia ▶ Bruits over the carotid artery ▶ Dysphasia ▶ Headaches ▶ Monocular vision disturbance or loss on the affected side ▶ Unilateral numbness ▶ Unilateral weakness or paralysis ▶ Ptosis ▶ Sensory changes ▶ Weakness
Middle cerebral artery	▶ Aphasia ▶ Dysgraphia (inability to write) ▶ Dyslexia (reading problems) ▶ Dysphasia ▶ Hemiparesis on the affected side that's more severe in the face and arm than in the leg ▶ Visual field cuts
Posterior cerebral artery	▶ Blindness from ischemia in the occipital area ▶ Coma ▶ Dyslexia ▶ Sensory impairment ▶ Visual field cuts
Vertebral or basilar artery	▶ Amnesia ▶ Ataxia ▶ Dizziness ▶ Dysphagia ▶ Mouth and lip numbness ▶ Poor coordination ▶ Slurred speech ▶ Vision deficits, such as color blindness, lack of depth perception, and diplopia

Nursing considerations

During the acute phase, efforts focus on survival needs and prevention of further complications. Effective care emphasizes continuing neurologic assessment, support of respiration, continuous monitoring of vital signs, careful positioning to prevent aspiration and contractures, management and prevention of GI problems, and careful monitoring of fluid, electrolyte, and nutritional status. Patient care must also include measures to prevent complications such as infection.

▶ Maintain patent airway and oxygenation. Keep the patient in a lateral position to allow secretions to drain naturally or suction secretions, as needed. Insert an artificial airway, and start mechanical ventilation or supplemental oxygen, if necessary.

▶ Monitor vital signs and neurologic status, record observations, and report any significant changes to the physician. Monitor blood pressure, level of consciousness, pupillary changes, motor function (voluntary and involuntary movements), sensory function, speech, skin color, temperature, signs of increased ICP, and nuchal rigidity or flaccidity.

▶ Monitor the patient after fibrinolytic therapy for signs and symptoms of bleeding.

▶ Watch for signs of pulmonary emboli from immobility. Monitor the patient for chest pain, shortness of breath, dusky color, tachycardia, fever, and changed sensorium.

▶ Monitor blood gases and alert the physician to increased partial pressure of carbon dioxide or decreased partial pressure of oxygen.

▶ Maintain fluid and electrolyte balance. Administer I.V. fluids as ordered. Monitor intake and output.

▶ Ensure adequate nutrition. Check for gag reflex before offering small oral feedings of semisolid foods. If oral feedings aren't possible, insert a nasogastric tube.

▶ Prevent GI problems. Be alert for signs that the patient is straining at elimination because this increases ICP. Modify diet and administer stool softeners, as ordered, and give laxatives, if necessary. If the patient vomits (usually during the first few days), keep him positioned on his side to prevent aspiration. Provide prophylaxis against GI ulcers as ordered.

▶ Provide careful mouth care.

▶ Provide meticulous eye care. Remove secretions with a cotton ball and sterile normal saline solution. Instill eyedrops as ordered. Patch the patient's affected eye if he can't close the lid.

▶ Position the patient and align his extremities correctly. To prevent pneumonia, turn the patient at least every 2 hours. Elevate the affected hand to control dependent edema, and place it in a functional position.

▶ Assist the patient with exercise. Perform range-of-motion exercises for both the affected and unaffected sides. Teach and encourage the patient to use his unaffected side to exercise his affected side. Encourage participation in physical and occupational therapy.

▶ Give medications as ordered, and watch for and report adverse effects.

▶ Provide psychological support. Set realistic short-term goals. Involve the patient's family in his care when possible, and explain his deficits and strengths.

▶ Establish and maintain communication with the patient. If he's aphasic, set up a simple method of communicating basic needs.

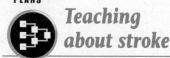

LESSON PLANS

Teaching about stroke

▶ Teach the patient and his family about the disease process, including the type of stroke that has occurred and signs and symptoms of reccurence. Review the treatment plan.

▶ Teach about prescribed drugs, including their names, indications, dosages, adverse effects, and special considerations.

▶ Discuss warning signs of complications that require immediate medical attention.

▶ Discuss risk factors for stroke, and help the patient identify those he can alter to reduce his risk of further stroke.

▶ If the patient is having surgery, explain the procedure and what he can expect before and after.

▶ Encourage participation in rehabilition. Refer the patient and family to support services as needed.

TESTS

Diagnostic testing to evaluate the nervous system typically includes laboratory tests, imaging studies, angiographic studies, and electrophysiologic studies. Other tests, such as lumbar puncture and transcranial Doppler studies, may also be used.

Laboratory tests

BACTERIAL MENINGITIS ANTIGEN

The bacterial meningitis antigen test can detect specific antigens of *Streptococcus pneumoniae, Neisseria meningitidis,* and *Haemophilus influenzae* type B, the principal etiologic agents in meningitis. It can be performed on samples of serum, cerebrospinal fluid (CSF), urine, pleural fluid, and joint fluid, but CSF and urine samples are preferred. Normally, results are negative for bacterial antigens. Positive results identify the specific bacterial antigen: *S. pneumoniae, N. meningitidis, H. influenzae* type B, or group B streptococci.

CEREBROSPINAL FLUID ANALYSIS

CSF, a clear substance that circulates in the subarachnoid space, has many vital functions. It protects the brain and spinal cord from injury and transports products of neurosecretion, cellular biosynthesis, and cellular metabolism through the central nervous system (CNS).

For qualitative analysis, CSF is most commonly obtained by lumbar puncture (LP) (usually between the third and fourth lumbar vertebrae) and, rarely, by cisternal or ventricular puncture. A CSF specimen may also be obtained during other neurologic tests such as myelography.

CSF analysis aids the diagnosis of viral or bacterial meningitis, subarachnoid or intracranial hemorrhage, tumors, brain abscesses, neurosyphilis, and chronic CNS infections.

Normally during LP, the CSF pressure is recorded and the appearance of the specimen is checked. Three tubes are collected routinely and are sent to the laboratory for protein, sugar, and cell analysis as well as for serologic testing such as the Venereal Disease Research Laboratory test for neurosyphilis. A separate specimen is also sent to the laboratory for culture and sensitivity testing. Electrolyte analysis and Gram stain may be ordered as supplementary tests. CSF electrolyte levels are of special interest in the patient with abnormal serum electrolyte levels or CSF infection and in the patient receiving hyperosmolar agents.

- Teach the importance of following a low-cholesterol, low-salt diet; achieving and maintaining an ideal weight; increasing activity; avoiding smoking and prolonged bed rest; and minimizing stress.
- Warn the patient and his family to seek emergency medical attention for any premonitory signs of a stroke, such as severe headache, drowsiness, confusion, and dizziness.
- Emphasize the importance of regular follow-up visits.
- Discuss alternate communication techniques, if indicated.
- Review dietary adjustments, such as semisoft foods for dysphagia and the use of assistive feeding devices.
- Review the safe use of a cane or walker and home safety tips.

Findings in cerebrospinal fluid analysis

Test	Normal	Abnormality	Implications
Pressure	50 to 180 mm H_2O	Increase	Increased intracranial pressure
		Decrease	Spinal subarachnoid obstruction above puncture site
Appearance	Clear, colorless	Cloudy	Infection
		Xanthochromic or bloody	Subarachnoid, intracerebral, or intraventricular hemorrhage; spinal cord obstruction; traumatic tap (usually noted only in initial specimen)
		Brown, orange, or yellow	Elevated protein levels, red blood cell (RBC) breakdown (blood present for at least 3 days)
Protein	15 to 50 mg/dl (SI, 0.15 to 0.5 g/L)	Marked increase	Tumors, trauma, hemorrhage, diabetes mellitus, polyneuritis, blood in cerebrospinal fluid (CSF)
		Marked decrease	Rapid CSF production
Gamma globulin	3% to 12% of total protein	Increase	Demyelinating disease, neurosyphilis, Guillain-Barré syndrome
Glucose	50 to 80 mg/dl (SI, 2.8 to 4.4 mmol/L)	Increase	Systemic hyperglycemia
		Decrease	Systemic hypoglycemia, bacterial or fungal infection, meningitis, mumps, postsubarachnoid hemorrhage
Cell count	0 to 5 white blood cells	Increase	Active disease: meningitis, acute infection, onset of chronic illness, tumor, abscess, infarction, demyelinating disease
	No RBCs	RBCs	Hemorrhage or traumatic lumbar puncture
Venereal Disease Research Laboratories, test for syphilis, and other serologic tests	Nonreactive	Positive	Neurosyphilis
Chloride	118 to 130 mEq/L (SI, 118 to 130 mmol/L)	Decrease	Infected meninges
Gram stain	No organisms	Gram-positive or gram-negative organisms	Bacterial meningitis

Imaging studies

The most common imaging studies used to detect neurologic disorders include computed tomography (CT) scan, magnetic resonance imaging (MRI), positron emission tomography (PET) scan, and skull and spinal X-rays.

COMPUTED TOMOGRAPHY SCAN

CT scanning of intracranial structures combines radiology and computer analysis of tissue density (determined by contrast dye absorption). CT scanning doesn't show blood vessels as well as an angiogram does; however, it carries less risk of complications and causes fewer traumas than cerebral angiography.

CT scanning of the spine is used to assess such disorders as herniated disk, spinal cord tumors, and spinal stenosis.

CT scanning of the brain is used to detect brain contusion, brain calcifications, cerebral atrophy, hydrocephalus, inflammation, space-occupying lesions (tumors, hematomas, edema, and abscesses), and vascular anomalies (arteriovenous malformation [AVM], infarctions, blood clots, and hemorrhage).

MAGNETIC RESONANCE IMAGING

MRI generates detailed pictures of body structures. The test may involve the use of a contrast medium such as gadolinium.

Compared with conventional X-rays and CT scans, MRI provides superior contrast of soft tissues, sharply differentiating healthy, benign, and cancerous tissue and clearly revealing blood vessels. In addition, MRI permits imaging in multiple planes, including sagittal and coronal views in regions where bones normally hamper visualization.

MRI is especially useful for studying the CNS because it can reveal structural and biochemical abnormalities associated with such conditions as transient ischemic attack (TIA), tumors, multiple sclerosis (MS), cerebral edema, and hydrocephalus.

POSITRON EMISSION TOMOGRAPHY SCAN

PET scanning provides colorimetric information about the brain's metabolic activity. It works by detecting how quickly tissues consume radioactive isotopes.

PET scanning is used to reveal cerebral dysfunction associated with tumors, seizures, TIA, head trauma, Alzheimer's disease, Parkinson's disease, MS, and some mental illnesses. In addition, a PET scan can be used to evaluate the effect of drug therapy and neurosurgery.

SKULL AND SPINAL X-RAYS

Skull X-rays are typically taken from two angles: anteroposterior and lateral. The physician may order other angles, including Waters view, or occipitomental projection, to examine the frontal and maxillary sinuses, facial bones, and eye orbits.

Skull X-rays are used to detect fractures; bony tumors or unusual calcifications; pineal displacement, which indicates a space-occupying lesion; skull or sella turcica erosion, which indicates a space-occupying lesion; and vascular abnormalities.

The physician may order anteroposterior and lateral spinal X-rays when:
▶ spinal disease is suspected
▶ injury to the cervical, thoracic, lumbar, or sacral vertebral segments exists.

Depending on the patient's condition, other X-ray images may be taken from special angles, such as the open-mouth view (to confirm odontoid fracture).

Spinal X-rays are used to detect spinal fracture; displacement and subluxation due to partial dislocation; destructive lesions, such as primary and metastatic bone tumors; arthritic changes or spondylolisthesis; structural abnormalities, such as kyphosis, scoliosis, and lordosis; and congenital abnormalities.

Angiographic studies

Angiographic studies include cerebral angiography and digital subtraction angiography (DSA).

CEREBRAL ANGIOGRAPHY

During cerebral angiography, the physician injects a radiopaque contrast medium, usually into the brachial artery (through retrograde brachial injection) or femoral artery (through catheterization).

This procedure highlights cerebral vessels, making it easier to:
▶ detect stenosis or occlusion associated with thrombus or spasm
▶ identify aneurysms and arteriovenous malformations
▶ locate vessel displacement associated with tumors, abscesses, cerebral edema, hematoma, or herniation
▶ assess collateral circulation.

DIGITAL SUBTRACTION ANGIOGRAPHY

Like cerebral angiography, DSA highlights cerebral blood vessels. DSA is done this way:
▶ Using computerized fluoroscopy, a technician takes an image of the se-

lected area, which is then stored in a computer's memory.
▶ After administering a contrast medium, the technician takes several more images.
▶ The computer produces high-resolution images by manipulating the two sets of images.

Arterial DSA requires more contrast medium than cerebral angiography but, because the dye is injected I.V., DSA doesn't increase the patient's risk of stroke and, therefore, the test can be done on an outpatient basis.

Comparing normal and abnormal cerebral angiograms

The angiograms below show the differences between normal and abnormal cerebral vasculature. The cerebral angiogram on the left is normal. The cerebral angiogram on the right shows occluded blood vessels caused by a large arteriovenous malformation.

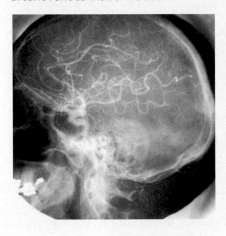 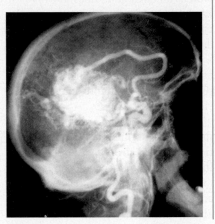

Electrophysiologic studies

Common electrophysiologic studies include EEG and evoked potential studies.

ELECTRO-ENCEPHALOGRAPHY

An EEG records the brain's electrical activity through electrodes attached to the patient's scalp. Then, this information is transmitted to an electroencephalograph, which records the resulting brain waves on recording paper. The procedure may be performed in a special laboratory or by a portable unit at the bedside.

Ambulatory recording EEGs are available for the patient to wear at home or the workplace to record brain activity as he performs his normal daily activities. Continuous-video EEG recording is available on an inpatient basis for identifying epileptic discharges during clinical events or for localization of a seizure focus during surgical evaluation of epilepsy. Intracranial electrodes are surgically implanted to record EEG changes for localization of the seizure focus. An EEG can help determine the presence and type of seizure disorder; aid in the diagnosis of intracranial lesions, such

as abscesses and tumors; evaluate the brain's electrical activity in those with metabolic disease, cerebral ischemia, head injury, meningitis, encephalitis, mental retardation, or psychological disorders or who are receiving drug therapy; and evaluate altered states of consciousness or brain death.

EEG records a portion of the brain's electrical activity as waves; some are irregular, whereas others demonstrate frequent patterns. Among the basic waveforms are the alpha, beta, theta, and delta rhythms.

Looking at an EEG

The generation of large EEG signals by synchronous activity. (a) In a population of pyramidal cells under an EEG electrode, each neuron receives many synaptic inputs. (b) If the inputs fire at irregular intervals, the pyramidal cell responses aren't synchronized, and EEG sum is small. (c) If the same number of inputs fire in a narrow time window so that the pyramidal cell responses are synchronized, the resulting EEG sum is much larger.

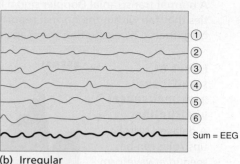

EEG electrode

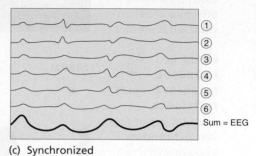

(b) Irregular

Sum = EEG

(c) Synchronized

Sum = EEG

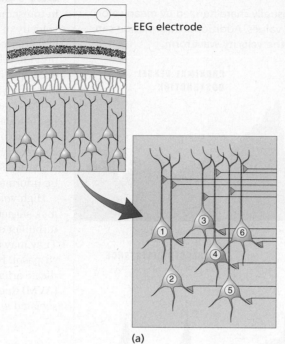

(a)

EVOKED POTENTIAL STUDIES

Evoked potential studies are used to measure the nervous system's electrical response to a visual, auditory, or sensory stimulus. The results are used to detect subclinical lesions such as tumors of cranial nerve VIII and complicating lesions in a patient with multiple sclerosis.

Evoked potential studies are also useful in diagnosing blindness and deafness in infants.

Other tests

Other neurologic tests include lumbar puncture, myelography, and transcranial Doppler studies.

LUMBAR PUNCTURE

During lumbar puncture, a sterile needle is inserted into the subarachnoid space of the spinal canal, usually between the third and fourth lumbar vertebrae. A physician does the lumbar puncture, with a nurse assisting. It requires sterile technique and careful patient positioning.

Lumbar puncture is used to:
▶ detect blood in cerebrospinal fluid (CSF)
▶ obtain CSF specimens for laboratory analysis

▶ inject dyes or gases for contrast in radiologic studies.

It's also used to administer drugs or anesthetics.

Lumbar puncture is contraindicated in patients with lumbar deformity or infection at the puncture site.

MYELOGRAPHY

Myelography uses fluoroscopy and radiography to evaluate the spinal subarachnoid space after injection of a contrast medium. Because the contrast medium is heavier than CSF, it flows through the subarachnoid space to the dependent area when the patient, lying prone on a fluoroscopic table, is tilted up or down. The fluoroscope al-

lows the physician to see the flow of the contrast medium and the outline of the subarachnoid space. X-rays are taken to provide a permanent record.

Myelography can help evaluate and determine the cause of neurologic symptoms (numbness, pain, weakness), identify lesions, such as tumors and herniated intervertebral disks that partially or totally block the flow of CSF in the subarachnoid space, and help detect arachnoiditis, spinal nerve root injury, or tumors in the posterior fossa of the skull. It may be performed to confirm the need for surgery.

Comparing velocity waveforms

A normal transcranial Doppler signal is usually characterized by mean velocities that fall within the normal reported values. Additional information can be gathered by evaluating the shape of the velocity waveform.

Effect of significant proximal vessel obstruction

A delayed systolic upstroke can be seen in a waveform when significant proximal vessel obstruction is present.

Effect of increased cerebrovascular resistance

Changes in cerebrovascular resistance, as occur with increased intracranial pressure, cause a decrease in diastolic flow.

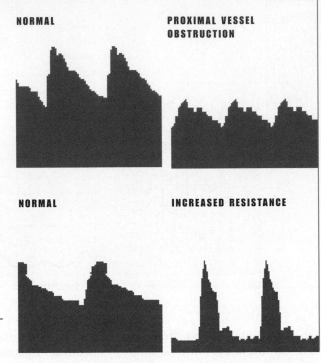

NORMAL

PROXIMAL VESSEL OBSTRUCTION

NORMAL

INCREASED RESISTANCE

TRANSCRANIAL DOPPLER STUDIES

In transcranial Doppler studies, the velocity of blood flow through cerebral arteries is measured. The results provide information about the presence, quality, and changing nature of blood flow to an area of the brain.

The types of waveforms and velocities obtained by testing indicate whether disease exists. Test results commonly aren't definitive, but this is a noninvasive way to obtain diagnostic information.

High velocities are typically abnormal, suggesting that blood flow is too turbulent or the vessel is too narrow. They may also indicate stenosis or vasospasm. High velocities may also indicate arteriovenous malformation (AVM) due to the extra blood flow associated with stenosis or vasospasm.

TREATMENTS AND PROCEDURES

Treatments for patients with neurologic dysfunction may include medication therapy, surgery, and other forms of treatment.

Medication therapy

For many of your patients with neurologic disorders, medication or drug therapy is essential. For example:
▶ thrombolytics are used to treat patients with acute ischemic stroke
▶ anticonvulsants are used to control seizures
▶ corticosteroids are used to reduce inflammation.

Types of drugs commonly used to treat patients with neurologic disorders include: analgesics, anticonvulsants, anticoagulants and antiplatelets, barbiturates, benzodiazepines, calcium channel blockers, corticosteroids, diuretics, and thrombolytics.

When caring for a patient receiving medication, stay alert for severe adverse reactions and interactions with other drugs. Some drugs such as barbiturates also carry a high risk of toxicity.

Successful therapy hinges on strict adherence to the medication schedule. Compliance is especially critical for drugs that require steady blood levels for therapeutic effectiveness such as anticonvulsants.

ANALGESICS
▶ May be opioid or nonopioid
▶ Used for mild to moderate pain
▶ Examples: morphine and codeine (opioid) and acetaminophen (Tylenol) (nonopioid)

ANTICONVULSANTS
▶ Used to treat seizure disorders or seizures during surgery or non-epileptic seizures after head trauma
▶ Examples: phenytoin (Dilantin), fosphenytoin (Cerebyx), carbamazepine (Tegretol), phenobarbital, gabapentin (Neurontin) and primidone (Mysoline), valproic acid (Depakene), clonazepam (Klonopin), and ethosuximide (Zarontin)

ANTICOAGULANTS
▶ Used for embolism prophylaxis after cerebral thrombosis
▶ Example: heparin

ANTIPLATELETS
▶ Used for thrombolytic stroke prophylaxis, transient ischemic attacks, and thromboembolic disorders
▶ Example: clopidogrel (Plavix)

BARBITURATES
▶ Used for seizure disorders and febrile seizures in children; may also be used for sedation and drug withdrawal
▶ Example: phenobarbital

BENZODIAZEPINES
▶ Used for seizures disorders, alcohol withdrawal, anxiety, and agitation
▶ Examples: clonazepam, diazepam (Valium), lorazepam (Ativan)

CALCIUM CHANNEL BLOCKERS
▶ Used for neurologic deficits caused by cerebral vasospasm after congenital aneurysm rupture
▶ Example: nimodipine (Nimotop)

CORTICOSTEROIDS
▶ Used to treat cerebral edema and severe inflammation
▶ Examples: dexamethasone (Decadron), methylprednisolone (Medrol)

DIURETICS
▶ Loop diuretics used to treat edema and hypertension
▶ Osmotic diuretics used to treat cerebral edema and increased intracranial pressure (ICP)
▶ Examples: furosemide (Lasix [loop diuretic]) and mannitol (Osmitrol [osmotic diuretic])

THROMBOLYTICS
▶ Used to treat acute ischemic stroke
▶ Examples: alteplase (Activase) and streptokinase (Streptase)

OTHER MEDICATION THERAPY
Antibiotics
▶ Prophylaxis to neurosurgical treatments or to treat existing infection, as with a brain or spinal abscess, or meningitis
▶ Treat another existing infection such as a urinary tract infection
▶ Type based on patient allergies and type of infection

Barbiturate coma
▶ Ordered when conventional treatments, such as fluid restriction, diuretic or corticosteroid therapy, or ventricular shunting, don't correct sustained or acute episodes of increased ICP
▶ Drug reduces the patient's metabolic rate and cerebral blood flow
▶ Goal is to relieve increased ICP and protect cerebral tissue by increasing cerebral perfusion pressures
▶ Last resort for patients with:
– acute ICP elevation (greater than 40 mm Hg)
– persistent ICP elevation (greater than 20 mm Hg)
– rapidly deteriorating neurologic status that's unresponsive to other treatments
▶ Example: I.V. phenobarbital (Luminal)

Chemotherapy
▶ May be used in conjunction with surgery and radiation therapy to treat brain tumors
▶ Chemotherapeutic agents are specific for the individual based on the type of cancer being treated

Neuromuscular blockade
▶ May be necessary when ICP can't be controlled through other measures
▶ May also be necessary to increase cerebral perfusion pressures in the patient with acute respiratory failure whose oxygenation isn't improving secondary to inverted inspiratory: expiratory ratio
▶ Examples: rocuronium (Zemuron), cisatracurium (Nimbex)

Surgery

Surgery is commonly the only viable treatment when a neurologic disorder is life-threatening. Instances such as brain tumors may be nonemergent. Surgery may need to be emergent in such circumstances as cerebral hemorrhage.

You may be responsible for the patient's care before and after surgery. The prospect of surgery usually causes fear and anxiety, so provide emotional support to the patient and his family. Answer their questions as completely as possible. Postoperative care may include teaching about diverse topics, such as ventricular shunt care and tips about cosmetic care after craniotomy.

Clipping a cerebral aneurysm

The clip, which is made of materials that won't affect metal detectors and that won't rust, is placed at the base of the aneurysm to stop the blood supply. The clip remains in place permanently.

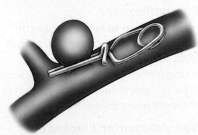

CEREBRAL ANEURYSM REPAIR

Surgical intervention is the only sure way to prevent rupture or rebleeding of a cerebral aneurysm.

With cerebral aneurysm repair, a craniotomy is performed to expose the aneurysm. Depending on the shape and location of the aneurysm, the surgeon then uses one of several corrective techniques, such as:
- clamping the affected artery
- wrapping the aneurysm wall with a biological or synthetic material
- clipping or ligating the aneurysm.

CRANIECTOMY

A craniectomy is a surgical procedure that removes part of the skull. It's performed to remove bone fragments from a skull fracture, or for decompression of the brain. It's usually performed after a traumatic head injury.

CRANIOTOMY

During craniotomy, a surgical opening into the skull exposes the brain. This procedure allows various treatments, such as ventricular shunting, excision of a tumor or abscess, hematoma aspiration, and aneurysm clipping (placing one or more surgical clips on the neck of an aneurysm to destroy it).

DEEP BRAIN STIMULATION

Deep brain stimulation (DBS) is a surgical procedure done to insert a neurotransmitter that delivers electrical stimulation to a targeted area to help control disabling neurological symptoms, such as essential tremors. The device is similar to a pacemaker. It's used to treat Parkinson's disease in the patient whose symptoms aren't adequately controlled by medication. The DBS system is made up of an electrode, an extension, and a neurotransmitter. The electrode is implanted into the targeted area of the brain through a small hole. The extension is threaded under the skin of the neck and shoulder and connected to the neurotransmitter, which is implanted under the collarbone.

SPINAL SURGERY

Surgery on the spine is performed when a herniated disk causes sensory loss, paresis, loss of sphincter control, compression of the spinal cord, severe, unrelenting pain, or sciatica that interferes with lifestyle. Spinal surgery may be performed with spinal trauma when there's evidence of spinal cord compression, penetrating wound or bone fragment in the spinal canal, or compound fracture of the vertebrae. The procedures that are performed may include:
- laminoplasty or posterior, anterior, or lateral laminectomy
- diskectomy
- hemilaminectomy
- spinal fusion
- foraminotomy
- microdiskectomy.

VENTRICULAR SHUNT

A ventricular shunt is a tube that's surgically inserted into one of the ventricles of the brain in order to drain cerebrospinal fluid (CSF) to reduce or prevent increased intracranial pressure (ICP). It's used to treat hydrocephalus. The shunt system is composed of a catheter, a reservoir, a one-way valve, and a terminal catheter. The catheter is inserted into the ventricle, with the reservoir resting on the mastoid bone. The reservoir is used to obtain CSF samples and to perform "pumping" of the shunt, which flushes the catheter of exudates that could cause obstruction. The one-way valve prevents CSF reflux and is set to open and drain CSF when the ICP reaches a level determined by the neurologist. The terminal catheter drains the CSF into the subarachnoid space, abdomen, or vena cava.

Looking at craniotomy

In a craniotomy, the surgeon makes an incision into the skull to expose the brain for such procedures as aneurysm clipping, tumor or abscess excision, hematoma aspiration, or ventricular shunting.

A window to the brain

To perform a craniotomy, the surgeon incises the skin, clamps the aponeurotic layer, and retracts the skin flap. Then he incises and retracts the muscle layer and scrapes the periosteum off the skull.

Using an air-driven or electric drill, the surgeon drills a series of burr holes in the corners of the skull incision. During drilling, warm saline solution is dripped into the burr holes, and the holes are suctioned to remove bone dust.

For a more complex lesion, such as a tumor or an aneurysm, the surgeon uses a dural elevator to separate the dura from the bone around the margin of each burr hole. Then he saws between burr holes to create a bone flap. He either leaves this flap attached to the muscle and retracts it or detaches the flap completely and removes it. In either case, the flap is wrapped to keep it moist and protected.

Finally, the surgeon incises and retracts the dura, exposing the brain.

INITIAL INCISION

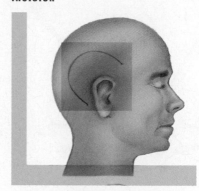

BURR HOLES DRILLED TO CREATE BONE FLAP

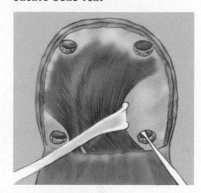

DURA EXPOSED

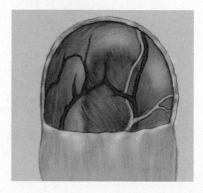

BRAIN EXPOSED

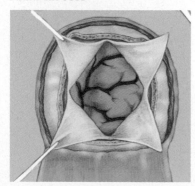

Understanding deep brain stimulation

The deep brain stimulation system consists of the stimulating lead (which is implanted to the desired target), the extension cable (which is tunneled under the scalp and soft tissues of the neck to the anterior chest wall), and the pulse generator (which is the programmable source of the electrical impulses). This illustration shows the placement of the stimulator in the patient's body.

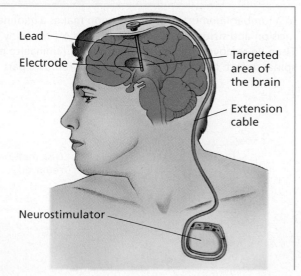

Lead

Electrode

Targeted area of the brain

Extension cable

Neurostimulator

Looking at laminoplasty

During laminoplasty, the surgeon removes the damaged lamina (see illustrations 1 and 2). The lamina is repaired using an allographic bone material and then secured with titanium screws and plates (see illustrations 3 and 4).

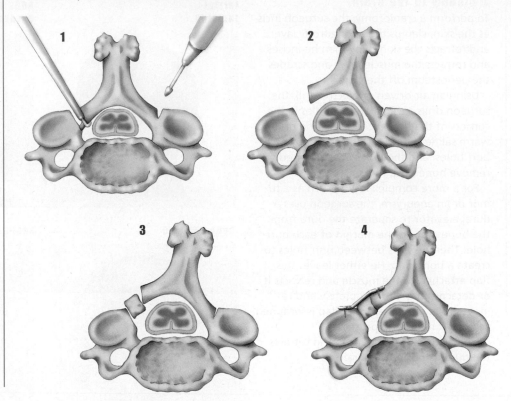

Removing disk material during a lumbar laminectomy

In a lumbar laminectomy, the surgeon makes a midline vertical incision and strips the fascia and muscles off the bony laminae. Then he removes one or more sections of laminae to expose the spinal defect. If the disk is herniated, he removes part or all of it.

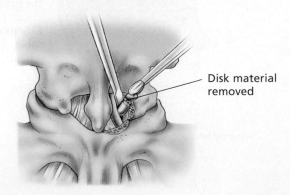

Disk material removed

Microdiskectomy

Microdiskectomy is a minimally invasive procedure performed with the aid of a surgical microscope. In a lumbar microdiskectomy, the surgeon makes a small incision in the patient's back for passage of the microscope and microsurgical instruments. Using a microsurgical grasping device, he carefully retracts the nerve root and removes disk fragments.

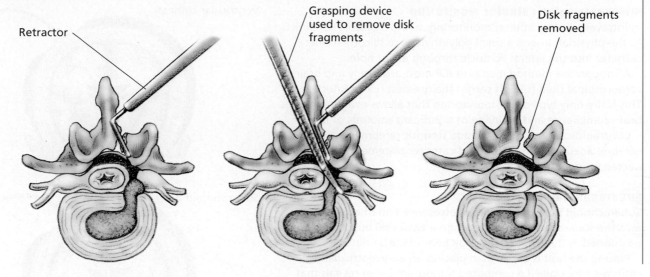

Retractor

Grasping device used to remove disk fragments

Disk fragments removed

Other treatments

Other treatments include cerebrospinal fluid (CSF) drainage, intracranial pressure (ICP) monitoring, plasmapheresis, and stereotactic radiosurgery.

CEREBROSPINAL FLUID DRAINAGE

The goal of CSF drainage is to reduce ICP to the desired level and keep it at that level. Fluid is withdrawn from the lateral ventricle through ventriculostomy.

To place the ventricular drain, a physician inserts a ventricular catheter through a burr hole in the patient's skull. This is usually done in the operating room but can be done at the bedside in the emergency department or the intensive care unit.

INTRACRANIAL PRESSURE MONITORING

With ICP monitoring, pressure exerted by the brain, blood, and CSF against the inside of the skull is measured. ICP monitoring enables prompt intervention, which can avert damage caused by cerebral hypoxia and shifts of brain mass.

Indications for ICP monitoring include:

▸ head trauma with bleeding or edema
▸ overproduction or insufficient absorption of CSF
▸ cerebral hemorrhage
▸ space-occupying lesions.

There are four basic types of ICP monitoring systems. Regardless of which system is used, the insertion procedure is always performed by a neurosurgeon in the operating room,

emergency department, or critical care unit. Insertion of an ICP monitoring device requires sterile technique to reduce the risk of central nervous system infection.

The physician inserts a ventricular catheter or subarachnoid screw through a twist-drill hole created in the skull. Some devices have built-in transducers that convert ICP to electrical impulses that allow constant monitoring.

Understanding ICP monitoring systems

Intracranial pressure (ICP) can be monitored using one of four systems.

Intraventricular catheter monitoring

In intraventricular catheter monitoring, which monitors ICP directly, the physician inserts a small polyethylene or silicone rubber catheter into the lateral ventricle through a burr hole.

Although this method measures ICP most accurately and drains cerebrospinal fluid (CSF), it carries the greatest risk of infection. This is the only type of ICP monitoring that allows evaluation of brain compliance and drainage of significant amounts of CSF.

Contraindications usually include stenotic cerebral ventricles, cerebral aneurysms in the path of catheter placement, and suspected vascular lesions.

Ventricular catheter

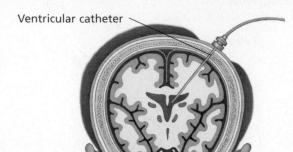

Subarachnoid bolt monitoring

Subarachnoid bolt monitoring involves insertion of a special bolt into the subarachnoid space through a twist-drill burr hole that's positioned in the front of the skull behind the hairline.

Placing the bolt is easier than placing an intraventricular catheter, especially if a computed tomography scan reveals that the cerebrum has shifted or the ventricles have collapsed. This type of ICP monitoring also carries less risk of infection and parenchymal damage because the bolt doesn't penetrate the cerebrum.

Subarachnoid bolt

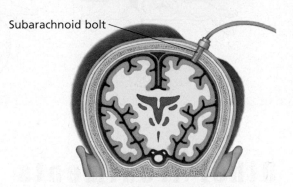

Epidural or subdural sensor monitoring

ICP can also be monitored from the epidural or subdural space. For epidural monitoring, a fiber-optic sensor is inserted into the epidural space through a burr hole. This system's main drawback is its questionable accuracy because ICP isn't being measured directly from a CSF-filled space.

For subdural monitoring, a fiber-optic transducer-tipped catheter is tunneled through a burr hole, and its tip is placed on brain tissue under the dura mater. The main drawback to this method is its inability to drain CSF.

Epidural sensor

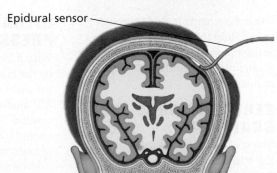

Intraparenchymal monitoring

In intraparenchymal monitoring, the physician inserts a catheter through a small subarachnoid bolt and, after puncturing the dura, advances the catheter a few centimeters into the brain's white matter. There's no need to balance or calibrate the equipment after insertion.

Although this method doesn't provide direct access to CSF, measurements are accurate because brain tissue pressures correlate well with ventricular pressures. Intraparenchymal monitoring may be used to obtain ICP measurements in patients with compressed or dislocated ventricles.

Dura mater
Arachnoid
White matter

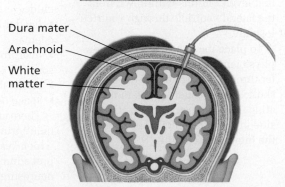

Setting up an ICP monitoring system

To set up an intracranial pressure (ICP) monitoring system, follow these steps.

▸ Begin by opening a sterile towel. On the sterile field, place a 20-ml luer-lock syringe, an 18G needle, a 250-ml bag filled with normal saline solution (with outer wrapper removed), and a disposable transducer.
▸ Put on sterile gloves and gown as per your facility's policy, and fill the 20-ml syringe with normal saline solution from the I.V. bag.
▸ Remove the injection cap from the patient line and attach the syringe. Turn the system stopcock off to the short end of the patient line, and flush through to the drip chamber (as shown). Allow a few drops to flow through the flow chamber (the manometer), the tubing, and the one-way valve into the drainage bag. (Fill the tubing and the manometer slowly to minimize air bubbles. If any air bubbles surface, be sure to force them from the system.) In some systems, the drainage system will prime itself with the patient's cerebrospinal fluid (CSF).

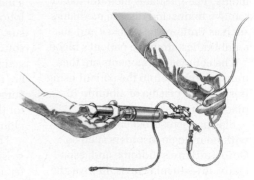

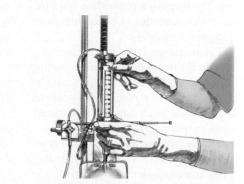

▸ Attach the manometer to the I.V. pole at the head of the bed.
▸ Slide the drip chamber onto the manometer, and align the chamber to the zero point (as shown), which should be at the inner canthus of the patient's eye.
▸ Next, connect the transducer to the monitor.
▸ Put on a clean pair of sterile gloves.
▸ Keeping one hand sterile, turn the patient stopcock off to the patient.

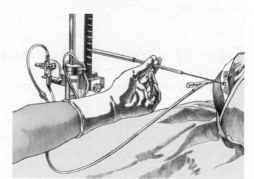

▸ Align the zero point with the center line of the patient's head, level with the middle of the ear (as shown).
▸ Lower the flow chamber to zero, and turn the stopcock off to the dead-end cap. With a clean hand, balance the system according to monitor guidelines.

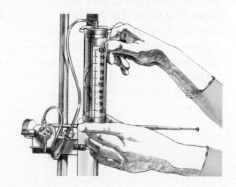

▸ Turn the system stopcock off to drainage, and raise the flow chamber to the ordered height (as shown).
▸ Return the stopcock to the ordered position, and observe the monitor for the return of ICP patterns.

PLASMAPHERESIS

Plasmapheresis is the process of plasma exchange, in which blood from the patient flows into a cell separator and it separates plasma from formed elements. The plasma is then filtered to remove toxins and disease mediators, such as immune complexes and autoantibodies, from the patient's blood.

The cellular components are then transfused back into the patient using fresh frozen plasma or albumin in place of the plasma removed.

Plasmapheresis benefits patients with neurologic disorders such as Guillain-Barré syndrome and, especially, myasthenia gravis. In myasthenia gravis, plasmapheresis is used to remove circulating antiacetylcholine receptor antibodies.

Plasmapheresis is used most commonly for patients with long-standing neuromuscular disease, but it can also be used to treat patients with acute exacerbations. Some acutely ill patients require treatment up to four times per week; others, about once every 2 weeks. When it's successful, treatment may relieve symptoms for months, but results vary.

STEREOTACTIC RADIOSURGERY

Stereotactic radiosurgery is a noninvasive procedure that uses radiation to treat brain tumors and other brain abnormalities, and as postsurgery follow-up to treat leftover tumor tissue. Three-dimensional computer software is used to plan specific targeting of the radiation beams. There are three types of stereotactic radiosurgery: gamma knife, linear accelerator (LINAC), and proton beam or cyclotron.

This treatment may involve a single session or multiple small sessions often completed in one day. If the patient requires fractionated treatment (sessions completed over weeks or months), it's called *stereotactic radiotherapy.*

Because this surgery is noninvasive, risks and complications are decreased. It provides a treatment option in cases where invasive surgery isn't recommended due to lesion location or the patient's age or condition.

Types of stereotactic radiosurgery

The three types of stereotactic radiosurgery differ in the type of instrument used and the source of radiation.

Gamma knife surgery

Gamma knife surgery is used to treat brain tumors that are 3.5 cm or less, arteriovenous malformations, and other brain dysfunctions, such as trigeminal neuralgia and seizures. It uses 201 beams of highly focused gamma radiation that targets the lesion, leaving surrounding tissue unharmed. One dose causes the lesion to slowly reduce in size and eventually dissolve.

Linear accelerator (LINAC)

LINAC machines deliver high-energy photons or electrons in curving paths around the patient's head. This type of radiation is effective on large tumors and can be used for fractionation of treatment. LINAC machines are also used for Intensity-Modulated Radiation Therapy (IMRT). IMRT is an advanced type of high-precision radiotherapy that conforms to the shape of the target and utilizes higher radiation doses.

Proton beam radiosurgery

Proton beam radiosurgery uses the quantum wave properties of protons (through use of a cyclotron) to reduce the amount of radiation to tissue surrounding the target to zero. It can be used for unusual-shaped tumors, skull base tumors, and vascular malformations of the brain.

Chapter 5

Gastrointestinal care

DISEASES
Appendicitis

Appendicitis, the most common major surgical disease, is an inflammation of the vermiform appendix, a small, fingerlike projection attached to the cecum just below the ileocecal valve. This disorder occurs at any age, affecting both sexes equally; however, between puberty and age 25, it's more prevalent in men. Since the advent of antibiotics, the incidence and mortality of appendicitis have declined. If untreated, this disease is fatal.

Appendicitis occurs when the appendix becomes inflamed from ulceration of the mucosa or obstruction of the lumen. It may result from an obstruction of the appendiceal lumen, caused by a fecal mass, stricture, barium ingestion, or viral infection. This obstruction sets off an inflammatory process that can lead to infection, thrombosis, necrosis, and perforation.

PICTURING PATHO

Appendix obstruction and inflammation

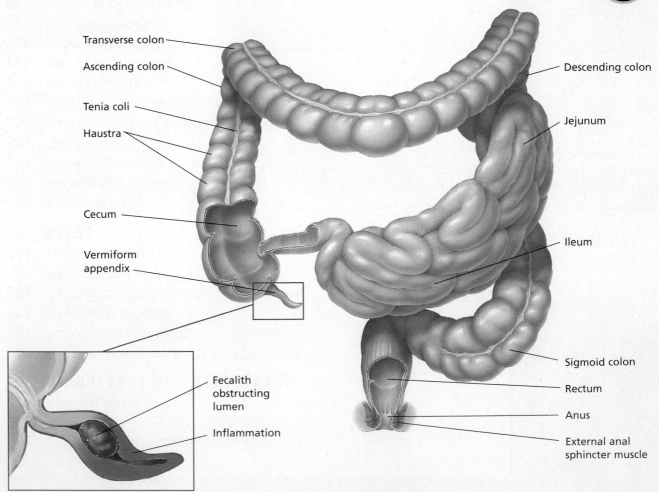

- Transverse colon
- Ascending colon
- Tenia coli
- Haustra
- Cecum
- Vermiform appendix
- Descending colon
- Jejunum
- Ileum
- Sigmoid colon
- Rectum
- Anus
- External anal sphincter muscle

- Fecalith obstructing lumen
- Inflammation

Signs and symptoms

▸ Abdominal pain (initially generalized but within a few hours becomes localized in the right lower abdomen [McBurney point]; worsens on gentle percussion and when the patient coughs)
▸ Anorexia
▸ Nausea
▸ Vomiting (one or two episodes)
▸ Low-grade fever
▸ Malaise
▸ Constipation
▸ Walking bent over to reduce right lower quadrant pain
▸ Sleeping or lying supine, keeping right knee bent up to decrease pain
▸ Normal bowel sounds
▸ Rebound tenderness and spasm of abdominal muscles common (pain in the right lower quadrant from palpating the lower left quadrant)
▸ Abdominal tenderness completely absent, if appendix positioned retrocecally or in the pelvis; instead, flank tenderness revealed by rectal or pelvic examination
▸ Abdominal rigidity and tenderness that worsen as condition progresses; sudden cessation of abdominal pain signaling perforation or infarction

HANDS ON

Eliciting abdominal pain

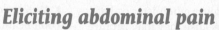

A positive response to the following tests helps diagnose appendicitis. Rebound tenderness and the iliopsoas and obturator signs can indicate such conditions as appendicitis and peritonitis.

Rebound tenderness

▸ Help the patient into a supine position with his knees flexed to relax the abdominal muscles.
▸ Place your hands gently on the right lower quadrant at the McBurney point (located about midway between the umbilicus and the anterior superior iliac spine).
▸ Slowly and deeply dip your fingers into the area; then release the pressure in a quick, smooth motion.
▸ Pain on release—rebound tenderness—is a positive sign. The pain may radiate to the umbilicus.

Iliopsoas sign

▸ Help the patient into a supine position with his legs straight.
▸ Instruct him to raise his right leg upward as you exert slight downward pressure with your hand on his right thigh.
▸ Repeat the maneuver with the left leg.
▸ When testing either leg, increased abdominal pain is a positive result, indicating irritation of the psoas muscle.

Obturator sign

▸ Help the patient into a supine position with his right leg flexed 90 degrees at the hip and knee.
▸ Hold the leg just above the knee and at the ankle; then rotate the leg laterally and medially.
▸ Pain in the hypogastric region is a positive sign, indicating irritation of the obturator muscle.

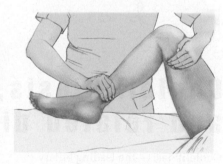

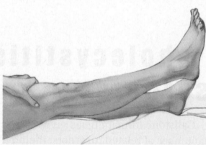

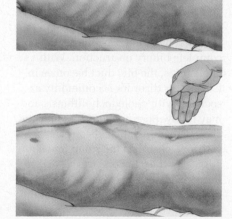

Treatment
▶ Appendectomy
▶ GI intubation, parenteral fluid and electrolyte replacement, and antibiotics (for peritonitis)

Nursing considerations
▶ Make sure the patient with suspected or known appendicitis receives nothing by mouth until surgery is performed.
▶ Administer I.V. fluids to prevent dehydration. Never administer cathartics or enemas because they may rupture the appendix.
▶ Don't administer analgesics until the diagnosis is confirmed because they mask symptoms.
▶ Place the patient in Fowler's position to reduce pain. (This is also helpful postoperatively.)
▶ Never apply heat to the right lower abdomen; this can cause the appendix to rupture.
▶ Provide preoperative care, including giving prescribed medications.

After appendectomy
▶ Monitor vital signs and intake and output.
▶ Give analgesics as ordered.
▶ Administer I.V. fluids, as needed, to maintain fluid and electrolyte balance.
▶ Document bowel sounds, passing of flatus, or bowel movements (signs of peristalsis). These signs in a patient whose nausea and boardlike abdominal rigidity have subsided indicate readiness to resume oral fluids.
▶ Watch closely for possible surgical complications, such as an abscess or wound dehiscence.
▶ If peritonitis occurs, nasogastric drainage may be necessary to decompress the stomach and reduce nausea and vomiting. If so, record drainage. Provide mouth and nose care.

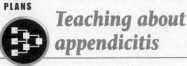

LESSON PLANS

Teaching about appendicitis

▶ Explain to the patient what happens in appendicitis.
▶ Help the patient understand the required surgery and its possible complications. If time allows, provide preoperative teaching.
▶ Teach the patient how to care for the incision. If he has a surgical dressing, demonstrate how to change it properly. Instruct him to observe the incision daily and to report any swelling, redness, bleeding, drainage, or warmth at the site.
▶ Review the proper use of all prescribed medications. Make sure the patient knows how to administer each drug and understands the desired effects and possible adverse reactions.
▶ Discuss postoperative activity limitations. Tell the patient to follow the practitioner's orders for driving, returning to work, and resuming physical activity.

Cholelithiasis, cholecystitis, and related disorders

Cholelithiasis—the leading biliary tract disease—is the formation of stones or calculi (also called *gallstones*) in the gallbladder. The prognosis is usually good with treatment; however, if infection occurs, the prognosis depends on the infection's severity and its response to antibiotics. Generally, gallbladder and duct diseases occur during middle age. Between ages 20 and 50, they're six times more common in women, but the incidence in men and women equalizes after age 50, increasing with each succeeding decade.

Gallstone formation can give rise to a number of related disorders, including cholecystitis, choledocholithiasis, cholangitis, and gallstone ileus. The type of disorder that develops depends on where in the gallbladder or biliary tract the calculi collect. Although the exact cause of gallstone formation is unknown, abnormal metabolism of cholesterol and bile salts clearly plays an important role.

With cholecystitis, the gallbladder becomes acutely or chronically inflamed, usually because a gallstone becomes lodged in the cystic duct, causing painful gallbladder distention. In choledocholithiasis, gallstones pass out of the gallbladder and lodge in the common bile duct, causing partial or complete biliary obstruction. With cholangitis, the bile duct becomes infected; this disorder is commonly associated with choledocholithiasis and may follow percutaneous transhepatic cholangiography. In gallstone ileus, a gallstone obstructs the small bowel. Typically, the gallstone travels through a fistula between the gallbladder and small bowel and lodges at the ileocecal valve.

How gallstones form

Gallstone formation (or cholecystitis) happens when cholesterol and bile salts are abnormally metabolized. A normal liver continuously produces bile that's concentrated and stored in the gallbladder until the duodenum needs it to help digest fat. If changes in bile composition or the gallbladder's lining occur, gallstones form. Cholecystitis may be acute or chronic. Acute cholecystitis is usually due to partial or complete obstruction of bile flow. The figures below illustrate how gallstones form.

Liver function

Certain conditions, such as age, obesity, and estrogen imbalance, cause the liver to secrete bile that's abnormally high in cholesterol or lacking the proper concentration of bile salts.

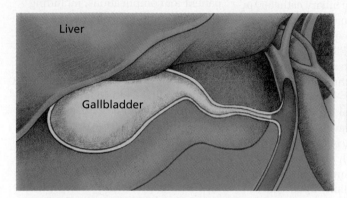

Gallstone obstruction

If a stone lodges in the common bile duct, the bile can't flow into the duodenum. Bilirubin is absorbed into the blood and causes jaundice.

Biliary narrowing and swelling of the tissue around the stone can also cause irritation and inflammation of the common bile duct.

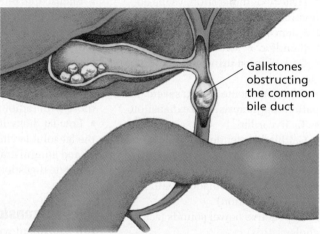

Gallstone formation

When the gallbladder concentrates this bile, inflammation may occur. Excessive reabsorption of water and bile salts makes the bile less soluble. Cholesterol, calcium, and bilirubin precipitate into gallstones.

Fat entering the duodenum causes the intestinal mucosa to secrete the hormone cholecystokinin, which stimulates the gallbladder to contract and empty. If a stone lodges in the cystic duct, the gallbladder contracts but can't empty.

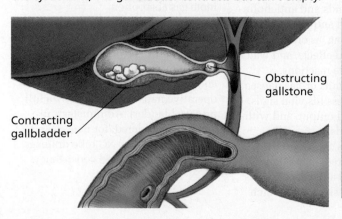

Common bile duct inflammation

Inflammation can progress up the biliary tree into any of the bile ducts. This causes scar tissue, fluid accumulation, cirrhosis, portal hypertension, and bleeding.

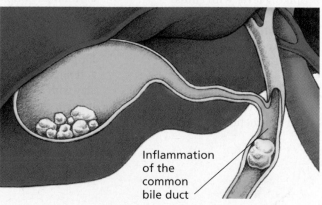

Signs and symptoms
◗ Possibly no symptoms, even when X-rays reveal gallstones

Cholecystitis
◗ Sudden onset of severe steady or aching pain in the midepigastric region or right upper abdominal quadrant
◗ Pain that radiates to the back, between the shoulder blades or over the right shoulder blade, or just to the shoulder area (known as *biliary colic*)
◗ Attack that occurs suddenly after eating a fatty meal or a large meal after fasting for an extended time
◗ Nausea, vomiting, chills, and a low-grade fever
◗ History of indigestion, vague abdominal discomfort, belching, and flatulence after eating high-fat foods
◗ Jaundice
◗ Dark-colored urine and clay-colored stools
◗ During an acute attack, severe pain, pallor, diaphoresis, and exhaustion
◗ Tachycardia
◗ Gallbladder tenderness that increases on inspiration
◗ A painless, sausagelike mass (in calculus-filled gallbladder without ductal obstruction)
◗ Hypoactive bowel sounds (acute cholecystitis)

Cholangitis
◗ History of choledocholithiasis and classic symptoms of biliary colic
◗ Jaundice and pain
◗ Spiking fever with chills

Gallstone ileus
◗ Colicky pain that persists for several days
◗ Nausea and vomiting
◗ Abdominal distention
◗ Absent bowel sounds (complete bowel obstruction)

Treatment
◗ Surgery, including cholecystectomy (laparoscopic or abdominal), cholecystectomy with operative cholangiography, choledochostomy, or exploration of the common bile duct
◗ Gallstone dissolution therapy in high-risk patients with small gallstones (if gallstones are radiolucent and consist all or in part of cholesterol) with oral chenodeoxycholic acid or ursodeoxycholic acid to partially or completely dissolve gallstones
◗ Visualization and removal of calculi using a basket-shaped tool (Dormia basket) that's inserted via percutaneous transhepatic biliary catheter under fluoroscopic guidance
◗ Endoscopic retrograde cholangiopancreatography (ERCP) to remove calculi with a balloon or basketlike tool that's passed through an endoscope
◗ Lithotripsy (breaking up gallstones using ultrasonic waves); successful in those with radiolucent calculi
◗ Low-fat diet with replacement of the fat-soluble vitamins A, D, E, and K, and administration of bile salts to facilitate digestion and vitamin absorption

Nursing considerations
◗ If the patient will be managed without invasive procedures, provide a low-fat diet and small, frequent meals to help prevent attacks of biliary colic. Also replace vitamins A, D, E, and K, and administer bile salts, as ordered.
◗ Administer opioids and anticholinergics for pain, and antiemetics for nausea and vomiting, as ordered. Monitor for desired effects, and watch for possible adverse reactions.
◗ If the patient vomits or has nausea, stay with him, assess his vital signs, monitor intake and output, and withhold food and fluids.
◗ If the patient has cholangitis, give antibiotics as ordered and watch for desired effects and adverse reactions. Also monitor vital signs, and watch for signs of severe toxicity, including confusion, septicemia, and septic shock.
◗ If surgery is scheduled, provide appropriate preoperative care, which may include insertion of a nasogastric (NG) tube.

After surgery
◗ After percutaneous transhepatic biliary catheterization or ERCP to remove gallstones, assess vital signs. Allow the patient nothing by mouth until the gag reflex returns. Monitor intake and output, keeping in mind that urine retention can be a problem. Observe the patient for complications, including cholangitis and pancreatitis.
◗ Be alert for signs of bleeding, infection, or atelectasis. Evaluate the incision site for bleeding. Serosanguineous and bile drainage is common during the first 24 to 48 hours if the patient has a wound drain, such as a Jackson-Pratt or Penrose drain. If, after a choledochostomy, a T tube drain is placed in the duct and attached to a drainage bag, make sure the drainage tube has no kinks. Also make sure the connecting tubing from the T tube is well secured to the patient to prevent dislodgment. Measure and record drainage daily (200 to 300 ml is normal).
◗ If the patient underwent laparoscopic cholecystectomy, assess for "free-air" pain caused by carbon dioxide insufflation. Encourage ambulation soon after the procedure to promote gas absorption.
◗ Monitor intake and output. Provide appropriate I.V. fluid intake. Allow the patient nothing by mouth for 24 to 48 hours or until bowel sounds resume and nausea and vomiting cease (postoperative nausea may indicate a full urinary bladder). Administer antiemetics, as ordered, for nausea and vomiting. Monitor NG tube drainage for color, amount, and consistency.

▶ When peristalsis resumes, remove the NG tube and begin a clear liquid diet, advancing diet as tolerated. If the patient doesn't void within 8 hours (or if he voids an inadequate amount based on I.V. fluid intake), percuss over the symphysis pubis for bladder distention (especially in patients receiving anticholinergics). Avoid catheterization, if possible.

▶ Encourage leg exercises every hour. The patient should ambulate the evening after surgery. Encourage hourly coughing and deep breathing. Discourage sitting in a chair. Provide antiembolism stockings to support leg muscles and promote venous blood flow, thus preventing stasis and possible clot formation. Have the patient rest in semi-Fowler's position as much as possible to direct any abdominal drainage into the pelvic cavity rather than allowing it to accumulate under the diaphragm.

LESSON PLANS

Teaching about cholecystitis

▶ Teach the patient about cholecystitis and the reasons for his symptoms.

▶ Explain scheduled diagnostic tests, reviewing pretest instructions and necessary aftercare.

▶ If a low-fat diet is prescribed, suggest ways to implement it and how the changes help to prevent biliary colic. If necessary, ask the dietitian to reinforce your instructions.

▶ Review the proper use of prescribed medications, explaining their desired effects. Point out possible adverse effects, especially those that warrant a call to the practitioner.

▶ Reinforce the practitioner's explanation of the ordered treatment, such as surgery, endoscopic retrograde cholangiopancreatography, or lithotripsy. Make sure the patient fully understands the possible complications, if any, associated with his treatment.

Before and after surgery

▶ Before surgery, teach the patient to breathe deeply, cough, expectorate, and perform leg exercises that are necessary after surgery. Also teach splinting, repositioning, and ambulation techniques.

▶ Explain the procedures that will be performed before, during, and after surgery to help ease the patient's anxiety and ensure his cooperation. Teach the patient who will be discharged with a T tube how to empty it, change the dressing, and provide skin care.

▶ On discharge (usually 4 to 7 days after traditional surgery), advise the patient against heavy lifting or straining for 6 weeks. Urge him to walk daily. Tell him that food restrictions are unnecessary unless he has intolerance to a specific food or some underlying condition (diabetes, atherosclerosis, or obesity) that requires such restriction.

Cirrhosis

Cirrhosis is a chronic hepatic disease characterized by diffuse destruction and fibrotic regeneration of hepatic cells. As necrotic tissue yields to fibrosis, this disease alters liver structure and normal vasculature, impairs blood and lymph flow, and ultimately causes hepatic insufficiency. Obstruction to venous flow leads to portal hypertension, ascites, esophageal varices, and gastric varices. As the liver becomes cirrhotic, it can no longer change ammonia (waste product of protein metabolism) to urea so that it can be eliminated by the kidney. Elevated ammonia levels in the blood are thought to contribute to hepatic encephalopathy.

Most cases are a result of alcoholism, but toxins, biliary destruction, hepatitis, and a number of metabolic conditions may stimulate the destruction process. There are many types of cirrhosis; causes differ with each type and include:

Laënnec's cirrhosis—also called *portal, nutritional, or alcoholic cirrhosis*—is the most common type.

Cirrhosis is characterized by irreversible chronic injury of the liver, extensive fibrosis, and nodular tissue growth. These changes result from:
▶ liver cell death (hepatocyte necrosis)
▶ collapse of the liver's purporting structure (the reticulin network)
▶ distortion of the vascular bed (blood vessels throughout the liver)
▶ nodular regeneration of the remaining liver tissue.

Signs and symptoms
▶ Abdominal pain
▶ Diarrhea
▶ Fatigue
▶ Nausea and vomiting
▶ Chronic dyspepsia
▶ Constipation
▶ Pruritus
▶ Weight loss
▶ Tendency for frequent nosebleeds, easy bruising, and bleeding gums
▶ Changes in level of consciousness

▶ Telangiectasis on the cheeks; spider angiomas on the face, neck, arms, and trunk; gynecomastia; umbilical hernia; distended, abdominal blood vessels; ascites; testicular atrophy; palmar erythema; clubbed fingers; thigh and leg edema; ecchymosis; and jaundice
▶ Large, firm liver with a sharp edge (early phase)
▶ Decreased liver size and nodular edge due to scar tissue (late phase)
▶ Enlarged spleen

Cirrhotic changes

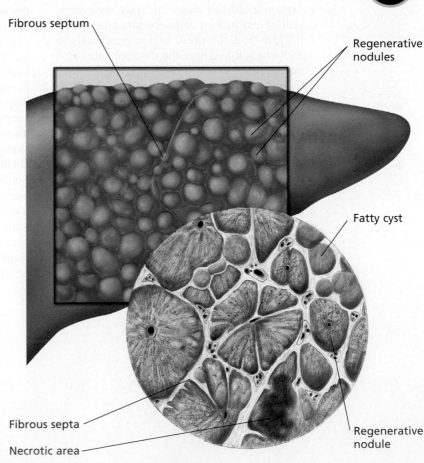

Fibrous septum

Regenerative nodules

Fatty cyst

Fibrous septa

Regenerative nodule

Necrotic area

Treatment

▶ Vitamins and nutritional supplements to promote healing of damaged hepatic cells and improve nutritional status

▶ Restricted sodium consumption (500 mg/day)

▶ Limited liquid intake (1,500 ml/day) to help manage ascites and edema

▶ Antacids and histamine antagonists to reduce gastric distress and decrease the potential for GI bleeding

▶ Potassium-sparing diuretics, such as furosemide (Lasix), to reduce ascites and edema

▶ Vasopressin for esophageal varices

▶ Rifaximin to treat acute hepatic encephalopathy

▶ Lactulose to reduce a high ammonia level

▶ Paracentesis to relieve abdominal pressure (for ascites)

▶ Peritoneovenous shunt to divert ascites into venous circulation

▶ Gastric intubation and esophageal balloon tamponade to control bleeding from esophageal varices or other GI hemorrhage

▶ Esophageal balloon tamponade to compress and stop bleeding from esophageal varices

▶ Sclerotherapy for repeated hemorrhagic episodes despite conservative treatment

▶ Blood transfusions for massive hemorrhage; crystalloid or colloid volume expanders given to maintain blood pressure

Nursing considerations

▶ Monitor vital signs, intake and output, and electrolyte levels to determine fluid volume status.

▶ To assess fluid retention, measure and record abdominal girth every shift. Weigh the patient daily and document his weight.

▶ Administer diuretics, potassium, and protein or vitamin supplements, as ordered. Restrict sodium and fluid intake as ordered.

▶ Provide or assist with oral hygiene before and after meals.

▶ Determine food preferences, and provide them within the patient's prescribed diet limitations. Provide patients with alcoholic cirrhosis small, frequent interval feedings, including a nighttime and morning snack, to improve nitrogen balance.

▶ Observe and document the degree of sclerae and skin jaundice.

▶ Provide frequent skin care, bathe the patient without soap, and massage with emollient lotions. Turn and reposition often to keep the skin intact.

▶ Observe for bleeding gums, ecchymoses, epistaxis, and petechiae. Administer blood products as ordered.

▶ Inspect stools for amount, color, and consistency. Test stools and vomitus for occult blood.

▶ Increase the patient's exercise tolerance by decreasing fluid volume and providing rest periods before exercise.

▶ Address the patient by name and tell him your name. Mention time, place, and date frequently throughout the day. Place a clock and a calendar where he can easily see them.

▶ Use appropriate safety measures to protect the patient from injury. Avoid physical restraints, if possible.

▶ Watch for signs of anxiety, epigastric fullness, restlessness, and weakness.

▶ Observe closely for signs of behavioral or personality changes. Report increasing stupor, lethargy, hallucinations, or neuromuscular dysfunction. Monitor level of consciousness. Watch for asterixis, a sign of developing encephalopathy.

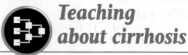

LESSON PLANS

Teaching about cirrhosis

▶ To minimize the risk of bleeding, warn the patient against taking aspirin or nonsteroidal anti-inflammatory drugs, straining to defecate, and blowing his nose or sneezing too vigorously. Suggest using an electric razor and a soft toothbrush.

▶ Advise the patient that rest and good nutrition conserve energy and decrease metabolic demands on the liver. Urge him to eat frequent, small meals. Teach him to alternate periods of rest and activity to reduce oxygen demand and prevent fatigue.

▶ Tell the patient how he can conserve energy while performing activities of daily living. For example, suggest that he sit on a bench while bathing or dressing.

▶ Stress the need to abstain from alcohol. Refer the patient to Alcoholics Anonymous, if appropriate.

Colorectal cancer

Colorectal cancer is the third most common form of cancer and the second leading cause of cancer-related deaths in the United States.

Malignant tumors of the colon or rectum are almost always adenocarcinomas. About half of these are sessile lesions of the rectosigmoid area; the rest are polypoid lesions.

Colorectal cancer progresses slowly, remaining localized for a long time. The 5-year survival rate varies based on the stage of the disease. It's poten-tially curable in 75% of patients if an early diagnosis allows resection before nodal involvement.

Although the exact cause of colorectal cancer is unknown, studies show a greater incidence in areas of higher economic development, suggesting a relationship to a diet that includes excess animal fat, especially from beef, and low fiber. Other factors that magnify the risk of developing colorectal cancer include diseases of the digestive tract, a history of ulcerative colitis, familial polyposis, and ethnicity. Blacks have the highest incidence of colorectal cancer of any race.

Signs and symptoms
Right side of colon
▶ History of black, tarry stools
▶ Anemia
▶ Abdominal aching and pressure
▶ Dull cramps
▶ Weakness
▶ Diarrhea
▶ Obstipation
▶ Anorexia
▶ Weight loss
▶ Vomiting

Left side of colon
▶ Rectal bleeding (due to hemor-rhoids)
▶ Intermittent abdominal fullness or cramping
▶ Rectal pressure
▶ Obstipation
▶ Diarrhea
▶ Ribbon- or pencil-shaped stools
▶ Passage of flatus or stool relieving pain
▶ Bleeding during defecation
▶ Dark or bright red blood in feces and mucus in or on stool

Rectal tumor
▶ Change in bowel habits
▶ Urgent need to defecate on arising (morning diarrhea) or obstipation alternating with diarrhea
▶ Blood or mucus in stool
▶ Sense of incomplete evacuation
▶ Pain that begins as a feeling of rectal fullness and progresses to a dull, sometimes constant ache confined to the rectum or sacral region
▶ Abdominal distention or visible, palpable masses
▶ Abdominal veins that appear enlarged and visible from portal obstruction
▶ Enlarged inguinal and supraclavicular nodes
▶ Abnormal bowel sounds

Types of colorectal cancer

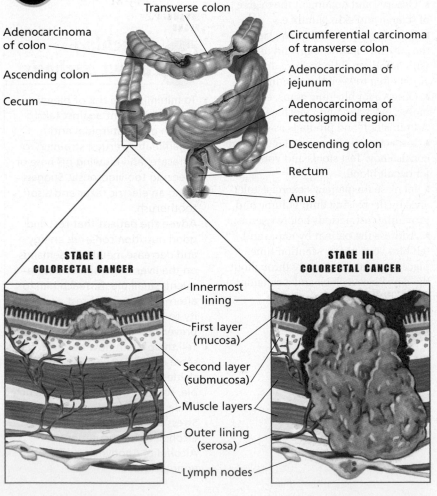

Transverse colon

Adenocarcinoma of colon

Ascending colon

Cecum

Circumferential carcinoma of transverse colon

Adenocarcinoma of jejunum

Adenocarcinoma of rectosigmoid region

Descending colon

Rectum

Anus

STAGE I COLORECTAL CANCER

STAGE III COLORECTAL CANCER

Innermost lining

First layer (mucosa)

Second layer (submucosa)

Muscle layers

Outer lining (serosa)

Lymph nodes

‣ Bulky right-sided tumors; tumors of the transverse portion more easily detected

Treatment
Cecum and ascending colon
‣ Right hemicolectomy
‣ Resection of the terminal segment of the ileum, cecum, ascending colon, and right half of the transverse colon with corresponding mesentery

Proximal and middle transverse colon
‣ Right colectomy that includes the transverse colon and mesentery corresponding to midcolic vessels, or segmental resection of the transverse colon and associated midcolic vessels

Sigmoid colon
‣ Surgery usually limited to the sigmoid colon and mesentery

Upper rectum
‣ Anterior or low anterior resection
‣ Surgery that involves the staple resection method (allows for much lower resections than previously possible)

Lower rectum
‣ Abdominoperineal resection and permanent sigmoid colostomy
‣ Chemotherapy, if metastasis has occurred or if the patient has residual disease or a recurrent inoperable tumor
‣ Fluorouracil combined with levamisole or leucovorin
‣ Fluorouracil with recombinant interferon alfa-2a (under research)
‣ Radiation therapy used preoperatively and postoperatively to induce tumor regression

Nursing considerations
‣ Before colorectal surgery, monitor the patient's diet modifications and administer laxatives, enemas, and antibiotics, as ordered.

‣ After surgery, monitor the patient's vital signs, intake and output, and fluid and electrolyte balance. Also monitor for complications.
‣ Care for the patient's incision and, if appropriate, the stoma.
‣ Encourage the patient to participate in stoma care as soon as possible. Teach hygiene and skin care.
‣ Consult with an enterostomal therapist, if available, to set up a postoperative regimen for the patient.
‣ Watch for adverse effects of radiation therapy and chemotherapy (nausea, vomiting, hair loss, malaise), and provide comfort measures and reassurance.
‣ Watch for complications of chemotherapy, such as infection and anemia.
‣ Listen to the patient's fears and concerns, and stay with him during periods of severe stress and anxiety.
‣ Whenever possible, include the patient and his family in care decisions.

LESSON PLANS

Teaching about colorectal cancer

‣ Throughout therapy, answer the patient's questions and tell him what to expect from surgery and other therapy.
‣ If appropriate, explain that the stoma will be red, moist, and swollen; reassure the patient that postoperative swelling eventually subsides.
‣ Prepare the patient for the I.V. lines, nasogastric tube, and indwelling urinary catheter he'll have postoperatively.
‣ Explain to the patient's family that their positive reactions foster the patient's adjustment.
‣ Direct the patient to follow a high-fiber diet.
‣ If flatus, diarrhea, or constipation occurs, tell the patient to eliminate suspected causative foods from his

diet. Explain that he may reintroduce them later.
‣ If diarrhea is a problem, advise the patient to eat applesauce, bananas, or rice. Caution him to take laxatives or antidiarrheal medications only as prescribed by his practitioner.
‣ When appropriate, explain that after several months, many patients with an ostomy establish control with irrigation and no longer need to wear a pouch. A stoma cap or gauze sponge placed over the stoma protects it and absorbs mucoid secretions.
‣ Tell the patient to avoid heavy lifting, which can cause herniation or prolapse through weakened muscles in the abdominal wall.

‣ Emphasize the need for keeping follow-up appointments.
‣ If the patient is to undergo radiation therapy or chemotherapy, explain the treatment to him. Make sure he understands the adverse effects that typically occur and the measures he can take to decrease their severity or prevent their occurrence.

Crohn's disease

Crohn's disease, a type of inflammatory bowel disease, may affect any part of the GI tract but usually involves the terminal ileum. The disease extends through all layers of the intestinal wall and may involve regional lymph nodes and the mesentery. When it affects only the small bowel, the disease is also known as *regional enteritis*. If it also involves the colon or only affects the colon, it's known as *Crohn's disease of the colon*. (Crohn's disease of the colon also has been termed *granulomatous colitis,* an inaccurate term because not all patients develop granulomas.)

Crohn's disease is an autoimmune disease. It's thought that an antigen initiates the inflammation, but the actual tissue damage is due to an overactive but inappropriate sustained inflammation. Genetic factors may also play a role: Crohn's disease sometimes occurs in monozygotic twins, and 10% to 20% of patients with the disease have one or more affected relatives. The first susceptibility gene, cardis, was recently discovered. Smoking doubles the risk of developing the disease and worsens the clinical course.

Inflammation spreads slowly and progressively, beginning with lymphadenia and obstructive lymphedema in the submucosa, where Peyer's patches develop in the intestinal mucosa. Lymphatic obstruction causes edema, with mucosal ulceration and development of fissures, abscesses and, sometimes, granulomas. The mucosa may acquire a characteristic "cobblestone" look.

As the disease progresses, fibrosis occurs, thickening the bowel wall and narrowing the lumen. Serositis (serosal inflammation) also develops, causing inflamed bowel loops to adhere to other diseased or normal loops. This may result in bowel shortening. Because inflammation usually occurs segmentally, the bowel may become a patchwork of healthy and diseased segments. Eventually, the diseased parts of the bowel become thicker, narrower, and shorter.

Signs and symptoms
- Fatigue, fever
- Abdominal pain
- Frequent diarrhea (usually without obvious bleeding)
- Weight loss
- Diarrhea that worsens after emotional upset or ingestion of poorly tolerated foods, such as milk, fatty foods, and spices
- Anorexia, nausea, and vomiting with abdominal pain that's steady, colicky, or cramping and that occurs in the right lower abdominal quadrant (with regional enteritis)
- Right lower abdominal quadrant tenderness
- Abdominal mass indicating adherent bowel loops

PICTURING PATHO

Bowel changes in Crohn's disease

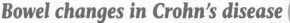

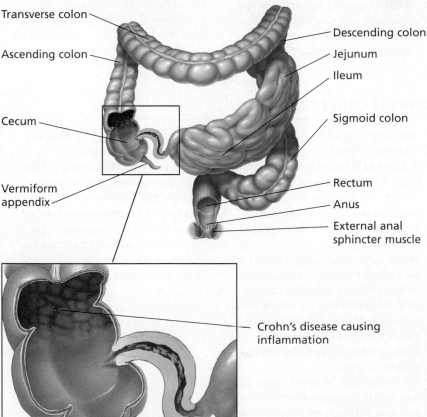

Transverse colon

Ascending colon

Cecum

Vermiform appendix

Descending colon

Jejunum

Ileum

Sigmoid colon

Rectum

Anus

External anal sphincter muscle

Crohn's disease causing inflammation

Mucosal surface of the bowel in Crohn's disease

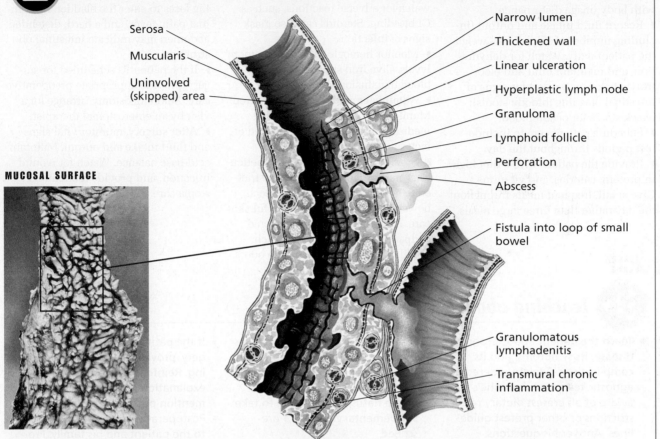

MUCOSAL SURFACE

Labels:
- Serosa
- Muscularis
- Uninvolved (skipped) area
- Narrow lumen
- Thickened wall
- Linear ulceration
- Hyperplastic lymph node
- Granuloma
- Lymphoid follicle
- Perforation
- Abscess
- Fistula into loop of small bowel
- Granulomatous lymphadenitis
- Transmural chronic inflammation

Treatment

▶ Corticosteroids, such as prednisone, to reduce signs and symptoms of diarrhea, pain, and bleeding by decreasing inflammation
▶ Immunosuppressant antimetabolite agents, such as azathioprine (Imuran), mercaptopurine (Purinethol), and methotrexate (Trexal) to suppress the body's response to antigens
▶ Sulfasalazine or mesalamine (alone or together) to reduce inflammation

▶ Metronidazole (Flagyl) to treat exacerbations and perianal complications
▶ Antidiarrheals, such as diphenoxylate and atropine, to combat diarrhea (contraindicated in patients with significant bowel obstruction)
▶ Biological agents, such as adalimumab (Humira), certolizumab (Cimzia), and infliximab (Remicade), to induce and maintain remission
▶ Opioids to control pain and diarrhea
▶ Lifestyle changes, such as stress reduction and reduced physical activity, to help rest the bowel, giving it time to heal

▶ Dietary modifications that include elimination of high-fiber foods (fruits or vegetables) and foods that irritate the mucosa (dairy products, and spicy and fatty foods); avoidance of foods that stimulate excessive intestinal activity (carbonated or caffeine-containing beverages)
▶ Vitamin B_{12} injections to compensate for the bowel's inability to absorb nutrients
▶ Surgery, if complications develop (indications include bowel perforation, massive hemorrhage, fistulas, or acute intestinal obstruction)
▶ Colectomy with ileostomy in patients with extensive disease of large intestine and rectum

Nursing considerations

▶ Provide emotional support to the patient and his family. Listen to the patient's concerns, and help him cope with body image disturbance.

▶ Record fluid intake and output (including number of stools), and weigh the patient daily. Watch for dehydration, and maintain fluid and electrolyte balance. Be alert for signs of intestinal bleeding (bloody stools); check stools for occult blood.

▶ Schedule patient care to include rest periods throughout the day.

▶ Provide the patient with a diet high in protein, calories, and vitamins. Give small, frequent meals throughout the day rather than three large meals.

▶ Carefully monitor the patient on total parenteral nutrition, and provide meticulous site care.

▶ If the patient is receiving steroids, watch for adverse reactions, such as GI bleeding. Steroids can also mask signs of infection.

▶ Monitor hemoglobin and hematocrit levels. Give iron supplements and blood transfusions, as ordered.

▶ Administer medications as ordered. Monitor the patient to ensure that medications are producing desired effects without adverse reactions.

▶ Provide patient hygiene and meticulous oral care if the patient is restricted to nothing by mouth. After each bowel movement, provide careful skin care. Always keep a clean, covered bedpan within the patient's reach. Ventilate the room to eliminate odors.

▶ Monitor the patient for fever and pain on urination, which may signal a bladder infection. Fistulas can form between the colon and bladder, allowing feces to enter the bladder. Abdominal pain, fever, and a hard, distended abdomen may indicate intestinal obstruction.

▶ If the patient is scheduled for surgery, provide appropriate preoperative care. Before ileostomy, arrange for a visit by an enterostomal therapist.

▶ After surgery, monitor vital signs and fluid intake and output. Maintain acid-base balance. Watch for wound infection, and provide meticulous stoma care.

LESSON PLANS

 Teaching about Crohn's disease

▶ Teach the patient about Crohn's disease, its symptoms, and its complications. Explain ordered diagnostic tests; make sure he's aware of all pretest dietary restrictions or other pretest guidelines. Answer his questions.

▶ Emphasize the importance of adequate rest. Explain that it helps to reduce intestinal motility and promote healing.

▶ Encourage the patient to identify and reduce sources of stress in his life, and teach him stress-management techniques or refer him for counseling.

▶ Make sure the patient understands prescribed dietary restrictions. Refer him to a dietitian for further instruction, if necessary.

▶ Give the patient a list of foods to avoid, including milk products, spicy or fried high-residue foods, raw vegetables and fruits, and whole-grain cereals. Advise him to avoid carbonated, caffeine-

containing, or alcoholic beverages (because they increase intestinal activity) and extremely hot or cold foods or fluids (because they increase flatus). Remind him to take supplemental vitamins, if prescribed.

▶ Be sure the patient understands the desired actions and possible adverse effects of his prescribed medications. Urge him to call his practitioner if adverse reactions occur.

▶ If the patient smokes, encourage him to join a smoking cessation program.

▶ Instruct the patient to notify his practitioner if he experiences signs and symptoms of complications, such as fever, fatigue, weakness, a rapid heart rate, abdominal cramping or pain, vomiting, and acute diarrhea.

▶ If the patient is scheduled for surgery, provide preoperative teaching. Reinforce the practitioner's explanation of the surgery, and mention possible complications.

▶ Postoperatively, teach stoma care to the patient and his family. Provide reassurance and emotional support.

▶ Refer the patient and family members to the local chapter of the Crohn's and Colitis Foundation of America for further support. If the patient has an ostomy, put him in touch with the United Ostomy Association.

Diverticular disease

Diverticular disease occurs when bulging pouches (diverticula) in the GI wall push the mucosal lining through the surrounding muscle. The most common site for diverticula is in the sigmoid colon, but they may develop anywhere, from the proximal end of the pharynx to the anus. Other typical sites are the duodenum, near the pancreatic border or the ampulla of Vater, and the jejunum. Diverticular disease of the stomach is rare and may be a precursor of peptic or neoplastic disease. Diverticular disease of the ileum (Meckel's diverticulum) is the most common congenital anomaly of the GI tract.

Although a definite cause is unknown, experts suspect that diverticula form because inadequate dietary fiber produces small stools that require high intraluminal pressure to move through the colon. Diverticular disease has two clinical forms. In *diverticulosis,* diverticula are present but don't cause symptoms.

Diverticulitis occurs when retained undigested food mixed with bacteria accumulates in the diverticulum, forming a hard mass (fecalith). This substance cuts off the blood supply to the diverticulum's thin walls, increasing its susceptibility to attack by colonic bacteria. Inflammation follows bacterial infection. Diet, especially highly refined foods, may be a contributing factor. Lack of fiber reduces fecal residue, narrows the bowel lumen, and leads to higher intra-abdominal pressure during defecation.

Signs and symptoms
Diverticulosis
▶ Intermittent pain in left lower abdominal quadrant relieved by defecation or passage of flatus
▶ Alternating bouts of constipation and diarrhea or altered bowel function
▶ Abdominal tenderness in left lower quadrant (rare)

PICTURING PATHO

Diverticulosis of the colon

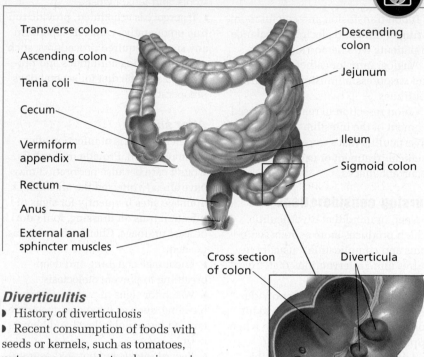

- Transverse colon
- Ascending colon
- Tenia coli
- Cecum
- Vermiform appendix
- Rectum
- Anus
- External anal sphincter muscles
- Descending colon
- Jejunum
- Ileum
- Sigmoid colon

Cross section of colon   Diverticula

Diverticulitis
▶ History of diverticulosis
▶ Recent consumption of foods with seeds or kernels, such as tomatoes, nuts, popcorn, and strawberries, or indigestible roughage, such as celery and corn
▶ Moderate pain in left lower abdominal quadrant that's dull or steady
▶ Straining, lifting, or coughing that aggravates pain
▶ Mild nausea
▶ Flatus
▶ Intermittent bouts of constipation, sometimes accompanied by rectal bleeding
▶ Diarrhea
▶ Distress
▶ Low-grade fever
▶ Muscle spasms and peritoneal irritation (acute form)
▶ Guarding and rebound tenderness
▶ Tender, inflamed mass close to the rectum

Treatment
Asymptomatic diverticulosis
▶ High-fiber, low-fat diet; stool softeners; and mineral oil (for intestinal diverticulosis that causes pain, mild GI distress, constipation, or difficult defecation)
▶ Increased water consumption (eight glasses per day) and bulk medication, such as psyllium, after pain subsides

Mild diverticulitis (without signs of perforation)
▶ Bed rest
▶ Liquid diet advancing to a low-residue diet
▶ Stool softeners
▶ Broadspectrum antibiotic
▶ Meperidine to control pain and relax smooth muscle
▶ Antispasmodic, such as propantheline (Pro-Banthine), to control muscle spasms

Severe diverticulitis
▶ Above measures and I.V. therapy
▶ Nasogastric (NG) tube to relieve intraabdominal pressure with nothing by mouth
▶ Blood transfusion and careful monitoring of fluid and electrolyte balance in patients who hemorrhage
▶ Angiography for catheter placement and vasopressin infusion if bleeding continues
▶ Colon resection to remove diseased segment of the intestine to treat diverticulitis that's unresponsive to medical treatment or causes severe recurrent attacks

Nursing considerations
▶ Keep in mind that diverticulitis, which produces more serious symptoms and complications, usually requires more interventions than diverticulosis.
▶ If the patient is anxious, provide psychological support. Listen to his concerns, and offer reassurance when appropriate.
▶ Administer medications (antibiotics, stool softeners, antispasmodics) as ordered. Monitor the patient for the desired effects, and observe for possible adverse reactions. If pain is severe, administer analgesics, such as meperidine, as ordered.
▶ Inspect all stools carefully for color and consistency. Note the frequency of bowel movements.
▶ Maintain bed rest for the patient with acute diverticulitis. Don't permit him to perform any actions that increase intra-abdominal pressure, such as lifting, straining, bending, and coughing.
▶ Maintain the diet as ordered. Maintain the patient experiencing an acute attack of diverticulitis on a liquid diet. If symptoms are severe, or if the patient experiences nausea and vomiting or abdominal distention, an NG tube may be ordered and attached to intermittent suction. Make sure this patient receives nothing by mouth, and administer ordered I.V. fluids. As symptoms subside, gradually advance the diet.
▶ Watch for temperature elevation, increasing abdominal pain, blood in stools, and leukocytosis.
▶ If surgery is scheduled, provide routine preoperative care. Also, perform any special required procedures, such as administering antibiotics and providing a specific diet for several days preoperatively.

After surgery
▶ Watch for signs of infection after colon resection. Provide meticulous wound care because perforation may have already infected the area. Check drainage sites frequently for signs of infection (pus on dressing, foul odor) or fecal drainage. Change dressings as needed.
▶ Encourage coughing and deep breathing to prevent atelectasis.
▶ Watch for signs of postoperative bleeding, such as hypotension and decreased hemoglobin level and hematocrit.
▶ Record intake and output accurately. Administer I.V. fluids and medications as ordered.
▶ Keep the NG tube patent. If it dislodges, notify the surgeon immediately; don't attempt to reposition it. After the NG tube is removed, advance the patient's diet, as ordered and note how he tolerates diet changes.
▶ If the patient has a colostomy, provide care and give the patient an opportunity to express his feelings.

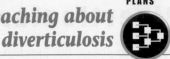

Teaching about diverticulosis

▶ With uncomplicated diverticulosis, patient teaching focuses on bowel and dietary habits.
▶ Explain what diverticula are and how they form. Teach the patient about necessary diagnostic tests and prescribed treatments.
▶ Make sure the patient understands the desired actions and possible adverse effects of his prescribed medications.
▶ Review recommended dietary changes. Encourage the patient to drink 2 to 3 qt (2 to 3 L) of fluid per day. Emphasize the importance of dietary roughage and the harmful effects of constipation and straining during a bowel movement. Advise increasing intake of foods high in undigestible fiber, such as fresh fruits and vegetables, whole grain breads, and wheat or bran cereals. Warn that a high-fiber diet may temporarily cause flatulence.
▶ Advise the patient to relieve constipation with stool softeners or bulk-forming cathartics.
▶ Instruct the patient to take bulk-forming cathartics with plenty of water. Be aware that if swallowed dry, they may absorb enough moisture in the mouth and throat to swell and obstruct the esophagus or trachea.
▶ Tell the patient to notify the practitioner if he experiences such complications as a temperature over 101° F (38.3° C); abdominal pain that's severe or that lasts for more than 3 days; or blood in his stool.
▶ Provide preoperative teaching, reinforce the practitioner's explanation of the surgery, and discuss possible complications.
▶ Postoperatively, teach the patient to care for his colostomy as needed. Arrange for a visit by an enterostomal therapist.

Esophageal cancer

Esophageal cancer is most common in males older than age 65 and is nearly always fatal.

Esophageal tumors are usually fungating and infiltrating. In most cases, the tumor partially constricts the lumen of the esophagus. Regional metastasis occurs early in disease progression in submucosal lymphatics, commonly fatally invading adjacent vital intrathoracic organs. If the patient survives primary extension, the liver and lungs are the usual sites of distant metastases. Unusual metastasis sites include the bones, kidneys, and adrenal glands.

Most cases arise in squamous cell epithelium, although a few are adenocarcinomas. About half the squamous cell cancers occur in the lower portion of the esophagus, 40% in the midportion, and the remaining 10% in the upper or cervical esophagus. Prognosis for esophageal cancer depends on the stage of the cancer. The 5-year survival rate of those with metastasis is 3%.

Although the cause of esophageal cancer is unknown, several predisposing factors have been identified. These include heavy smoking or excessive use of alcohol; Barrett's esophagus and long-standing gastroesophageal reflux disease; stasis-induced inflammation, as in achalasia or stricture; human papillovirus infection; sclerotherapy; previous head and neck tumors; and nutritional deficiency, as in untreated sprue and Plummer-Vinson syndrome.

Signs and symptoms

▶ Feeling of fullness or pressure
▶ Indigestion
▶ Antacid use to relieve GI upset
▶ Dysphagia (first occurs only after eating solid foods, especially meat; later causes difficulty swallowing coarse foods and, in some cases, liquids)
▶ Weight loss
▶ Hoarseness
▶ Chronic cough
▶ Anorexia
▶ Vomiting
▶ Pain on swallowing
▶ Pain that radiates to the back

PICTURING PATHO

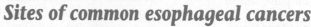
Sites of common esophageal cancers

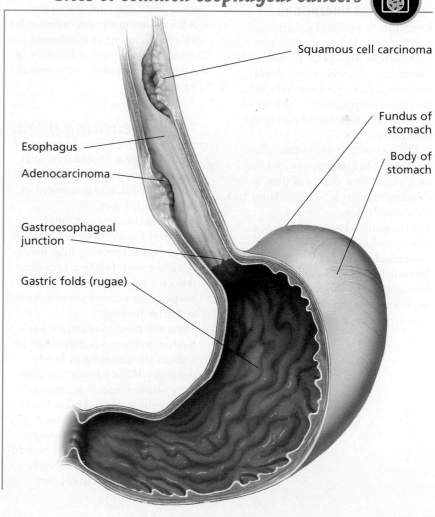

Squamous cell carcinoma

Fundus of stomach

Body of stomach

Esophagus

Adenocarcinoma

Gastroesophageal junction

Gastric folds (rugae)

Treatment

▶ Palliative therapy to keep the esophagus open, including dilation of the esophagus, laser therapy, radiation therapy, and placement of an endoluminal stent

▶ Radical surgery to excise the tumor and resect either the esophagus alone or the stomach and esophagus

▶ Chemotherapy and radiation therapy to slow tumor growth

▶ Gastrostomy or jejunostomy to help provide adequate nutrition

▶ A prosthesis to seal any fistula that develops

▶ Endoscopic laser treatment and bipolar electrocoagulation to restore swallowing by vaporizing cancerous tissue

▶ Analgesics for pain control

Nursing considerations

▶ Monitor the patient's nutritional and fluid status, and provide him with high-calorie, high-protein foods. If he's having trouble swallowing solids, puree or liquefy his food and offer a nutritional supplement. As ordered, provide tube feedings or parenteral nutrition.

▶ To prevent food aspiration, place the patient in Fowler's position for meals and allow plenty of time to eat. If he regurgitates food after eating, provide mouth care.

▶ If the patient has a gastrostomy tube, give food slowly—by gravity—in prescribed amounts (usually 200 to 500 ml). Offer him food to chew before each feeding to promote gastric secretions and provide some semblance of normal eating.

▶ Administer ordered analgesics for pain relief as needed. Provide comfort measures, such as repositioning and distractions.

▶ After surgery, monitor vital signs, fluid and electrolyte balance, and intake and output. Immediately report unexpected changes in the patient's condition. Monitor for such complications as infection, fistula formation, pneumonia, empyema, and malnutrition.

▶ If an anastomosis to the esophagus was performed, position the patient flat on his back to prevent tension on the suture line. Watch for signs of an anastomotic leak.

▶ If the patient had a prosthetic tube inserted, make sure it doesn't become blocked or dislodged, which could cause a perforation of the mediastinum or precipitate tumor erosion.

▶ After radiation therapy, monitor for such complications as esophageal perforation, pneumonitis and fibrosis of the lungs, and myelitis of the spinal cord.

▶ After chemotherapy, take steps to decrease adverse effects, such as providing normal saline mouthwash to help prevent mouth ulcers. Allow the patient plenty of rest, and administer medications, as ordered, to reduce adverse effects.

▶ Protect the patient from infection.

▶ Throughout therapy, answer the patient's questions and tell him what to expect from surgery and other therapies. Listen to his fears and concerns, and stay with him during periods of severe anxiety.

▶ Encourage the patient to identify actions and care measures that promote his comfort and relaxation. Try to perform these measures, and encourage the patient and family members to do so as well.

▶ Whenever possible, include the patient in care decisions.

LESSON PLANS

Teaching about esophageal cancer

▶ Explain surgical procedures, such as closed chest drainage, nasogastric suctioning, and placement of gastrostomy tubes.

▶ If appropriate, instruct family members in gastrostomy tube care. This includes checking tube patency before each feeding, providing skin care around the tube, and keeping the patient upright during and after feeding.

▶ Stress the need to maintain adequate nutrition. Ask a dietitian to instruct the patient and family members. If the patient has difficulty swallowing solids, instruct him to puree or liquefy his food and to follow a high-calorie, high-protein diet to minimize weight loss. Also, recommend that he add a commercially available, high-calorie supplement to his diet.

▶ Encourage the patient to follow as normal a routine as possible after recovery from surgery and during radiation therapy and chemotherapy. Tell him that this will help him maintain a sense of control.

▶ Advise the patient to rest between activities and to stop activity that tires him or causes pain.

▶ Refer the patient and family members to appropriate organizations such as the American Cancer Society.

Gastric cancer

Although gastric cancer is common worldwide, its incidence exhibits unexplained geographic, cultural, and gender differences. Mortality is high in Japan, Iceland, Chile, and Austria. Incidence is also higher in males older than age 40.

During the past 25 years in the United States, the incidence of gastric cancer has decreased 50%, with the resulting death rate now one-third of what it was 30 years ago. This decrease has been attributed, without proof, to the improved, well-balanced diets and to refrigeration, which reduces the number of nitrate-producing bacteria.

Gastric cancer occurs more commonly in some parts of the stomach than in others; the pyloric area accounts for 50% and the lesser curvature for 25% of the incidence. This adenocarcinoma rapidly infiltrates the regional lymph nodes, omentum, liver, and lungs by way of the walls of the stomach, duodenum, and esophagus; the lymphatic system; adjacent organs; the bloodstream; and the peritoneal cavity.

Helicobacter pylori infection is the most common cause of stomach cancer. Autoimmune gastritis is also a risk factor. Genetic factors also have been implicated. People with type A blood have a 10% increased risk, and the disease occurs more commonly in people with a family history of such cancer. Dietary factors also seem to have an effect. For instance, certain types of food preparation and preservation (especially smoked foods, pickled vegetables, and salted fish and meat) and physical properties of some foods increase the risk. High alcohol consumption and smoking increase the chances of developing gastric cancer.

Signs and symptoms

▶ Back pain or pain in epigastric or retrosternal areas that's relieved with nonprescription medications
▶ Vague feeling of fullness, heaviness, and moderate abdominal distention after meals
▶ Weight loss
▶ Nausea and vomiting (coffee-ground vomitus with tumor of the cardia)
▶ Weakness
▶ Fatigue
▶ Dysphagia (tumor located in proximal area of stomach)
▶ Abdominal mass
▶ Enlarged lymph nodes, especially the supraclavicular and axillary nodes

PICTURING PATHO

Adenocarcinoma of the stomach

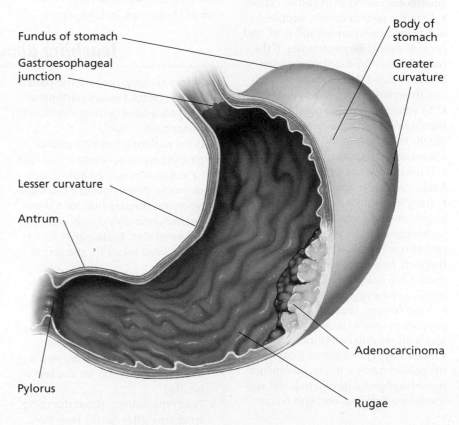

Fundus of stomach

Gastroesophageal junction

Lesser curvature

Antrum

Pylorus

Body of stomach

Greater curvature

Adenocarcinoma

Rugae

Treatment

‣ Gastroduodenostomy, gastrojejunostomy, partial gastric resection, and total gastrectomy
‣ Removal of the omentum and spleen (for metastasis)
‣ Chemotherapy for GI tumors (including fluorouracil, carmustine, doxorubicin, and mitomycin)
‣ Antiemetics to control nausea, which intensifies as the tumor grows
‣ Sedatives and tranquilizers to control overwhelming anxiety
‣ Opioid analgesics to relieve severe and unremitting pain
‣ Radiation therapy with chemotherapy for nonresectable or partially resectable tumor
‣ Antispasmodics and antacids to relieve GI distress

Nursing considerations

‣ Provide a high-protein, high-calorie diet to help the patient avoid or recover from weight loss, malnutrition, and anemia associated with gastric cancer.
‣ Give the patient dietary supplements, such as vitamins and iron, and provide small, frequent meals. If the patient has an iron deficiency, give him iron-rich foods, such as spinach and dried fruit.
‣ To stimulate a poor appetite, administer steroids or antidepressants, as ordered. Wine or brandy may also help stimulate the appetite.
‣ If the patient can't tolerate oral foods, provide parenteral nutrition.
‣ Administer an antacid to relieve heartburn and gastric acid and a histamine-receptor antagonist, such as cimetidine (Tagamet) or famotidine (Pepcid), to decrease gastric secretions. Give opioid analgesics, as ordered, to relieve pain.
‣ After surgery, provide meticulous supportive care to promote recovery and help prevent complications.
‣ After any type of gastrectomy, turn the patient every 2 hours, administer opioid analgesics as ordered, and regularly assist the patient with cough-

ing, deep breathing, and turning to help prevent respiratory problems.
‣ After total gastrectomy, support the patient during episodes of dumping syndrome. Keep an emesis basin at the bedside, and provide small meals six to eight times per day when the patient is allowed food by mouth.
‣ Monitor the patient's nasogastric tube for drainage. Expect little or no drainage from the tube because no secretions form after the stomach is removed.
‣ Watch for signs of vitamin B_{12} malabsorption (weakness, sore tongue, numbness, and tingling in the extremities), the result of an absence of intrinsic factor from gastric secretions.
‣ If the patient has poor digestion and absorption after a gastrectomy, provide a special diet. Provide frequent feedings of small amounts of clear liquids, increasing to small, frequent feedings of bland food. If necessary, administer pancreatin and sodium bicarbonate after meals to prevent or control steatorrhea and dyspepsia.

‣ Observe the surgical wound regularly for signs of infection (redness, swelling, warmth) and failure to heal. If needed, administer vitamin C to improve wound healing.
‣ During radiation treatment offer fluids such as ginger ale to minimize nausea and vomiting.
‣ During chemotherapy, watch for complications, such as infection, and expected adverse effects, such as nausea, vomiting, mouth ulcers, and alopecia.
‣ Throughout treatment, listen to the patient's fears and concerns and offer reassurance. Stay with him during periods of severe anxiety.
‣ Whenever possible, include the patient and family members in decisions related to the patient's care.

LESSON PLANS

Teaching about gastric cancer

‣ Before surgery, prepare the patient for its effects. Explain postoperative procedures such as insertion of a nasogastric tube.
‣ If the patient is having a partial gastric resection, reassure him that he eventually may be able to eat normally. If he's having a total gastrectomy, prepare him for a slow recovery and only partial return to a normal diet. Explain that he has to eat small meals for the rest of his life.
‣ After surgery, emphasize the importance of deep breathing and changing position every 2 hours.
‣ Stress the importance of good nutrition. Explain that the patient must take vitamins (to prevent B_{12} deficiency) and iron for the rest of his life.
‣ Teach the patient about dumping syndrome after gastric resection.

Early dumping syndrome, which may be mild or severe, occurs a few minutes after eating and lasts up to 45 minutes. Onset is sudden, with nausea, weakness, sweating, palpitations, dizziness, flushing, borborygmi, explosive diarrhea, and increased blood pressure and pulse rate. Late dumping syndrome, which is less serious, occurs 2 to 3 hours after eating.
‣ Explain the ordered treatments to the patient and his family. Describe the adverse effects the treatment may cause, and tell the patient to notify the practitioner if these effects persist.
‣ Prepare the patient for chemotherapy's adverse effects, such as nausea and vomiting, and suggest measures, such as drinking plenty of fluids, that may help relieve these problems.

Gastroesophageal reflux disease

Commonly known as *heartburn,* gastroesophageal reflux disease is the backflow of gastric or duodenal contents, or both, into the esophagus and past the lower esophageal sphincter (LES), without associated belching or vomiting. Reflux may cause symptoms or pathologic changes. Persistent reflux can cause reflux esophagitis, an inflammation of the esophageal mucosa. The prognosis varies with the underlying cause.

Normally, gastric contents don't back up into the esophagus because the LES creates enough pressure around the lower end of the esophagus to close it. Reflux occurs when LES pressure is deficient or pressure in the stomach exceeds LES pressure. When this happens, the LES relaxes, allowing gastric contents to regurgitate into the esophagus. Any of these predisposing factors can lead to reflux:

▶ pyloric surgery (alteration or removal of the pylorus), which allows reflux of bile or pancreatic juice
▶ nasogastric intubation for more than 4 days
▶ any agent that lowers LES pressure: food, alcohol, cigarettes, anticholinergics (atropine, belladonna, propantheline), and other drugs (morphine, diazepam, calcium channel blockers, meperidine)
▶ hiatal hernia with incompetent sphincter
▶ any condition or position that increases intra-abdominal pressure.

Understanding gastroesophageal reflux disease

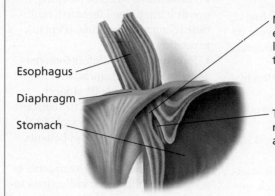

Esophagus
Diaphragm
Stomach

Normally, the LES maintains enough pressure around the lower end of the esophagus to close it and prevent reflux.

Typically, the sphincter relaxes after each swallow to allow food into the stomach.

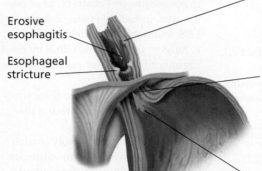

Erosive esophagitis
Esophageal stricture

The high acidity of the stomach contents causes pain and irritation when the contents enter the esophagus.

In gastroesophageal reflux disease, the sphincter doesn't remain closed (usually because of deficient LES pressure or pressure within the stomach that exceeds LES pressure).

The pressure in the stomach pushes the stomach contents into the esophagus.

Factors affecting LES pressure

Various dietary and lifestyle elements can increase or decrease lower esophageal sphincter (LES) pressure. Take these into account as you plan the patient's treatment program.

What increases LES pressure
▶ Carbohydrates
▶ Low-dose ethanol
▶ Nonfat milk
▶ Protein

What decreases LES pressure
▶ Antiflatulent (simethicone)
▶ Chocolate
▶ Cigarette smoking
▶ Coffee
▶ Fat
▶ High-dose ethanol
▶ Lying on right or left side
▶ Orange juice
▶ Sitting
▶ Soda
▶ Tomatoes
▶ Whole milk

Signs and symptoms

‣ Heartburn and regurgitation that worsens with vigorous exercise, bending, or lying down (relieved by using antacids or sitting upright)
‣ Regurgitating without associated nausea or belching
‣ A feeling of warm fluid traveling up the throat that's followed by a sour or bitter taste in the mouth if fluid reaches the pharynx
‣ A feeling of fluid accumulation in the throat
‣ Odynophagia, possibly followed by a dull substernal ache
‣ Bright red or dark brown blood in vomitus
‣ Chronic pain that may mimic angina pectoris, radiating to the neck, jaw, and arm
‣ Nocturnal hypersalivation

Treatment

‣ Drug therapy to strengthen the LES
‣ Neutralizing gastric contents
‣ Reducing intra-abdominal pressure
‣ Lifestyle or dietary habit changes

‣ Weight loss
‣ Smoking cessation
‣ Positional therapy (sleeping with the head of the bed elevated and avoiding lying down after meals and late-night snacks)
‣ Histamine-2 receptor blocking agents (cimetidine [Tagamet], ranitidine [Zantac], famotidine [Pepcid], nizatidine [Axid])
‣ Proton pump inhibitors (omeprazole [Prilosec], lansoprazole [Prevacid], pantoprazole [Protonix], esomeprazole (Nexium), dexlansoprazole (Dexilant), or rabeprazole [Aciphex]); heals up to 90% of patients with erosive esophagitis
‣ Surgery for refractory symptoms or serious complications; indications including pulmonary aspiration, hemorrhage, esophageal obstruction or perforation, intractable pain, incompetent LES, or associated hiatal hernia
‣ Surgery that reduces reflux by creating an artificial closure at the gastroesophageal junction
‣ Fundoplication that involves wrapping the gastric fundus around the esophagus
‣ Vagotomy or pyloroplasty (which may be combined with an antireflux regimen) to modify gastric contents

Nursing considerations

‣ Offer emotional and psychological support to help the patient cope with pain and discomfort.
‣ With a dietitian, develop a diet that takes the patient's food preferences into account but, at the same time, helps to minimize his reflux symptoms. If the patient is obese, place him on a weight reduction diet as ordered.
‣ To reduce intra-abdominal pressure, have the patient sleep in reverse Trendelenburg's position (with the head of the bed elevated 6″ to 12″ [15 to 30.5 cm]). Have him avoid lying down for 3 hours after meals and eating late-night snacks.
‣ After surgery, pay particular attention to the patient's respiratory status because the surgical procedure is performed close to the diaphragm. Administer prescribed analgesics, oxygen, and I.V. fluids. Monitor his intake and output, and check his vital signs. If surgery was performed using a thoracic approach, watch and record chest tube drainage. If needed, provide chest physiotherapy.

LESSON PLANS

Teaching about gastroesophageal reflux disease

‣ Teach the patient about the causes of gastroesophageal reflux disease, and review his antireflux regimen of medication, diet, and positional therapy.

‣ Discuss recommended dietary changes. Advise the patient to sit upright after meals and snacks and to eat small, frequent meals. Explain that he should eat meals at least 2 to 3 hours before lying down. Tell him to avoid highly seasoned food, acidic juices, alcoholic drinks, bedtime snacks, and high-fat foods because these reduce lower esophageal sphincter pressure.

‣ Instruct the patient to avoid situations or activities that increase intra-abdominal pressure, such as bending, coughing, vigorous exercise, obesity, constipation, and wearing tight clothing. Caution him to refrain from using any substance that reduces sphincter control, including cigarettes, alcohol, fatty foods, and certain drugs.
‣ Encourage compliance with the drug regimen. Review the desired drug actions and potential adverse effects. If the patient is taking an antacid, advise him not to take it with his other mediations because it will decrease their absorption.

Irritable bowel syndrome

Irritable bowel syndrome (IBS) (also called *spastic colon, spastic colitis,* or *mucous colitis*) is a common condition marked by chronic or periodic diarrhea alternating with constipation. It's accompanied by straining and abdominal cramps. The disorder occurs mostly in women, with symptoms first emerging before age 40. The prognosis is good.

Although the precise etiology is unclear, IBS involves a change in bowel motility, reflecting an abnormality in the neuromuscular control of intestinal smooth muscle.

Contributing or aggravating factors include anxiety and stress. Initial episodes occur early in life; psychological stress probably causes most exacerbations. In fact, a history of sexual or physical abuse is one of the strongest predictors of a poor clinical outcome. IBS may also result from dietary factors, such as fiber, fruits, coffee, alcohol, and foods that are cold, highly seasoned, or laxative in nature. Other possible triggers include hormones, laxative abuse, and allergy to certain foods or drugs.

Signs and symptoms

▶ Chronic constipation, diarrhea, or both
▶ Lower abdominal pain (usually in the left lower quadrant) that's commonly relieved by defecation or passage of gas
▶ Bouts of diarrhea, typically occur during the day; alternating with constipation or normal bowel function
▶ Small stools with visible mucus or small, pasty, and pencil-like stools
▶ Dyspepsia
▶ Abdominal bloating
▶ Heartburn, faintness
▶ Weakness
▶ Anxiety, fatigue
▶ Normal bowel sounds
▶ Relaxed abdomen
▶ Tympany over a gas-filled bowel

PICTURING PATHO

Effects of irritable bowel syndrome

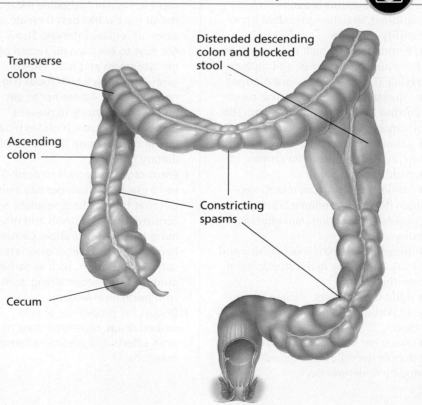

Transverse colon

Ascending colon

Cecum

Distended descending colon and blocked stool

Constricting spasms

Treatment
▶ Medications for severe symptoms
▶ Elimination of citrus fruits, coffee, corn, dairy products, tea, and wheat, to identify what triggers symptoms
▶ Elimination of sorbitol (artificial sweetener that causes diarrhea, abdominal distention, and bloating)
▶ Elimination of nonabsorbable carbohydrates, such as beans and cabbage, and lactose-containing foods, which cause flatulence
▶ Addition of 15 g per day of bulky foods, such as wheat bran, oatmeal, oat bran, rye cereals, prunes, dried apricots, and figs, to control diarrhea, minimize abdominal pain, and help promote stool formation
▶ Increased water intake (eight glasses per day)
▶ Counseling to explain the relationship between stress and illness; instruction in stress-management techniques
▶ Anticholinergic, antispasmodic drugs, such as dicyclomine (Bentyl) and propantheline bromide (Pro-Banthine), to reduce intestinal hypermotility and pain
▶ Antidiarrheals, such as loperamide (Imodium) and atropine and diphenoxylate (Lomotil), to control diarrhea
▶ Alosetron (Lotronex) to treat severe diarrhea in diarrhea-predominant IBS in women.
▶ Osmotic laxatives for constipation; lubiprostone (amitiza) for chronic idiopathic constipation
▶ Antiemetics, such as metoclopramide (Reglan), to relieve heartburn, epigastric discomfort, and after-meal fullness
▶ Simethicone to relieve belching and bloating from gas in the stomach and intestines
▶ Mild tranquilizers, such as diazepam (Valium), to reduce psychological stress
▶ Selective serotonin reuptake inhibitors or tricyclic antidepressants for anxiety or depression

Nursing considerations
Because the patient with IBS isn't hospitalized, nursing interventions almost always focus on patient teaching.

LESSON PLANS

Teaching about IBS

▶ Explain irritable bowel syndrome (IBS) to the patient, and reassure her that it can be relieved. Point out, however, that IBS is chronic with no known cure.
▶ Help the patient understand ordered diagnostic tests. Review all pretest guidelines. Explain that these tests can't specifically diagnose IBS but can rule out other disorders.
▶ Help the patient develop a dietary plan, and suggest ways to implement it. Help her schedule meals; the GI tract works best if meals are eaten at regular intervals. Show her how to keep a daily record of her symptoms and food intake, carefully noting which foods trigger symptoms. Advise her to eat slowly and carefully to prevent swallowing air, which causes bloating, and to increase her intake of dietary fiber.
▶ Encourage the patient to drink 8 to 10 glasses of fluid per day. Point out that this will help regulate the consistency of her stools and promote balanced hydration. Caution her to avoid beverages associated with GI discomfort, such as carbonated or caffeine-containing drinks, fruit juices, and alcohol.
▶ Discuss the proper use of prescribed drugs, reviewing their desired effects and possible adverse reactions.

▶ Help the patient to implement lifestyle changes that reduce stress. Teach her to set priorities in her daily activities and, if possible, to delegate some responsibilities to other family members. Encourage her to schedule more time for rest and relaxation. Provide instruction in such relaxation techniques as guided imagery, biofeedback, yoga, and deep-breathing exercises, and advise her to perform them regularly. If appropriate, instruct her to seek professional counseling for stress management.
▶ Remind the patient that regular exercise is important to relieve stress and promote regular bowel function; even a 20- or 30-minute walk each day is helpful.
▶ Discourage smoking. If the patient smokes, warn her that this habit can aggravate her symptoms by altering bowel motility.
▶ Explain the need for regular physical examinations. For patients over age 40, emphasize the need for colorectal cancer screening, including annual proctosigmoidoscopy and rectal examinations.

Liver cancer

Primary liver cancer accounts for roughly 2% of all cancers in North America, though its incidence is rising. It's most prevalent in males, particularly those older than age 60, and the incidence increases with age.

Most primary liver tumors (90%) originate in the parenchymal cells and are hepatomas. Some primary tumors originate in the intrahepatic bile ducts and are known as cholangiomas.

Staging of liver cancer is complicated by the fact that no particular staging system exists. The prognosis is almost always poor since many patients don't develop symptoms until the advanced stages of the disease. If advanced, the disease progresses rapidly, with death usually occurring within 6 months of diagnosis from GI hemorrhage, progressive cachexia, liver failure, or metastatic spread. When cirrhosis is present, the prognosis is especially grim, with death resulting from liver failure.

Liver cancer in adults may result from environmental exposure to carcinogens, including the chemical compound aflatoxin (a mold that grows on rice and peanuts), and thorium dioxide (a contrast medium used for liver radiography in the past), and heavy alcohol use. Cirrhosis and obesity are also risk factors along with hepatitis B and C.

PICTURING PATHO

Common sites of liver cancer

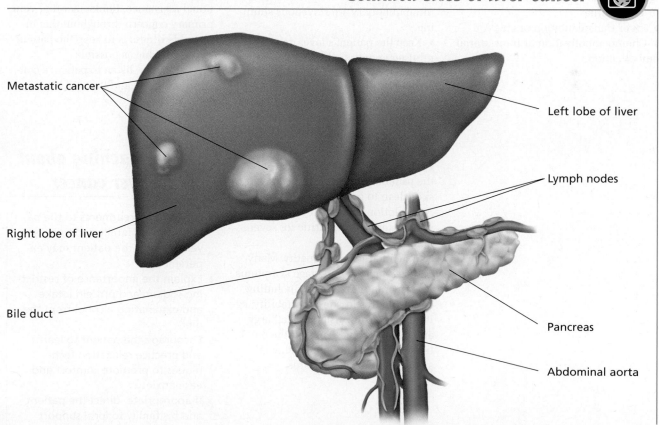

Metastatic cancer

Left lobe of liver

Lymph nodes

Right lobe of liver

Bile duct

Pancreas

Abdominal aorta

Signs and symptoms
▶ Weight loss resulting from anorexia
▶ Weakness, fatigue
▶ Fever
▶ Severe pain in epigastrium or right upper quadrant (palpable mass)
▶ Jaundice (including scleral icterus)
▶ Dependent edema
▶ Bruit, hum, or rubbing sound if the tumor involves a large part of the liver
▶ Enlarged liver that's tender and nodular
▶ Ascites

Treatment
▶ Lobectomy or partial hepatectomy of a tumor that's solitary and not accompanied by cirrhosis, jaundice, or ascites
▶ Radiation therapy (alone or with chemotherapy) or radioembolization
▶ Fluorouracil, doxorubicin, methotrexate, streptozocin, and lomustine I.V. or regular infusion of fluorouracil or floxuridine
▶ Liver transplantation or ablation
▶ Chemoembolization or transarterial embolization

Nursing considerations
▶ Give analgesics as ordered, and encourage the patient to identify care measures that promote comfort.
▶ Monitor the patient's diet throughout his illness. Most patients need a special diet that restricts sodium, fluids, and protein and prohibits alcohol. Weigh the patient daily, and note intake and output accurately.
▶ Control ascites; if signs develop—peripheral edema, orthopnea, and dyspnea on exertion—measure and record the patient's abdominal girth daily.
▶ To increase venous return and prevent edema, elevate the patient's legs whenever possible.
▶ Monitor respiratory function. Note shortness of breath or increase in respiratory rate. Bilateral pleural effusion (evident on chest X-ray) and metastasis to the lungs are common. Watch carefully for signs of hypoxemia from intrapulmonary arteriovenous shunting.
▶ Keep the patient's fever down. Administer sponge baths and aspirin suppositories if the patient has no signs of GI bleeding. Avoid acetaminophen; the diseased liver can't metabolize it. If a high fever develops, the patient has an infection and needs antibiotics.
▶ Provide meticulous skin care. Turn the patient frequently, and keep his skin clean to prevent pressure ulcers. Apply lotion to prevent chafing, and administer an antipruritic for severe itching.
▶ Watch for encephalopathy. Many patients develop end-stage symptoms of ammonia intoxication, including confusion, restlessness, irritability, agitation, delirium, asterixis, lethargy and, finally, coma. Monitor the patient's serum ammonia level, vital signs, and neurologic status.

▶ As ordered, control ammonia accumulation with sorbitol (to induce osmotic diarrhea), neomycin (to reduce bacterial flora in the GI tract), lactulose (to control bacterial elaboration of ammonia), and sodium polystyrene sulfonate (to lower the potassium level).
▶ If the patient has a transhepatic catheter in place to relieve obstructive jaundice, irrigate it frequently with the prescribed solution (0.9% sodium chloride or, sometimes, 5,000 units of heparin in 500 ml dextrose 5% in water). Monitor vital signs frequently for bleeding or infection.
▶ After surgery, watch for intraperitoneal bleeding and sepsis, which may precipitate coma. Watch for renal failure by monitoring the patient's urine output, blood urea nitrogen, and serum creatinine levels.
▶ Throughout therapy, provide comprehensive supportive care and emotional assistance. Remember that your primary concern throughout this intractable illness is to keep the patient as comfortable as possible.
▶ At all times, listen to patient's concerns and fears and those of his family.

LESSON PLANS

Teaching about liver cancer
▶ Explain the treatments to the patient and his family, including adverse effects the patient may experience.
▶ Explain the importance of restricting sodium and protein intake and eliminating alcohol from the diet.
▶ Encourage the patient to learn and practice relaxation techniques to promote comfort and ease anxiety.
▶ If appropriate, direct the patient and his family to local support groups and services.

Pancreatic cancer

Pancreatic cancer is the fourth most lethal of all carcinomas. It occurs most commonly among blacks, particularly in males between ages 35 and 70. Prognosis is poor, with most patients dying within 1 year of diagnosis.

Evidence suggests that pancreatic cancer is linked to inhalation or absorption of carcinogens that are then excreted by the pancreas. Examples of such carcinogens include:

▶ cigarette smoke
▶ excessive fat and protein
▶ food additives
▶ industrial chemicals, such as beta-naphthalene, benzidine, and urea.

Other possible predisposing factors include chronic pancreatitis, diabetes mellitus, and chronic alcohol abuse.

Tumors of the pancreas are almost always adenocarcinomas. They arise most frequently (67% of the time) in the head of the pancreas. Tumors in this location commonly obstruct the ampulla of Vater and common bile duct and metastasize directly to the duodenum. Adhesions anchor the tumor to the spine, stomach, and intestines. Less frequently, tumors arise in the body and tail of the pancreas. When this happens, large nodular masses become fixed to retropancreatic tissues and the spine. The spleen, left kidney, suprarenal gland, and diaphragm are directly invaded, and the celiac plexus becomes involved, resulting in splenic vein thrombosis and spleen infarction.

In pancreatic cancer, two main tissue types form fibrotic nodes: Cylinder cells arise in ducts and degenerate into cysts, and large, fatty, granular cells arise in parenchyma.

Signs and symptoms

▶ Dull, intermittent epigastric pain (early)
▶ Continuous pain that radiates to the right upper quadrant or dorsolumbar area (late)
▶ Epigastric pain aggravated by meals
▶ Anorexia
▶ Nausea and vomiting
▶ Rapid, profound weight loss
▶ Jaundice
▶ Palpable, well-defined, large mass in subumbilical or left hypochondrial region (in cancer of the tail of the pancreas)
▶ Pulsating mass caused by adherence to large vessels or the vertebral column
▶ Abdominal bruit of the left hypochondrium if the tumor has involved or compressed the splenic artery

PICTURING PATHO

Pancreatic adenocarcinoma

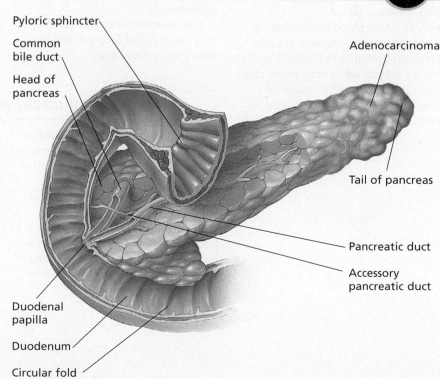

Pyloric sphincter

Common bile duct

Head of pancreas

Adenocarcinoma

Tail of pancreas

Pancreatic duct

Accessory pancreatic duct

Duodenal papilla

Duodenum

Circular fold

Treatment

▶ Total pancreatectomy, cholecystojejunostomy, choledochoduodenostomy, and choledochojejunostomy; gastrojejunostomy, and the Whipple procedure or radical pancreatoduodenectomy
▶ Gemcitabine (Gemzar)—the standard chemotherapeutic agent currently in use; also fluorouracil
▶ Radiation therapy used as an adjunct to fluorouracil chemotherapy (may prolong survival time)
▶ Antibiotics, anticholinergics (propantheline bromide [Pro-Banthine]), antacids, diuretics, insulin, opioid analgesics, and pancreatic enzymes

Nursing considerations

▶ Monitor the patient's fluid balance, abdominal girth, metabolic state, and weight daily.
▶ Serve small, frequent meals. Consult the dietitian to ensure proper nutrition, and make mealtimes as pleasant as possible. Administer an oral pancreatic enzyme at mealtimes, if needed. As ordered, give an antacid to prevent stress ulcers.
▶ Administer blood transfusions (to combat anemia), vitamin K (to overcome prothrombin deficiency), antibiotics (to prevent postoperative complications), and gastric lavage (to maintain gastric decompression), as ordered.

▶ After surgery, watch for and report complications, such as fistula, pancreatitis, fluid and electrolyte imbalance, infection, hemorrhage, skin breakdown, nutritional deficiency, liver failure, renal insufficiency, and diabetes.
▶ If the patient is receiving chemotherapy, watch for and symptomatically treat its toxic effects.
▶ To prevent constipation, administer laxatives, stool softeners, and cathartics, as ordered. Also, modify the patient's diet and increase his fluid intake. To increase GI motility, position him properly during and after meals and assist him with walking.
▶ Ensure adequate rest and sleep (with a sedative, if necessary). Assist with range-of-motion (ROM) and isometric exercises, as appropriate.
▶ Administer analgesics for pain, and antibiotics and antipyretics for fever, as ordered.
▶ Watch for signs of hypoglycemia or hyperglycemia, and give glucose or an antidiabetic agent (such as tolbutamide) as ordered. Monitor blood glucose levels and the patient's response to treatment.
▶ Provide scrupulous skin care to prevent pruritus and necrosis, and keep the skin clean and dry.

▶ Watch for signs of upper GI bleeding. Test stools and emesis for blood, and maintain a flow sheet of frequent hemoglobin and hematocrit determinations.
▶ Ease discomfort from pyloric obstruction with a nasogastric tube.
▶ To prevent thrombosis, apply antiembolism stockings and assist with ROM exercises. If thrombosis occurs, elevate the patient's legs and apply moist heat to the thrombus site. Give an anticoagulant, such as enoxaparin, as ordered, to prevent further clot formation and pulmonary embolus.
▶ Throughout therapy, answer the patient's questions and tell him what to expect from surgery and other therapies. Listen to his fears and concerns, and stay with him during periods of severe stress and anxiety.
▶ Encourage the patient to identify actions and care measures that promote his comfort and relaxation.
▶ Whenever possible, include the patient and family members in care decisions.

Teaching about pancreatic cancer

▶ Describe expected postoperative procedures and adverse effects of radiation therapy and chemotherapy.
▶ If appropriate, provide information on diabetes.
▶ Encourage the patient to follow as normal a routine as possible. Explain that leading a near-normal life helps foster feelings of independence and control.

▶ Help the patient and his family cope with the impending reality of death.
▶ Refer the patient to resource and support services, such as the social service department, local home health care agencies, hospices, and the American Cancer Society.

Peptic ulcer disease

Peptic ulcers, which are circumscribed lesions in the mucosal membrane, can develop in the lower esophagus, stomach, duodenum, or jejunum. The major forms are duodenal ulcer and gastric ulcer; both are chronic conditions.

Duodenal ulcers, which account for about 80% of peptic ulcers, affect the proximal part of the small intestine. These ulcers, which occur most commonly in men between ages 20 and 50, follow a chronic course characterized by remissions and exacerbations.

Gastric ulcers, which affect the stomach mucosa, are most common in middle-aged and elderly men, especially among those who are poor and undernourished. This kind of ulcer also tends to occur in chronic users of aspirin or alcohol.

Researchers have identified a bacterial infection with *Helicobacter pylori* (formerly known as *Campylobacter pylori*) as a leading cause of peptic ulcer disease. They also found that *H. pylori* releases a toxin that promotes mucosal inflammation and ulceration. In a peptic ulcer resulting from *H. pylori,* acid seems to be mainly a contributor to the consequences of the bacterial infection rather than its dominant cause. Other risk factors include the use of certain medications—nonsteroidal anti-inflammatory drugs, for example—and pathologic hypersecretory states, such as Zollinger-Ellison syndrome.

PICTURING PATHO

Common ulcer types and sites

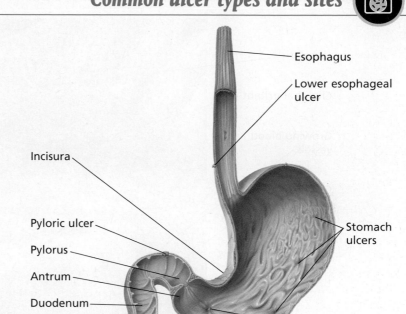

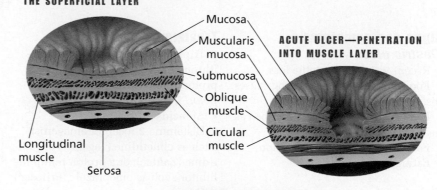

EROSION—PENETRATION OF ONLY THE SUPERFICIAL LAYER

ACUTE ULCER—PENETRATION INTO MUSCLE LAYER

PERFORATING ULCER—PENETRATION OF WALL

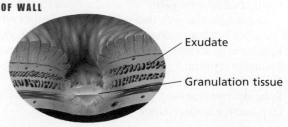

A closer look at H. pylori

The bacteria *Helicobacter pylori* are a contributing factor in chronic gastritis (chronic inflammation of stomach mucosa) and in ulcer formation. They're typically seen within the muscular layers and between cells that line the gastric pits. These bacteria cause tissue inflammation, which can lead to ulcers.

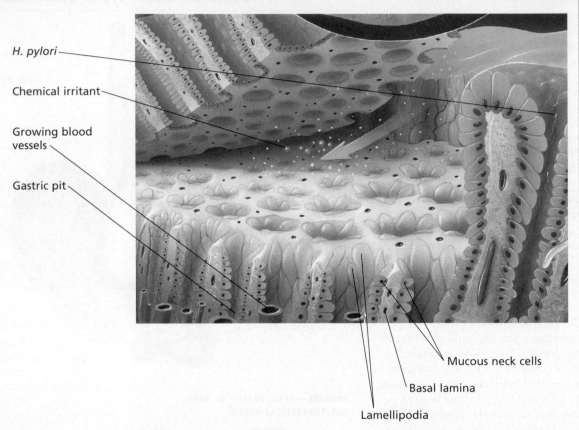

H. pylori

Chemical irritant

Growing blood vessels

Gastric pit

Mucous neck cells

Basal lamina

Lamellipodia

Signs and symptoms
Gastric ulcer
▶ Recent weight or appetite loss
▶ Food aversion because eating causes discomfort
▶ Pain in left epigastrium described as heartburn or indigestion
▶ Feeling of fullness or distention
▶ Eating that triggers pain

Duodenal ulcer
▶ Eating that relieves pain
▶ Nocturnal pain or pain that occurs 90 minutes to 3 hours after eating
▶ Epigastric pain described as sharp, gnawing, or burning
▶ Pallor (with anemia)
▶ Epigastric tenderness
▶ Hyperactive bowel sounds

Treatment
▶ Triple therapy consisting of clarithromycin and amoxicillin with a proton pump inhibitor to treat *H. pylori* infection
▶ Antacids
▶ Histamine-2 receptor antagonists, such as cimetidine (Tagamet) or ranitidine (Zantac), or a proton pump inhibitor such as omeprazole (Prilosec)
▶ Coating agents such as sucralfate for duodenal ulcers
▶ Antisecretory agents such as misoprostol (Cytotec)
▶ Sedatives and tranquilizers, such as chlordiazepoxide and phenobarbital
▶ Anticholinergics such as propantheline

▶ Physical rest and decreased activity to help decrease gastric secretion
▶ Diet therapy that consists of eating six small meals daily (or small hourly meals) rather than three regular meals
▶ Emergency treatment for GI bleeding that begins with the passage of a nasogastric (NG) tube to allow iced saline lavage, possibly containing norepinephrine
▶ Gastroscopy that allows visualization of the bleeding site and coagulation by laser or cautery to control bleeding
▶ Surgery for perforation; type dependent on the location and extent of the disorder
▶ Bilateral vagotomy, pyloroplasty, and gastrectomy

Nursing considerations

▸ Administer prescribed medications. Monitor the patient for the desired effects, and watch for adverse reactions.

▸ Provide six small meals or small hourly meals, as ordered.

▸ Continuously monitor the patient for complications: hemorrhage (sudden onset of weakness, fainting, chills, dizziness, thirst, the desire to defecate, and passage of loose, tarry, or even red stools); perforation (acute onset of epigastric pain followed by lessening of the pain and the onset of a rigid abdomen, tachycardia, fever, or rebound tenderness); obstruction (feeling of fullness or heaviness, copious vomiting containing undigested food after meals); and penetration (pain radiating to the back, night distress). If any of the above occurs, notify the practitioner immediately.

After surgery

▸ Keep the NG tube patent. If the tube isn't functioning, don't reposition it; you could damage the suture line or anastomosis. Notify the surgeon promptly.

▸ Monitor intake and output, including NG tube drainage. Also, check bowel sounds. Allow the patient nothing by mouth until peristalsis resumes and the NG tube is removed or clamped.

▸ Replace fluids and electrolytes. Assess for signs of dehydration, sodium deficiency, and metabolic alkalosis, which can occur secondary to gastric suction. Provide parenteral nutrition, if ordered.

▸ Control postoperative pain with narcotics and analgesics as ordered.

▸ Watch for such complications as hemorrhage; shock; iron, folate, or vitamin B_{12} deficiency anemia; and dumping syndrome.

LESSON PLANS

 Teaching about peptic ulcer disease

▸ Teach the patient about peptic ulcer disease, and help him to recognize its signs and symptoms. Explain scheduled diagnostic tests and prescribed therapies. Review symptoms associated with complications, and urge him to notify the practitioner if any of these occur. Emphasize the importance of complying with treatment, even after his symptoms are relieved.

▸ Review the proper use of prescribed medications, discussing the desired actions and possible adverse reactions of each drug.

▸ Instruct the patient to take antacids 1 hour after meals. If he follows a sodium-restricted diet, advise him to take only low-sodium antacids.

▸ Check all medications the patient is using. Antacids inhibit the absorption of many other drugs, including digoxin. Work out a schedule for taking medications.

▸ Warn against excessive intake of coffee and alcoholic beverages during exacerbations.

▸ Encourage the patient to make appropriate lifestyle changes. Explain that emotional tension can precipitate an ulcer attack and prolong healing.

▸ If the patient smokes, urge him to stop because smoking stimulates gastric acid secretion. Refer him to a smoking cessation program.

▸ Tell the patient to read labels of nonprescription medications and to avoid preparations that contain corticosteroids, aspirin, or other nonsteroidal anti-inflammatory drugs such as ibuprofen.

▸ Tell the patient that, although cimetidine, famotidine, and other histamine-receptor antagonists are available over the counter, he shouldn't take them without consulting his practitioner. These drugs may duplicate prescribed medications or suppress important symptoms.

▸ To avoid dumping syndrome after gastric surgery, advise the patient to lie down after meals, drink fluids between meals rather than with meals, avoid eating large amounts of carbohydrates, and eat four to six small, high-protein, low-carbohydrate meals daily.

Viral hepatitis

Viral hepatitis is a fairly common systemic disease. It's marked by hepatic cell destruction, necrosis, and autolysis, leading to anorexia, jaundice, and hepatomegaly. In most patients, hepatic cells eventually regenerate with little or no residual damage, allowing recovery. However, old age and serious underlying disorders make complications more likely. The prognosis is poor if edema and hepatic encephalopathy develop. Today, six types of viral hepatitis are recognized.

Type A

Type A hepatitis is usually self-limiting and without a chronic form.

Type A hepatitis is highly contagious and is usually transmitted by the fecal-oral route, commonly within institutions or families. Hepatitis A usually results from ingestion of contaminated food, milk, or water. Outbreaks of this type are commonly traced to ingestion of seafood from polluted water.

Type B

Type B, or serum or long-incubation, hepatitis is also increasing among human immunodeficiency virus (HIV) positive individuals. Hepatitis B is considered a sexually transmitted disease because of its high incidence and rate of transmission by this route. Routine screening of donor blood for the hepatitis B surface antigen has decreased the incidence of posttransfusion cases, but transmission by needles shared by drug abusers remains a major problem.

Type B hepatitis, once thought to be transmitted only by the direct exchange of contaminated blood, is now known to be transmitted also by contact with contaminated human secretions and stools. As a result, nurses, physicians, laboratory technicians, and dentists are frequently exposed to type B hepatitis, commonly as a result of wearing defective gloves. Today, hepatitis B vaccination is mandatory for military personnel, health care workers, and school children. Transmission of this type also occurs during intimate sexual contact and through perinatal transmission.

Type C

Type C accounts for about 20% of all viral hepatitis cases. It's primarily transmitted through sharing dirty needles or illicit drug use. It can also be spread by tatooing if the ink or needles are contaminated. Sexual transmission is rare.

Type D

Type D, or delta hepatitis, is responsible for about 50% of all cases of fulminant hepatitis, which has a high mortality. Fulminant hepatitis causes unremitting liver failure with encephalopathy. It progresses to coma and commonly leads to death within 2 weeks.

In the United States, type D hepatitis is confined to people who are frequently exposed to blood and blood products, such as I.V. drug users and hemophiliacs. It's transmitted parenterally and, less commonly, sexually.

Type D hepatitis is found only in patients who have had hepatitis B. Type D infection requires the presence of the hepatitis B surface antigen; the type D virus depends on the double-shelled type B virus to replicate. Hepatitis B vaccination protects against hepatitis D because hepatitis D can only occur with prior or concurrent infection with hepatitis B.

Type E

Type E occurs primarily in people who have recently returned from an endemic area (such as India, Africa, Asia, or Central America); it's more common in young adults and more severe in pregnant women. Type E hepatitis is transmitted enterically and is commonly waterborne, much like type A. Because this virus is inconsistently shed in stools, detection is difficult. Outbreaks of type E hepatitis have occurred in developing countries.

Type G

Type G commonly occurs in those who receive blood transfusions. It's thought to be blood-borne, with transmission similar to that of hepatitis C.

PICTURING PATHO

Viral hepatitis

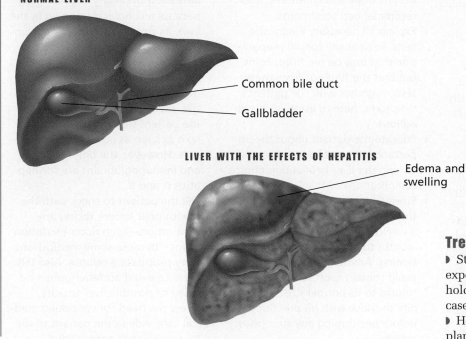

NORMAL LIVER

— Common bile duct

— Gallbladder

LIVER WITH THE EFFECTS OF HEPATITIS

— Edema and swelling

Signs and symptoms

Assessment findings are similar for the different types of hepatitis. Typically, signs and symptoms progress in several stages. Hepatitis C is usually mild or asymptomatic in the acute phase.

Prodromal (preictal) stage

▶ Easy fatigue
▶ Anorexia
▶ Mild weight loss
▶ Depression
▶ Headache
▶ Weakness
▶ Arthralgia
▶ Myalgia
▶ Photophobia
▶ Nausea with vomiting
▶ Changes in sense of taste and smell
▶ Fever (100° to 102° F [37.8° to 38.9° C])

Clinical jaundice stage

▶ Pruritus
▶ Abdominal pain or tenderness
▶ Indigestion
▶ Anorexia (later appetite may return)
▶ Jaundice that can last for 1 to 2 weeks
▶ Dark-colored urine
▶ Clay-colored stools
▶ Abdominal tenderness, an enlarged and tender liver, and splenomegaly and cervical adenopathy

Recovery or posticteric stage

▶ Decreased or subsided symptoms
▶ Decreased liver size
▶ Generally lasting from 2 to 12 weeks

Treatment

▶ Standard immunoglobulin for those exposed to hepatitis A and the household contacts of those with confirmed cases
▶ Hepatitis A vaccine for travelers planning visits to areas known to harbor such viruses
▶ Hepatitis B immunoglobulin and hepatitis B vaccine for individuals exposed to blood or body secretions of infected individuals
▶ Hepatitis B vaccine for people at risk for exposure, which includes neonates of hepatitis B virus (HBV)–positive mothers, sexual contacts of HBV-positive individuals, hemodialysis patients, health care workers, and male homosexuals
▶ Combination therapy with peginterferon alfa-2b (PEG-Intron) and ribavirin for chronic hepatitis C
▶ Rest and small, high-calorie, high-protein meals to combat anorexia
▶ Parenteral nutrition for persistent vomiting and those unable to maintain oral intake
▶ Antiemetics (trimethobenzamide [Tigan]) given half an hour before meals to relieve nausea and prevent vomiting
▶ Resin cholestyramine (Questran) for severe pruritus

Nursing considerations

▶ Observe standard precautions to prevent transmission of the disease. Make sure that visitors also observe these precautions.

▶ Provide rest periods throughout the day. Schedule treatments and tests so that the patient can rest between activities.

▶ Because inactivity may make the patient anxious, include diversional activities as part of his care. Gradually add activities to his schedule as he begins to recover.

▶ Take care not to overmedicate, which may cause loss of appetite. Determine his food preferences, and try to include his favorite foods in the meal plan.

▶ Administer supplemental vitamins and commercial feedings, as ordered. If symptoms are severe and the patient can't tolerate oral intake, provide I.V. therapy and parenteral nutrition, as ordered.

▶ Provide adequate fluid intake. The patient should consume at least 4 qt (4 L) of liquid per day to maintain adequate hydration. To help him meet or exceed this goal, provide him with fruit juices, soft drinks, ice chips, and water.

▶ Administer antiemetics as ordered. Observe the patient for the desired effects, and note any adverse reactions.

▶ Record weight daily, and keep accurate intake and output records. Observe the stools for color, consistency, and amount. Also note the frequency of defecation.

▶ Watch for signs of complications, such as changes in level of consciousness, ascites, edema, dehydration, respiratory problems, myalgia, and arthralgia.

▶ Report all cases of hepatitis to health officials. Ask the patient to name anyone he came in contact with recently.

Teaching about viral hepatitis

▶ Teach the patient about viral hepatitis, its signs and symptoms, and recommended treatments.

▶ Explain all necessary diagnostic tests. Review any special preparation that may be required. Point out that the findings from these tests, together with the patient's symptoms, help to establish his diagnosis.

▶ Educate the patient about the importance of rest and a proper diet to help the liver heal and minimize complications.

▶ Stress that complete recovery takes time. Point out that the liver takes 3 weeks to regenerate and up to 4 months to return to normal functioning. Advise the patient to avoid contact sports until his liver returns to its normal size. Instruct him to check with his practitioner before performing any strenuous activity.

▶ Emphasize the importance of good nutrition in promoting liver regeneration. Advise him to eat several small meals rather than three large meals. Also, stress the importance of drinking adequate fluids every day.

▶ Tell the patient recuperating at home to weigh himself every day and to report any weight loss greater than 5 lb (2.3 kg) to his practitioner.

▶ Warn the patient to abstain from alcohol. If necessary, explain that, because alcohol is detoxified in the liver, its consumption could put undue stress on the liver during the illness.

▶ Explain to the patient and family members that anyone exposed to the disease through contact with the patient should receive prophylaxis as soon as possible after exposure. However, the only vaccines and immunoglobulins are for hepatitis A and B.

▶ Tell the patient to check with the practitioner before taking any medication—even nonprescription drugs—because some medications can precipitate a relapse. Also tell them to avoid acetaminophen because of possible liver toxicity.

▶ Stress the need for continued medical care. Advise the patient to see his practitioner again about 2 weeks after the diagnosis is made. Mention the probable need for follow-up visits every month for up to 6 months after diagnosis. Also, explain that if chronic hepatitis develops, he'll have to visit his practitioner regularly so that the disease can be monitored.

TESTS
Laboratory tests

Common laboratory tests used to diagnose GI disorders include studies of stool, urine, and esophageal, gastric, and peritoneal contents as well as percutaneous liver biopsy.

ACID PERFUSION TEST

To distinguish the pain of esophagitis from that caused by angina pectoris or other disorders, normal saline and acidic solutions are perfused separately into the esophagus through a nasogastric (NG) tube to determine whether the lower esophageal sphincter (which normally prevents gastric reflux) is competent.

Intraesophageal pH monitoring has largely replaced the acid perfusion test because it offers continuous measurement of esophageal pH for up to 48 hours. It's especially useful in monitoring nocturnal symptoms. The test is done by placing a pH capsule through the nose or mouth with the Bravo delivery system. It records pH continuously over a set period. The patient may perform regular activities with the monitor in place. The patient should record symptoms of reflux and dyspepsia while being monitored to help correlate activity with pH.

FECAL CONTENT STUDIES

Fecal content studies examine the content (fat, blood), condition (soft, hard, liquid, ribbonlike), and color (tan, white, yellow, green, red, black) of stool to determine certain disorders for further investigation. Normal stool appears brown and formed but soft. Narrow, ribbonlike stool signals spastic or irritable bowel, or partial bowel or rectal obstruction. Diarrhea may indicate spastic bowel or viral infection. Soft stool mixed with blood and mucus can signal bacterial infection; mixed with blood and pus, colitis.

Yellow or green stool suggests severe, prolonged diarrhea; black stool suggests GI bleeding or intake of iron supplements or raw-to-rare meat. Tan or white stool shows hepatic-duct or gallbladder-duct blockage, hepatitis, or cancer. Red stool may signal colon or rectal bleeding, but some drugs and foods can also cause this coloration. Pasty or greasy stool, which contains higher fat content, is a possible sign of intestinal malabsorption or pancreatic disease.

PERCUTANEOUS LIVER BIOPSY

A percutaneous liver biopsy involves the needle aspiration of a core of liver tissue for histologic analysis. It's done under local or general anesthesia. This biopsy can identify hepatic disorders and cancer after ultrasonography, computed tomography (CT) scans, and radionuclide studies have failed. Because many patients with hepatic disorders have clotting defects, a clotting profile (prothrombin time, partial thromboplastin time) along with type and crossmatching should precede liver biopsy.

PERITONEAL FLUID ANALYSIS

The peritoneal fluid analysis series includes examination of gross appearance, erythrocyte and leukocyte counts, cytologic studies, microbiological studies for bacteria and fungi, and determinations of protein, glucose, amylase, ammonia, and alkaline phosphatase levels. A sample of peritoneal fluid is obtained by paracentesis, which involves inserting a trocar and cannula through the abdominal wall with the patient under a local anesthetic. If the sample of fluid is being removed for therapeutic purposes, the cannula can be connected to a drainage system.

URINE TESTS

Urinalysis provides valuable information about hepatic and biliary function. Urinary bilirubin and urobilinogen tests are commonly used to evaluate liver function.

Bilirubin is normally excreted in bile as its principal pigment, but it occurs abnormally in urine. Conjugated bilirubin is present in urine when serum levels rise, as in biliary tract obstruction or hepatocellular damage, and is accompanied by jaundice.

Urobilinogen is primarily excreted in stool, producing its characteristic brown color. A small amount is reabsorbed by the portal system and is mainly reexcreted in bile, although the kidneys do excrete some. As a result, elevated urine urobilinogen levels may be an early indication of hepatic damage. With biliary obstruction, urine urobilinogen levels decline.

Endoscopy

Using a fiber-optic endoscope, the physician can directly view hollow visceral linings to diagnose inflammatory, ulcerative, and infectious diseases; benign and malignant neoplasms; and other esophageal, gastric, and intestinal mucosal lesions. Endoscopy can also be used for therapeutic interventions or to obtain biopsy specimens.

CAMERA ENDOSCOPY

With camera endoscopy, a tiny video camera with a light source and transmitter inside a capsule allows for recording of images along its path. After swallowing the capsule, the patient can leave the health care facility and resume work or other activities of daily living.

ENDOSCOPIC RETROGRADE CHOLANGIO-PANCREATOGRAPHY

In endoscopic retrograde cholangio-pancreatography, the physician passes an endoscope into the duodenum and injects dye through a cannula inserted into the ampulla of Vater. This test helps to determine the cause of jaundice; evaluate tumors and inflammation of the pancreas, gallbladder, or liver; and locate obstructions in the pancreatic duct and hepatobiliary tree.

LOWER GI ENDOSCOPY

Lower GI endoscopy, also called *colonoscopy,* aids diagnosis of inflammatory and ulcerative bowel disease, pinpoints lower GI bleeding, and detects lower GI abnormalities, such as tumors, polyps, hemorrhoids, and abscesses.

Abbreviated versions of a lower GI endoscopy include flexible sigmoidoscopy and proctosigmoidoscopy.

Camera endoscopy

With camera endoscopy, the patient swallows the capsule, which then travels through the body by the natural movement of the digestive tract. A receiver worn outside the body records the images. The strength of the signal indicates the capsule's location.

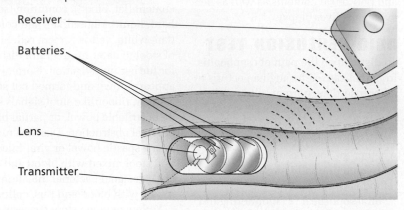

Receiver
Batteries
Lens
Transmitter

Abnormal ERCP

This endoscopic retrograde cholangiopancreatographic (ERCP) view shows a dilated pancreatic duct secondary to stenosis. Stenosis was caused by carcinoma at the head of the pancreas.

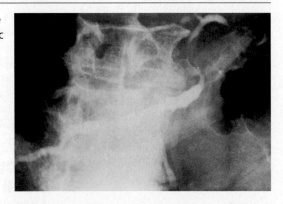

Abnormal colonoscopy

These two views, taken with a fiber-optic colonoscope, show ulcerative colitis (left) and diverticulosis (right).

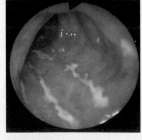

ULCERATIVE COLITIS

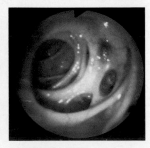

DIVERTICULOSIS

UPPER GI ENDOSCOPY

Upper GI endoscopy, also called *esophagogastroduodenoscopy,* identifies abnormalities of the esophagus, stomach, and small intestine, such as esophagitis, inflammatory bowel disease, Mallory-Weiss tear, lesions, tumors, gastritis, and polyps. During endoscopy, biopsies may be taken to detect the presence of *Helicobacter pylori* or to rule out gastric carcinoma.

Colon abnormalities

These abnormal views of the colon were taken with a proctosigmoidoscope. The view on the left demonstrates familial polyposis—multiple adenomatous growths and high malignancy potential. The view on the right shows diverticular orifices of the colon associated with muscle hypertrophy, which almost obscures the slitlike lumen at the far right of this photograph.

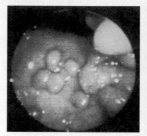 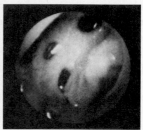

Nuclear imaging and ultrasonography

Nuclear imaging methods, which include liver-spleen scanning and magnetic resonance imaging, analyze concentrations of injected or ingested radiopaque substances to enhance visual evaluation of possible disease processes. Nuclear imaging methods are used to study the liver, spleen, and other abdominal organs.

Ultrasonography is used to create images of internal organs, such as the gallbladder, spleen, and liver. Gas-filled structures, such as the intestines, can't be seen with this technique.

LIVER-SPLEEN SCAN

With a liver-spleen scan, a scanner or gamma camera records the distribution of radioactivity within the liver and spleen after I.V. injection of a radioactive colloid. Most of this colloid is taken up by Kupffer cells in the liver, and smaller amounts lodge in the spleen and bone marrow. By registering the extent of this absorption, the imaging device detects such abnormalities as tumors, cysts, and abscesses. Because the test demonstrates disease nonspecifically (as an area that fails to take up the colloid, or a cold spot), test results usually require confirmation by ultrasonography, computed tomography scan, gallium scan, or biopsy.

Comparing normal and abnormal images of the pancreas

The ultrasound view on the top shows a normal pancreas (shown in color). The ultrasound view on the bottom shows a diffusely enlarged pancreas caused by pancreatitis. The color indicates the extent of enlargement.

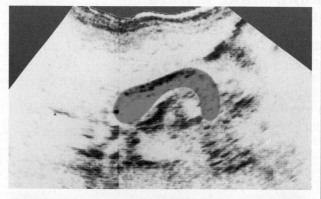

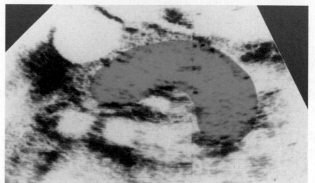

MAGNETIC RESONANCE IMAGING

Magnetic resonance imaging (MRI) is used in imaging the liver and abdominal organs. The image is generated by energizing protons into a strong magnetic field. Radio waves emitted as protons return to former equilibrium state and are recorded. No ionizing radiation is transmitted during the scan. Disadvantages to MRI are the closed, tubelike space that's required for the scan. Newer MRI centers offer a less confining "open-MRI" scan. The test can't be performed on patients with metal or implanted devices. MRI is useful in evaluating liver disease to help characterize tumors, masses, or cysts found on previous studies.

ULTRASONOGRAPHY

Ultrasonography uses a focused beam of high-frequency sound waves to create echoes, which then appear as spikes and dots on a monitor. Echoes vary with tissue density. The test helps differentiate between obstructive and nonobstructive jaundice and diagnoses cholelithiasis, cholecystitis, and certain metastases and hematomas. When used with liver-spleen scanning, it can clarify the nature of cold spots, such as tumors, abscesses, and cysts. The technique also aids diagnosis of pancreatitis, pseudocysts, pancreatic cancer, ascites, and splenomegaly. When Color Doppler is added (duplex scan), the speed, direction, and patterns of blood flow throughout the vessels and organs can be determined.

Radiographic tests

Radiographic tests include abdominal X-rays, computed tomography scans, various contrast medium studies, and virtual colonoscopy.

ABDOMINAL X-RAYS

An abdominal X-ray, also called *flat plate of the abdomen* or *kidney-ureter-bladder radiography,* helps detect and evaluate tumors, kidney stones, abnormal gas collection, and other abdominal disorders. The test consists of two plates: one taken with the patient supine and the other taken while he stands. On X-ray, air appears black, adipose tissue appears gray, and bone appears white.

Although a routine X-ray won't reveal most abdominal organs, it will show the contrast between air and fluid. For example, intestinal blockage traps large amounts of detectable fluids and air inside organs. When an intestinal wall tears, air leaks into the abdomen and becomes visible on the X-ray.

COMPUTED TOMOGRAPHY SCAN

In computed tomography (CT) scanning, a computer translates the action of multiple X-ray beams into three-dimensional oscilloscope images of the biliary tract, liver, and pancreas. The test can be done without a contrast medium, but contrast is preferred unless the patient is allergic. This test:
▶ helps distinguish between obstructive and nonobstructive jaundice
▶ identifies abscesses, cysts, hematomas, tumors, and pseudocysts
▶ helps evaluate the cause of weight loss
▶ detects occult malignancy
▶ helps diagnose and evaluate pancreatitis.

Normal CT scan of the pancreas

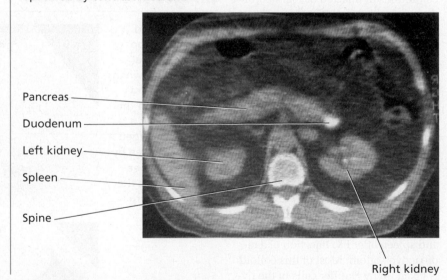

This normal pancreatic computed tomography (CT) scan shows the pancreas opacified by contrast medium.

Pancreas

Duodenum

Left kidney

Spleen

Spine

Right kidney

Contrast radiography

Some X-ray tests require contrast media to more accurately assess the GI system because the media accentuate differences among densities of air, fat, soft tissue, and bone. These tests include barium enema, barium swallow test, cholangiography, small-bowel series and enema, and upper GI series.

BARIUM ENEMA

The barium enema is most commonly used to evaluate suspected lower intestinal disorders. It helps diagnose inflammatory disorders, colorectal cancer, polyps, diverticula, and large-intestine structural changes such as intussusception.

BARIUM SWALLOW TEST

The barium swallow test allows examination of the pharynx and esophagus to detect strictures, ulcers, tumors, polyps, diverticula, hiatal hernia, esophageal webs, gastroesophageal reflux disease, motility disorders and, sometimes, achalasia.

CHOLANGIOGRAPHY

In cholangiography (percutaneous and postoperative), a contrast agent is injected into the biliary tree through a flexible needle. In percutaneous transhepatic cholangiography, a radiopaque dye is injected directly into the liver through the eighth or ninth mid-axillary intercostal space. If done postoperatively, the dye is injected via a T tube. In an oral cholangiogram, the patient is given the contrast medium by mouth. These tests are used to determine the cause of upper abdominal pain that persists after cholecystectomy, to evaluate jaundice, and to determine the location, the extent and, usually, the cause of mechanical obstructions.

Abnormal percutaneous cholangiogram

In this percutaneous cholangiogram, the dilated hepatic ducts indicate obstruction of the common bile duct by a tumor. The catheter tip has been passed through the tumor into the duodenum.

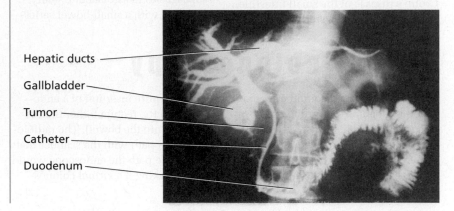

Hepatic ducts
Gallbladder
Tumor
Catheter
Duodenum

Normal T tube cholangiogram

This T tube cholangiogram shows homogeneous filling of biliary ducts. The ducts are of normal diameter, and the presence of contrast medium in the duodenum shows that the ducts are also patent.

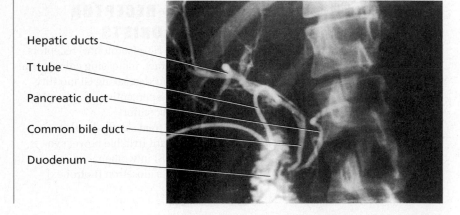

Hepatic ducts
T tube
Pancreatic duct
Common bile duct
Duodenum

SMALL-BOWEL SERIES

Results of a small-bowel series or enema, which follow the contrast agent through the small intestine, may suggest sprue, obstruction, motility disorders, malabsorption syndrome, Hodgkin's disease, lymphosarcoma, ischemia, bleeding, inflammation, or Crohn's disease of the small intestine. Although the enema study is longer and more uncomfortable than the small-bowel series, it better distends the bowel, making lesion identification easier.

UPPER GI SERIES

In an upper GI series, the physician follows the barium's passage from the esophagus to the stomach. Usually combined with a small-bowel series, the upper GI series helps diagnose gastritis, cancer, hiatal hernia, diverticula, strictures, and (most commonly) gastric and duodenal ulcers. It may also suggest motility disorders.

Virtual colonoscopy

Virtual colonoscopy combines computed tomography scanning and X-ray images with sophisticated image processing computers to generate three-dimensional images of the patient's colon. It's a noninvasive approach that doesn't require insertion of a endoscope into the rectum (other than to inject air into the bowel). The radiologist plots a path with the scanner that mimics the path the endoscope would follow, making it a virtual colonoscopy. The scan takes about 10 minutes, and the images are assembled in a computer program that can be viewed on a screen.

TREATMENTS AND PROCEDURES

Treatments for GI disorders include drug therapy, surgery, and related procedures.

Drug therapy

The most commonly used GI drugs include 5-HT$_3$-receptor antagonists, adsorbents, antacids, anticholinergics, antidiarrheals, antiemetics, antiflatulents, digestants, histamine-2 (H$_2$) receptor antagonists, laxatives, and proton pump inhibitors. Some of these drugs, such as antacids and antiemetics, provide immediate relief. Others, such as laxatives and H$_2$-receptor antagonists, may take several days or longer to treat the problem.

5-HT$_3$-RECEPTOR ANTAGONISTS

▶ Block 5-HT$_3$ (serotonin) receptors in the GI tract, increasing colonic transit time and decreasing GI motility
▶ Decrease perception of pain and GI tract discomfort
▶ Used to treat severe diarrhea-predominant irritable bowel syndrome (IBS) in women
▶ Example: alosetron (Lotronex)

ADSORBENT DRUGS

▶ Attract and bind to toxins in the GI tract, which prevents absorption
▶ Used as antidote for oral ingestion of toxins that can lead to poisoning or overdose
▶ Example: activated charcoal

ANTACIDS

▶ Used for heartburn, acid indigestion, and adjunct therapy with peptic ulcer disease
▶ Work locally in the stomach by neutralizing gastric acid
▶ Example: aluminum hydroxide (Amphogel)

ANTICHOLINERGICS

▶ Relax the GI tract and inhibit gastric acid secretion
▶ Example: propantheline (Pro-Banthine)

ANTIDIARRHEALS

▶ Opioid-related drugs that decrease peristalsis in the intestines
▶ Example: loperamide (Imodium)

ANTIEMETICS

▶ Prevent and treat nausea
▶ Examples: ondansetron (Zofran), granisetron (Kytril)

ANTIFLATULENTS

▶ Create foaming action in the GI tract, creating a film on the intestines that helps to disperse mucus-enclosed gas pockets
▶ Help prevent the formation of gas pockets
▶ Treat excessive amounts of air or gas in the stomach or intestines, such as gastric bloating, diverticular disease, or spastic or irritable colon
▶ Example: simethicone (Flatulex, Gas-X, Maalox Anti-Gas, Mylanta Gas, Mylicon, Phazyme)

DIGESTANTS

▶ Resemble that of the substance they're replacing
▶ Bile acids used to increase output of bile in the liver; pancreatic enzymes, to replace normal pancreatic enzymes

▶ Dehydrocholic acid used to treat constipation and promote bile flow; pancreatic enzymes used in patients with a deficiency of natural pancreatic enzymes, such as in pancreatitis or cystic fibrosis
▶ Examples: dehydrocholic acid, pancreatic enzymes (pancreatin, pancrelipase, lipase, protease, and amylase)

H₂-RECEPTOR ANTAGONISTS

▶ Block histamine from stimulating acid-secreting parietal cells of the stomach to decrease hydrochloric acid
▶ Examples: cimetidine (Tagamet), ranitidine (Zantac), famotidine (Pepcid), nizatidine (Axid)

LAXATIVES

▶ Stimulate defecation and include hyperosmolar laxatives, bulk-forming laxatives, emollients, stimulants, and lubricants
▶ Hyperosmolar laxatives: draw water into the intestine, thereby promoting bowel distention and peristalsis; example: lactulose (Chronulac)
▶ Bulk-forming laxatives: resemble dietary fiber and contain natural and semisynthetic polysaccharides and cellulose; examples: psyllium (Metamucil) and polycarbophil (Equalactin)

▶ Emollient laxatives (stool softeners): emulsify fat and water components of feces in the small and large intestine, allowing water to penetrate stool, making it softer and easier to eliminate; example: docusate (Colace)
▶ Stimulant laxatives: stimulate peristalsis and produce a bowel movement by irritating the intestinal mucosa or stimulating nerve endings of the intestinal smooth muscle; examples: bisacodyl (Dulcolax), senna (Senokot)
▶ Lubricants: lubricate the intestinal mucosa and prevent water absorption from the bowel lumen, increasing the fluid content of the feces and increasing peristalsis; example: mineral oil

PROTON PUMP INHIBITORS

▶ Disrupt chemical binding in stomach cells to reduce acid production, lessening irritation
▶ Examples: omeprazole (Prilosec), lansoprazole (Prevacid), pantoprazole (Protonix), or esomeprazole (Nexium)

Surgery

Surgical procedures can involve the stomach (gastric surgery), bowel (with ostomy; resection and anastomosis), appendix (appendectomy), gallbladder, and liver (transplantation and resection or repair).

GASTRIC SURGERY

Gastric surgery can take various forms, depending on the location and extent of the disorder. For example, a partial gastrectomy reduces the amount of acid-secreting mucosa. A bilateral vagotomy relieves ulcer symptoms and eliminates vagal nerve stimulation of gastric secretions. A pyloroplasty improves drainage and prevents obstruction. Most commonly, however, two gastric surgeries are combined, such as vagotomy with gastroenterostomy or vagotomy with antrectomy. In cases of morbid obesity, gastric reduction surgery may be performed to aid in weight loss.

Types of gastric surgery

Note: Dotted lines below show the areas removed.

Gastroduodenostomy

Also called *Billroth I*, gastroduo-denostomy may be done to remove a pyloric tumor. The surgeon resects the distal one-third to one-half of the stomach and anastomoses the remaining stomach portion to the duodenum.

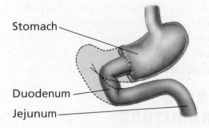

Gastrojejunostomy

In gastrojejunostomy (Billroth II), the surgeon removes the distal portion of the antrum, anastomoses the remaining stomach to the jejunum, and closes the duodenal stump.

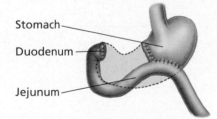

Partial gastric resection

For a tumor in a defined stomach area, the surgeon performs partial gastric resection by removing the diseased stomach portion and attaching the remaining stomach to the jejunum.

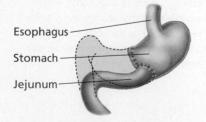

Total gastrectomy

Total gastrectomy may be done if the tumor is in the cardia or high in the fundus. The surgeon removes the entire stomach and attaches the lower end of the esophagus to the jejunum (esophagojejunostomy) at the entrance to the small intestine.

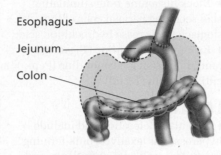

Vagotomy with gastroenterostomy

In this procedure, the surgeon resects the vagus nerve and creates a stoma for gastric drainage. He'll perform selective, truncal, or parietal cell vagotomy, depending on the degree of decreased gastric acid secretion required.

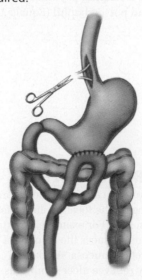

Vagotomy with antrectomy

After resecting the vagus nerves, the surgeon removes the antrum. Then he anastomoses the remaining stomach segment to the jejunum and closes the duodenal stump.

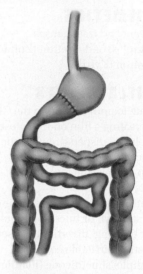

Vagotomy with pyloroplasty

In this procedure, the surgeon resects the vagus nerves and refashions the pylorus to widen the lumen and aid gastric emptying.

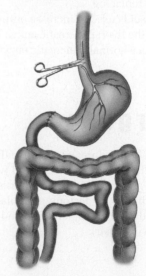

BOWEL SURGERY WITH OSTOMY

In bowel surgery with ostomy, the surgeon removes diseased colonic and rectal segments and creates a stoma on the outer abdominal wall to allow fecal elimination. This surgery is performed for such intestinal maladies as inflammatory bowel disease, familial polyposis, diverticulitis, and advanced colorectal cancer if conservative surgery and other treatments aren't successful or if the patient develops acute complications, such as obstruction, abscess, and fistula.

The surgeon can choose from several types of surgery.

‣ Permanent colostomy and removal of affected bowel segments—for intractable obstruction of the ascending, transverse, descending, or sigmoid colon.

Types of intestinal stomas

End stoma

To form an end stoma, the surgeon pulls a section of the intestine through the outer abdominal wall, everts the section, and sutures it to the skin.

‣ Abdominoperineal resection—for cancer of the rectum and lower sigmoid colon, which involves creation of a permanent colostomy and removal of the remaining colon, rectum, and anus.

‣ Temporary colostomy—for perforated sigmoid diverticulitis, Hirschsprung's disease, rectovaginal fistula, and penetrating trauma, which interrupts intestinal flow and allows inflamed and injured bowel segments to heal. After healing occurs (usually within 8 weeks), the divided segments are anastomosed to restore bowel integrity and function.

Loop stoma

To create a loop stoma, the surgeon brings a loop of intestine out through an abdominal incision to the abdominal surface and supports it with a rod or bridge (usually removed in 5 to 7 days). Then he opens the anterior wall of the bowel loop with a small incision to provide fecal diversion. The result is a stoma with a proximal, functioning limb and a distal, nonfunctioning limb. The surgeon then closes the wound around the exposed intestinal loop.

‣ Double-barrel colostomy—which divides the transverse colon and brings both ends out through the abdominal wall to create a proximal stoma for fecal drainage and a distal stoma that leads to the nonfunctioning bowel.

‣ Loop colostomy—performed to relieve acute obstruction in an emergency—involves creating proximal and distal stomas from a loop of intestine that has been pulled through an abdominal incision and supported with a plastic or glass rod.

Double-barrel stoma

For a double-barrel stoma, the surgeon divides the intestine and brings both the proximal and distal ends through the abdominal incision to the abdominal surface. He makes a small incision in the proximal stoma for fecal drainage. The distal stoma (also called a *mucous fistula*) leads to the inactive intestine and is left intact.

Later, when the intestinal injury has healed or the inflammation has subsided, the colostomy is reversed and the divided ends of the intestine are anastomosed to restore intestinal integrity.

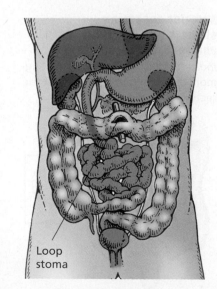

End stoma

Loop stoma

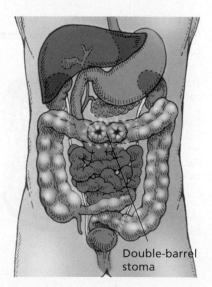

Double-barrel stoma

▶ Ileostomy—total or near-total removal of the colon and rectum, creating an ileostomy from the proximal ileum, for severe, widespread colonic obstruction. A permanent ileostomy requires that the patient wear a drainage pouch or bag over the stoma to receive the constant fecal drainage. In contrast, a continent, or Kock, ileostomy doesn't require an external pouch.

BOWEL RESECTION AND ANASTOMOSIS

Surgical bowel resection of diseased intestinal tissue and anastomosis (connection) of the remaining segments are used to treat localized obstructive disorders, such as acute diverticulosis, adhesions, and benign or malignant intestinal tumors. Resection is also the preferred treatment for localized bowel cancer.

The surgeon excises diseased colonic tissue and then connects the remaining bowel segments to restore patency. He may use one of two anastomosis techniques:

▶ End-to-end anastomosis (in which the ends of two structures are joined) is faster and produces a more physiologically sound junction but requires bowel segments large enough to prevent postoperative obstruction.

▶ Side-to-side anastomosis (in which structures positioned next to each other are joined) reduces the danger of obstruction but takes longer to perform.

Types of bowel resection

The shaded areas indicate the portions of bowel that are removed. Boxed illustrations show the structure of the anastomosed bowel.

Right hemicolectomy
Indications: Disease of the cecum and lower ascending colon

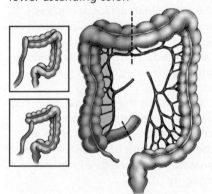

Left hemicolectomy
Indications: Disease of the descending and upper sigmoid colon

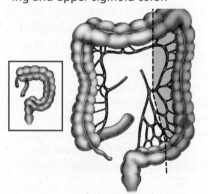

Sigmoid colectomy
Indications: Disease of the lower sigmoid colon or upper rectum

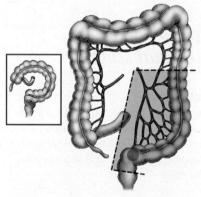

Transverse colectomy
Indications: Disease of the transverse colon

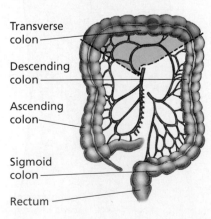

Transverse colon

Descending colon

Ascending colon

Sigmoid colon

Rectum

Anterior resection of the sigmoid colon and rectosigmoidostomy
Indications: Disease of the lower sigmoid or rectosigmoid portion of the rectum

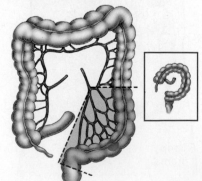

Abdominoperineal resection (Miles' resection)
Indications: Disease of the lower sigmoid colon, rectum, and anus. *Note:* In this procedure, these parts are removed and a permanent colostomy is formed.

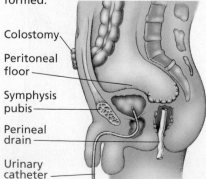

Colostomy

Peritoneal floor

Symphysis pubis

Perineal drain

Urinary catheter

APPENDECTOMY

With rare exception, the only effective treatment for acute appendicitis is to remove the inflamed vermiform appendix. A common emergency surgery, an appendectomy aims to prevent imminent rupture or perforation of the appendix. When completed before these complications occur, it's usually effective and uneventful. However, if the appendix ruptures or perforates before surgery, its infected contents spill into the peritoneal cavity, possibly causing peritonitis, which is the most common and fatal complication of appendicitis, with a mortality rate of 10%. Most appendectomies are now done laparoscopically, except in cases where rupture is suspected.

Laparoscopic appendectomy

In laparoscopic appendectomy, the surgeon makes three small incisions in the abdomen for trocar placement and the introduction of the laparoscope (with attached video camera) and surgical instruments. He then insufflates the abdominal cavity with carbon dioxide to aid visualization. He uses grasping forceps and stapling instruments to transect the appendix. Then the surgeon cauterizes the appendiceal stump and removes the appendix through the umbilical incision. He irrigates and suctions the abdomen and closes the incisions.

GALLBLADDER SURGERY

Gallbladder surgery, or *cholecystectomy,* is the removal of the gallbladder and any gallstones to restore biliary flow in patients with gallstone disease (cholecystitis or cholelithiasis). It's one of the most commonly performed surgeries, relieving symptoms in 90% of patients. Open cholecystectomy requires a large incision, produces considerable discomfort, and results in weeks of recovery time. Alternatively, laparoscopic cholecystectomy allows gallbladder removal without major abdominal surgery, thereby speeding recovery and reducing the risk of

Laparoscopic appendectomy

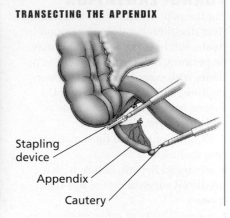

TROCAR PLACEMENT

Port
Umbilical port
Port

TRANSECTING THE APPENDIX

Stapling device
Appendix
Cautery

Laparoscopic cholecystectomy

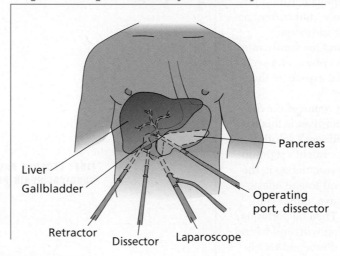

Liver
Gallbladder
Retractor
Dissector
Laparoscope
Pancreas
Operating port, dissector

complications, such as infection and herniation.

In patients who aren't good candidates for cholecystectomy, cholecystostomy (incision into the fundus of the gallbladder to remove and drain any retained gallstones or inflammatory debris) or choledochotomy (incision into the common bile duct to remove any gallstones or other obstructions) is sometimes performed.

In laparoscopic cholecystectomy, the surgeon makes a small incision at the umbilicus for the laparoscope and its attached camera. Then he insuf-

flates the abdomen with carbon dioxide so he can visualize the structures. He'll make three more incisions to introduce additional instruments. Then he retracts the gallbladder, exposing the cystic duct. Intraoperative cholangiography may be performed. Next, the surgeon clips and divides the cystic duct and dissects the cystic artery and gallbladder. He suctions out bile and stones and removes the gallbladder through the umbilical port. He may use a specimen bag to secure the gallbladder.

LIVER TRANSPLANTATION

For the patient with a life-threatening liver disorder that doesn't respond to treatment, liver transplantation may be performed. Candidates include patients with congenital biliary abnormalities, chronic hepatitis B or C, inborn errors of metabolism, or end-stage liver disease.

Criteria for referral for transplantation include:

▶ advanced hepatic failure with a predicted survival rate of less than 2 years
▶ unavailability of other medical or surgical therapies that offer long-term survival
▶ absence of contraindicated conditions, such as extrahepatic carcinoma, severe cardiac disease, and current active alcohol or drug addiction
▶ that the patient and his family must fully understand the physical, psychological, and financial aspects of the transplant process.

After the surgeon removes the diseased liver, the donor liver is flushed with cold lactated Ringer's solution and placed in the recipient's right upper abdomen. To revascularize it, the surgeon performs end-to-end anastomoses of the vena cava, portal vein, and hepatic artery. Then he performs biliary reconstruction with end-to-end anastomosis of the donor and recipient common bile ducts and inserts a T tube.

If end-to-end anastomosis can't be done, an end-to-side anastomosis is made between the common bile duct of the donor liver and a loop (Roux-en-Y portion) of the recipient's jejunum. With this procedure, the surgeon places internal surgical drains and closes the wound.

Transplanting a liver

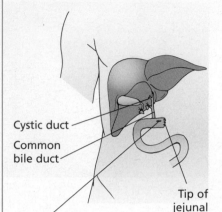

ROUX-EN-Y HEPATOJEJUNOSTOMY

Cystic duct
Common bile duct
Enterotomy for choledochojejunostomy
Tip of jejunal Roux-en-Y loop

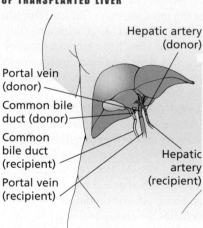

FINAL APPEARANCE OF TRANSPLANTED LIVER

Hepatic artery (donor)
Portal vein (donor)
Common bile duct (donor)
Common bile duct (recipient)
Portal vein (recipient)
Hepatic artery (recipient)

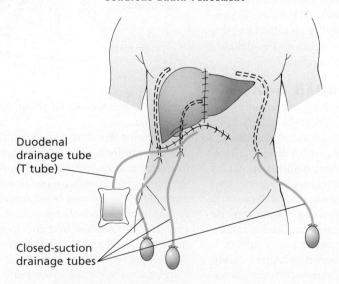

FINAL CLOSURE AND SURGICAL DRAIN PLACEMENT

Duodenal drainage tube (T tube)
Closed-suction drainage tubes

Managing liver transplantation complications

This table gives possible complications of liver transplantation and the assessment and nursing interventions for each complication.

Complication	Assessment and intervention
Effects of immunosuppressant therapy	▶ Note any signs or symptoms of opportunistic infection, including fever, tachycardia, chills, leukocytosis, leukopenia, and diaphoresis. ▶ Report drug adverse reactions. ▶ Check the patient's weight daily.
Hemorrhage and hypovolemic shock	▶ Assess the patient's vital signs and other indicators of fluid volume hourly, and note trends indicating hypovolemia; hypotension; weak, rapid, irregular pulse; oliguria; decreased level of consciousness; and signs of peripheral vasoconstriction. ▶ Monitor the patient's hematocrit and hemoglobin levels daily. ▶ Maintain patency of all I.V. lines, and reserve 2 units of blood in case the patient needs a transfusion.
Hepatic failure	▶ Monitor nasogastric tube drainage for upper GI bleeding. ▶ Frequently assess the patient's neurovascular status. ▶ Note development of peripheral edema and ascites. ▶ Monitor the patient's renal function by checking urine output, blood urea nitrogen levels, and serum creatinine and potassium levels. Monitor serum amylase levels daily.
Pulmonary insufficiency or failure	▶ Maintain ventilation at prescribed levels. ▶ Monitor the patient's arterial blood gas levels daily, and change ventilator settings, as ordered. ▶ Auscultate for abnormal breath sounds every 2 to 4 hours. ▶ Suction the patient as needed.
Vascular obstruction	▶ Be alert for signs and symptoms of acute vascular obstruction in the right upper quadrant—cramping pain or tenderness, nausea, and vomiting. Notify the physician immediately if any occur. ▶ If ordered, prepare for emergency thrombectomy. Maintain I.V. infusions, check and document the patient's vital signs, and maintain airway patency.
Wound infection or abscess	▶ Assess the incision site daily, and report any inflammation, tenderness, drainage, or other signs and symptoms of infection. ▶ Change the dressing daily or as needed. ▶ Note and report any signs or symptoms of peritonitis or abscess, including fever, chills, leukocytosis (or leukopenia with bands), and abdominal pain, tenderness, and rigidity. ▶ Take the patient's temperature every 4 hours. ▶ Swab the wound for culture and sensitivity studies. Document the color, amount, odor, and consistency of drainage. ▶ Assess the patient for signs of infection in other areas, such as the urinary tract, respiratory system, and blood. Document and report any signs of infection.

LIVER RESECTION OR REPAIR

Resection or repair of diseased or damaged liver tissue may be indicated for various hepatic disorders, icluding cysts, abscesses, tumors, and lacerations or crush injuries from blunt or penetrating trauma. Usually, surgery is performed only after conservative measures prove ineffective. For instance, if aspiration fails to correct a liver abscess, resection may be necessary.

Liver resection procedures include a partial or subtotal hepatectomy (excision of a portion of the liver) and lobectomy (excision of an entire lobe). Lobectomy is the surgery of choice for primary liver tumors, but partial hepatectomy may be effective for small tumors. Even so, because liver cancer is typically advanced at diagnosis, few tumors are resectable. In fact, only single tumors confined to one lobe are usually considered resectable, and then only if the patient is free from complicating cirrhosis, jaudice, or ascites. Because of the liver's anatomic location, surgery is usually performed through a thoracoabdominal incision.

Other treatments and procedures

Other treatments and procedures include abdominal compartment pressure monitoring, colostomy and ileostomy care, feeding tube insertion, gastric lavage, gastrostomy feeding button care, nasogastric (NG) tube care, NG tube insertion and removal, transabdominal tube feeding and care, and tube feeding.

Abdominal compartment pressure monitoring

Abdominal compartment pressure monitoring, also known as *intra-abdominal pressure (IAP) monitoring*, indirectly measures the pressure within the abdominal compartment. The abdominal wall creates a closed, fixed compartment containing the abdominal and pelvic organs and vasculature. Intra-abdominal hypertension (IAH) is caused by conditions that increase the pressure within the abdominal compartment and results in impaired capillary perfusion and reduced venous blood flow to the heart. Abdominal compartment syndrome develops when IAH progresses to organ and tissue ischemia and infarction. Early recognition and treatment of IAH can prevent multisystem organ failure and death.

IAH may be caused by such conditions as massive fluid resuscitation, intraperitoneal bleeding, major abdominal surgery or trauma, liver dysfunction and ascites, pancreatitis, gastroparesis or ileus, burns, and obesity.

Various systems may be used to indirectly determine IAP in the patient with an indwelling urinary catheter. Pressure within the bladder is measured and reflects the pressure within the abdominal compartment. Commonly, a system that connects a pressure transducer, normal saline I.V. fluid, and a 25- or 30-ml syringe to the sampling port of the urinary catheter is used. Normal saline solution is instilled in the bladder; the catheter tubing is clamped, preventing the fluid from exiting the bladder; and pressure is measured. An IAP greater than 12 mm Hg is associated with IAH. An IAP of 20 mm Hg or more is associated with new organ dysfunction or failure.

IAP should be measured:
▶ with the patient supine if possible
▶ with the transducer zeroed at the iliac crest, midaxillary line
▶ after 25 ml of saline is instilled into the bladder
▶ at end expiration
▶ without active contractions of the abdominal muscles.

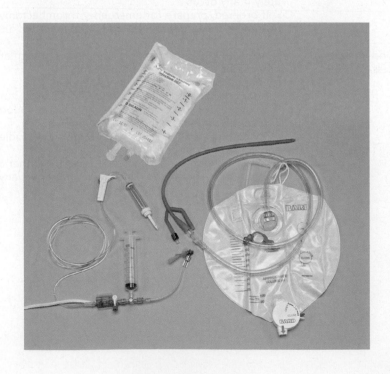

COLOSTOMY AND ILEOSTOMY CARE

A patient with an ascending or transverse colostomy or an ileostomy must wear an external pouch to collect emerging fecal matter, which will be watery or pasty. Besides collecting waste matter, the pouch helps to control odor and to protect the stoma and peristomal skin. Most disposable pouching systems can be used for 2 to 7 days; some models last even longer.

All pouching systems need to be changed immediately if a leak develops, and every pouch needs emptying when it's one-third to one-half full. The patient with an ileostomy may need to empty his pouch four or five times daily. Naturally, the best time to change the pouching system is when the bowel is least active, usually between 2 and 4 hours after meals. After a few months, most patients can predict the best changing time.

The selection of a pouching system should take into consideration which system provides the best adhesive seal and skin protection for the individual patient. The type of pouch selected also depends on the stoma's location and structure, availability of supplies, wear time, consistency of effluent, personal preference, and finances.

Comparing ostomy pouching systems

Disposable pouches

The patient who must empty his pouch often (because of diarrhea or a new colostomy or ileostomy) may prefer a one-piece, drainable, disposable pouch with a closure clamp attached to a skin barrier (as shown below at left). These transparent or opaque, odor-proof, plastic pouches come with attached adhesive or karaya seals. Some pouches have microporous adhesive or belt tabs. The bottom opening allows for easy draining. This pouch may be used permanently or temporarily, until stoma size stabilizes.

One-piece pouches

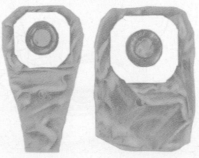

Open-end   Closed-end
pouch   pouch

Also disposable and also made of transparent or opaque odor-proof plastic, a one-piece, disposable, closed-end pouch (as shown on the right, above) may come in a kit with an adhesive seal, belt tabs, a skin barrier, or a carbon filter for gas release. A patient with a regular bowel elimination pattern may choose this style for additional security and confidence.

A two-piece, drainable, disposable pouch with a separate skin barrier (as shown top of next column) permits frequent changes and also minimizes skin breakdown. Also made of transparent or opaque, odor-proof

plastic, this style comes with belt tabs and usually snaps to the skin barrier with a flange mechanism.

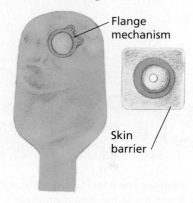

Flange
mechanism

Skin
barrier

Reusable pouches

Typically manufactured from sturdy, opaque, hypoallergenic plastic, the reusable pouch comes with a separate custom-made faceplate and O-ring, (as shown below). Some pouches have a pressure valve for releasing gas. The device has a 1- to 2-month life span, depending on how frequently the patient empties the pouch.

Reusable equipment may benefit a patient who needs a firm faceplate or who wishes to minimize cost. However, many reusable ostomy pouches aren't odor-proof.

Reusable pouches

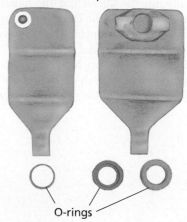

O-rings

Applying a skin barrier and pouch

Fitting a skin barrier and ostomy pouch properly can be done in a few steps. Shown below is a two-piece pouching system with flanges, which is in common use.

1. Measure the stoma using a measuring guide.

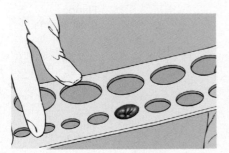

2. Trace the appropriate circle carefully on the back of the skin barrier.

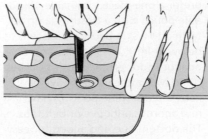

3. Cut the circular opening in the skin barrier. Bevel the edges to keep them from irritating the patient.

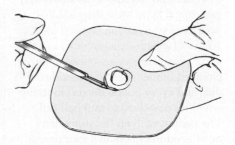

4. Remove the backing from the skin barrier, and moisten it or apply barrier paste, as needed, along the edge of the circular opening.

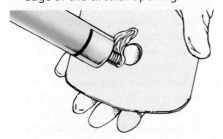

5. Center the skin barrier over the stoma, adhesive side down, and gently press it to the skin.

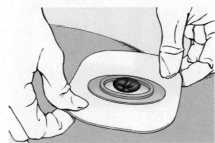

6. Gently press the pouch opening onto the ring until it snaps into place.

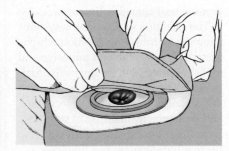

FEEDING TUBE INSERTION

Inserting a feeding tube nasally or orally into the stomach or duodenum allows a patient who can't or won't eat to receive nourishment. The tube also permits supplemental feedings in a patient who has very high nutritional requirements, such as one who's unconscious or who has extensive burns.

Typically, tube insertion is done by a nurse, as ordered. The preferred route is nasal, but the oral route may be used for patients with such conditions as a head injury, a deviated septum, or another nose injury.

The physician also may order duodenal feeding when the patient can't tolerate gastric feeding or when he expects gastric feeding to produce aspiration. Absence of bowel sounds or possible intestinal obstruction contraindicates using a feeding tube.

Feeding tubes differ somewhat from standard nasogastric tubes. Made of silicone, rubber, or polyurethane, feeding tubes have small diameters and great flexibility. These small-bore tubes usually have radiopaque markings and a water-activated coating, which provides a lubricated surface. These features help to reduce oropharyngeal irritation, necrosis from pressure on the tracheoesophageal wall, distal esophageal irritation, and discomfort from swallowing. To facilitate passage, some feeding tubes are weighted with tungsten, and some need a guide wire to keep them from curling in the back of the throat.

Managing tube feeding problems

Complication	Interventions
Aspiration of gastric secretions	▸ Discontinue feeding immediately. ▸ Perform tracheal suction of aspirated contents, if possible. ▸ Notify the physician. Prophylactic antibiotics and chest physiotherapy may be ordered. ▸ Check tube placement before feeding to prevent complication. ▸ Keep the head of the bed elevated during feedings.
Constipation	▸ Provide additional fluids if the patient can tolerate them. ▸ Have the patient participate in an exercise program, if possible. ▸ Administer a bulk-forming laxative. ▸ Review medications, and discontinue those that have a tendency to cause constipation.
Electrolyte imbalance	▸ Monitor serum electrolyte levels. ▸ Notify the physician. He may want to adjust the formula content to correct the deficiency. ▸ Replace electrolytes as needed.
Hyperglycemia	▸ Monitor blood glucose levels. ▸ Notify the physician of elevated levels. ▸ Administer insulin, if ordered. ▸ Be aware that the physician may adjust the sugar content of the formula.
Oral, nasal, or pharyngeal irritation or necrosis	▸ Provide frequent oral hygiene using mouthwash or sponge-tipped swabs. Use petroleum jelly on cracked lips. ▸ If oral, change the tube's position. If necessary, replace the tube.
Tube obstruction	▸ Flush the tube with warm water. If necessary, replace the tube. ▸ Flush the tube with 50 ml of water after each feeding to remove excess sticky formula, which could occlude the tube. ▸ When possible, use liquid forms of medications. Otherwise, crush medications well, if not contraindicated.
Vomiting, bloating, diarrhea, or cramps	▸ Reduce the flow rate. ▸ Verify tube placement. ▸ Warm the formula to prevent GI distress. ▸ For 30 minutes after feeding, position the patient on his right side with his head elevated to facilitate gastric emptying. ▸ Notify the physician. He may want to reduce the amount of formula being given during each feeding.

GASTRIC LAVAGE

After poisoning or a drug overdose, especially in patients who have central nervous system depression or an inadequate gag reflex, gastric lavage flushes the stomach and removes ingested substances through a gastric lavage tube. The procedure is also used to empty the stomach in preparation for endoscopic examination. For patients with gastric or esophageal bleeding, lavage with tepid or iced water or normal saline solution may be used to stop bleeding. However, some controversy exists over the effectiveness of iced lavage for this purpose. Most experts question the effectiveness of iced lavage to treat GI bleeding because iced irrigating solutions stimulate the vagus nerve, which triggers increased hydrochloric acid secretion. In turn, this stimulates gastric motility, which can irritate the bleeding site.

Most physicians prefer to use unchilled normal saline solution (which may prevent rapid electrolyte loss) or even water if the patient must avoid sodium. No research exists to support the use of iced irrigant to stop acute GI bleeding.

Gastric lavage can be continuous or intermittent. Typically, this procedure is done in the emergency department or intensive care unit by a physician, gastroenterologist, or nurse; a widebore lavage tube is almost always inserted by a gastroenterologist. Gastric lavage is contraindicated after ingestion of a corrosive substance (such as lye, petroleum distillates, ammonia, alkalis, or mineral acids) because the lavage tube may perforate the already compromised esophagus.

GASTROSTOMY FEEDING BUTTON CARE

A gastrostomy feeding button serves as an alternative feeding device for an ambulatory patient who's receiving long-term enteral feedings. Approved by the U.S. Food and Drug Administration for 6-month implantation, feeding buttons can be used to replace gastrostomy tubes, if necessary.

The button has a mushroom dome at one end and two wing tabs and a flexible safety plug at the other. When inserted into an established stoma, the button lies almost flush with the skin, with only the top of the safety plug visible.

The button can usually be inserted into a stoma in less than 15 minutes. Besides its cosmetic appeal, the device is easily maintained, reduces skin irritation and breakdown, and is less likely to become dislodged or to migrate than an ordinary feeding tube. A one-way, antireflux valve mounted just inside the mushroom dome prevents accidental leakage of gastric contents. The device usually requires replacement after 3 to 4 months, typically because the antireflux valve wears out.

HANDS ON

Preparing for gastric lavage

Follow these steps when preparing a lavage setup:
▸ Connect one of the three pieces of the large-lumen tubing to the irrigant container.
▸ Insert the Y-connector stem in the other end of the tubing.
▸ Connect the remaining two pieces of tubing to the free ends of the Y-connector.
▸ Place the unattached end of one of the tubes into one of the drainage containers. (Later, you'll connect the other piece of tubing to the patient's gastric tube.)
▸ Clamp the tube leading to the irrigant.
▸ Suspend the entire setup from the I.V. pole, hanging the irrigant container at the highest level.

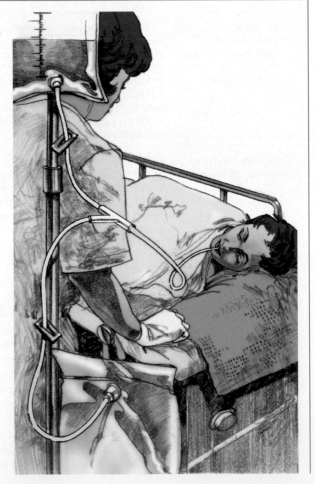

Reinserting a gastrostomy feeding button

If your patient's gastrostomy feeding button pops out (with coughing, for instance), either you or he will need to reinsert the device. Here are some steps to follow.

Prepare the equipment

Collect the feeding button, an obturator, and water-soluble lubricant. If the button will be reinserted, wash it with soap and water and rinse it thoroughly.

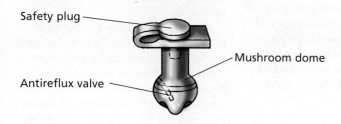

Insert the button

▸ Check the depth of the patient's stoma to make sure you have a feeding button of the correct size. Then clean around the stoma.
▸ Lubricate the obturator with a water-soluble lubricant, and distend the button several times to ensure patency of the antireflux valve within the button.
▸ Lubricate the mushroom dome and the stoma. Gently push the button through the stoma into the stomach.

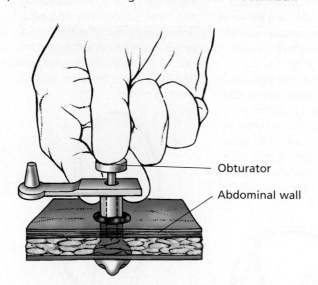

▸ Remove the obturator by gently rotating it as you withdraw it to keep the antireflux valve from adhering to it. If the valve sticks nonetheless, gently push the obturator back into the button until the valve closes.
▸ After removing the obturator, make sure the valve is closed. Then close the flexible safety plug, which should be relatively flush with the skin surface.

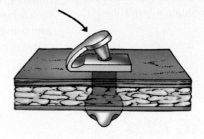

▸ If you need to administer a feeding right away, open the safety plug and attach the feeding adapter and feeding tube. Deliver the feeding as ordered.

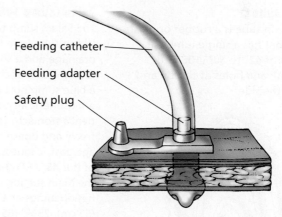

NASOGASTRIC TUBE CARE

Providing effective nasogastric (NG) tube care requires meticulous monitoring of the patient and the equipment. Monitoring the patient involves checking drainage from the NG tube and assessing GI function. Monitoring the equipment involves verifying correct tube placement and irrigating the tube to ensure patency and to prevent mucosal damage.

Specific care varies only slightly for the most commonly used NG tubes: the single-lumen Levin tube and the double-lumen Salem sump tube.

NASOGASTRIC TUBE INSERTION AND REMOVAL

Usually inserted to decompress the stomach, an NG tube can prevent vomiting after major surgery. It's typically in place for 48 to 72 hours after surgery, by which time peristalsis usually resumes. It may remain in place for shorter or longer periods, however, depending on its use.

The NG tube has other diagnostic and therapeutic applications, especially in assessing and treating upper GI bleeding, collecting gastric contents for analysis, performing gastric lavage, aspirating gastric secretions, and administering medications and nutrients.

Inserting an NG tube requires close observation of the patient and verification of proper placement. Removing the tube requires careful handling to prevent injury or aspiration. The tube must be inserted with extra care in a pregnant patient and in one with an increased risk of complications. For example, the physician will order an NG tube for a patient with aortic aneurysm, gastric hemorrhage, or esophageal varices only if he believes that the benefits outweigh the risks of intubation.

Most NG tubes have a radiopaque marker or strip at the distal end so that the tube's position can be verified by X-ray. If the position can't be confirmed, the physician may order fluoroscopy to verify placement. The most common NG tubes are the Levin tube, Salem sump tube, and Moss tube.

Types of NG tubes

The physician will choose the type and diameter of nasogastric (NG) tube that best suits the patient's needs, including lavage, aspiration, enteral therapy, or stomach decompression. Tube choices may include the Levin, Salem sump, and Moss.

Levin tube

The Levin tube is a rubber or plastic tube that has a single lumen, a length of 42″ to 50″ (106.5 to 127 cm), and holes at the tip and along the side.

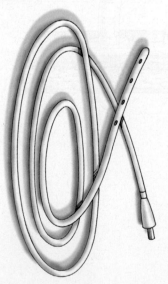

Salem sump tube

The Salem sump tube is a double-lumen tube (one for suction and drainage and a smaller one for ventilation) made of clear plastic and has a blue sump port (pigtail) that allows atmospheric air to enter the patient's stomach. Thus, the tube floats freely and doesn't adhere to or damage gastric mucosa. The larger port of this 48″ (121.9-cm) tube serves as the main suction conduit. The tube has openings at 17¾″ (45 cm), 21⅝″ (55 cm), 25⅝″ (65 cm), and 29½″ (75 cm) as well as a radiopaque line to verify placement.

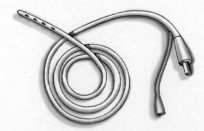

Moss tube

The Moss tube (usually inserted during surgery) has a radiopaque tip and three lumens. The first, positioned and inflated in the cardia, serves as a balloon inflation port. The second is an esophageal aspiration port. The third is a duodenal feeding port.

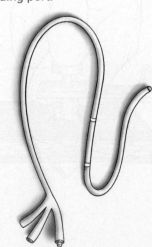

Determining NG tube length

To determine how long the NG tube must be to reach the stomach, hold the end of the tube at the tip of the patient's nose. Extend the tube to the patient's earlobe and then down to the xiphoid process.

Inserting tube placement

After you have determined tube length, lubricate the first 3″ (7.6 cm) with a water-soluble gel to minimize injury to the nasal passages. Next, instruct the patient to hold his head straight and upright. Grasp the tube with the end pointing downward, curve it if necessary, and carefully insert it into the more patent nostril. Aim the tube downward and toward the ear closer to the chosen nostril, and advance it slowly. When the tube reaches the nasopharynx, you'll feel resistance. Instruct the patient to lower his head slightly to close the trachea and open the esophagus. Then

rotate the tube 180 degrees toward the opposite nostril to redirect it so that the tube won't enter the patient's mouth.

Unless contraindicated, offer the patient a cup or glass of water with a straw. Direct him to sip and swallow as you slowly advance the tube. (If you aren't using water, ask the patient to swallow.)

Ensuring proper tube placement

To ensure proper tube placement, use a tongue blade and penlight to examine the patient's mouth and throat for signs of coiled tubing (especially in an unconscious patient). As you carefully advance the tube and the patient swallows, watch for respiratory distress signs, which may mean the tube is in the bronchus and must be removed immediately. Stop advancing the tube when the tape mark or the tube marking reaches the patient's nostril.

Attach a catheter-tip or bulb syringe to the tube, and try to aspirate stomach contents. If you don't obtain stomach contents, position the patient on his left side to move the contents into the stomach's greater curvature, and aspirate again. Gently aspirate stomach contents. Examine the aspirate, and place a small amount on the pH test strip. Proper gastric placement reveals aspirate with a typical gastric fluid appearance (grassy green, clear and colorless with mucus shreds, or brown) and pH of less than or equal to 5.0.

TRANSABDOMINAL TUBE FEEDING AND CARE

To access the stomach, duodenum, or jejunum, the physician may place a tube through the patient's abdominal wall. This may be done surgically or percutaneously. A gastrostomy or jejunostomy tube is usually inserted during intra-abdominal surgery. The tube may be used for feeding during the immediate postoperative period or it may provide long-term enteral access, depending on the type of surgery.

In contrast, a percutaneous endoscopic gastrostomy (PEG) or percutaneous endoscopic jejunostomy (PEJ) tube can be inserted endoscopically without the need for laparotomy or general anesthesia. Typically, the insertion is done in the endoscopy suite or at the patient's bedside. A PEG or PEJ tube may be used for nutrition, drainage, and decompression. Contraindications to endoscopic placement include obstruction (such as an esophageal stricture or duodenal blockage), previous gastric surgery, morbid obesity, and ascites. These conditions would necessitate surgical placement. With either type of tube placement, feedings may begin after 24 hours (or when peristalsis resumes).

HANDS ON

Measuring nasogastric tube length

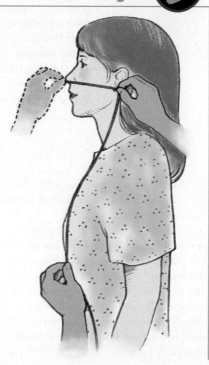

Mark the distance from the tip of the patient's nose to the ear and then to the xiphoid process on the tubing with tape, or note the marking already on the tube. (Average measurements for an adult range from 22″ to 26″ [56 to 66 cm].) It may be necessary to add 2″ (5.1 cm) to this measurement in tall individuals to ensure entry into the stomach.

Caring for a PEG or PEJ site

The exit site of a percutaneous endoscopic gastrostomy (PEG) tube or percutaneous endoscopic jejunostomy (PEJ) tube requires routine observation and care. Follow these care guidelines:

▶ Change the dressing daily while the tube is in place.
▶ After removing the dressing, carefully slide the tube's outer bumper away from the skin (as shown below) about ½" (1.3 cm).

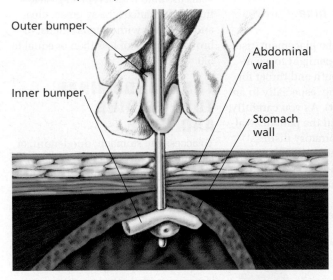

Outer bumper

Inner bumper

Abdominal wall

Stomach wall

▶ Examine the skin around the tube. Look for redness and other signs of infection or erosion.
▶ Gently depress the skin surrounding the tube, and inspect for drainage (as shown below). Expect minimal wound drainage initially after implantation. This should subside in about 1 week.

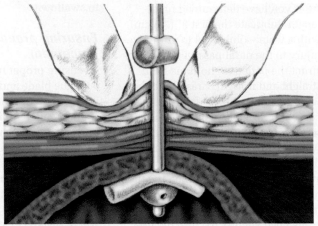

▶ Inspect the tube for wear and tear. (A tube that wears out will need replacement.)
▶ Clean the site with the prescribed cleaning solution.
▶ Rotate the outer bumper 90 degrees to avoid repeating the same tension on the same skin area, and slide the outer bumper back over the exit site.
▶ If leakage appears at the PEG site, or if the patient risks dislodging the tube, apply a sterile gauze dressing over the site. Don't put sterile gauze underneath the outer bumper. Loosening the anchor this way allows the feeding tube free play, which could lead to wound abscess.
▶ Write the date and time of the dressing change on the tape.

TUBE FEEDING

Tube feeding is delivery of a liquid feeding formula directly to the stomach (known as *gastric gavage*), duodenum, or jejunum. Gastric gavage typically is indicated for a patient who can't eat normally because of dysphagia or oral or esophageal obstruction or injury. Gastric feedings may also be given to an unconscious or intubated patient or to a patient recovering from GI tract surgery who can't ingest food orally.

Enteral feeding is preferable to parenteral therapy provided there are no contraindications, access can be safely attained, and oral intake isn't possible. For short-term (less than 30-day) feeding, nasogastric (NG) or nasoenteric tubes are preferable to gastrostomy or jejunostomy tubes. Tube feeding is

contraindicated in patients who have no bowel sounds or a suspected intestinal obstruction.

Duodenal or jejunal feedings decrease the risk of aspiration because the formula bypasses the pylorus. Jejunal feedings result in reduced pancreatic stimulation; thus, patients may require an elemental diet. Patients usually receive gastric feedings on an intermittent schedule. For duodenal or jejunal feedings, however, most pa-

tients seem to better tolerate a continuous slow drip.

Liquid nutrient solutions come in various formulas for administration through an NG tube, a small-bore feeding tube, gastrostomy or jejunostomy tube, a PEG or PEJ tube, or a gastrostomy feeding button.

Chapter 6

Musculoskeletal Care

DISEASES
Arm and leg fractures

An arm or a leg fracture is a break in the continuity of the bone, usually caused by trauma. A fracture can result in substantial muscle, nerve, and other soft-tissue damage. The prognosis varies with the extent of disability or deformity, the amount of tissue and vascular damage, the adequacy of reduction and immobilization, and the patient's age, health, and nutritional status. Children's bones usually heal rapidly and without deformity; the bones of adults in poor health or those with osteoporosis or impaired circulation may never heal properly.

Most arm and leg fractures result from trauma, such as a fall on an outstretched arm, a skiing or motor vehicle accident, and child, spouse, or elder abuse (shown by multiple or repeated episodes of fractures). However, in a person with a bone-weakening disease, such as osteoporosis, bone tumor, or metabolic disease, a mere cough or sneeze can cause a pathological fracture. Prolonged standing, walking, or running can cause stress fractures of the foot and ankle—usually in nurses, postal workers, soldiers, and joggers.

Possible complications of fractures include arterial damage, nonunion, fat embolism, infection, shock, avascular necrosis, peripheral nerve damage, and compartment syndrome. Severe fractures, especially of the femoral shaft, may cause substantial blood loss and life-threatening hypovolemic shock.

Signs and symptoms
- Crepitus
- Deformity or shortening of the injured limb
- Discoloration over the fracture site
- Dislocation
- Loss of pulses distal to the injury (arterial compromise)
- Numbness distal to the injury and cool skin at the extremity's end (nerve and vessel damage)
- Pain that increases with movement and an inability to intentionally move part of the arm or leg distal to the injury
- Soft-tissue edema
- Skin wound and bleeding (open fracture)
- Tingling sensation distal to the injury, possibly indicating nerve and vessel damage
- Warmth at the injury site

Identifying peripheral nerve injuries

This table lists signs and symptoms that can help you pinpoint where a patient has nerve damage. Keep in mind that you won't be able to rely on these signs and symptoms in a patient with severed extension tendons or severe muscle damage.

Nerve	Associated injury	Sign or symptom
Radial	Fracture of the humerus (especially the middle and distal thirds)	The patient can't extend his thumb.
Ulnar	Fracture of the medial humeral epicondyle	The patient can't perceive pain in the tip of his little finger.
Median	Elbow dislocation or wrist or forearm injury	The patient can't perceive pain in the tip of his index finger.
Peroneal	Tibia or fibula fracture or dislocation of the knee	The patient can't extend his foot (this also may indicate sciatic nerve injury).
Sciatic and tibial	Rare with fractures or dislocations	The patient can't perceive pain in his sole.

Understanding common fractures

FRACTURES OF THE ELBOW

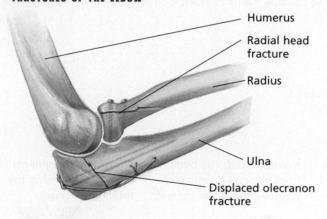

Humerus

Radial head
fracture

Radius

Ulna

Displaced olecranon
fracture

FRACTURE OF THE HAND AND WRIST

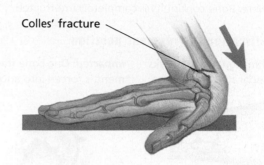

Colles' fracture

FRACTURES OF THE HIP

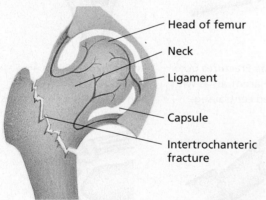

Head of femur

Neck

Ligament

Capsule

Intertrochanteric
fracture

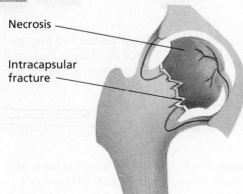

Necrosis

Intracapsular
fracture

FRACTURES OF THE FOOT AND ANKLE

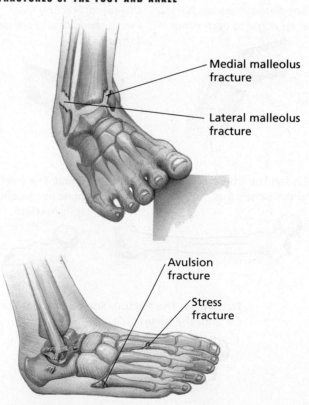

Medial malleolus
fracture

Lateral malleolus
fracture

Avulsion
fracture

Stress
fracture

Classifying fractures

One of the best-known systems for classifying fractures uses a combination of general terms to describe the fracture (for example, a simple, nondisplaced, oblique fracture).

Here are definitions of the classifications and terms used to describe fractures along with illustrations of fragment positions and fracture lines.

General classification of fractures

Simple (closed): Bone fragments don't penetrate the skin.
Compound (open): Bone fragments penetrate the skin.
Incomplete (partial): Bone continuity isn't completely interrupted.
Complete: Bone continuity is completely interrupted.

Classification of fragment position

Comminuted: Bone breaks into separate small pieces.

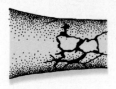

Impacted: One bone fragment is forced into another.

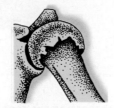

Nondisplaced: The two sections of bone maintain essentially normal alignment.

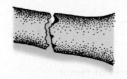

Overriding: Fragments overlap, shortening the total bone length.

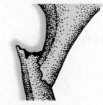

Angulated: Fragments lie at an angle to each other.

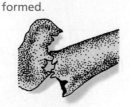

Displaced: Fracture fragments separate and are deformed.

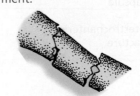

Segmental: Fractures occur in two adjacent areas with an isolated central segment.

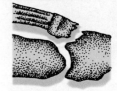

Avulsed: Fragments are pulled from normal position by muscle contractions or ligament resistance.

Linear: The fracture line runs parallel to the bone's axis.

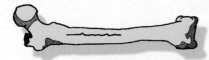

Spiral: The fracture line crosses the bone at an oblique angle, creating a spiral pattern.

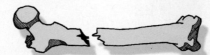

Longitudinal: The fracture line extends in a longitudinal (but not parallel) direction along the bone's axis.

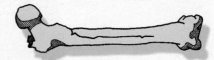

Transverse: The fracture line forms a right angle with the bone's axis.

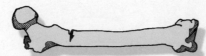

Oblique: The fracture line crosses the bone at roughly a 45-degree angle to the bone's axis.

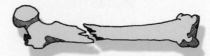

Treatment

▶ Reduction of edema and pain by splinting the limb above and below the suspected fracture, applying a cold pack, and elevating the limb
▶ Direct pressure to control bleeding (for severe fracture) to prevent blood loss
▶ Fluid replacement (including blood products) to prevent or treat hypovolemic shock (for severe fracture)
▶ Reduction (restoring displaced bone segments to their normal position) after confirmed fracture
▶ Closed reduction (manual manipulation): a local anesthetic, such as lidocaine, and an analgesic, such as morphine I.M., to minimize pain; a muscle relaxant, such as diazepam I.V., or a sedative, such as midazolam, to facilitate muscle stretching that's necessary for bone realignment
▶ Open reduction: rods, plates, or screws placed during surgery to reduce and immobilize the fracture (if closed reduction isn't possible); followed by casting
▶ Immobilization: requires skin or skeletal traction, using a series of weights and pulleys (when the splint or cast fails to maintain reduction)
▶ Careful wound cleaning, tetanus prophylaxis, prophylactic antibiotics and, possibly, additional surgery to repair soft-tissue damage (for an open fracture)

Nursing considerations

▶ Know that the severity of pain depends on the fracture type.
▶ Reassure the patient with a fracture, who will probably be frightened and in pain. Ease pain with analgesics as needed.
▶ If the patient has a severe open fracture of a large bone, such as the femur, watch for signs of shock. Monitor his vital signs; a rapid pulse, decreased blood pressure, pallor, and cool, clammy skin may indicate shock. Administer I.V. fluids and blood products as ordered.
▶ If the fracture requires long-term immobilization, reposition the patient often to increase comfort and prevent pressure ulcers. Assist with active range-of-motion exercises to prevent muscle atrophy. Encourage deep breathing and coughing to avoid hypostatic pneumonia.
▶ In long-term immobilization, urge adequate fluid intake to prevent urinary stasis and constipation. Watch for signs of renal calculi (flank pain, nausea, vomiting, and constipation).
▶ Provide for diversional activity. Allow the patient to express his concerns over lengthy immobilization and the problems it creates.
▶ Provide cast care. While the plaster cast is wet, support it with pillows. Observe for skin irritation near the cast edges, and check for foul odors or discharge, particularly after open reduction, compound fracture, or skin

lacerations and wounds on the affected limb.
▶ Encourage the patient to start moving around as soon as he can, and help him with walking.
▶ After cast removal, refer the patient for physical therapy to restore limb mobility.
▶ Know that arm and leg fractures may produce any or all of the "5 Ps": pain and joint tenderness, pallor, pulse loss, paresthesia, and paralysis. The last three are distal to the fracture site.
▶ Monitor the patient's white blood cell count, hemoglobin level, and hematocrit, and report any abnormal values to the practitioner.
▶ Be sure the patient with immobility from the fracture has adequate deep vein thrombosis prophylaxis.

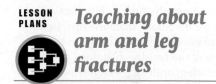

LESSON PLANS
Teaching about arm and leg fractures

▶ Help the patient set realistic goals for recovery.
▶ Show the patient how to use his crutches properly.
▶ Tell the patient with a cast to report signs of impaired circulation (skin coldness, numbness, tingling, or discoloration) immediately. Warn him against getting the cast wet, and instruct him not to insert foreign objects under the cast.
▶ Teach the patient to exercise joints above and below the cast as ordered.
▶ Advise the patient not to walk on a leg cast or foot cast without the physician's permission. If the patient has a fiberglass cast, he may be able to walk immediately. Plaster casts require 48 hours to dry and harden.
▶ Emphasize the importance of returning for follow-up care.

Carpal tunnel syndrome

Carpal tunnel syndrome, a form of repetitive stress injury, is the most common nerve entrapment syndrome. It results from compression of the median nerve in the wrist, where it passes through the carpal tunnel.

The median nerve controls motions in the forearm, wrist, and hand, such as turning the wrist toward the body, flexing the index and middle fingers, and many thumb movements. It also supplies sensation to the index, middle, and ring fingers. Compression of this nerve causes loss of movement and sensation in the wrist, hand, and fingers.

Carpal tunnel syndrome usually occurs in women between ages 30 and 60 and may pose a serious occupational health problem. It may also occur in people who move their wrists continuously, such as butchers, computer operators, machine operators, and concert pianists. Any strenuous use of the hands—sustained grasping, twisting, or flexing—aggravates the condition.

Signs and symptoms

▶ Fingernails that may be atrophied, with surrounding dry, shiny skin
▶ Inability to make a fist
▶ Pain, burning, numbness, or tingling in one or both hands
▶ Pain relieved by shaking hands vigorously or dangling arms at the side
▶ Pain that spreads to the forearm and, in severe cases, as far as the shoulder
▶ Paresthesia that may affect the thumb, forefinger, middle finger, and half of the ring finger; worsening at night and in the morning
▶ Weakness in the hand or wrist

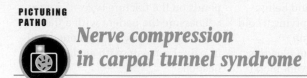

PICTURING PATHO

Nerve compression in carpal tunnel syndrome

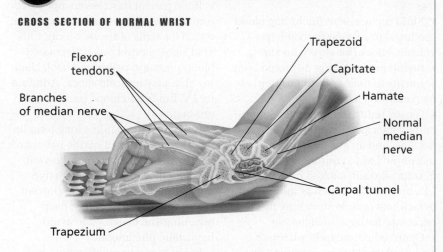

CROSS SECTION OF NORMAL WRIST

- Flexor tendons
- Branches of median nerve
- Trapezium
- Trapezoid
- Capitate
- Hamate
- Normal median nerve
- Carpal tunnel

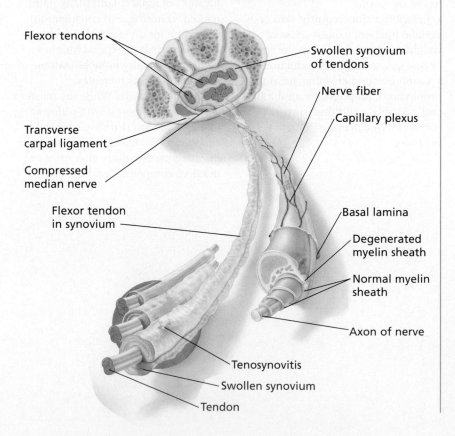

CROSS SECTION OF WRIST WITH CARPAL TUNNEL SYNDROME

- Flexor tendons
- Transverse carpal ligament
- Compressed median nerve
- Flexor tendon in synovium
- Swollen synovium of tendons
- Nerve fiber
- Capillary plexus
- Basal lamina
- Degenerated myelin sheath
- Normal myelin sheath
- Axon of nerve
- Tenosynovitis
- Swollen synovium
- Tendon

Treatment
▶ Wrist splinting for 1 to 2 weeks
▶ Possible occupational changes
▶ Correction of any underlying disorder
▶ Oral nonsteroidal anti-inflammatory drugs, such as indomethacin (Indocin), mefenamic acid (Ponstel), or naproxen
▶ Injectable corticosteroids
▶ Pyridoxine for vitamin B_6 deficiency
▶ Surgical decompression of the nerve by sectioning the entire transverse carpal tunnel ligament
▶ Neurolysis (freeing the nerve fibers)

Nursing considerations
▶ Encourage the patient to express his concerns. Listen and offer your support and encouragement.
▶ Have him perform as much self-care as his immobility and pain allow. Provide him with adequate time to perform these activities at his own pace.
▶ Administer mild analgesics as needed. Encourage the patient to use his hands as much as possible; if the condition has impaired his dominant hand, you may have to assist with eating and bathing.
▶ After surgery, monitor vital signs and regularly check the color, sensation, and motion of the affected hand.
▶ Be aware that the patient's history may disclose that his occupation or hobby requires strenuous or repetitive use of the hands. It may also reveal a hormonal condition, wrist injury, rheumatoid arthritis, or another condition that causes swelling in carpal tunnel structures.

HANDS ON

Testing for carpal tunnel syndrome

Tinel's sign
▶ Lightly percuss the transverse carpal ligament over the median nerve where the patient's palm and wrist meet.
▶ If this action produces numbness and tingling shooting into the palm and finger, the patient has Tinel's sign and may have carpal tunnel syndrome.

Phalen's maneuver
▶ Have the patient put the backs of his hands together and flex his wrists downward at a 90-degree angle.
▶ Pain or numbness in his hand or fingers during this maneuver indicates a positive Phalen's sign. The more severe the carpal tunnel syndrome, the more rapidly the symptoms develop.

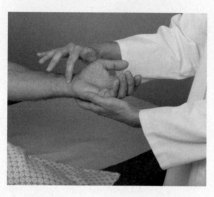

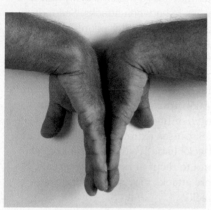

LESSON PLANS

Teaching about carpal tunnel syndrome

▶ Teach the patient how to apply a splint. Advise him not to make it too tight. Show him how to remove the splint to perform gentle range-of-motion exercises (which should be done daily).
▶ Advise the patient who's about to be discharged to occasionally exercise his hands in warm water. If he's using a sling, tell him to remove it several times a day to exercise his elbow and shoulder.
▶ If the patient requires surgery, explain preoperative and postoperative care procedures.

▶ Review the prescribed medication regimen. Emphasize that drug therapy may require 2 to 4 weeks before maximum effectiveness is achieved. If the regimen includes nonsteroidal anti-inflammatory drugs, advise taking the drug with food or antacids to decrease stomach upset. List possible adverse reactions. Instruct the patient regarding which adverse reactions require immediate medical attention.
▶ If the patient is pregnant, advise her to avoid nonsteroidal anti-inflammatory drugs because of possible teratogenic effects.

Gout

Gout—also known as *gouty arthritis*—is a metabolic disease marked by monosodium urate deposits that cause red, swollen, and acutely painful joints. Gout can affect any joint but mostly affects those in the feet, especially the great toe, ankle, and midfoot.

Primary gout typically occurs in men over age 30 and in postmenopausal women who take diuretics. It follows an intermittent course that may leave patients symptom-free for years between attacks. Secondary gout occurs in older people.

In asymptomatic patients, serum urate levels rise but produce no symptoms. In symptom-producing gout, the first acute attack strikes suddenly and peaks quickly. Although it may involve only one or a few joints, this attack causes extreme pain. Mild, acute attacks usually subside quickly yet tend to recur at irregular intervals. Severe attacks may persist for days or weeks.

Intercritical periods are the symptom-free intervals between attacks. Most patients have a second attack between 6 months and 2 years after the first; in some patients, the second attack is delayed for 5 to 10 years. Delayed attacks, which may be polyarticular, are more common in untreated patients. These attacks tend to last longer and produce more symptoms than initial episodes. A migratory attack strikes various joints and the Achilles tendon sequentially and may be associated with olecranon bursitis.

Secondary gout can be the result of other diseases such as obesity, diabetes mellitus, polycythemia, and sickle cell anemia.

Eventually, chronic polyarticular gout sets in. This final, unremitting stage of the disease (also known as tophaceous gout) is marked by persistent painful polyarthritis. An increased concentration of uric acid leads to urate deposits—called tophi—in cartilage, synovial membranes, tendons, and soft tissue. Tophi form in the fingers, hands, knees, feet, ulnar sides of the forearms, pinna of the ear, and Achilles tendon and, rarely, in such internal organs as the kidneys and myocardium. Renal involvement may adversely affect renal function.

Patients who receive treatment for gout have a good prognosis.

Gout of the knee and foot

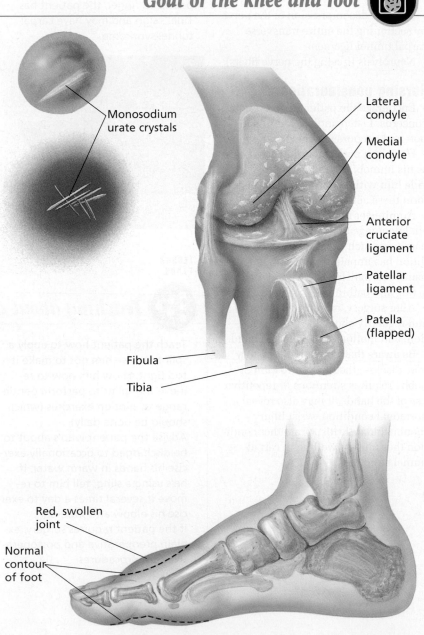

Monosodium urate crystals

Lateral condyle

Medial condyle

Anterior cruciate ligament

Patellar ligament

Patella (flapped)

Fibula

Tibia

Red, swollen joint

Normal contour of foot

Signs and symptoms
◗ Chills and a mild fever
◗ Erosions, deformity, and disability
◗ History of a sedentary lifestyle and hypertension and renal calculi
◗ Pain in the great toe or another location in the foot
◗ Pain that becomes so intense that eventually the patient can't bear the weight of bed sheets or the vibrations of a person walking across the room
◗ Skin over the tophi that ulcerates and releases a chalky white exudate or pus
◗ Swollen, dusky red or purple joint with limited movement
◗ Tophi, especially in the outer ears, hands, and feet
◗ Warmth over the joint and extreme tenderness
◗ Hypertension

Treatment
Correct management has three goals:
◗ First, terminate the acute attack.
◗ Next, treat hyperuricemia to reduce urine uric acid levels.
◗ Finally, prevent recurrent gout and renal calculi.

Acute gout
◗ Bed rest
◗ Immobilization and protection of the inflamed, painful joints
◗ Local application of cold
◗ Analgesics such as acetaminophen (for mild attacks)
◗ Nonsteroidal anti-inflammatory drugs or I.M. corticotropin (for acute attacks)
◗ Corticosteroids given orally or by intra-articular injection
◗ Colchicine (Colcrys) (for acute attacks and for prophylaxis)

Looking at gout

Gout is a metabolic disorder in which uric acid deposits in the joints cause the joints to become painful, arthritic, red, and swollen. Skin temperature may be elevated because of the irritation and inflammation.

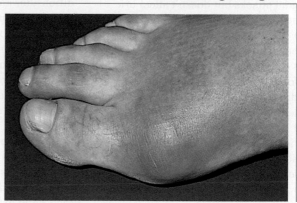

Understanding pseudogout

Pseudogout—also known as *calcium pyrophosphate disease*—results when calcium pyrophosphate crystals collect in periarticular joint structures.

Signs and symptoms
Like true gout, pseudogout causes sudden joint pain and swelling—most commonly of the knee, wrist, ankle, or other peripheral joints.

Pseudogout attacks are self-limiting and are triggered by stress, trauma, surgery, severe dieting, thiazide therapy, or alcohol abuse. Associated symptoms resemble those of rheumatoid arthritis.

Diagnosis
Diagnosis of pseudogout involves joint aspiration and synovial biopsy to detect calcium pyrophosphate crystals. X-rays show calcium deposits in the fibrocartilage and linear markings along the bone ends. Blood tests may detect an underlying endocrine or metabolic disorder.

Treatment
Management of pseudogout may include aspirating the joint to relieve pressure; instilling corticosteroids and administering analgesics or nonsteroidal anti-inflammatory drugs to treat inflammation; and, if appropriate, treating the underlying disorder.

Without treatment, pseudogout leads to permanent joint damage in about half of those it affects, most of whom are elderly people.

Chronic gout

▸ Decrease of serum uric acid level to less than 6.5 mg/dl
▸ Allopurinol (Aloprim) (for overexcretion of uric acid)
▸ Uricosuric agents (probenecid) that promote uric acid excretion and inhibit accumulation of uric acid
▸ Colchicine, which prevents acute gout attacks but doesn't affect uric acid levels
▸ Avoidance of alcohol (especially beer and wine)
▸ Limiting the use of purine-rich foods, such as anchovies, liver, sardines, kidneys, sweetbreads, and lentils
▸ Weight loss program for obese patients (weight reduction decreases uric acid levels and eases stress on painful joints)
▸ Surgery to improve joint function or correct deformities
▸ Excision and drainage of infected or ulcerated tophi to prevent further ulceration, improve the patient's appearance, or make it easier for him to wear shoes or gloves

Nursing considerations

▸ To diffuse anxiety and promote coping mechanisms, encourage the patient to express his concerns about his condition. Listen supportively. Include him and family members in all phases of care and decision making. Answer questions about the disorder as completely as possible.

▸ Urge the patient to perform as much self-care as his immobility and pain allow. Provide him with adequate time to perform these activities at his own pace.
▸ Encourage bed rest, but use a bed cradle to keep bed linens off of sensitive, inflamed joints.
▸ Carefully evaluate the patient's condition after joint aspiration. Provide emotional support during diagnostic tests and procedures.
▸ Give pain medication as needed, especially during acute attacks. Monitor the patient's response to this medication. Apply cold packs to inflamed joints to ease discomfort and reduce swelling.
▸ To promote sleep, administer pain medication at times that allow for maximum rest. Provide the patient with sleep aids, such as a bath, massage, or an extra pillow.
▸ Help the patient identify techniques and activities that promote rest and relaxation. Encourage him to perform them.
▸ Administer anti-inflammatory medication and other drugs as ordered. Watch for adverse reactions. Be alert for GI disturbances if the patient takes colchicine.
▸ Encourage fluids, and record intake and output accurately. Be sure to monitor serum uric acid levels regularly. As ordered, administer sodium bicarbonate or other agents to alkalinize the patient's urine.
▸ Provide a nutritious diet without purine-rich foods.
▸ Watch for acute gout attacks 24 to 96 hours after surgery. Even minor surgery can trigger an attack. Before and after surgery, administer colchicine to help prevent gout attacks, as ordered.

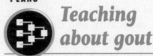

LESSON PLANS

Teaching about gout

▸ Urge the patient to drink plenty of fluids (up to 2 qt [2 L] per day) to prevent renal calculi.
▸ Explain all treatments, tests, and procedures. Warn the patient before his first needle aspiration that it will be painful.
▸ Make sure the patient understands the rationale for evaluating serum uric acid levels periodically.
▸ Teach the patient relaxation techniques. Encourage him to perform them regularly.
▸ Instruct the patient to avoid purine-rich foods, such as anchovies, liver, sardines, kidneys, and lentils, because these substances raise the urate level.
▸ Discuss the principles of gradual weight reduction with the obese patient. Explain the advantages of a diet containing moderate amounts of protein and little fat.
▸ If the patient receives allopurinol or other drugs, instruct him to report immediately any adverse reactions, such as nausea, vomiting, drowsiness, dizziness, urinary frequency, and dermatitis. Warn the patient taking probenecid or sulfinpyrazone to avoid aspirin or other salicylates. Their combined effect causes urate retention.
▸ Inform the patient that long-term colchicine therapy is essential during the first 3 to 6 months of treatment with uricosuric drugs or allopurinol. Stress the importance of compliance.
▸ Urge the patient to control hypertension, especially if tophaceous renal deposits are present. Keep in mind that diuretics aren't advised for the patient with gout; alternative antihypertensives are preferred.

Hallux valgus

Hallux valgus is a common, painful foot condition that involves lateral deviation of the great toe at the metatarsophalangeal joint. It occurs with medial enlargement of the first metatarsal head and bunion formation (bursa and callus formation at the bony prominence). It's more common in women.

With congenital hallux valgus, abnormal bony alignment (an increased space between the first and second metatarsal known as *metatarsus primus varus*) causes bunion formation. With acquired hallux valgus, bony alignment is normal at the outset of the disorder.

Signs and symptoms

▶ A flat, splayed forefoot with severely curled toes (hammertoes)
▶ Characteristic tender bunion covered by deformed, hard, erythematous skin and palpable bursa, typically distended with fluid
▶ Chronic pain over a bunion
▶ Family history of hallux valgus, degenerative arthritis, or both
▶ Small bunion on the fifth metatarsal
▶ Laterally deviated great toe
▶ Pain over the second or third metatarsal heads

Treatment

▶ Proper shoes and foot care to eliminate the need for further treatment
▶ Felt pads to protect the bunion
▶ Foam pads or other devices to separate the first and second toes at night
▶ A supportive pad and exercises to strengthen the metatarsal arch
▶ Bunionectomy
▶ Warm compresses, soaks, exercises, and analgesics to relieve pain and stiffness

Nursing considerations

▶ Encourage the patient to perform as much self-care as his immobility and pain allow. Give him time to perform these activities at his own pace.
▶ Administer analgesics, as ordered, to relieve pain.

PICTURING PATHO

Understanding hammertoe

With hammertoe, the toe assumes a clawlike position caused by hyperextension of the metatarsophalangeal joint, flexion of the proximal interphalangeal joint, and hyperextension of the distal interphalangeal joint, usually under pressure from hallux valgus displacement.

Signs and symptoms
The combined pressure that causes hammertoe results in a painful corn on the back of the interphalangeal joint and on the bone end and a callus on the sole of the foot, both of which make walking painful. Hammertoe may be mild or severe and can affect one or all toes.

Diagnosis
Hammertoe can be congenital and familial or acquired from repeatedly wearing short, narrow shoes, which puts pressure on the end of the long toe. Acquired hammertoe is usually bilateral and commonly develops in children who rapidly outgrow their shoes and socks.

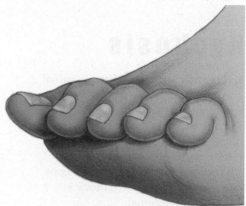

▶ Before surgery, assess the foot's neurovascular status (temperature, color, sensation, and blanching sign).
▶ After bunionectomy, apply ice to reduce swelling. Increase negative venous pressure and reduce edema by elevating the foot or supporting it with pillows.

Treatment
In young children or adults with early deformity, repeated foot manipulation and splinting of the affected toe relieve discomfort and may correct the deformity. Other treatment includes protection of protruding joints with felt pads, corrective footwear (open-toed shoes and sandals or special shoes that conform to the shape of the foot), a metatarsal arch support, and exercises such as passive manual stretching of the proximal interphalangeal joint. Severe deformity requires surgical fusion of the proximal interphalangeal joint in a straight position.

▶ Record the neurovascular status of the patient's toes, including the ability to move them (taking into account the inhibiting effect of the dressing). Perform this check every hour for the first 24 hours, then every 4 hours. Report any change in neurovascular status to the physician immediately.

▶ Prepare the patient for walking by having him dangle his foot over the bedside briefly before he gets up. This increases venous pressure gradually.

▶ Encourage the patient to express concerns about limited mobility, and offer support when appropriate. Answer any questions. Give positive reinforcement and, whenever possible, include the patient in care decisions.

Teaching about hallux valgus

▶ Teach the patient how to use crutches if they are needed. Make sure the proper cast shoe or boot is used to protect the cast or dressing.
▶ Before discharge, instruct the patient to limit activities, to rest frequently with feet elevated (especially with pain or edema), and to wear wide-toed shoes and sandals after the dressings are removed.
▶ Teach the patient proper foot care, including cleanliness and massages. Show her how to cut toenails straight across to prevent ingrown nails and infection.
▶ Demonstrate exercises the patient can do at home to strengthen foot muscles, such as standing at the edge of a step on the heel and then raising and inverting the top of the foot.
▶ Stress the importance of follow-up care and prompt medical attention for painful bunions or corns.
▶ If the patient needs surgery, explain all preoperative and postoperative procedures and treatments.

Kyphosis

Kyphosis is an anteroposterior spinal curve that causes the back to bow, commonly at the thoracic level but sometimes at the thoracolumbar or sacral level. It was once known as "*roundback*" or "*dowager's hump.*" The normal spine has a slightly convex shape, but excessive thoracic kyphosis is abnormal.

Kyphosis occurs in children and adults. Symptomatic adolescent kyphosis affects more girls than boys and is most common between ages 12 and 16.

Disk lesions (Schmorl's nodes) may develop in this disorder. These small fingers of nuclear material (from the nucleus pulposus) protrude through the cartilage plates and into the spongy bone of the vertebral bodies. If the protrusion destroys the anterior portions of cartilage, bridges of new bone may form at the intervertebral space and cause ankylosis.

Recognizing kyphosis

If the patient has pronounced kyphosis, the thoracic curve is abnormally rounded, as shown here.

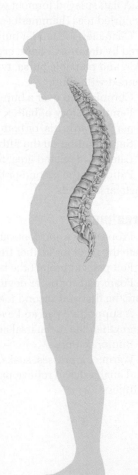

Signs and symptoms
▶ A history of excessive athletic activity (in adolescents)
▶ Compensatory lordosis
▶ Fatigue, tenderness, or stiffness in the involved area or along the entire spine
▶ Increased thoracic curvature when the patient stands or bends forward
▶ Poor posture
▶ Mild pain at the apex of the spinal curve

Treatment

▸ Bed rest on a firm mattress (with or without traction) and a brace to correct the spinal curve until the patient stops growing

▸ Pelvic tilt to decrease lumbar lordosis, hamstring stretch to overcome muscle contractures, and thoracic hyperextension to flatten the kyphotic curve

▸ Spinal arthrodesis (rarely necessary unless kyphosis causes neurologic damage, a spinal curve greater than 60 degrees, or intractable and disabling back pain in a skeletally mature patient)

▸ Posterior spinal fusion (with spinal instrumentation, iliac bone grafting, and plaster casting for immobilization) or an anterior spinal fusion (followed by casting) if kyphosis produces a spinal curve greater than 70 degrees

Nursing considerations

▸ After surgery, check the patient's neurovascular status every 2 to 4 hours for the first 48 hours and report any changes immediately. Turn the patient often, using the logroll method.

▸ If patient-controlled analgesia isn't used, offer an analgesic every 3 to 4 hours.

▸ Maintain fluid balance and monitor for ileus.

▸ Maintain adequate ventilation and oxygenation.

▸ Encourage family support. For an adolescent patient, suggest that family members supply diversional activities. For an adult patient, arrange for alternating periods of rest and activity.

▸ If the patient requires a brace, check its condition daily. Look for worn or malfunctioning parts. Carefully assess how the brace fits the patient. Keep in mind that weight changes may alter proper fit.

▸ Give meticulous skin care. Check the skin at the cast edges several times daily; use heel and elbow protectors to prevent skin breakdown. Remove antiembolism stockings, if ordered, at least three times per day for at least 30 minutes. Change dressings as ordered.

▸ Provide emotional support and encourage communication. Urge the patient and family members to voice their concerns, and answer their questions completely. Expect more mood changes and depression in the adolescent patient than in the adult patient. Offer frequent encouragement and reassurance.

▸ Include the patient in care-related decisions. If possible, include family members in all phases of patient care.

▸ Assist during suture removal and new cast application (usually about 10 days after surgery). Encourage gradual ambulation (usually beginning with a tilt table in the physical therapy department). As needed, arrange for follow-up care with a social worker and a home health nurse.

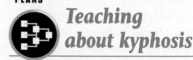

LESSON PLANS

Teaching about kyphosis

▸ For the adolescent patient with kyphosis, outline the fundamentals of good posture and demonstrate prescribed exercises. Have the patient perform a return demonstration, if appropriate. Suggest bed rest to relieve severe pain. Encourage him to use a firm mattress, preferably with a bed board.

▸ If the patient has a cast, provide detailed, written care instructions for the cast at discharge. Tell him to immediately report pain, burning, skin breakdown, loss of feeling, tingling, numbness, or cast odor. Urge him to drink plenty of liquids to avoid constipation and to report any illness (especially abdominal pain or vomiting) immediately. Show him how to use proper body mechanics to minimize strain on the spine. Warn him not to lie on his stomach or on his back with his legs flat.

▸ If the patient is discharged with a brace, explain its purpose and tell him how and when to wear it. Make sure he understands how to check it daily for proper fit and function. Teach him to perform proper skin care. Advise against using lotions, ointments, or powders that can irritate the skin where it comes in contact with the brace. Warn that only the physician or orthotist should adjust the brace.

Muscular dystrophy

Muscular dystrophy is a group of hereditary disorders characterized by progressive symmetrical wasting of skeletal muscles but no neural or sensory defects. Four main types of muscular dystrophy occur: Duchenne's (pseudohypertrophic) muscular dystrophy, which accounts for 50% of all cases; Becker's (benign pseudohypertrophic) muscular dystrophy; Landouzy-Dejerine (facioscapulohumeral) dystrophy; and Erb's (limb-girdle) dystrophy. Duchenne's and Becker's muscular dystrophies affect males almost exclusively. The other two types affect both sexes about equally.

Depending on the type, the disorder may affect vital organs and lead to severe disability, even death. Early in the disease, muscle fibers necrotize and regenerate in various states. Over time, regeneration slows and degeneration dominates. Fat and connective tissue replace muscle fibers, causing weakness.

The prognosis varies. Duchenne's muscular dystrophy typically begins during early childhood and causes death within 10 to 15 years. Patients with Becker's muscular dystrophy may live into their 40s. Landouzy-Dejerine and Erb's dystrophies usually don't shorten life expectancy.

Signs and symptoms

▸ Family history that points to evidence of genetic transmission
▸ If another family member has muscular dystrophy, clinical characteristics that indicate the type of dystrophy and how he may be affected
▸ Progressive muscle weakness that varies with the type of dystrophy

Muscles affected in muscular dystrophy

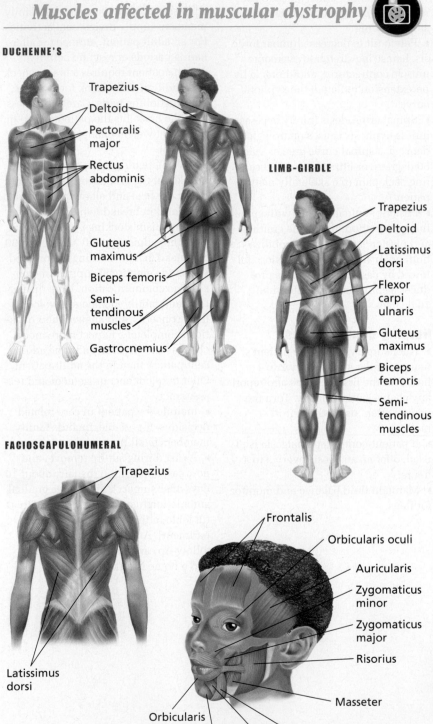

DUCHENNE'S

Trapezius
Deltoid
Pectoralis major
Rectus abdominis
Gluteus maximus
Biceps femoris
Semi-tendinous muscles
Gastrocnemius

Trapezius
Deltoid

LIMB-GIRDLE

Trapezius
Deltoid
Latissimus dorsi
Flexor carpi ulnaris
Gluteus maximus
Biceps femoris
Semi-tendinous muscles

FACIOSCAPULOHUMERAL

Trapezius

Latissimus dorsi

Frontalis
Orbicularis oculi
Auricularis
Zygomaticus minor
Zygomaticus major
Risorius
Masseter
Orbicularis oris
Depressor anguli oris
Mentalis
Depressor labii inferioris

HANDS ON

Testing for Gowers' sign

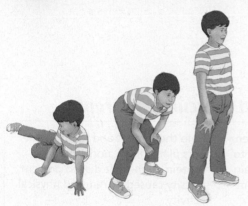

A positive Gowers' sign—an inability to lift the trunk without using the hands and arms to brace and push—indicates pelvic muscle weakness, as occurs in muscular dystrophy and spinal muscle atrophy. To check for Gowers' sign, place the patient in the supine position and ask him to rise.

Duchenne's muscular dystrophy
▶ Begins insidiously
▶ Gowers' sign when rising from a sitting or supine position
▶ Onset that typically occurs between ages 3 and 5
▶ Rapid progression; by age 12, child usually unable to walk
▶ Weakness that begins in the pelvic muscles and interferes with ability to run, climb, and walk
▶ Wide stance and a waddling gait

Becker's muscular dystrophy
▶ Gowers' sign
▶ Resemble those of Duchenne's but progress more slowly
▶ Beginning after age 5, but patient can still walk well beyond age 15 and, in some cases, into his 40s
▶ Wide stance and a waddling gait

Landouzy-Dejerine dystrophy
▶ Abnormal facial movements
▶ Absence of facial movements when laughing or crying
▶ Diffuse facial flattening that leads to a masklike expression
▶ Inability to pucker the lips or whistle
▶ Inability to raise arms over the head or close eyes completely

▶ Pelvic muscles weaken as the disease progresses
▶ Pendulous lower lip
▶ Symptoms that develop during adolescence
▶ Nasolabial fold that disappears
▶ Typically beginning before age 10
▶ Weakness of the eye, face, and shoulder muscles
▶ Inability to suckle (in infants)
▶ Scapulae that develop a winglike appearance

Erb's dystrophy
▶ Slow course and commonly causes only slight disability
▶ Inability to raise the arms
▶ Lordosis with abdominal protrusion
▶ Muscle weakness (first appears in the upper arm and pelvic muscles)
▶ Muscle wasting
▶ Onset between ages 6 and 10 but may occur in early adulthood
▶ Poor balance
▶ Waddling gait
▶ Winging of the scapulae

Detecting muscular dystrophy

With muscular dystrophy, the trapezius muscle typically rises, creating a stepped appearance at the shoulder's point.

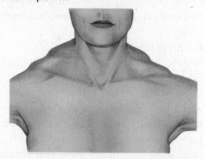

From the posterior view, the scapulae ride over the lateral thoracic region, giving them a winged appearance. With Duchenne's and Becker's dystrophies, this winglike sign appears when the patient raises his arms. With other dystrophies, the sign is obvious without arm raising. (In fact, the patient can't raise his arms.)

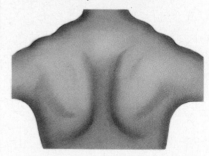

Treatment

▸ Currently, no treatment that can stop progressive muscle impairment
▸ Orthopedic appliances, exercise, physical therapy, and surgery to correct contractures that can help preserve the patient's mobility and independence

Nursing considerations

▸ If a patient with Duchenne's or Becker's muscular dystrophy develops respiratory involvement, encourage coughing and deep-breathing exercises.
▸ Help the patient to preserve joint mobility and prevent muscle atrophy by encouraging and assisting with active and passive range-of-motion exercises.
▸ The patient may need splints, braces, grab bars, and overhead slings. For comfort and to prevent footdrop, use a footboard or high-topped shoes and a foot cradle.
▸ Because inactivity can cause constipation, encourage adequate fluid intake, increase dietary bulk, and obtain an order for a stool softener. Because the patient is prone to obesity from reduced physical activity, provide him with a low-calorie, high-protein, high-fiber diet.
▸ Allow the patient plenty of time to perform even simple physical tasks.

LESSON PLANS

Teaching about muscular dystrophy

▸ Facilitate communication between family members and the patient to help them handle emotional strain and cope with changes in body image.
▸ Encourage the patient and family members to express their concerns. Listen to them and answer their questions.
▸ Help a child with Duchenne's muscular dystrophy maintain peer relationships and realize his intellectual potential by encouraging the parents to keep him in a regular school as long as possible.
▸ Teach the patient and parents ways to maintain his mobility and independence for as long as possible.
▸ Inform the patient and parents about possible complications and steps they can take to prevent them.
▸ Explain the possibility of respiratory tract infections, signs to watch for, and what to do if the patient develops a respiratory infection. Urge the patient and the parents to report signs of infection to the physician immediately.
▸ When the patient becomes confined to a wheelchair, help him and family members to see the chair as a way to preserve his independence. Have an occupational therapist teach the patient about his wheelchair and other supportive devices that can help him with activities of daily living.

▸ Help the patient and family members plan a low-calorie, high-protein, high-fiber diet to prevent obesity caused by reduced physical activity.
▸ Advise the patient to avoid long periods of bed rest and inactivity.
▸ If appropriate, refer adult patients for sexual counseling.
▸ Refer the patient for physical therapy, vocational rehabilitation, social services, and financial assistance. Suggest the Muscular Dystrophy Association as a source of information and support.
▸ Refer family members who carry the muscular dystrophy trait for genetic counseling so they understand the risk of transmitting this disorder.

Osteoarthritis

Osteoarthritis is the most common form of arthritis. It causes deterioration of the joint cartilage and formation of reactive new bone at the margins and subchondral areas of the joints. This chronic degeneration results from a breakdown of chondrocytes, most commonly in the hips and knees.

Osteoarthritis occurs in both sexes, after age 40, with the earliest symptoms occurring in middle age and progressing with advancing age.

Depending on the site and severity of joint involvement, disability can range from minor limitation of the fingers to near immobility in people with hip or knee disease. Progression rates vary; joints may remain stable for years in the early stage of deterioration.

Signs and symptoms

▶ Aching with changes in weather
▶ A grating feeling with joint movement
▶ Contractures
▶ Crepitus of joint during motion
▶ Deep, aching joint pain, particularly after exercise or weight bearing on the affected joint
▶ Deformity of the involved areas
▶ Fingers that become numb and lose their dexterity
▶ Gait abnormalities (when arthritis affects hips or knees)
▶ Joint instability, swelling, tenderness, and warmth without redness
▶ Limited movement
▶ Muscle atrophy and spasms
▶ Hard nodes called *Heberden's nodes* on the distal and *Bouchard's nodes* on the proximal interphalangeal joints; beginning as painless, then becoming red, swollen, and tender
▶ Predisposing event such as a traumatic injury
▶ Rest that relieves pain
▶ Stiffness in the morning and after exercise
▶ Crepitus of joint during motion

Osteoarthritis of the hand, knee, and hip

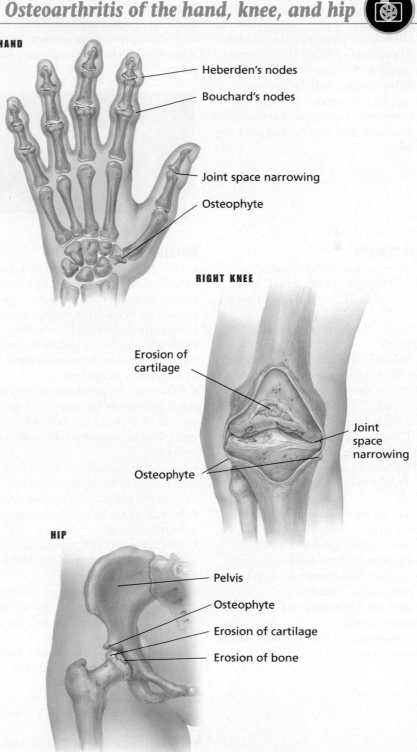

HAND

Heberden's nodes

Bouchard's nodes

Joint space narrowing

Osteophyte

RIGHT KNEE

Erosion of cartilage

Joint space narrowing

Osteophyte

HIP

Pelvis

Osteophyte

Erosion of cartilage

Erosion of bone

Detecting Heberden's and Bouchard's nodes

Heberden's and Bouchard's nodes are typically seen in patients with osteoarthritis, a chronic deterioration of the joint cartilage that commonly occurs in the hips, knees, and joints of the fingers. Initially, the nodes may be red, swollen, and painful. Eventually, they become painless but are associated with limited joint mobility.

Heberden's nodes

Heberden's nodes are hard, bony, and cartilaginous enlargements that appear on the distal interphalangeal joints.

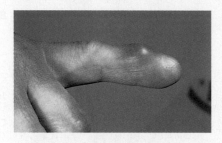

Bouchard's nodes

Bouchard's nodes are similar but less common and appear on the proximal interphalangeal joints.

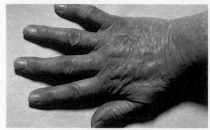

Treatment

▶ Nonsteroidal anti-inflammatory drugs, including COX-2 inhibitors
▶ Intra-articular corticosteroid injections
▶ Adequate rest that's balanced with activity
▶ Massage, moist heat, paraffin dips for the hands, supervised exercise to decrease muscle spasms and atrophy, and protective techniques for preventing undue joint stress
▶ Crutches, braces, a cane, a walker, a cervical collar, or traction to reduce stress and increase stability
▶ Weight reduction (for obese patients)
▶ For severe disability or uncontrollable pain:
– arthroplasty (partial or total)—replacement of the deteriorated part of a joint with a prosthetic appliance
– arthrodesis—surgical fusion of bones, used primarily in the spine (laminectomy)
– osteoplasty—scraping and lavage of deteriorated bone from the joint.

Nursing considerations

▶ Provide emotional support and reassurance to help the patient cope with limited mobility. Give the patient opportunities to voice his feelings about immobility and nodular joints. Include him and family members in all phases of his care. Answer questions as completely as you can.
▶ Encourage the patient to perform as much self-care as his immobility and pain allow. Provide him with adequate time to perform activities at his own pace.
▶ To help promote sleep, adjust pain medications to allow maximum rest. Provide the patient with normal sleep aids, such as a bath, massage, or an extra pillow.
▶ Assess the patient's pain pattern, and give analgesics as needed. Monitor his response.
▶ Help the patient identify techniques and activities that promote rest and relaxation. Encourage him to perform them.
▶ Administer anti-inflammatory medication and other drugs as ordered. Watch for adverse reactions.
▶ For joints in the hand, provide hot soaks and paraffin dips to relieve pain, as ordered.
▶ For lumbosacral spinal joints, provide a firm mattress (or bed board) to decrease morning pain.

▶ For cervical spinal joints, adjust the patient's cervical collar to avoid constriction; watch for irritated skin with prolonged use.
▶ For the hip, use moist heat pads to relieve pain. Administer antispasmodic drugs as ordered.
▶ For the knee, assist with prescribed range-of-motion exercises twice daily to maintain muscle tone. Help perform progressive resistance exercises to increase the patient's muscle strength.
▶ Provide elastic supports or braces, if needed.
▶ Check crutches, a cane, braces, or a walker for proper fit. A patient with unilateral joint involvement should use an orthopedic appliance (such as a cane or walker) on the unaffected side.

Teaching about osteoarthritis

- Instruct the patient to plan for adequate rest during the day, after exertion, and at night. Encourage him to learn and use energy conservation methods, such as pacing, simplifying work procedures, and protecting joints.
- Instruct him to take medications exactly as prescribed. Tell him which adverse reactions to report immediately.
- Advise against overexertion. Tell the patient that he should take care to stand and walk correctly, to minimize weight-bearing activities, and to be especially careful when stooping or picking up objects.

- Tell the patient to wear well-fitting support shoes and to repair worn heels.
- Recommend having safety devices installed in the home, such as grab bars in the bathroom.
- Teach the patient to perform range-of-motion exercises, performing them as gently as possible.
- Advise maintaining proper body weight to minimize strain on joints.
- Teach the patient how to use crutches or other orthopedic devices properly. Stress the importance of proper fitting and regular professional readjustment of such

devices. Warn that impaired sensation might allow tissue damage from these aids without discomfort.
- Recommend using cushions when sitting (for hip and knee involvement). Also suggest using an elevated toilet seat. Both reduce stress when rising from a seated position.
- Positively reinforce the patient's efforts to adapt. Point out improving or stabilizing physical functioning.
- As necessary, refer the patient to an occupational therapist or a home health nurse to help him cope with activities of daily living.

Osteomyelitis

Osteomyelitis is a pyogenic bone infection that may be chronic or acute. The disease commonly results from combined traumatic injury—usually minor but severe enough to cause a hematoma—and acute infection originating elsewhere in the body. Osteomyelitis usually remains a local infection, but it can spread through the bone to the marrow, cortex, and periosteum. The most common infecting organism is *Staphylococcus aureus*.

Acute osteomyelitis is typically a blood-borne disease that most commonly affects rapidly growing children, particularly boys. Multiple draining sinus tracts and metastatic lesions characterize the rarer chronic osteomyelitis. The incidence of both types of osteomyelitis is declining, except in drug abusers.

In children, the most common disease sites include the lower end of the femur and the upper end of the tibia,

humerus, and radius. In adults, the disease commonly localizes in the pelvis and vertebrae and usually results from contamination related to surgery or trauma.

The prognosis for a patient with acute osteomyelitis is good if he receives prompt treatment. The prognosis for a patient with chronic osteomyelitis (more prevalent in adults) is poor.

**PICTURING
PATHO**

Stages of osteomyelitis

INITIAL INFECTION

Initial site of infection

Fibula

Periosteum

Tibia

FIRST STAGE

Blood supply blocked

Subperiosteal abscess (pus)

SECOND STAGE

Sequestrum (dead bone)

Pus drainage

Involucrum (new bone formation)

Signs and symptoms

▶ Sudden, severe pain in affected bone (unrelieved by rest and worsening with motion)
▶ Chills
▶ Fever
▶ Malaise
▶ Nausea
▶ Persistent pus drainage from an old pocket in a sinus tract (chronic infection)
▶ Tachycardia
▶ Swelling, restricted movement, tenderness, and warmth over the infection site
▶ Patient history that reveals previous injury, surgery, or primary infection

Treatment

▶ High doses of I.V. antibiotics, such as a penicillinase-resistant agent like nafcillin or oxacillin
▶ Surgical drainage of the infected site
▶ Cast, traction, or bed rest to immobilize infected bone
▶ Analgesics and I.V. fluids as needed

For abscess

▶ Incision and drainage
▶ Culture of the drainage
▶ Systemic antibiotics
▶ Intracavitary instillation of antibiotics through closed-system continuous irrigation with low intermittent suction
▶ Limited irrigation with a blood drainage system equipped with suction, such as a Hemovac
▶ Packed, wet, antibiotic-soaked dressings applied locally
▶ Hyperbaric oxygen therapy for chronic abscesses
▶ Free tissue transfers and local muscle flaps to fill in dead space and increase blood supply
▶ Sequestrectomy to remove dead bone and saucerization to promote drainage and decrease pressure (for chronic osteomyelitis)
▶ Amputation of arm or leg (for unrelieved chronic osteomyelitis)
▶ Use of wound vacuum for draining areas

Nursing considerations

▶ Encourage the patient to verbalize his concerns about his disorder. Offer support and encouragement. Include the patient and family members in all phases of his care. Answer questions as honestly as you can.
▶ Encourage the patient to perform as much self-care as his condition allows. Give him adequate time to perform these activities at his own pace.
▶ Use aseptic technique when changing dressings and irrigating wounds.
▶ If the patient is in skeletal traction for compound fractures, cover the pin insertion points with small, dry dressings. Tell the patient not to touch the skin around the pins and wires.
▶ Provide a diet high in protein and vitamin C to promote healing.
▶ Assess vital signs, wound appearance, and new pain (which may indicate secondary infection) daily.
▶ Carefully monitor drainage and suctioning equipment. Keep containers nearby that are filled with the irrigation solution being instilled. Monitor the amount of solution instilled and drained.
▶ Provide thorough skin care. Turn the patient gently every 2 hours, and watch for signs of developing pressure ulcers.

▶ Provide complete cast care. Support the cast with firm pillows, and petal the edges with pieces of adhesive tape or moleskin to smooth rough edges. Check circulation and drainage. If a wet spot appears on the cast, circle it with a marking pen and note the time of appearance on the cast. Be aware of how much drainage to expect. Check the circled spot at least every 4 hours. Assess increasing drainage, and report as appropriate. Monitor vital signs for excessive blood loss.
▶ Protect the patient from mishaps, such as jerky movements and falls. Tell him to report sudden pain, unusual bone sensations and noises (crepitus), or deformity immediately. Watch for any sudden malpositioning of the limb, which may indicate fracture.
▶ Assess the patient's pain pattern. Give analgesics as needed. Monitor his response.
▶ Instruct the patient to protect the area from pathological fractures.

LESSON PLANS

Teaching about osteomyelitis

▶ Explain all test and treatment procedures.
▶ Review prescribed medications. Discuss possible adverse reactions to drug administration, and instruct the patient to report them to the physician.
▶ Before surgery, explain all preoperative and postoperative procedures to the patient and family members.
▶ Teach the patient techniques for promoting rest and relaxation. Encourage him to perform them.

▶ Before discharge, teach the patient how to protect and clean the wound site and, most important, how to recognize signs of recurring infection (elevated temperature, redness, localized heat, and swelling).
▶ Urge the patient to schedule follow-up examinations and to seek treatment for possible sources of recurrent infection, such as blisters, boils, sties, and impetigo.
▶ As necessary, refer the patient to an occupational therapist or a home health nurse to help him manage activities of daily living.

Osteoporosis

With osteoporosis, a metabolic bone disorder, the rate of bone resorption accelerates and the rate of bone formation decelerates. The result is decreased bone mass. Bones affected by this disease lose calcium and phosphate and become porous, brittle, and abnormally vulnerable to fracture. Osteoporosis may be primary or secondary to an underlying disease.

Primary osteoporosis can be classified as idiopathic, type I, or type II. Idiopathic osteoporosis affects children and adults. Type I (or postmenopausal) osteoporosis usually affects women ages 51 to 75. Related to the loss of estrogen's protective effect on bone, type I osteoporosis results in trabecular bone loss and some cortical bone loss. Vertebral and wrist fractures are common. Type II (or senile) osteoporosis occurs most commonly between ages 70 and 85. Trabecular and cortical bone loss and consequent fractures of the proximal humerus, proximal tibia, femoral neck, and pelvis characterize type II osteoporosis.

Signs and symptoms

▶ Backache and pain radiating around the trunk (vertebral collapse)
▶ Decreased spinal movement with flexion more limited than extension
▶ Kyphosis (humped back)
▶ Loss of height
▶ Markedly aged appearance
▶ Muscle spasm
▶ Pain that developed slowly over several years
▶ Snapping sound with sudden pain in the lower back when bending to lift

Calcium metabolism in osteoporosis

Normally, blood absorbs calcium from the digestive system and deposits it in the bones. If calcium absorption is impaired or if calcium intake is inadequate, calcium may move from the bones. This may occur more frequently during times of rapid bone growth (for example, teenage years) or when rapid bone loss occurs after menopause.

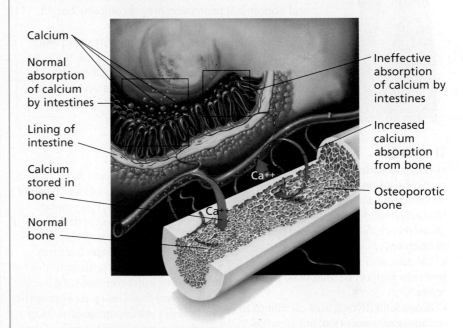

Calcium
Normal absorption of calcium by intestines
Lining of intestine
Calcium stored in bone
Normal bone
Ineffective absorption of calcium by intestines
Increased calcium absorption from bone
Osteoporotic bone
Ca++
Ca++

Bone formation and resorption

The organic portion of bone, called *osteoid,* acts as the matrix or framework for the mineral portion.

Bone cells called *osteoblasts* produce the osteoid matrix. The mineral portion, which consists of calcium and other minerals, hardens the osteoid matrix.

Large bone cells called *osteoclasts* reshape mature bone by resorbing the mineral and organic components. However, in osteoporosis, osteoblasts continue to produce bone but resorption by osteoclasts exceeds bone formation.

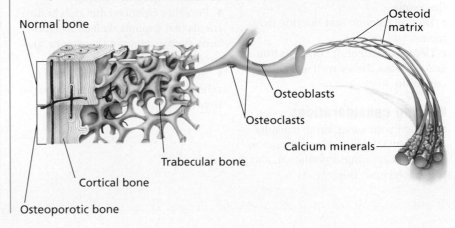

Normal bone
Osteoid matrix
Osteoblasts
Osteoclasts
Calcium minerals
Trabecular bone
Cortical bone
Osteoporotic bone

Detecting height loss

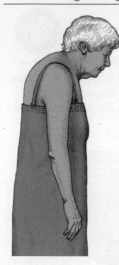

A patient with osteoporosis typically loses height gradually. A condition known as *dowager's hump* (shown at left) develops when repeated vertebral fractures increase the spinal curvature. (Although a hallmark of osteoporosis, this malformation may occur apart from the disease.)

Reduced thoracic and abdominal volumes, decreased exercise tolerance, pulmonary insufficiency, and abdominal protrusion may accompany height loss.

To assess height loss, have the patient stand with her arms raised laterally and parallel to the floor. A measured difference exceeding 1½" (3.8 cm) between the patient's height and the distance across the outstretched arms (from longest fingertip to longest fingertip) suggests height loss.

Treatment

▶ Weight-bearing exercise
▶ Bisphosphonates, such as alendronate (Fosamax), ibandronate (Boniva), and risedronate (Actonel), to prevent bone loss and reduce the risk of fractures
▶ Calcium and vitamin D supplements to support normal bone metabolism
▶ Raloxifene (Evista) and calcitonin to reduce bone resorption and slow decline in bone mass
▶ Teniparatide (Forteo) to help form new bone for patients at high risk for fractures
▶ Back brace to support weakened vertebrae
▶ Open reduction and internal fixation to correct pathologic fractures of the femur
▶ Dietary calcium and fluoride treatments
▶ Decreased alcohol consumption and caffeine use as well as smoking cessation

Nursing considerations

▶ Design your care plan to consider the patient's fragility. Concentrate on careful positioning, ambulation, and prescribed exercises.

▶ Include the patient and family members in all phases of care. Answer questions as completely as you can.
▶ Check the patient's skin daily for redness, warmth, and new sites of pain, which may indicate fractures.
▶ Provide the patient with activities that involve mild exercise; help her to walk several times daily. As appropriate, perform passive range-of-motion exercises or encourage her to perform active exercises. Make sure she attends scheduled physical therapy sessions.
▶ Impose safety precautions. Move the patient gently and carefully at all times. Discuss with ancillary facility personnel how easily an osteoporotic patient's bones can fracture.
▶ Provide a balanced diet rich in nutrients that support skeletal metabolism, such as vitamin D, calcium, and protein.
▶ Administer analgesics and heat to relieve pain as ordered. Assess the patient's response.

LESSON PLANS

Teaching about osteoporosis

▶ Explain all treatments, tests, and procedures. If the patient is undergoing surgery to repair a fracture, explain all preoperative and postoperative procedures and treatments to the patient and family members.
▶ Make sure the patient and family members clearly understand the prescribed drug regimen. Tell them how to recognize significant adverse reactions and to report them immediately.
▶ Demonstrate or explain which weight-bearing exercises would improve bone strength and balance.
▶ If the patient takes a calcium supplement, encourage liberal fluid intake to help maintain adequate urine output and thereby avoid renal calculi, hypercalcemia, and hypercalciuria.
▶ Make sure the calcium supplement includes vitamin D, which helps with calcium absorption.
▶ Advise the patient to eat a calcium-rich diet; provide a list of calcium-rich foods.
▶ Tell the patient to report new pain sites immediately, especially after trauma.
▶ Reinforce the patient's efforts to adapt, and show her how her condition is improving or stabilizing. As necessary, refer her to an occupational therapist or a home health nurse to help her cope with activities of daily living.

Primary malignant bone tumors

Primary malignant bone tumors (sarcomas of the bone) are rare, constituting less than 1% of all malignant tumors. Most bone tumors result from metastasis from another malignant tumor.

Primary bone tumors occur more commonly in males than in females, especially in children and adolescents, although some types occur in people between ages 35 and 60.

Although the cause of primary malignant bone tumors remains unknown, it's believed that they arise in centers of rapid skeletal growth because children and young adults with these tumors seem to be much taller than average. Other theories point to heredity factors, trauma, and excessive radiotherapy as causes.

Prior exposure to carcinogens, an underlying condition such as Paget's disease, and radiation exposure have been linked with the development of osteogenic sarcomas, chondrosarcomas, and fibrosarcomas.

Primary malignant bone tumors may originate in osseous or non-osseous tissue. Osseous tumors arise from the bony structure as well as from cartilage, fibrous tissue, and bone marrow. They include osteogenic sarcoma (the most common), parosteal osteogenic sarcoma, chondrosarcoma (malignant cartilage tumor), and malignant giant cell tumor. Together, these make up about 60% of all malignant bone tumors.

Nonosseous tumors arise from hematopoietic, vascular, and neural tissues. They include Ewing's sarcoma, fibrosarcoma, and chordoma. Osteogenic and Ewing's sarcomas are the most common bone tumors in children.

Types of bone tumors

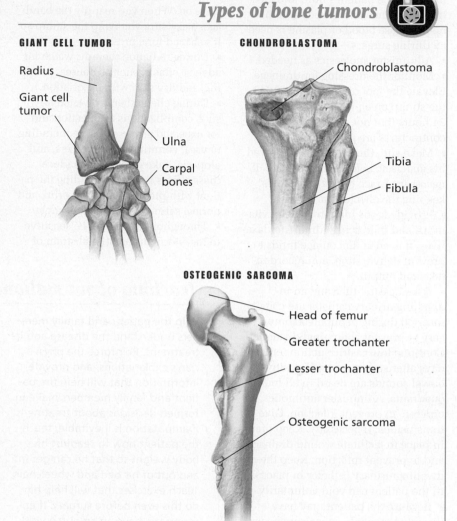

GIANT CELL TUMOR

Radius

Giant cell tumor

Ulna

Carpal bones

CHONDROBLASTOMA

Chondroblastoma

Tibia

Fibula

OSTEOGENIC SARCOMA

Head of femur

Greater trochanter

Lesser trochanter

Osteogenic sarcoma

Signs and symptoms

▸ Pathologic fracture
▸ Bone pain that's described as a dull ache
▸ Mass or tumor, possibly accompanied by swelling
▸ Movement that doesn't aggravate the pain
▸ Pain that's more intense at night
▸ Limp when walking
▸ Cachexia, with fever and impaired mobility (in late stages)
▸ Localized or referred pain from the hip or spine
▸ Weakness in the affected limb

Treatment

▸ Surgical resection of the tumor usually with preoperative radiation (or chemotherapy for large tumors) and postoperative chemotherapy, which saves many limbs from amputation
▸ Radical surgery such as hemipelvectomy
▸ Intensive chemotherapy that combines cyclophosphamide, cisplatin (Platinol), vincristine, doxorubicin (Doxil), methotrexate (Trexall), bleomycin (Blenoxane), and dacarbazine (may be done intra-arterially into the long bones of the legs)

Nursing considerations

▶ Before surgery, start I.V. infusions to maintain the patient's fluid and electrolyte balance and to keep a vein open in case blood or plasma is needed during surgery.

▶ Administer analgesics as needed.

▶ Monitor the dressing for drainage. Elevate the foot of the bed, or place the stump on a pillow, for the first 24 hours (but not more than 48 hours; contractures are possible).

▶ Make sure the patient has received his analgesic before morning care. If necessary, brace him with pillows, keeping the affected part at rest.

▶ Provide foods high in protein, vitamins, and folic acid. Administer laxatives, if needed. Encourage fluids to prevent dehydration, and record intake and output.

▶ A nasogastric tube and an indwelling urinary catheter are usually inserted during hemipelvectomy surgery to prevent abdominal distention. Continue low gastric suction for 2 days after surgery or until positive bowel sounds are heard in all four quadrants. Administer antibiotics, as ordered, to prevent infection. Give transfusions, if necessary. Keep drains in place to facilitate wound drainage and to prevent infection. Keep the indwelling urinary catheter in place until the patient can void voluntarily.

▶ Because the patient may have thrombocytopenia, make sure he uses a soft toothbrush and an electric razor to avoid bleeding. Don't give I.M. injections or take rectal temperatures. Be careful not to bump the patient's arms or legs; low platelet count causes bruising.

▶ To encourage rehabilitation, start physical therapy 24 hours postoperatively.

▶ The patient usually doesn't have severe pain after amputation. If he does, check for such wound complications as hematoma, excessive stump edema, and infection.

▶ Wash the stump, massage it gently, and keep it dry until it heals. Make sure the bandage is firm and always stays on. When you reapply the bandage, make sure you wrap the stump so it's shaped for a prosthesis.

▶ During radiation therapy, watch for adverse effects, such as nausea, vomiting, and dry skin with excoriation.

▶ During chemotherapy, watch for such complications as infection and for expected adverse effects, including nausea, vomiting, mouth ulcers, and alopecia. Take measures to reduce these effects, such as providing the patient with plenty of fluids to drink and normal saline mouthwash to gargle.

▶ Throughout treatment, be sensitive to the enormous emotional strain of amputation. Encourage communication, and help the patient set realistic goals.

▶ Listen to the patient's fears and concerns, and offer reassurance when appropriate. Stay with the patient during periods of severe stress and anxiety.

▶ Whenever possible, include the patient and family members in care decisions.

▶ Be alert for phantom limb pain.

LESSON PLANS

Teaching about malignant bone tumors

▶ Help the patient and family members understand the disease and its treatment. Reinforce the physician's explanations, and provide information that will help the patient and family members make informed decisions about treatment.

▶ If amputation is inevitable, teach the patient how to readjust his body weight so that he can get in and out of his bed and wheelchair. Teach exercises that will help him do this even before surgery. If appropriate, have an amputee visit the patient.

▶ Emphasize the importance of deep breathing and turning every 2 hours immediately after surgery.

▶ Teach the patient about phantom limb syndrome. Explain that he may sense an itch or tingling in the amputated extremity. Reassure him this sensation is normal after amputation and usually subsides within several hours. Explain, however, that the sensation may recur off and on for years.

▶ To avoid contractures and ensure the best conditions for wound healing, teach the patient not to dangle the stump over the edge of the bed; sit in a wheelchair with the stump flexed; place a pillow under his hip, knee, or back, or between his thighs; lie with knees flexed; rest an above-the-knee stump on the crutch handle; or abduct an above-the-knee stump.

▶ Teach the patient and a family member how to care for the stump. Stress the need for following aseptic technique to prevent infection.

▶ Emphasize the importance of sound nutrition. Ask the dietitian to provide instruction for the patient.

▶ Refer the patient and family to the social service department, home health care agencies, and support groups such as the American Cancer Society, as appropriate.

Scoliosis

With scoliosis, a lateral curvature of the spine, the vertebrae rotate into the convex part of the curve. This rotation causes rib prominence along the thoracic spine and waistline asymmetry in the lumbar spine. Scoliosis can affect the spine at any level, but right thoracic curves are most common.

Idiopathic scoliosis affects less than 1% of school-age children and is most common during the growth spurt between ages 10 and 13. It affects boys and girls equally, but spinal curve progression is more common in girls.

This disorder can be classified as nonstructural or structural. In nonstructural scoliosis, the spinal curve appears flexible, straightening temporarily when the patient leans sideways. In contrast, structural scoliosis is a fixed deformity that doesn't correct itself when the patient leans sideways.

Scoliosis is also classified by age of onset as infantile, juvenile, adolescent, or adult. Infantile scoliosis is most common in boys ages 1 to 3. It may resolve spontaneously, or it may progress and require treatment. Juvenile scoliosis equally affects boys and girls ages 3 to 10. This disorder usually requires long-term follow-up and treatment during the peak growing years. Adolescent scoliosis occurs after age 10 and during adolescence. Adult scoliosis occurs after age 18.

Signs and symptoms

▶ Appearance of uneven hemlines, unequal length of pant legs, one hip rising higher than the other (as noticed by a parent)
▶ Family history of scoliosis
▶ Backache, fatigue, and dyspnea

Looking at scoliosis

In a patient with scoliosis, lateral deviation of the spine is present and the patient leans to the side (shown at right). Other findings include:
▶ uneven shoulder blade height and shoulder blade prominence
▶ unequal distance between the arms and the body
▶ asymmetrical waistline
▶ uneven hip height.

HANDS ON

Testing for scoliosis

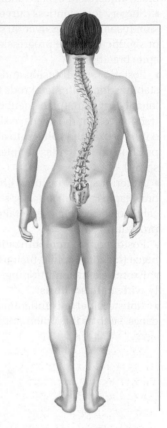

When assessing your patient for an abnormal spinal curve, use this screening test for scoliosis. Have the patient remove her shirt and stand as straight as she can with her back to you. Instruct her to distribute her weight evenly on each foot. While the patient does this, observe both sides of her back from neck to buttocks. Look for these signs:
▶ uneven shoulder height and shoulder blade prominence
▶ unequal distance between the arms and body
▶ asymmetrical waistline
▶ uneven hip height
▶ a sideways lean.

With the patient's back still facing you, ask her to do the "forward-bend" test. In this test, the patient places her palms together and slowly bends forward, remembering to keep her head down. As she complies, check for these signs:
▶ asymmetrical thoracic spine or prominent rib cage (rib hump) on either side
▶ asymmetrical waistline.

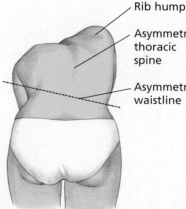

Rib hump

Asymmetrical thoracic spine

Asymmetrical waistline

Treatment

▶ Spinal bracing with follow-up and brace adjustment every 3 months
▶ Surgery for relentless curve progression (usually curves over 40 degrees) or significant curve progression despite bracing
▶ Posterior spinal fusion and internal stabilization with metal rods to correct lateral curvature (placement of a distraction rod on the concave side of the curve "jacks" the spine into a straight position and provides an internal splint)
▶ Anterior spinal fusion with vertebral staples and an anterior stabilizing cable to correct curvature (alternative procedure)
▶ Postoperative immobilization in a brace (for some spinal fusions)
▶ Exercise and conditioning, especially with adult scoliosis
▶ Nonsteroidal anti-inflammatory drugs, such as ibuprofen or naproxen

Nursing considerations

▶ Allow the patient to verbalize her concerns about the disorder, and answer her questions completely. Include the patient and family members in all phases of care.
▶ Encourage the patient to perform as much self-care as her immobility and pain allow. Provide her with adequate time to perform these activities at her own pace.
▶ If the patient needs a body cast, remember that its application can be traumatic because it's done on a special frame with the patient's head and face covered throughout the procedure.
▶ Check the skin around the cast edge daily. Keep the cast clean and dry. Petal the edges of the cast.
▶ After corrective surgery, provide the patient with pain medications, as ordered, and assess the patient's response to them.
▶ Check sensation, movement, color, and blood supply in all extremities every 2 to 4 hours for the first 48 hours and then several times per day to detect neurovascular deficit (a serious complication following spinal surgery). Logroll the patient often.
▶ Measure intake, output, and urine specific gravity to monitor the effects of blood loss, which may be substantial.
▶ Monitor abdominal distention and bowel sounds.
▶ Encourage deep-breathing exercises to avoid pulmonary complications.
▶ Promote active range-of-motion (ROM) arm exercises to help maintain muscle strength. Any exercise, even brushing the hair or teeth, is helpful. Encourage the patient to perform quadriceps-setting, calf-pumping, and active ROM exercises with the feet.
▶ Watch for skin breakdown and signs and symptoms of cast syndrome.
▶ Apply sequential compression device as indicated.

LESSON
PLANS

Teaching about scoliosis

▶ If the patient needs a brace, explain what it does and how to care for it (for example, how to check the screws for tightness and how to pad the uprights to prevent excessive wear on clothing). Suggest loose-fitting, oversized clothes for greater comfort.
▶ Instruct the patient to wear the brace 23 hours per day and to remove it only for bathing and exercise.
▶ To prevent skin breakdown, advise the patient not to use lotions, ointments, or powders on areas where the brace contacts the skin.
▶ Instruct the patient to turn her whole body instead of just her head when looking to the side.
▶ If the patient has a cast, make sure she and her family members understand proper cast care.
▶ If the patient is having surgery, explain preoperative and postoperative procedures. After surgery, make sure she knows how to recognize complications and the measures to take to prevent them. Before discharge, check with the surgeon about activity limitations and make sure the patient understands them.
▶ Discuss all prescribed medications and any adverse reactions with the patient. Advise the patient to notify the physician if these reactions persist.

Tendinitis and bursitis

With tendinitis, inflammation affects the tendons and tendon-muscle attachments to bone, usually in the shoulder rotator cuff, hip, Achilles tendon, hamstring, or elbow.

Tendinitis is more common in older people, but it can afflict anyone who performs an activity that overstresses a tendon or repeatedly stresses a joint. The disorder causes localized pain around the affected area and restricts joint movement. Initially, swelling results from fluid accumulation. As the disorder progresses, calcium deposits form in and around the tendon, causing further swelling and immobility.

Bursitis is a painful inflammation of one or more bursae. These closed sacs hold lubricating synovial fluid and facilitate the movement of muscles and tendons over bony prominences. Bursitis causes sudden or gradual pain and limits joint motion. Usually, the disorder occurs in the subdeltoid, subacromial, olecranon, trochanteric, calcaneal, or prepatellar bursae. It may be septic, calcific, acute, or chronic.

Understanding epicondylitis

Epicondylitis (also called *tennis elbow*) is one of several activity-related joint disorders. It occurs when the forearm extensor supinator tendon fibers become inflamed at their common attachment to the lateral humeral epicondyle.

Epicondylitis may produce acute or subacute pain. It probably begins as a partial tear and is common among tennis players or people whose activities require a forceful grasp, wrist extension against resistance, or frequent forearm rotation.

Signs and symptoms

The patient may initially have elbow pain that gradually increases, radiating to the forearm and back of the hand whenever he grasps an object or twists his elbow. Rarely, the elbow is red, swollen, warm, or restricted in range of motion. The patient may have tenderness over the involved lateral or medial epicondyle or over the head of the radius.

Selective tissue tension assessment may reproduce the pain by wrist extension and supination with lateral involvement or by flexion and pronation with medial epicondyle involvement. Neuromuscular test results may reveal a weak grasp.

Treatment

The patient may receive a local injection of a corticosteroid and anesthetic and systemic nonsteroidal anti-inflammatory drugs, such as aspirin or ibuprofen, to relieve pain. Supportive treatment includes:
▶ immobilization with a splint from the distal forearm to the elbow, which may relieve pain in 2 to 3 weeks
▶ heat therapy with warm compresses, short wave diathermy, or ultrasound (alone or with diathermy)
▶ a "tennis elbow strap" wrapped snugly around the forearm about 1″ (2.5 cm) below the epicondyle to relieve the strain on affected forearm muscles and tendons.

If medical and careful physical therapy and supportive measures fail, surgical release of the tendon at the epicondyle may be necessary.

Anatomy of tendons and bursae

Tendons, like stiff rubber bands, hold the muscles in place and enable them to move the bones. Bursae are located at friction points around joints and between tendons, cartilage, or bone. Bursae keep these body parts lubricated so they move freely.

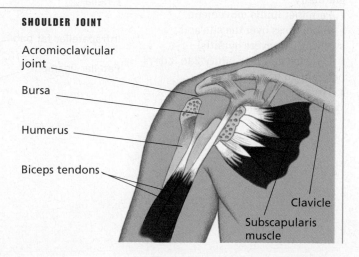

SHOULDER JOINT

Acromioclavicular joint

Bursa

Humerus

Biceps tendons

Clavicle

Subscapularis muscle

Signs and symptoms
Tendinitis
▶ Palpable tenderness over the affected site, referred tenderness in a related segment, or both
▶ Traumatic injury or strain associated with athletic activity

Tendinitis of the shoulder
▶ Heat that aggravates shoulder pain rather than provides relief
▶ Localized pain that's most severe at night and commonly interferes with sleep
▶ Restricted shoulder movement (especially abduction)

Tendinitis of the elbow (epicondylitis)
▶ Tenderness over the lateral epicondyle and pain when grasping objects or twisting the elbow

Tendinitis of the hamstring
▶ Pain in the posterolateral aspect of the knee
▶ Tenderness with the knee flexed at a 90-degree angle

Tendinitis of the foot
▶ Crepitus when moving the foot
▶ Pain over the Achilles tendon and on dorsiflexion

Bursitis
▶ Pain that develops suddenly or gradually
▶ Pain that limits movement
▶ Tenderness over the site and swelling (in severe bursitis)
▶ Unusual strain or injury 2 to 3 days before pain begins
▶ Work or leisure activity that involves repetitive action

Bursitis of the hip and knee

HIP

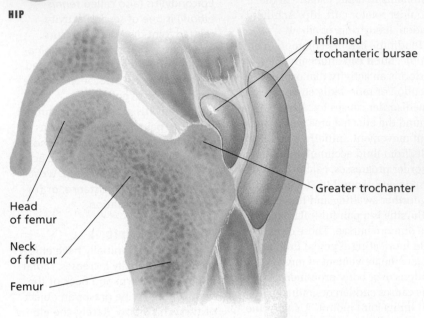

Inflamed trochanteric bursae

Greater trochanter

Head of femur

Neck of femur

Femur

KNEE

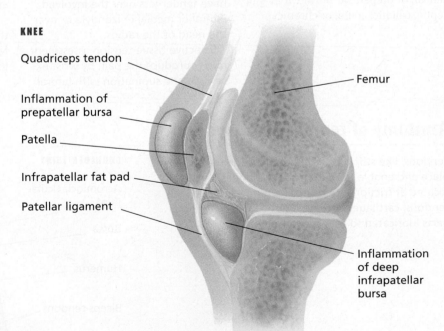

Quadriceps tendon

Inflammation of prepatellar bursa

Patella

Infrapatellar fat pad

Patellar ligament

Femur

Inflammation of deep infrapatellar bursa

Treatment

- Joint immobilization
- Nonsteroidal anti-inflammatory drugs
- Cold, heat, or ultrasound applications
- Possible injection of a local anesthetic (such as lidocaine) and corticosteroids for immediate relief
- Extended-release corticosteroids, such as triamcinolone or prednisolone, for longer relief
- Oral anti-inflammatory agents and short-term analgesics
- Needle aspiration to remove fluid
- Physical therapy to preserve motion and prevent frozen joints
- Lifestyle changes for long-term control of chronic bursitis and tendinitis

Nursing considerations

- Assess the severity of the patient's pain. Also assess range of motion in the affected joint to determine the effectiveness of the treatment.
- Encourage the patient to verbalize his concerns about his disorder. Listen, answer his questions, and offer support and encouragement. Include the patient and family members in all phases of his care.
- Encourage the patient to perform as much self-care as his immobility and pain allow. Provide him with adequate time to perform these activities at his own pace.
- Give medications, as ordered, and assess the patient's response to them.
- Before injecting corticosteroids or local anesthetics, ask the patient whether he has any drug allergies.
- Assist with intra-articular injection. Scrub the patient's skin thoroughly with povidone-iodine (or a comparable solution), and shave the injection site if necessary. After the injection, massage the area to ensure penetration through the tissue and joint space. Apply ice intermittently for about 4 hours to minimize pain. Avoid applying heat to the area for 2 days.

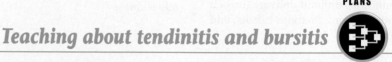

Teaching about tendinitis and bursitis

- Instruct the patient to take anti-inflammatory agents with food to minimize GI distress. Direct him to report any signs or symptoms of GI distress immediately.
- Help the patient identify and perform activities that promote rest and relaxation.
- Teach the patient how to perform strengthening exercises, and encourage him to follow the prescribed exercise regimen. To maintain joint mobility and prevent muscle atrophy, urge him to perform exercises or physical therapy regularly when he's free from pain.
- Advise the patient to wear a sling during the first few days of an attack of subdeltoid bursitis or tendinitis to support the arm and protect the shoulder, particularly at night. Demonstrate how to apply and wear the sling to relieve weight on the shoulder. To protect the shoulder during sleep, a splint may be worn instead of a sling. Instruct the patient to remove the splint during the day.

- Tell the patient with sports-related bursitis or tendinitis to evaluate his sports equipment, shoes, and playing surfaces.
- If the patient has Achilles tendinitis, recommend that he wear cushioned shoes, lose excess weight, and choose non-weight-bearing activities such as swimming.
- If the patient needs cold treatments to relieve swelling and pain, show him how to use a commercial cold pack or how to make an ice pack. If he needs heat applications, show him how to apply dry and moist heat. With either therapy, caution him to limit treatments to 20 minutes to prevent skin damage.
- To prevent recurrence, teach the patient to use proper body mechanics to minimize joint stress.
- Review all medications, including drug administration and possible adverse effects.

Torticollis

With torticollis, a neck deformity also known as *wryneck*, spastic or shortened sternocleidomastoid neck muscles cause the head to tilt to the affected side and the chin to rotate to the opposite side. The disorder may be acquired or congenital. Acquired torticollis usually develops either before age 10 or after age 40. It may be acute, spasmodic, or hysterical. Congenital (muscular) torticollis mostly affects infants after difficult delivery (breech presentation), firstborn infants, and girls.

Signs and symptoms
Acquired torticollis
▶ An enlarged, firm, and tender sternocleidomastoid muscle
▶ Gradual onset of painful neck deformity
▶ Pain followed by a drawing sensation and a momentary twitching or contraction that pulls the head to the side
▶ Recurring and unilateral neck muscle stiffness

Congenital torticollis
▶ An enlarged sternocleidomastoid muscle visible at birth and for several weeks afterward
▶ Permanent contracture due to incomplete regression
▶ Flattened face and head from sleeping on the affected side (severe deformity)
▶ Muscle that slowly shrinks (or regresses) over 6 months

PICTURING PATHO

Looking at torticollis

ACQUIRED TORTICOLLIS

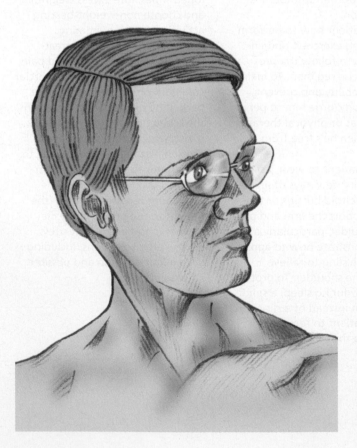

CONGENITAL (MUSCULAR) TORTICOLLIS

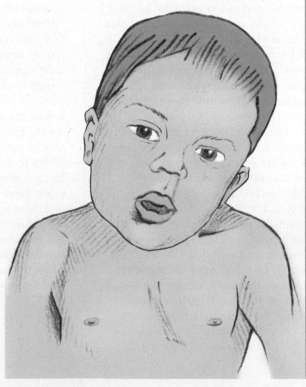

Treatment

Acquired torticollis

▶ Heat, cervical traction, and gentle massage to relieve pain
▶ Stretching exercises and a neck brace to relieve symptoms (for spasmodic and hysterical forms)
▶ Carbidopa-levodopa, carbamazepine, and haloperidol (for elderly patients)
▶ Botulinum toxin A (Botox) injected directly into the neck muscles
▶ Muscle relaxants
▶ Deep brain stimulation
▶ Nonsteroidal anti-inflammatory drugs

Congenital torticollis

▶ Passive neck stretching and proper positioning during sleep
▶ Active stretching exercises (for an older child)
▶ Surgical correction during preschool years and only if other therapies fail

Nursing considerations

▶ To aid early diagnosis of congenital torticollis, observe the infant for limited neck movement.
▶ Provide passive stretching and massage for an infant and encourage active stretching for the older child and adult.
▶ Prepare the patient for surgery. Also prepare him for possible immobilization with a brace.
▶ After corrective surgery, monitor the patient closely for nausea or signs of respiratory complications, especially if he's in cervical traction. Keep suction equipment available to manage possible aspiration.
▶ If the patient has an immobilization device such as a brace, monitor circulation, sensation, and color around the device. Inspect the skin around the device for signs of breakdown.
▶ Provide emotional support for the patient and family members to relieve their anxiety caused by fear, pain, an altered body image, and limitations imposed by treatments.
▶ Help the patient begin stretching exercises, as ordered, as soon he can tolerate them.

▶ Help the patient identify causes of stress, which may worsen signs and symptoms.

LESSON PLANS

Teaching about torticollis

▶ Teach parents how to perform stretching exercises with the child. Suggest placing toys or hanging mobiles on the side of the crib opposite the affected side of the child's neck. This encourages the child to move his head and stretch his neck in that direction.
▶ Before discharge, emphasize to the patient or his parents the importance of continuing daily heat applications, massages, and stretching exercises, as prescribed.
▶ Explain that physical therapy is essential to recovery.
▶ Teach relaxation skills to reduce stress.
▶ Explain the need for adequate rest to help reduce signs and symptoms.

TESTS
Laboratory tests

Common laboratory tests used to diagnose musculoskeletal disorders include serum calcium and serum phosphorus, alkaline phosphatase (ALP), and serum muscle enzymes (aldolase [ALD], aspartate aminotransferase [AST], creatine kinase [CK], and lactate dehydrogenase [LD]).

ALD

ALD is an enzyme found particularly in muscles. It's needed by muscles to turn glucose into energy. Elevated ALD levels may indicate muscular dystrophy.

ALP

ALP is an enzyme that influences bone calcification as well as lipid and metabolite transport. Although skeletal and hepatic diseases can raise ALP levels, this test is most useful for diagnosing metabolic bone disease.

AST

AST is found in the cytoplasm and mitochondria of many cells, including skeletal muscles. It's released into serum in proportion to cellular damage.

AST levels fluctuate in response to the extent of cellular necrosis, being transiently and minimally increased early in the disease process and extremely increased during the most acute phase. Depending on when the initial sample is drawn, AST levels may increase, indicating increasing disease severity and tissue damage, or decrease, indicating disease resolution and tissue repair. Elevated AST levels may indicate progressive muscular dystrophy or skeletal muscle trauma.

CK

CK is an enzyme that catalyzes the creatine-creatinine metabolic pathway in muscle cells and brain tissue. Isoenzyme CK-MM (CK_3) is the only isoenzyme found in skeletal muscle. Elevatated CK levels may indicate muscle trauma or progressive muscular dystrophy.

LD

Also a serum muscle enzyme, elevations of LD may indicate extensive cancer, progressive muscular dystrophy, or skeletal muscle necrosis.

SERUM CALCIUM

Serum calcium levels measure the total amount of calcium in the blood, and ionized calcium measures the fraction of serum calcium that's in the ionized form. Elevated serum calcium levels may indicate metastatic cancer of the bone or bone fractures in the healing stage.

SERUM PHOSPHORUS

Phosphates are essential in the storage and utilization of energy, calcium regulation, red blood cell function, acid-base balance, the formation of bone, and the metabolism of carbohydrates, protein, and fat. Elevated serum phosphorus levels may indicate bone fractures in the healing stage or bone tumors.

Aspiration tests

Fluid may be aspirated from the joint capsule (arthrocentesis) or from the bone marrow to detect various disorders.

ARTHROCENTESIS

Arthrocentesis is a joint puncture that's used to collect fluid for analysis to identify the cause of pain and swelling, to assess for infection, and to distinguish forms of arthritis, such as pseudogout and infectious arthritis. The knee may be used for this procedure, but synovial fluid may also be obtained from the wrist, ankle, elbow, or first metatarsophalangeal joint.

With joint infection, synovial fluid looks cloudy and contains more white blood cells and less glucose than normal. When trauma causes bleeding into a joint, synovial fluid contains red blood cells. In specific types of arthritis, crystals can confirm the diagnosis—for instance, urate crystals indicate gout.

Arthrocentesis also has therapeutic value. For example, in symptomatic joint effusion, removing excess synovial fluid relieves pain.

BONE MARROW ASPIRATION

Bone marrow aspiration can help diagnose many abnormalities, including rheumatoid arthritis, tuberculosis, amyloidosis, syphilis, bacterial or viral infection, parasitic infestation, tumors, and hematologic problems.

Aspiration usually involves the sternum or iliac crests. The site is prepared as for any minor surgical procedure and then infiltrated with a local anesthetic such as lidocaine. A marrow needle, with stylet in place is inserted through the cortex into the marrow cavity. Marrow cavity penetration causes the patient to feel a collapsing sensation. Then the stylet is removed and attached to a syringe and 0.2 to 0.5 ml of fluid is aspirated.

Endoscopic tests

Endoscopic studies allow direct visualization of joint problems. Arthroscopy is a common endoscopic procedure.

ARTHROSCOPY

Arthroscopy is usually used to evaluate the knee. It helps the physician assess joint problems, plan surgical approaches, and document disease.

After inserting a large-bore needle into the suprapatellar pouch, the physician injects sterile saline solution to distend the joint. Then he passes a fiber-optic scope through puncture sites lateral or medial to the tibial plateau, allowing direct visualization. With a large scope, he can remove articular debris and small, loose bodies or repair a torn meniscus.

Radiographic and imaging studies

Radiographic and imaging studies include bone densitometry, bone scans, computed tomography (CT) scans, magnetic resonance imaging (MRI), ultrasonography, and X-rays.

BONE DENSITOMETRY

Bone densitometry assesses bone mass quantitatively. This noninvasive technique, also known as *dual energy X-ray absorptiometry* (DEXA), uses an X-ray tube to measure bone mineral density but exposes the patient to only minimal radiation. The images detected are computer analyzed to determine bone mineral status. The computer calculates size and thickness of the bone as well as volumetric density to determine potential resistance to mechanical stress. It's used to help diagnose osteoporosis, especially before a fracture occurs.

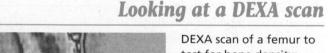

Looking at a DEXA scan

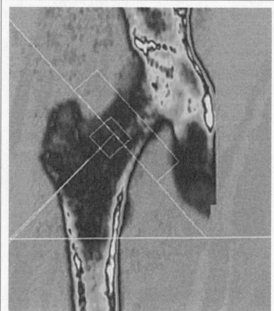

DEXA scan of a femur to test for bone density; warmer colors (yellows, reds) indicate areas of low bone density.

BONE SCAN

A bone scan helps detect bony metastasis, benign disease, fractures, avascular necrosis, and infection.

After I.V. introduction of a radioactive material, such as the radioisotope technetium pyrophosphate, the isotope collects in areas of increased bone activity or active bone formation. A scintillation counter detects the gamma rays, indicating abnormal areas of increased uptake (positive findings). The radioisotope has a short half-life and soon passes from the patient's body.

CT SCAN

A CT scan aids diagnosis of bone tumors and other abnormalities. It helps assess questionable cervical or spinal fractures, fracture fragments, bone lesions, and intra-articular loose bodies.

Multiple X-ray beams from a computerized body scanner are directed at the body from different angles. The beams pass through the body and strike radiation detectors, producing electrical impulses. A computer then converts these impulses into digital information, which is displayed as a three-dimensional image on a video monitor.

MRI

MRI can show irregularities of the spinal cord and is especially useful for diagnosing disk herniation.

The MRI scanner uses a powerful magnetic field and radiofrequency energy to produce images based on the hydrogen content of body tissues. The computer processes signals and displays the resulting high-resolution image on a video monitor. The patient can't feel the magnetic fields, and no harmful effects have been observed.

ULTRASONOGRAPHY

Ultrasonography may be used to determine soft-tissue injury or disorders, such as masses and fluid accumulation. It may also reveal traumatic joint injury and osteomyelitis.

X-RAYS

Anteroposterior, posteroanterior, and lateral X-rays allow three-dimensional visualization. They help diagnose:
▶ traumatic disorders, such as fractures and dislocations
▶ bone disease, including solitary lesions, multiple focal lesions in one bone, or generalized lesions involving all bones
▶ Joint disease, such as arthritis, infection, degenerative changes, synovio-sarcoma, osteochondromatosis, avascular necrosis, slipped femoral epiphysis, and inflamed tendons and bursae around a joint
▶ masses and calcifications.

If further clarification of standard X-rays is needed, a CT scan or MRI may be ordered.

Looking at a bone scan

The scan on the left shows areas of minimal isotope collection possibly indicating arthritis or a fracture.

The scan on the right shows areas of collection which may indicate increased bone activity or bone formation, possibly indicating cancer that has spread to multiple locations.

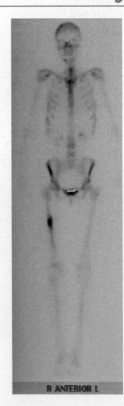

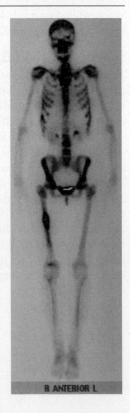

Other diagnostic tests

ELECTROMYOGRAPHY

Electromyography records the electrical activity of selected skeletal muscle groups at rest and during voluntary contraction. It involves percutaneous insertion of a needle electrode into a muscle. The electrical discharge of the muscle is then measured by an oscilloscope. Nerve conduction time is commonly measured simultaneously.

TREATMENTS AND PROCEDURES
Drug therapy

Drug therapy includes biphosphates, corticosteroids, nonsteroidal anti-inflammatory drugs (NSAIDs), and skeletal muscle relaxants, parathyroid hormone, selective estrogen receptor modulators (SERMs).

BIPHOSPHATES

▸ Inhibit bone reabsorption by binding with crystal elements found in bone
▸ Examples: alendronate (Fosamax), ibandronate (Boniva), risedronate (Actonel)

CORTICOSTEROIDS

▸ Local injection that's useful for some conditions (such as rotator cuff injuries); benefits lasting only weeks to months

NSAIDs

▸ Used for gouty arthritis, tendonitis, and bursitis and for mild to moderate pain associated with trauma
▸ Taken orally, are particularly useful, providing a combination of analgesic and anti-inflammatory effects in conditions with ongoing inflammation, such as arthropathies and strained ligaments
▸ Examples: ibuprofen (Advil, Nuprin), indomethacin (Indocin), etodolac (Lodine)

PARATHYROID HORMONE

▸ Treatment of osteoporosis in men and women
▸ Example: teriparatide (Forteo), subcutaneous injection

SERMs

▸ Mimic estrogen in some parts of the body while blocking the effect in other parts
▸ Used to treat or manage osteoporosis
▸ Example: raloxifene (Evista)

SKELETAL MUSCLE RELAXANTS

▸ Relieve musculoskeletal pain or spasms and spasticity
▸ Centrally or direct acting
▸ Centrally acting for treating muscle spasms caused by anxiety, inflammation, pain, or trauma; examples: carisoprodol (Soma), chlorzoxazone, tizanidine (Zanaflex)
▸ Direct-acting most effective for spasticity of cerebral origin in such disorders as muscle sclerosis, cerebral palsy, spinal cord injury, and stroke; example: dantrolene (Dantrium)

Nonsurgical treatments

Nonsurgical treatment may include closed reduction of a fracture, immobilization, and mechanical traction.

CLOSED REDUCTION

Closed reduction involves external manipulation of fracture fragments or dislocated joints to restore their normal position and alignment. It may be done under local, regional, or general anesthesia.

IMMOBILIZATION

Immobilization devices are commonly used to maintain proper alignment and limit movement. They also relieve pressure and pain.

Immobilization devices include:
▶ plaster and synthetic casts applied after closed or open reduction of fractures or after other severe injuries
▶ splints to immobilize fractures, dislocations, or subluxations
▶ slings to support and immobilize an injured arm, wrist, or hand, or to support the weight of a splint or hold dressings in place
▶ skin or skeletal traction, using a system of weights and pulleys to reduce fractures, treat dislocations, correct deformities, or decrease muscle spasms
▶ cervical collars to immobilize the cervical spine, decrease muscle spasms and, possibly, relieve pain.

Types of cervical collars

Cervical collars are used to support an injured or weakened cervical spine and to maintain alignment during healing.

Made of rigid plastic, the molded cervical collar holds the patient's neck firmly, keeping it straight, with the chin slightly elevated and tucked in.

The soft cervical collar, made of spongy foam, provides gentler support and reminds the patient to avoid cervical spine motion.

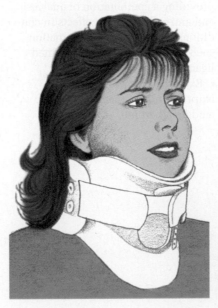
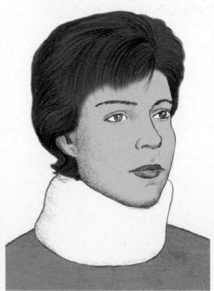

Types of cylindrical casts

Made of plaster, fiberglass, or synthetic material, casts may be applied almost anywhere on the body—to support a single finger or the entire body. Common casts are shown below.

HANGING ARM CAST

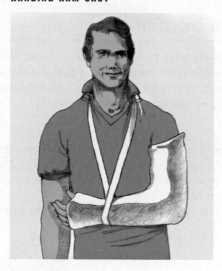

SHOULDER SPICA

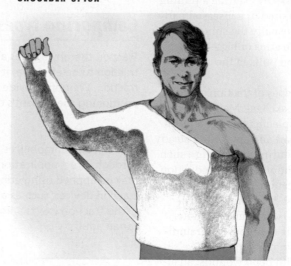

SHORT ARM CAST

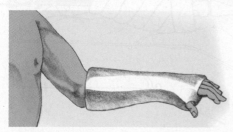

SINGLE HIP-SPICA

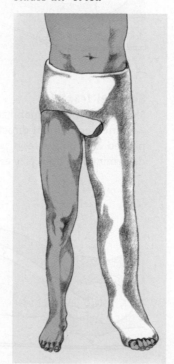

ONE AND ONE-HALF HIP-SPICA

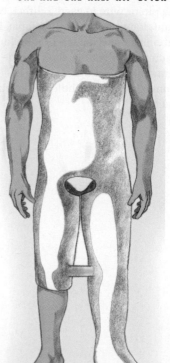

LONG LEG CAST

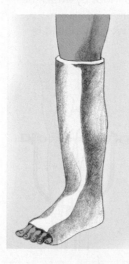

SHORT LEG CAST

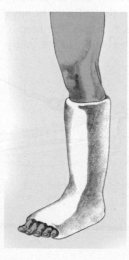

MECHANICAL TRACTION

Mechanical traction is used to reduce fractures, treat dislocations, correct or prevent deformities, improve or correct contractures, or decrease muscle spasms. It works by exerting a pulling force on an injured or a diseased part of the body—usually the spine, pelvis, or bones of the arms or legs—while countertraction pulls in the opposite direction.

The three types of traction are manual, skin, and skeletal. Manual traction involves placing hands on the affected body part and applying a steady pull, usually during a procedure such as cast application, fracture reduction, or halo application.

Skin traction is ordered when a light, temporary, or noncontinuous pulling force is required. Contraindications for skin traction include a severe injury with open wounds, an allergy to tape or other skin traction equipment, circulatory disturbances, dermatitis, and varicose veins.

For skeletal traction, an orthopedist inserts a pin or wire through the bone and attaches the traction equipment to the pin or wire to exert a direct, constant, longitudinal pulling force. Indications for skeletal traction include fractures of the tibia, femur, and humerus. Infections, such as osteomyelitis, contraindicate skeletal traction.

Comparing types of traction

Traction therapy applies a pulling force to an injured or diseased limb. For traction to be effective, it must be combined with an equal mix of countertraction. Weights provide the pulling force. Countertraction is produced by positioning the patient's body weight against the traction pull.

Skin traction

Skin traction immobilizes a body part intermittently over an extended period through direct application of a pulling force on the patient's skin. The force may be applied using adhesive or nonadhesive traction tape or other skin traction devices, such as a boot, belt, or halter.

This traction exerts a light pull and uses up to 8 lb (3.6 kg) per extremity for an adult.

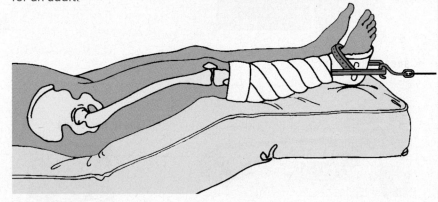

Skeletal traction

Skeletal traction immobilizes a body part for prolonged periods by attaching weighted equipment directly to the patient's bones. This may be accomplished with pins, screws, wires, or tongs. The amount of weight applied is determined by body size and the extent of the injury.

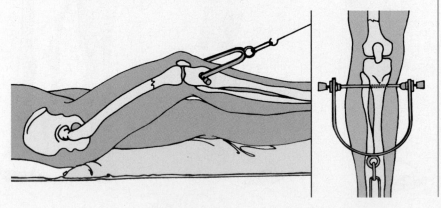

Surgery

For some patients with musculoskeletal disorders, surgery can offer an alternative to a life of chronic pain and disability. Surgical procedures include amputation, arthroplasty, arthroscopy, electrical bone growth stimulation, external fixation, and open reduction and internal fixation.

AMPUTATION

Amputation is the removal of a part of the body and can be surgical or traumatic. Surgical amputation can be performed as open (guillotine) or closed (flap method). An open method is usually performed in patients who have or are expected to develop an infection, because the wound remains open and can drain until the infection clears. With the closed method, the surgeon sutures the flap over the stump. With both methods, the surgeon tries to preserve as much of the body part as he can.

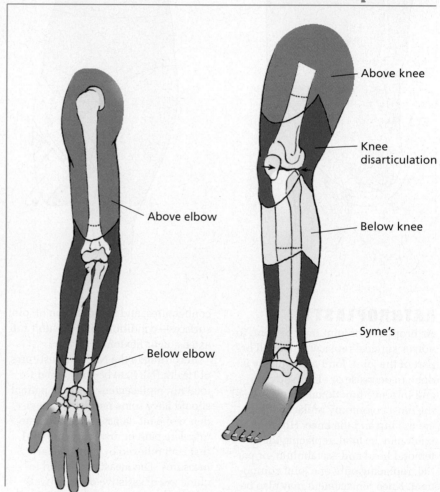

Levels of amputation

Above knee

Knee disarticulation

Below knee

Syme's

Above elbow

Below elbow

Wrapping a stump

Proper stump care helps protect the limb, reduces swelling, and prepares the limb for a prosthesis. As you perform the procedure, teach these steps to the patient.

Start by obtaining two 4″ (10.2-cm) elastic bandages. Center the end of the first 4″ bandage at the top of the patient's thigh. Unroll the bandage downward over the stump and to the back of the leg (as shown below).

Make three figure-eight turns to adequately cover the ends of the stump. As you wrap, be sure to include the roll of flesh in the groin area. Use enough pressure to ensure that the stump narrows toward the end so that it fits comfortably into the prosthesis.

Use the second 4″ bandage to anchor the first bandage around the waist. For a below-the-knee amputation, use the knee to anchor the bandage in place. Secure it with clips, safety pins, or adhesive tape. Check the stump bandage regularly, and rewrap it if it bunches at the end.

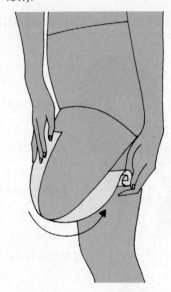

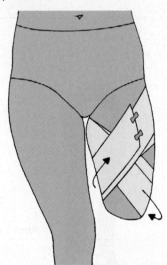

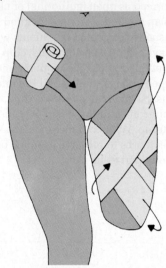

ARTHROPLASTY

Arthroplasty, or joint replacement, involves surgical replacement of all or part of the joint. Joint arthroplasty is done to decrease or eliminate pain and improve functional status. Two of the most commonly replaced joints are the hip and the knee. Hip replacement may be total, replacing the femoral head and acetabulum, or partial, replacing only one joint component. Knee replacement may also be partial, replacing either the medial or lateral compartment of the knee joint, or total, replacing the entire knee joint. Total knee replacement is commonly used to treat severe pain, joint

contractures, and deterioration of joint surfaces—conditions that prohibit full extension or flexion.

According to the National Institutes of Health (NIH), to be considered for total hip replacement (THR), a patient should have some radiographic evidence of joint damage and moderate to severe pain or disability (or both) that isn't relieved by nonsurgical measures. The measures should include use of assistive devices (walkers), analgesics and nonsteroidal anti-inflammatory drugs, physical therapy, and a reduction in physical activity. NIH statistics show that THR is most

commonly used for patients with osteoarthritis. Other indications include:

▶ ankylosing spondylitis
▶ arthritis associated with Paget's disease
▶ avascular necrosis
▶ benign and malignant bone tumors
▶ certain hip fractures
▶ juvenile rheumatoid arthritis
▶ rheumatoid arthritis
▶ sickle cell anemia
▶ traumatic arthritis.

Total knee replacement

With the patient in a supine position with his knee flexed slightly, a tourniquet is applied to the upper thigh. The surgeon makes a midline incision about 4″ (10.2 cm) above the patella, enters the joint capsule medially, and exposes the tibiofemoral joint. He resects and sizes the tibia and femur and then reams the tibia. Then he reassesses tibial size, sizes the patella, and inserts the knee prosthesis (with or without bone cement).

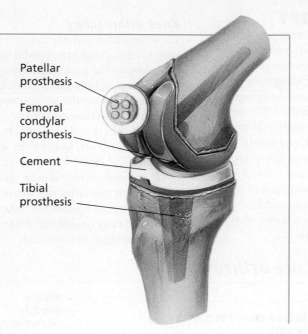

Patellar prosthesis

Femoral condylar prosthesis

Cement

Tibial prosthesis

Total hip replacement

With the patient in the lateral position, the surgeon makes an incision to expose the hip joint. He incises or excises the hip capsule and reams and shapes the acetabulum to accept the socket of the prosthesis. He repeats the process on the head of the femur for the ball of the prosthesis.

Next, he cements the femoral head prosthesis in place to articulate with a cup, which he cements into the deepened acetabulum. To avoid using cement, he may implant a prosthesis with a porous coating that promotes bony ingrowth.

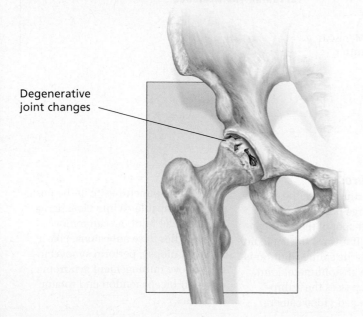

Degenerative joint changes

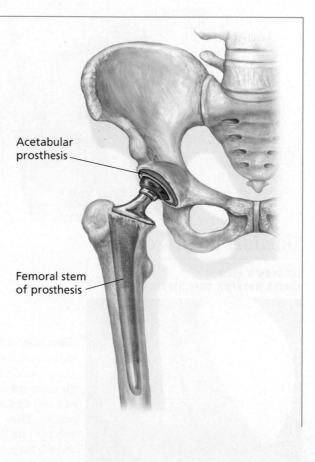

Acetabular prosthesis

Femoral stem of prosthesis

ARTHROSCOPY

A common endoscopic procedure, arthroscopy is used to visualize a joint, allowing the surgeon to assess for problems, plan surgical approaches, document disease, and diagnose and treat joint disorders. The procedure is most commonly performed on the knee, shoulder, and wrists.

The surgeon inserts the arthroscope into the patient's joint through a puncture. Through two additional punctures, he manipulates additional instruments, such as scissors, shaving knives, and forceps.

Knee arthroscopy

To perform knee arthroscopy, the surgeon inserts a large-bore needle into the suprapatellar pouch and injects sterile saline solution into the distended joint. He passes the arthroscope (with attached video camera) through puncture sites lateral or medial to the tibial plateau. Then he removes articular debris and small, loose bodies.

This procedure may also be done to repair a torn meniscus, reconstruct the anterior cruciate ligament, or take a synovial biopsy or shaving of the patella, cartilage, or meniscus.

Knee arthroscopy

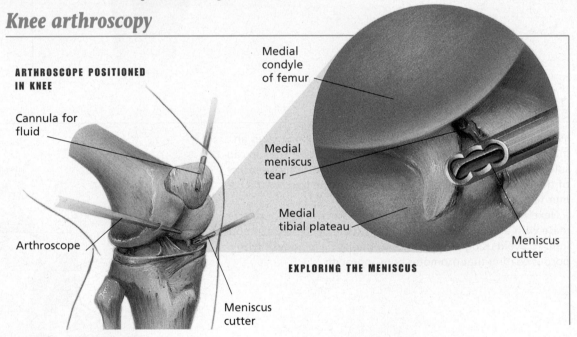

ARTHROSCOPE POSITIONED IN KNEE

Cannula for fluid

Arthroscope

Meniscus cutter

EXPLORING THE MENISCUS

Medial condyle of femur

Medial meniscus tear

Medial tibial plateau

Meniscus cutter

Shoulder arthroscopy

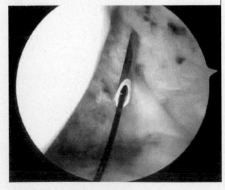

SURGEON'S VIEW DURING ROTATOR CUFF REPAIR

Shoulder arthroscopy

With shoulder arthroscopy, the surgeon inserts a large-bore needle into the posterior soft spot of the joint capsule and directs it toward the coracoid process. Then sterile saline solution is injected into the glenohumeral joint, and the surgeon passes the arthroscope (with attached video camera) through the puncture site of the posterior joint capsule. While visualizing the shoulder joint, he can remove loose bodies, lyse adhesions, take a synovial biopsy, perform synovectomy, relieve impingement syndrome, or repair biceps tendon and rotator cuff tears.

ELECTRICAL BONE GROWTH STIMULATION

Indications for the use of electrical bone growth stimulators include augmentation of open reduction with internal and external fixation, promotion of bone growth, treatment of infected nonunions and failed arthrodesis and, most recently, treatment of disuse osteoporosis. By limiting the body's natural electrical forces, this procedure initiates or accelerates the healing process.

Three basic electrical bone growth stimulation techniques are available: fully implantable direct current stimulation, semi-invasive percutaneous stimulation, and noninvasive electromagnetic coil stimulation. Choice of technique depends on the fracture type and location, the practitioner's preference, and the patient's ability and willingness to comply. The invasive device requires little or no patient involvement. With the other two methods, however, the patient must manage his own treatment schedule and maintain the equipment. Treatment time averages 3 to 6 months.

HANDS ON

Using an external bone growth stimulator

An external bone growth stimulator (EBGS) is a noninvasive and painless alternative to surgical bone grafting to promote healing. To use it, first gather the necessary equipment and familiarize the patient with the components of the EBGS system.

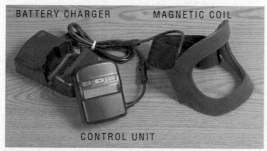

BATTERY CHARGER   MAGNETIC COIL

CONTROL UNIT

Teach the patient where and how to place the coil. Inform her that she may place the coil over her cast or against her skin. A layer of clothing between the coil and her skin will provide adequate protection against skin irritation. Show her how to secure the coil with the strap and connect the control unit to the coil.

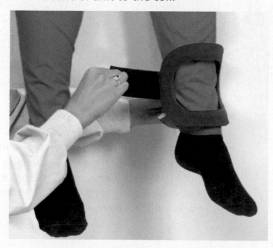

Pressing the button will start the unit, which will begin transmitting and recording. Be sure to show the patient when the battery needs changing. Depending on the type of unit, she may need to do this after each use or when the words "recharge battery" appear on the light-emitting diode (LED) screen. To charge the unit, tell her to plug it into an outlet at home and leave it plugged in for at least 2 hours.

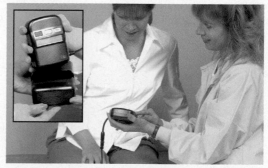

On the patient's return visits, turn on the control unit. The LED screen should display the hourly use per day and the number of days used and not used. Use these data to determine whether she has used the EBGS according to her prescribed regimen. Be sure to document the usage times in her medical record.

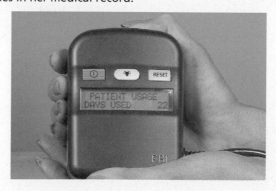

EXTERNAL FIXATION

External fixation is a system of percutaneous pins and wires that are inserted through the skin and muscle into the bone and affixed to an adjustable external frame, which maintains the bones in proper alignment. Specialized types of external fixators may be used to lengthen leg bones or immobilize the cervical spine.

An advantage of external fixation over other immobilization techniques is that it stabilizes the fracture while allowing full visualization and access to open wounds. It also facilitates early ambulation, thus reducing the risk of complications from immobilization.

The Ilizarov Fixator is a special type of external fixation device. This device is a combination of rings and tensioned transosseous wires used primarily in limb lengthening, bone transport, and limb salvage. Highly complex, it provides gradual distraction resulting in good-quality bone formation with a minimum of complications.

External fixation devices

The practitioner's selection of an external fixation device depends on the severity of the patient's fracture and on the type of bone alignment needed.

Universal day frame

A universal day frame is used to manage tibial fractures. The frame allows the practitioner to readjust the position of bony fragments by angulation and rotation. The compression-distraction device allows compression and distraction of bony fragments.

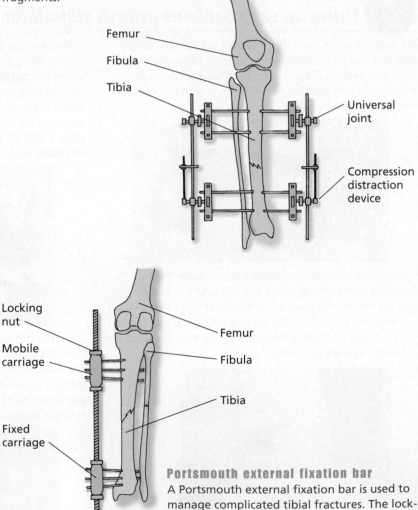

Femur
Fibula
Tibia
Universal joint
Compression distraction device

Locking nut
Mobile carriage
Fixed carriage
Femur
Fibula
Tibia

Portsmouth external fixation bar

A Portsmouth external fixation bar is used to manage complicated tibial fractures. The locking nut adjustment on the mobile carriage only allows bone compression, so the practitioner must accurately reduce bony fragments before applying the device.

OPEN REDUCTION AND INTERNAL FIXATION

Open reduction is a surgical procedure to realign a fracture; internal fixation is the addition of devices to stabilize the fracture. Internal fixation devices include nails, screws, pins, wires, and rods. They can be used individually or in combination with metal plates to attain stabilization.

Internal fixation devices

The choice of a specific internal fixation device depends on the location, type, and configuration of the fracture.

For an uncomplicated fracture of the femoral shaft, the surgeon may use an intramedullary rod. This device permits early ambulation with partial weight bearing.

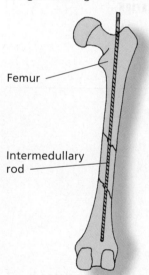

Femur

Intermedullary rod

Another choice for fixation of a long-bone fracture is a screw plate, shown below on the tibia.

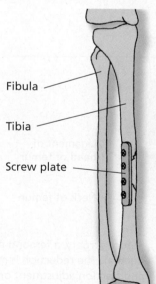

Fibula

Tibia

Screw plate

For an arm fracture, the surgeon may fix the involved bones with a plate, rod, screw, or nail. Most radial and ulnar fractures may be fixed with plates, whereas humeral fractures are commonly fixed with rods.

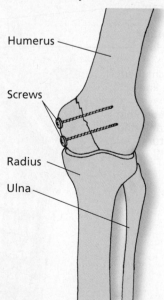

Humerus

Screws

Radius

Ulna

Internal fixation devices for hip fracture

The choice of internal fixation devices (screws and plates) for hip fracture repair depends on the type of fracture. The cannulated screw fixation device is used for nondisplaced femoral neck fractures.

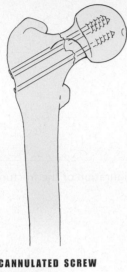

CANNULATED SCREW FIXATION

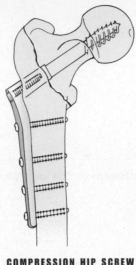

COMPRESSION HIP SCREW AND SIDE PLATE

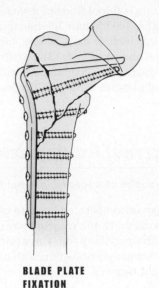

BLADE PLATE FIXATION

Repairing a femoral neck fracture

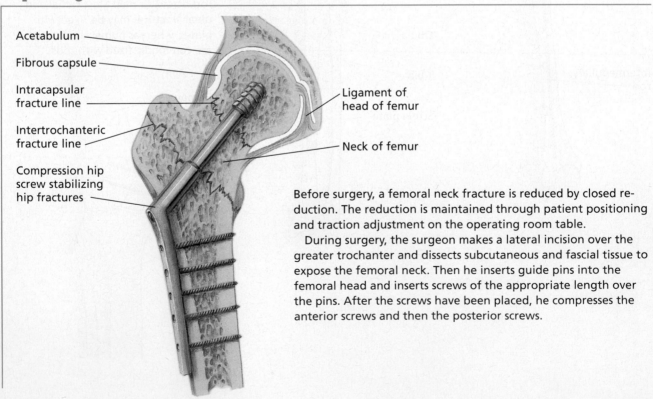

Acetabulum

Fibrous capsule

Intracapsular fracture line

Intertrochanteric fracture line

Compression hip screw stabilizing hip fractures

Ligament of head of femur

Neck of femur

Before surgery, a femoral neck fracture is reduced by closed reduction. The reduction is maintained through patient positioning and traction adjustment on the operating room table.

During surgery, the surgeon makes a lateral incision over the greater trochanter and dissects subcutaneous and fascial tissue to expose the femoral neck. Then he inserts guide pins into the femoral head and inserts screws of the appropriate length over the pins. After the screws have been placed, he compresses the anterior screws and then the posterior screws.

Chapter 7
Renal and urologic care

DISEASES
Acute pyelonephritis

Acute pyelonephritis (also called *acute interstitial nephritis*) is one of the most common renal diseases. With this disorder, sudden inflammation is caused by bacterial infection of the kidneys. It occurs mainly in the interstitial tissue and the renal pelvis, and occasionally in the renal tubules. It may affect one or both kidneys.

Typically, the infection spreads from the bladder to the ureters and then to the kidneys, commonly through vesicoureteral reflux. Vesicoureteral reflux may result from a congenital weakness at the junction of the ureter and the bladder. The infecting bacteria are usually normal intestinal and fecal flora that grow readily in urine. Infection may also result from procedures that involve the use of instruments (such as catheterization, cystoscopy, and urologic surgery) or from a hematogenic infection (such as septicemia and endocarditis).

Pyelonephritis may result from an inability to empty the bladder (for example, in patients with neurogenic bladder), urinary stasis, or urinary obstruction caused by tumors, strictures, or benign prostatic hyperplasia.

With treatment and continued follow-up care, the prognosis is good and extensive permanent damage is rare.

PICTURING
PATHO

Phases of pyelonephritis

ACUTE PYELONEPHRITIS AND PROGRESSIVE SCARRING FROM REPEATED INFECTION

3. END PHASE

Progressive scarring

Atrophied parenchyma

2. PROGRESSIVE PHASE

Focal parenchyma scarring

Narrowed calyx neck

1. EARLY PHASE (EDEMATOUS)

Signs and symptoms
◗ Pain over one or both kidneys
◗ Urinary urgency and frequency
◗ Burning during urination
◗ Dysuria
◗ Nocturia
◗ Hematuria (usually microscopic but possibly gross)
◗ Flank pain upon palpation
◗ Cloudy urine with an ammonia-like or fishy odor
◗ Temperature of 102° F (38.9° C) or higher
◗ Chills
◗ Anorexia
◗ General fatigue
◗ Occasional proteinuria

Treatment
◗ Antibiotic therapy appropriate to the specific infecting organism after identification by urine culture and sensitivity studies, such as:
– *Enterococcus* that requires ampicillin (Principen), penicillin G, or vancomycin
– *Staphylococcus* that requires penicillin G or semisynthetic penicillin such as nafcillin, or cephalosporin for resistant bacterium
– *Escherichia coli* that requires sulfisoxazole (Eryzole), nalidixic acid (NegGram), nitrofurantoin (Macrobid), or ciprofloxacin (Cipro)
– *Klebsiella* that requires cephalosporin, gentamicin, or tobramycin
– *Proteus* that requires ampicillin, sulfisoxazole, nalidixic acid, or cephalosporin
– *Pseudomonas* that requires ciprofloxacin (Cipro), gentamicin, tobramycin, or carbenicillin (Geocillin)
◗ Broad-spectrum antibiotic, such as ampicillin or cephalexin (Keflex) (for non-identifiable infecting organism)

Nursing considerations
◗ Administer antipyretics for fever.
◗ Encourage fluids to achieve a urine output of more than 2,000 ml/24 hours. This helps empty the bladder of contaminated urine and prevents calculus formation. Don't encourage intake of more than 2 to 3 qt (2 to 3 L) because this can decrease the effectiveness of the antibiotics.
◗ Provide an acid-ash diet to prevent calculus formation.
◗ Observe sterile technique during catheter insertion and care.
◗ Be sure to refrigerate or culture a urine specimen within 30 minutes of collection to prevent overgrowth of bacteria.

LESSON
PLANS

Teaching about pyelonephritis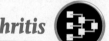

◗ Encourage the patient to urinate frequently to prevent stasis of urine.
◗ Instruct a female patient to avoid bacterial contamination by always wiping the perineum from front to back.
◗ Teach proper technique for collecting a clean-catch urine specimen.
◗ Stress the need to complete the prescribed antibiotic regimen, even after symptoms subside. Encourage long-term follow-up care for a high-risk patient.

◗ Advise routine checkups for a patient with a history of urinary tract infections. Teach him to recognize signs and symptoms of infection, such as cloudy urine, burning on urination, and urinary urgency and frequency, especially when accompanied by a low-grade fever and back pain.

Acute renal failure

About 5% of all hospitalized patients develop acute renal failure, the sudden interruption of renal function resulting from obstruction, reduced circulation, or renal parenchymal disease. This condition is classified as *prerenal*, *intrarenal*, or *postrenal* and normally passes through three distinct phases: *oliguric*, *diuretic*, and *recov-*ery. It may be reversible with medical treatment. If it progresses to end-stage renal disease and dialysis isn't initiated, uremia and death are probable.

The three types of acute renal failure each have separate causes. Prerenal failure results from conditions that diminish blood flow to the kidneys. Between 40% and 80% of all cases of acute renal failure are caused by prerenal azotemia. Intrarenal failure (also called *intrinsic* or *parenchymal renal failure*) results from damage to the kidneys themselves, usually from acute tubular necrosis. Postrenal failure results from bilateral obstruction of urine outflow.

Causes of acute renal failure

Acute renal failure can be classified as prerenal, intrarenal, or postrenal. All conditions that lead to prerenal failure impair renal perfusion, resulting in decreased glomerular filtration rate and increased proximal tubular reabsorption of sodium and water. Intrarenal failure results from damage to the kidneys themselves; postrenal failure results from obstruction of urine flow. Listed here are the possible causes of each type of acute renal failure.

Prerenal failure	Intrarenal failure	Postrenal failure
Cardiovascular disorders	**Acute tubular necrosis**	**Bladder obstruction**
▸ Arrhythmias	▸ Ischemic damage to renal parenchyma from unrecognized or poorly treated prerenal failure	▸ Anticholinergic drugs
▸ Cardiac tamponade		▸ Autonomic nerve dysfunction
▸ Cardiogenic shock		▸ Infection
▸ Heart failure	▸ Nephrotoxins—analgesics (such as phenacetin), anesthetics (such as methoxyflurane), antibiotics (such as gentamicin), heavy metals (such as lead), radiographic contrast media, organic solvents	▸ Tumor
▸ Myocardial infarction		
▸ Pulmonary embolism		**Ureteral obstruction**
		▸ Blood clots
Hypovolemia		▸ Calculi
▸ Burns		▸ Edema or inflammation
▸ Dehydration	▸ Obstetric complications—eclampsia, postpartum renal failure, septic abortion, uterine hemorrhage	▸ Necrotic renal papillae
▸ Diuretic abuse		▸ Retroperitoneal fibrosis or hemorrhage
▸ Hemorrhage		▸ Surgery (accidental ligation)
▸ Hypovolemic shock	▸ Pigment release—crush injury resulting in rhabdomyolysis, myopathy, sepsis, transfusion reaction	▸ Tumor
▸ Liver failure		▸ Uric acid crystals
▸ Trauma		
	Other parenchymal disorders	**Urethral obstruction**
Peripheral vasodilation	▸ Acute glomerulonephritis	▸ Prostatic hyperplasia or tumor
▸ Antihypertensive drugs	▸ Acute interstitial nephritis	▸ Strictures
▸ Sepsis	▸ Acute pyelonephritis	
	▸ Bilateral renal vein thrombosis	
Renovascular obstruction	▸ Malignant nephrosclerosis	
▸ Arterial embolism	▸ Papillary necrosis	
▸ Arterial or venous thrombosis	▸ Periarteritis nodosa	
▸ Tumor	▸ Renal myeloma	
▸ Disseminated intravascular coagulation	▸ Sickle cell disease	
	▸ Systemic lupus erythematosus	
Severe vasoconstriction	▸ Vasculitis	
▸ Eclampsia		
▸ Malignant hypertension		
▸ Vasculitis		

Signs and symptoms

▶ Recent history of fever
▶ Chills
▶ Headache
▶ GI problems, such as anorexia, nausea, vomiting, diarrhea, and constipation
▶ Irritability
▶ Drowsiness
▶ Confusion
▶ Seizures and coma (advanced stages)
▶ Oliguria (less than 500 ml/24 hours) or anuria (less than 100 ml/24 hours)
▶ Petechiae and ecchymoses
▶ Hematemesis
▶ Dry, pruritic skin
▶ Uremic frost (rare)
▶ Dry mucous membranes
▶ Uremic breath odor
▶ Muscle weakness (with hyperkalemia)
▶ Tachycardia
▶ Irregular heart rhythm
▶ Bibasilar crackles and peripheral edema (with heart failure)
▶ Abdominal pain (with pancreatitis or peritonitis)
▶ Edema in lower extremities or facial edema

PICTURING PATHO

Mechanisms of acute renal failure

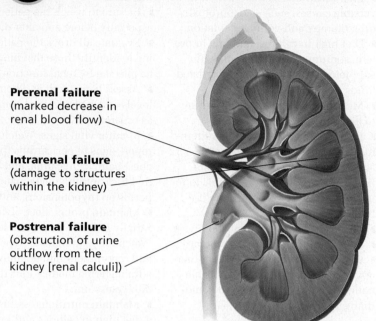

Prerenal failure (marked decrease in renal blood flow)

Intrarenal failure (damage to structures within the kidney)

Postrenal failure (obstruction of urine outflow from the kidney [renal calculi])

Stages of acute renal failure

Before assessing a patient with renal failure, review the stages of the condition and the characteristics as described here.

Stage	Characteristics
Onset (hours to several days)	Begins with the precipitating event, which is usually recognized in retrospect. Nitrogenous waste products (blood urea nitrogen [BUN] and creatinine) begin to accumulate in serum.
Oliguric* (usually 1 to 2 weeks)	Urine output is 100 to 400 ml/24 hours. Serum shows increasing levels of BUN, creatinine, potassium phosphate, and magnesium and decreasing levels of calcium and bicarbonate. Sodium is increased but is diluted by water retention.
Diuretic (2 to 6 weeks)	Kidneys lose ability to concentrate urine; urine is diluted with output of 3,000 to 10,000 ml/24 hours. BUN and creatinine levels begin to decrease. A return to normal BUN and creatinine levels signals the end of this stage. Normal renal tubular function is reestablished unless some residual damage remains.
Recovery (up to 1 year)	Renal function and electrolyte levels return to normal unless irreversible renal damage has occurred.

*Note: Some patients don't experience the oliguric phase of acute renal failure.

Treatment

▶ Maintaining fluid balance, blood volume, and blood pressure during and after surgery
▶ Identification and treatment of reversible causes, such as nephrotoxic drug therapy and volume depletion
▶ Diet high in calories and low in protein, sodium, and potassium, with supplemental vitamins and restricted fluids
▶ Meticulous electrolyte monitoring to detect hyperkalemia
▶ Hypertonic glucose-and-insulin infusions and sodium bicarbonate (I.V.) and sodium polystyrene sulfonate (Kayexalate) by mouth or enema to remove potassium from the body (for hyperkalemia)
▶ Hemodialysis or peritoneal dialysis
▶ Early initiation of diuretic therapy
▶ Continuous renal replacement therapy (for hemodynamically unstable patients or those refractory to hemodialysis or peritoneal dialysis)

Nursing considerations

▶ Measure and record intake and output of all fluids, including wound drainage, nasogastric tube output, and diarrhea.
▶ Be sure to weigh the patient daily especially before and after dialysis.
▶ Evaluate all drugs the patient is taking to identify those that may affect or be affected by renal function.
▶ Assess hematocrit and hemoglobin levels and replace blood components as ordered.
▶ Monitor vital signs. Watch for and report signs of pericarditis (pleuritic chest pain, tachycardia, and pericardial friction rub), inadequate renal perfusion (hypotension), and acidosis.
▶ Maintain proper electrolyte balance. Strictly monitor potassium levels. Watch for symptoms of hyperkalemia and report them immediately. Avoid administering medications that contain potassium.
▶ Maintain nutritional status. Provide a diet high in calories and low in protein, sodium, and potassium, with vitamin supplements.
▶ Monitor the patient for signs and symptoms of developing acidosis, such as decreased level of consciousness, development of cardiac arrhythmias, and changes in the rate and depth of respirations.

▶ Prevent complications of immobility by encouraging frequent coughing and deep breathing and by performing passive range-of-motion exercises.
▶ Provide mouth care frequently to lubricate dry mucous membranes.
▶ Monitor GI bleeding by testing all stools for occult blood.
▶ Provide meticulous perineal care to reduce the risk of ascending urinary tract infection (in women) and to protect skin integrity.
▶ If the patient requires hemodialysis, check the vascular access site (arteriovenous fistula or graft, subclavian or femoral catheter) every 2 hours for patency and signs of clotting. Don't use the arm with the graft or fistula for measuring blood pressure, inserting I.V. lines, or drawing blood.
▶ During hemodialysis, monitor vital signs, clotting times, blood flow, vascular access site function, and arterial and venous pressures.
▶ After hemodialysis, monitor vital signs, check the vascular access site, weigh the patient, and watch for signs of fluid and electrolyte imbalances.
▶ Provide emotional support to the patient and his family.
▶ Administer prescribed medications after hemodialysis is completed. Many medications are removed from the blood during treatment.

LESSON PLANS

Teaching about acute renal failure

▶ Reassure the patient and his family by clearly explaining all diagnostic tests, treatments, and procedures.
▶ Tell the patient about his prescribed medications, and stress the importance of complying with the regimen.
▶ Stress the importance of following the prescribed diet and fluid allowance.
▶ Instruct the patient to weigh himself daily and report changes of 3 lb (1.4 kg) or more immediately.

▶ Advise the patient against overexertion. If he becomes dyspneic or short of breath during normal activity, tell him to report this finding to his physician.
▶ Teach the patient how to recognize edema, and tell him to report this finding to the physician.

Acute tubular necrosis

Acute tubular necrosis (also called *acute tubulointerstitial nephritis*) is the most common cause of acute renal failure in critically ill patients or those who have undergone extensive surgery (accounting for about 75% of all cases). This disorder injures the tubular segment of the nephron, causing renal failure and uremic syndrome.

Acute tubular necrosis results from ischemic necrosis or nephrotoxic injury. In ischemic necrosis, disruption of blood flow to the kidneys may result from circulatory collapse, severe hypotension, trauma, hemorrhage, dehydration, cardiogenic or septic shock, surgery, anesthetics, or transfusion reactions. Nephrotoxic injury may follow ingestion or inhalation of certain chemicals, such as aminoglycoside antibiotics, amphotericin B (Abelcet), and radiographic contrast agents, or it may result from prolonged use of aspirin-containing agents or a hypersensitivity reaction of the kidneys.

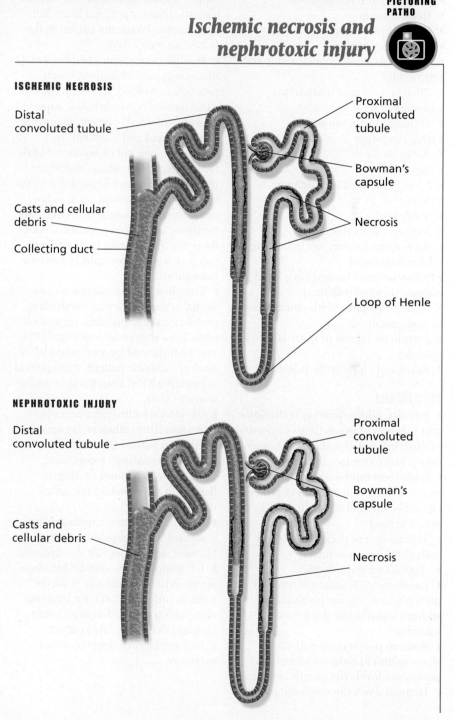

PICTURING PATHO

Ischemic necrosis and nephrotoxic injury

ISCHEMIC NECROSIS

Distal convoluted tubule

Proximal convoluted tubule

Bowman's capsule

Casts and cellular debris

Necrosis

Collecting duct

Loop of Henle

NEPHROTOXIC INJURY

Distal convoluted tubule

Proximal convoluted tubule

Bowman's capsule

Casts and cellular debris

Necrosis

Signs and symptoms

▶ History of an ischemic or a nephrotoxic injury
▶ Oliguria (less than 500 ml/24 hours)
▶ Petechiae and ecchymoses
▶ Hematemesis
▶ Dry and pruritic skin
▶ Uremic frost (rare)
▶ Dry mucous membranes and uremic breath odor
▶ Muscle weakness (with hyperkalemia)
▶ Lethargy and somnolence
▶ Disorientation
▶ Asterixis
▶ Agitation
▶ Myoclonic muscle twitching
▶ Seizures
▶ Tachycardia
▶ Irregular heart rhythm
▶ Pericardial friction rub indicating pericarditis (rare)
▶ Bibasilar crackles and peripheral edema (with heart failure)
▶ Abdominal pain (with pancreatitis or peritonitis)
▶ Peripheral edema (if heart failure is present)
▶ Fever and chills (with infection)

Treatment

▶ Initially, administration of diuretics and infusion of fluids (large amounts) to flush tubules of cellular casts and debris and to replace fluid loss
▶ Long-term fluid management that requires daily replacement of projected and calculated losses (including insensible loss)
▶ Transfusion of packed red blood cells (RBCs) (for anemia)
▶ Antibiotics (for infection)
▶ Emergency I.V. administration of 50% glucose, regular insulin, and sodium bicarbonate (for hyperkalemia)
▶ Sodium polystyrene sulfonate (Kayexalate) to reduce extracellular potassium levels (by mouth or enema)
▶ Hemodialysis (for catabolic patient)

Nursing considerations

▶ Maintain fluid balance and watch for fluid overload, a common complication of therapy. Record intake and output, including wound drainage, nasogastric tube output, and hemodialysis balances. Weigh the patient at the same time every day.
▶ Monitor hemoglobin (Hb) level and hematocrit, and administer blood products as needed. Use fresh packed RBCs instead of whole blood, especially in an elderly patient, to prevent fluid overload and heart failure.
▶ Maintain electrolyte balance. Monitor laboratory test results and report imbalances. Restrict foods that contain sodium and potassium, such as bananas, prunes, orange juice, chocolate, tomatoes, and baked potatoes. Check for potassium content in prescribed medications (for example, potassium penicillin).
▶ Provide adequate calories and essential amino acids while restricting protein intake to maintain an anabolic state. Total parenteral nutrition (TPN) may be indicated for a severely debilitated or catabolic patient. If the patient is receiving TPN, keep his skin meticulously clean.
▶ Use sterile technique, particularly when handling catheters, because the debilitated patient is vulnerable to infection. Immediately report fever, chills, delayed wound healing, or flank pain if the patient has an indwelling catheter.
▶ If anemia worsens, causing pallor, weakness, or lethargy with decreased Hb level, administer RBCs as ordered.
▶ For acidosis, give sodium bicarbonate or assist with dialysis in severe cases as ordered. Watch for hypotension, which diminishes renal perfusion and decreases urine output.
▶ Perform passive range-of-motion exercises.

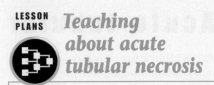

LESSON PLANS
Teaching about acute tubular necrosis

▶ Teach the patient the signs of infection, and tell him to report them to the physician immediately. Remind him to stay away from crowds and any infected person.
▶ Review the prescribed diet, including restrictions, and stress the importance of adhering to it.
▶ Teach the patient how to cough and perform deep breathing to prevent pulmonary complications.
▶ Fully explain each procedure to the patient and his family as often as necessary, and help them set goals that are realistic for the patient's prognosis.

Bladder cancer

Benign or malignant tumors may develop on the bladder wall surface or grow within the wall and quickly invade underlying muscles. About 90% of bladder cancers are transitional cell carcinomas, arising from the transitional epithelium of mucous membranes.

Bladder tumors are most prevalent in people older than age 50, are more common in males than in females, and occur more often in densely populated industrial areas.

Certain environmental carcinogens, such as tobacco, 2-naphthylamine, and nitrates are known to predispose a person to transitional cell tumors. Exposure to these carcinogens places certain industrial workers at higher risk for developing such tumors, including rubber workers, weavers, aniline dye workers, hairdressers, petroleum workers, spray painters, and leather finishers.

Signs and symptoms

▶ Gross, painless, intermittent hematuria (typically with clots)
▶ Suprapubic pain after voiding (suggesting invasive lesions)
▶ Bladder irritability
▶ Urinary frequency
▶ Nocturia
▶ Dribbling
▶ Flank pain (with obstructed ureter)

Looking at a bladder tumor

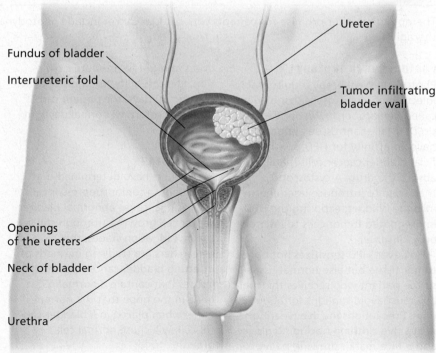

Ureter

Fundus of bladder

Interureteric fold

Tumor infiltrating bladder wall

Openings of the ureters

Neck of bladder

Urethra

Treatment
Superficial bladder tumors
▶ Cystoscopic transurethral resection and fulguration
▶ Intravesical chemotherapy to prevent recurrence (for tumors in many sites)
▶ Intravesical administration of live, attenuated bacille Calmette-Guérin vaccine (for primary and relapsed carcinoma in situ)
▶ Segmental bladder resection to remove a full-thickness section of the bladder (only for tumors not near bladder neck or ureteral orifices)
▶ Bladder instillations of thiotepa after transurethral resection

Infiltrating bladder tumors
▶ Radical cystectomy and urinary diversion (usually an ileal conduit)

Advanced bladder cancer
▶ Cystectomy
▶ Radiation therapy
▶ Combination systemic chemotherapy with cisplatin (Platinol) (most effective)
▶ Doxorubicin (Doxil), cyclophosphamide (Cytoxan), and fluorouracil (may arrest the cancer)

Nursing considerations
▶ Listen to the patient's fears and concerns. Stay with him during periods of severe stress and anxiety, and provide psychological support.
▶ To relieve discomfort, provide ordered pain medications as necessary.
▶ Before surgery, offer information and support when the patient and enterostomal therapist select a stoma site.

▶ After surgery, encourage the patient to look at the stoma.
▶ After ileal conduit surgery, watch for these complications: wound infection, enteric fistulas, urine leaks, ureteral obstruction, bowel obstruction, and pelvic abscesses.
▶ After radical cystectomy and construction of a urine reservoir, watch for these complications: incontinence, difficult catheterization, urine reflux, obstruction, bacteriuria, and electrolyte imbalances.
▶ If the patient is receiving chemotherapy, watch for complications resulting from the particular drug regimen.
▶ If the patient is having radiation therapy, watch for these complications: radiation enteritis, colitis, and skin reactions.

Bladder cancer treatments

Therapies that offer promise for patients with bladder cancer include photodynamic, gene, and immunotoxin therapies.

Photodynamic therapy
Photodynamic therapy requires I.V. injection of a photosensitizing agent called *hematoporphyrin derivative (HPD)*. Malignant tissue appears to have an affinity for HPD, so superficial bladder cancer cells readily absorb the drug. A cystoscope is then used to introduce laser energy into the bladder; exposing the HPD-impregnated tumor cells to laser energy kills them.

However, HPD sensitizes not only tumor tissue but also normal tissue, so the patient who receives this therapy must avoid sunlight for about 30 days. Precautions involve wearing protective clothing (including gloves and a face mask), drawing heavy curtains at home during the day, scheduling outdoor travel for night, and conducting exercises inside or out-

doors at night to promote circulation, joint mobility, and muscle activity. After 30 days, the patient can gradually return to normal daylight activities.

Gene therapy
Researchers have determined that mutations in tumor suppressor cells, such as p53, cause abnormal bladder cancer cell growth. Although still in the investigation stages, the researchers are studying methods of infecting bladder cancer cells with viruses that contain a normal p53 gene in the hope that the normal gene, when placed in a bladder cancer cell, will cause normal cell growth.

Immunotoxin therapy
Although still in investigational stages, researchers have hope that immunotoxin therapy will someday effectively treat bladder cancer. Immunotoxins are laboratory-manufactured antibodies with powerful toxins attached to them that can recognize cancer cells. After an antibody recognizes a cancer cell, it releases the toxin, which enters the cancer cell and kills it.

LESSON PLANS

 Teaching about bladder cancer

▶ Tell the patient what to expect from diagnostic tests. For example, make sure he understands that he may be anesthetized for cystoscopy. After the test results are known, explain the implications to the patient and his family.
▶ Provide complete preoperative teaching. Discuss equipment and procedures that the patient can expect postoperatively. Demonstrate essential coughing and deep-breathing exercises. Encourage the patient to ask questions.

For the patient with a urinary stoma:
▶ Teach the patient how to care for his urinary stoma. Encourage appropriate caregivers to attend the teaching session. Advise them beforehand that a negative reaction to the stoma can impede the patient's adjustment.

▶ If the patient is to wear a urine collection pouch, teach him how to prepare and apply it. First, find out whether he will wear a reusable pouch or a disposable pouch. If he chooses a reusable pouch, he needs at least two to wear alternately.
▶ Instruct the patient to remeasure the stoma after he goes home in case the size changes.
▶ Advise him to make sure the pouch has a push-button or twist-type valve at the bottom to allow for drainage.
▶ Tell him to empty the pouch when it's one-third full, or every 2 to 3 hours.
▶ Offer the patient tips on effective skin seal. Explain that urine tends to destroy skin barriers that contain mostly karaya (a natural skin barrier). Suggest that he select a barrier made of urine-resistant synthetics with little or no karaya. Advise him to check the pouch frequently to ensure that the skin seal remains intact. Tell the patient that the ileal conduit stoma should reach its permanent size about 2 to 4 months after surgery.

▶ Explain that the surgeon constructs the ileal conduit from the intestine, which normally produces mucus. For this reason, the patient will see mucus in the drained urine. Assure him that this finding is normal.
▶ Teach the patient how to keep the skin around the stoma clean and free from irritation. Instruct him to remove the pouch, wash the skin with water and mild soap, and rinse well with clear water to remove soapy residue. Tell him to gently pat the skin dry. Never rub.
▶ Demonstrate how to place a gauze sponge soaked in vinegar water (1 part vinegar to 3 parts water) over the stoma for a few minutes to prevent a buildup of uric acid crystals. When he cares for his skin, suggest that he place a rolled-up dry sponge over the stoma to collect (or wick) draining urine.
▶ Next, instruct him to coat his skin with a silicone skin protectant and then cover with the collection pouch. Advise him to apply hydrocolloid powder to irritated or eroded skin.
▶ Postoperatively, tell the patient with a urinary stoma to avoid heavy lifting and contact sports. Encourage him to participate in his usual athletic and physical activities.
▶ Before discharge, arrange for follow-up home nursing care. Also refer the patient for services provided by the enterostomal therapist.
▶ Provide contact information for the United Ostomy Association or American Cancer Society for additional education and support.

Chronic glomerulonephritis

Chronic glomerulonephritis is a slowly progressive disease characterized by inflammation of the glomeruli, which results in sclerosis, scarring and, eventually, renal failure. This condition normally remains subclinical until the progressive phase begins. By the time it produces symptoms, chronic glomerulonephritis is usually irreversible.

Common causes of chronic glomerulonephritis include primary renal disorders, such as membranoproliferative glomerulonephritis, membranous glomerulopathy, focal segmental glomerulosclerosis, rapidly progressive glomerulonephritis and, less commonly, poststreptococcal glomerulonephritis. Systemic disorders that may cause chronic glomerulonephritis include systemic lupus erythematosus, Goodpasture's syndrome, and hemolytic-uremic syndrome.

PICTURING PATHO

Immune complex deposits on a glomerulus

Endothelial cell swelling

White blood cell

Basement membrane

Subendothelial deposits

Subepithelial deposits

Signs and symptoms
▶ Insidious development without symptoms, typically occurring over many years
▶ Edema and hypertension (with sudden progression)
▶ Foamy urine (proteinuria)
▶ Dark urine
▶ Fatigue
▶ Decreased urination

Late stage
▶ Nausea
▶ Vomiting
▶ Pruritus
▶ Dyspnea
▶ Malaise
▶ Fatigue
▶ Mild to severe edema
▶ Severe hypertension and associated cardiac complications

Treatment
▶ Antihypertensives and a sodium-restricted diet to control hypertension
▶ Correction of fluid and electrolyte imbalances through restrictions and replacement
▶ Loop diuretics, such as furosemide (Lasix), to reduce edema and prevent heart failure
▶ Antibiotics for symptomatic urinary tract infection
▶ Dialysis
▶ Kidney transplantation

Nursing considerations
▶ Monitor vital signs, intake and output, and daily weight to evaluate fluid retention. Observe for signs of fluid, electrolyte, and acid-base imbalances.
▶ Ask the dietitian to help the patient plan low-sodium, high-calorie meals with adequate protein.
▶ Provide skin care to help prevent complications of pruritus, edema, and friability.
▶ Help the patient adjust to his illness by encouraging him to express his feelings and ask questions.
▶ Encourage adequate fluid intake to maintain adequate renal blood flow.

LESSON PLANS

Teaching about chronic glomerulonephritis

▶ Instruct the patient to take prescribed antihypertensives and diuretics as scheduled, even if he feels better. Advise him to take diuretics in the morning so that his sleep won't be disturbed.
▶ Teach the patient the signs of infection, particularly those of urinary tract infection, and warn him to report them immediately. Tell him to avoid contact with people who have communicable illnesses.
▶ Urge compliance with the prescribed diet.
▶ Stress the importance of keeping all follow-up examinations to assess renal function.

Hydronephrosis

Hydronephrosis is an abnormal dilation of the renal pelvis and the calyces of one or both kidneys. It's caused by an obstruction of urine flow in the genitourinary tract. A partial obstruction and hydronephrosis may not produce symptoms initially, but pressure that builds up behind the area of obstruction eventually results in symptoms of renal dysfunction.

The most common causes of hydronephrosis are benign prostatic hyperplasia (BPH), urethral strictures, and calculi. Less common causes include strictures or stenosis of the ureter or bladder outlet; congenital abnormalities; bladder, ureteral, or pelvic tumors; blood clots; and neurogenic bladder.

Signs and symptoms

◗ Dependent upon cause of obstruction, including:
– Mild pain and slightly decreased urine flow
– Severe, colicky renal pain or dull flank pain radiating to the groin
– Gross urinary abnormalities, such as hematuria, pyuria, dysuria, alternating oliguria and polyuria, and anuria
– Nausea
– Vomiting
– Abdominal fullness
– Pain on urination
– Dribbling
– Urinary hesitancy
– Pain on only one side, usually in the flank area, signaling unilateral obstruction

Renal damage in hydronephrosis

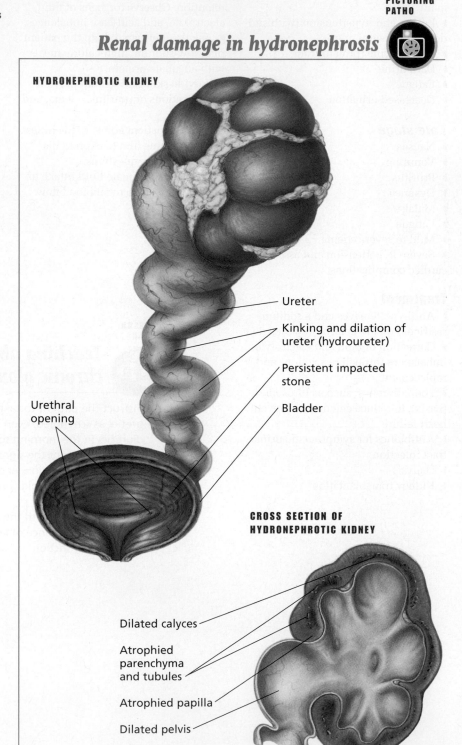

HYDRONEPHROTIC KIDNEY

Ureter

Kinking and dilation of ureter (hydroureter)

Persistent impacted stone

Bladder

Urethral opening

CROSS SECTION OF HYDRONEPHROTIC KIDNEY

Dilated calyces

Atrophied parenchyma and tubules

Atrophied papilla

Dilated pelvis

Treatment

▶ Dilatation (for urethral stricture)
▶ Ureteral stents to maintain patency
▶ Prostatectomy (for BPH)
▶ Diet low in protein, sodium, and potassium to stop renal failure progression before surgery (if renal function has already been affected)
▶ Decompression and drainage of the kidney, using a temporary or permanent nephrostomy tube placed in the renal pelvis (for inoperable obstructions)
▶ Antibiotic therapy (for concurrent infection)

Understanding postobstructive diuresis

Polyuria—urine output that exceeds 2,000 ml in 8 hours—and excessive electrolyte losses characterize postobstructive diuresis. Although usually self-limiting, this condition can cause vascular collapse, shock, and death if not treated with fluid and electrolyte replacement.

Prolonged pressure of retained urine damages renal tubules, limiting their ability to concentrate urine. Removing the obstruction relieves the pressure, but tubular function may not significantly improve for days or weeks, depending on the patient's condition.

Although diuresis typically abates in a few days, it persists if serum creatinine levels remain high. When these levels approach the normal range (0.7 to 1.4 mg/dl), diuresis usually subsides.

Nursing considerations

▶ Administer prescribed pain medication as needed and evaluate response.
▶ Monitor renal function studies daily, including blood urea nitrogen, serum creatinine, and serum potassium levels. Specific gravity tests can be done at the bedside.
▶ Postoperatively, closely monitor intake and output, vital signs, and fluid and electrolyte status. Watch for a rising pulse rate and cold, clammy skin, which can indicate impending hemorrhage and shock.
▶ Keep in mind that postobstructive diuresis may cause the patient to lose great volumes of dilute urine over hours or days. If this occurs, administer I.V. fluids at a constant rate, as ordered, plus an amount of I.V. fluid equal to a percentage of hourly urine output to safely replace intravascular volume.
▶ If a nephrostomy tube was inserted, frequently check it for bleeding and patency. Irrigate the tube only as ordered and don't clamp it. Provide meticulous skin care to the area surrounding the tube; if urine leaks, provide a protective skin barrier to decrease excoriation. Observe for signs of infection.

LESSON PLANS

Teaching about hydronephrosis

▶ Explain hydronephrosis to the patient and his family. Also explain the purpose of diagnostic tests and how they're performed.
▶ If the patient is scheduled for surgery, explain the procedure and postoperative care.
▶ If the patient is to be discharged with a nephrostomy tube in place, teach him how to care for it, including how to thoroughly clean the skin around the insertion site.

▶ If the patient must take antibiotics after discharge, tell him to take all of the prescribed medication even if he feels better.
▶ To prevent the progression of hydronephrosis to irreversible renal disease, urge the patient (especially a patient with a family history of benign prostatic hyperplasia or prostatitis) to have routine medical checkups. Teach him to recognize and report symptoms of hydronephrosis, such as colicky pain or hematuria, or urinary tract infection.

Polycystic kidney disease

Polycystic kidney disease is an inherited disorder characterized by multiple, bilateral, grapelike clusters of fluid-filled cysts that enlarge the kidneys, compressing and eventually replacing functioning renal tissue. The disease affects males and females equally and appears in two distinct forms: Autosomal recessive polycystic kidney disease (ARPKD), which affects infants, and autosomal dominant polycystic kidney disease (ADPKD), which affects adults. The adult form has an insidious onset but usually becomes obvious between ages 30 and 50; rarely, it may not cause symptoms until the patient is in his 70s. Renal deterioration is more gradual in the adult form than in the infantile form, but in both groups the disease progresses relentlessly to fatal uremia.

The prognosis in adults varies widely. Progression may be slow, even after symptoms of renal insufficiency appear. When uremic symptoms develop, polycystic disease usually is fatal within 4 years unless the patient receives dialysis or kidney transplantation.

Signs and symptoms

ADPKD:
▶ Asymptomatic until between ages 30 and 50 (common)
▶ Polyuria, polydipsia
▶ Gross hematuria
▶ Renal colic
▶ Urinary tract infection (UTI)
▶ Hypertension
▶ Lumbar pain
▶ Widening girth
▶ Abdominal swelling, tenderness, and pain (worsened by exertion and relieved by lying down)
▶ Grossly enlarged kidneys (advanced stages)

ARPKD:
▶ Large, palpable flank masses
▶ Abnormal extremities
▶ Abdominal distention

PICTURING PATHO

Recognizing a polycystic kidney

CROSS SECTION

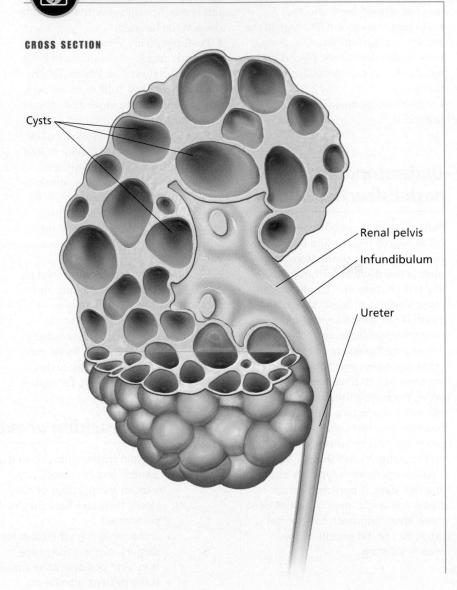

Cysts

Renal pelvis

Infundibulum

Ureter

▶ Polyuria, polydipsia
▶ Potter Facies: Flattened nose, recessed chin, low-set ears, prominent epicanthal folds

Treatment

▶ No cure, necessitating preservation of renal parenchyma and prevention of pyelonephritis
▶ Dialysis or, kidney transplantation (for progressive renal failure)
▶ Urine cultures and creatinine clearance tests every 6 months (for asymptomatic stage)
▶ Antibiotics (for infection even if asymptomatic)
▶ Surgical drainage (for cystic abscess, retroperitoneal bleeding, or intractable pain)
▶ Antihypertensives
▶ Nephrectomy and diuretics (for neonates)
▶ Iron and erythropoietin (for anemia)

Nursing considerations

▶ Provide supportive care to minimize any associated symptoms.
▶ Encourage the patient to rest, and help with activities of daily living when he has abdominal pain. Offer analgesics as needed.
▶ Administer antibiotics, as ordered, for UTI. Provide adequate hydration during antibiotic therapy.
▶ Screen urine for blood, cloudiness, and calculi or granules. Report any of these findings immediately.
▶ Monitor intake and output and daily weight to detect fluid imbalance.
▶ Before beginning excretory urography and other procedures that use an iodine-based contrast medium, ask the patient if he has ever had an allergic reaction to iodine or shellfish. Even if he says no, watch for a possible allergic reaction after the procedures.
▶ If the patient requires peritoneal dialysis, position him carefully, elevating the head of the bed to reduce pressure on the diaphragm and aid in respiration. Be alert for signs of infection, such as cloudy drainage, elevated temperature and, rarely, bleeding. If pain occurs, reduce the amount of dialysate. Periodically monitor the diabetic patient's blood glucose levels, and administer insulin as ordered. Watch for complications, such as peri-

tonitis, atelectasis, hypokalemia, pneumonia, and shock.
▶ If the patient requires hemodialysis, check the vascular access site (arteriovenous fistula or graft or subclavian or femoral catheter) every 4 hours for patency and signs of clotting. Don't use the arm with the graft or fistula for measuring blood pressure, inserting I.V. access devices, or drawing blood. Weigh the patient before and after dialysis.
▶ During hemodialysis, monitor vital signs, blood flow, vascular access site function, and arterial and venous pressures. Watch for complications, such as hypotension, air embolism, and rapid fluid and electrolyte losses.
▶ Provide adequate nutrition. Administer tube feedings and supplements to optimize nutritional intake.

LESSON PLANS

Teaching about polycystic kidney disease

▶ Discuss the patient's prognosis, including possible treatments, such as dialysis or transplantation. Answer all questions.
▶ Explain all diagnostic procedures to the patient or his family if he's an infant.
▶ Discuss prescribed medications and their possible adverse effects. Stress the need to take medications exactly as prescribed, even if symptoms are minimal or absent.
▶ Refer the young adult patient or the parents of an infant with polycystic kidney disease for genetic counseling. Parents usually have questions about the risk to other offspring.
▶ Review nutritional needs. Refer the patient to a nutritionist as indicated.

Renal calculi

Renal calculi can form anywhere in the urinary tract, but they most commonly develop in the renal pelvis or calices. Calculi form when substances that normally are dissolved in the urine (such as calcium oxalate, calcium phosphate, uric acid, cystine, and magnesium ammonium phosphate) precipitate. Renal calculi vary in size and may be solitary or multiple.

Annually, about 1 in 1,000 U.S. residents require hospitalization for renal calculi. They're more common in men than in women.

Types of renal calculi

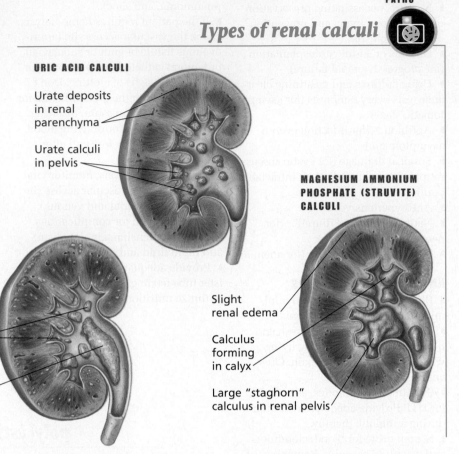

URIC ACID CALCULI

Urate deposits in renal parenchyma

Urate calculi in pelvis

MAGNESIUM AMMONIUM PHOSPHATE (STRUVITE) CALCULI

Slight renal edema

Calculus forming in calyx

Large "staghorn" calculus in renal pelvis

CALCIUM CALCULI

Small calcium calculi

Large calcium calculus

Causes of renal calculi

The exact cause of renal calculi is unknown, but predisposing factors include:

Dehydration
Decreased water excretion concentrates calculus-forming substances.

Infection
Infected, scarred tissue may be a site for calculus development. In addition, infected calculi (usually magnesium ammonium phosphate or staghorn calculi) may develop if bacteria serve as the nucleus in calculus formation. Struvite calculus formation commonly results from *Proteus* infections, which may lead to destruction of renal parenchyma.

Urine pH changes
Consistently acidic or alkaline urine may provide a favorable medium for calculus formation, especially for magnesium ammonium phosphate or calcium phosphate calculi.

Obstruction
Urinary stasis allows calculi constituents to collect and adhere, forming calculi. Obstruction also encourages infection, which compounds the obstruction.

Immobilization
Immobility from spinal cord injury or other disorders allows calcium to be released into the circulation and, eventually, to be filtered by the kidneys.

Metabolic factors
Hyperparathyroidism, renal tubular acidosis, elevated uric acid (usually with gout), defective metabolism of oxalate, a genetically caused defect in metabolism of cystine, and excessive intake of vitamin D or dietary calcium may predispose a person to renal calculi.

Other factors
Other possible causes of renal calculi include multiple myeloma, Paget's disease, bone cancer, Cushing's disease or syndrome (loss of bone calcium), and milk-alkali syndrome.

Signs and symptoms
◗ Severe pain that travels from the costovertebral angle, to the flank, to the upper outer quadrant of the abdomen on the affected side, and then to the suprapubic region and external genitalia (classic renal colic)
◗ Pain intensity that fluctuates and may be excruciating at its peak
◗ Constant, dull pain (in the renal pelvis and calices)
◗ Nausea
◗ Vomiting
◗ Fever and chills
◗ Hematuria
◗ Abdominal distention

Treatment
◗ Vigorous hydration (more than 3 qt [3 L]/24 hours) to encourage natural passage of small calculi
◗ Antimicrobial agents (for infection, varying with the cultured organism)
◗ Nonsteroidal anti-inflammatory drugs such as ketorolac (proven effective for renal coli pain)
◗ Analgesics, such as morphine (for pain)
◗ Diuretics to prevent urinary stasis and further calculus formation (thiazides decrease calcium excretion into the urine)
◗ Methenamine mandelate to suppress calculus formation (for infection)
◗ Diet of adequate calcium intake, commonly combined with oxalate-binding cholestyramine (for absorptive hypercalciuria)
◗ Parathyroidectomy (for hyperparathyroidism)
◗ Allopurinol (Alloprim) (for uric acid calculi)
◗ Daily oral doses of ascorbic acid to acidify urine
◗ Percutaneous ultrasonic lithotripsy and extracorporeal shock-wave lithotripsy (for calculi too large for natural passage)
◗ Ureteroscopy (for stones of 1 to 2 cm)
◗ Stents to maintain patency of the ureters and to facilitate urine passage

Nursing considerations
◗ To aid diagnosis, maintain a 24- to 48-hour record of urine pH using Nitrazine pH paper. Strain all urine through gauze or a tea strainer, and save all solid material recovered for analysis.
◗ To facilitate spontaneous passage of calculi, encourage the patient to walk, if possible. Also encourage fluids to maintain a urine output of 3,000 to 4,000 ml/24 hours. (Urine should be very dilute and colorless.)
◗ If the patient can't drink the required amount of fluid, give supplemental I.V. fluids.
◗ Record intake and output and daily weight to assess fluid status and renal function.
◗ Medicate for pain and evaluate response.
◗ If the patient had calculi surgically removed, he probably has an indwelling catheter or a nephrostomy tube. Unless one of his kidneys was removed, expect bloody drainage from the catheter. Immediately report excessive drainage or a rising pulse rate, symptoms of hemorrhage. Use sterile technique when changing dressings or providing catheter care.
◗ Watch for signs of infection, such as a rising fever or chills, and give antibiotics as ordered.

LESSON PLANS

 Teaching about renal calculi

◗ Encourage increased fluid intake. If appropriate, show the patient how to check his urine pH, and instruct him to keep a daily record. Tell him to immediately report symptoms of acute obstruction, such as pain or an inability to void.
◗ Urge the patient to follow a prescribed diet and comply with drug therapy to prevent recurrence of calculi. For example, if a hyperuricemic condition caused the patient's calculi, teach him which foods are high in purine (organ meats, cream). For calcium oxalate calculi, teach him to avoid foods high in oxalates (such as spinach, swiss chard, chocolate, peanuts, and pecans).
◗ If surgery is necessary, supplement and reinforce the physician's teaching. The patient is apt to be fearful, especially if he requires kidney removal, so emphasize that the body can adapt well to one kidney. If he's having an abdominal or flank incision, teach deep-breathing and coughing exercises.
◗ Explain how to strain urine and the importance of retaining any stones to submit for chemical analysis.

Renal cancer

About 85% of renal cancers—also called *nephrocarcinoma, renal carcinoma, hypernephroma,* and *Grawitz's tumor*—originate in the kidneys. Others are metastasis from various primary-site carcinomas.

Most renal tumors are large, firm, nodular, encapsulated, unilateral, and solitary. They may affect either kidney; occasionally they're bilateral or multifocal.

Renal cancer can be separated histologically into clear-cell, granular-cell, and spindle-cell types. Sometimes the prognosis is considered better for the clear-cell type than for the other types; in general, however, the prognosis depends more on the cancer's stage than on its type.

Although the cause of renal cancer is unknown, some studies implicate particular factors, including heavy cigarette smoking. Patients who receive chronic hemodialysis may also be at increased risk.

Signs and symptoms
▶ Hematuria
▶ Dull, aching flank pain
▶ Weight loss (uncommon)
▶ Smooth, firm, nontender abdominal mass

Treatment
▶ Open radical nephrectomy, with or without regional lymph node dissection, or laparoscopic radical nephrectomy
▶ Radiation (for cancer that has spread into the perinephric region or lymph nodes or when the primary tumor or metastatic sites can't be completely excised)
▶ Chemotherapy
▶ Biotherapy with lymphokine-activated killer cells plus recombinant interleukin-2 (can be expensive and causes many adverse reactions)
▶ Interferon and hormone therapy, such as medroxyprogesterone (Depo-Provera) and testosterone (Androderm) (for advanced disease)

Nursing considerations
▶ Before surgery, assure the patient that his body will adequately adapt to the loss of a kidney.
▶ Administer prescribed analgesics as necessary. Provide comfort measures, such as positioning and distractions, to help the patient cope with discomfort.
▶ After surgery, encourage diaphragmatic breathing and coughing.
▶ Assist the patient with leg exercises, and turn him every 2 hours to reduce the risk of phlebitis.
▶ Check dressings often for excessive bleeding. Watch for signs of internal bleeding, such as restlessness, sweating, and increased pulse rate.
▶ Position the patient on the operative side to allow the pressure of adjacent organs to fill the dead space at the operative site, improving dependent drainage.
▶ If possible, assist the patient with walking within 24 hours of surgery.
▶ Provide adequate fluid intake, and monitor intake and output.

Two forms of renal cancer

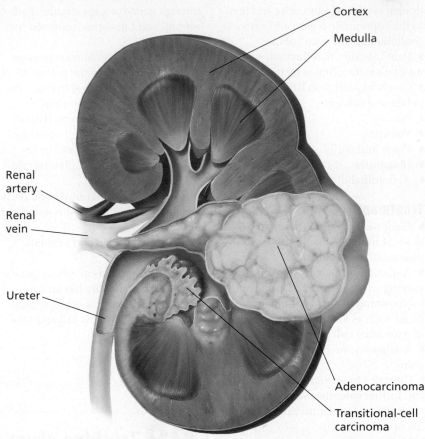

Cortex

Medulla

Renal artery

Renal vein

Ureter

Adenocarcinoma

Transitional-cell carcinoma

▶ Monitor laboratory test results for anemia, polycythemia, and abnormal blood chemistry values that may point to bone or hepatic involvement or may result from radiation therapy or chemotherapy.
▶ Provide symptomatic treatment for adverse effects of chemotherapeutic drugs.
▶ Encourage the patient to express his anxieties and fears, and remain with him during periods of severe stress and anxiety.

Teaching about renal cancer

▶ Tell the patient what to expect from surgery and other treatments.
▶ Before surgery, teach diaphragmatic breathing and effective coughing techniques such as how to splint the incision.
▶ Explain the possible adverse effects of radiation and drug therapy. Advise the patient how to prevent and minimize these problems.

▶ When preparing the patient for discharge, stress the importance of compliance with the prescribed outpatient treatment. This includes an annual follow-up chest X-ray to rule out lung metastasis and excretory urography every 6 to 12 months to check for contralateral tumors.
▶ If appropriate, refer the patient and his family to cancer support groups and hospice care.

Renovascular hypertension

Renovascular hypertension occurs when systemic blood pressure increases because of stenosis of the major renal arteries or their branches, or because of intrarenal atherosclerosis. This narrowing (stenosis) may be partial or complete, and the resulting blood pressure elevation may be benign or malignant. Critical renal artery stenosis is defined as at least a 70% narrowing of the renal artery. About 5% to 15% of patients have high blood pressure related to renal artery stenosis.

In about 95% of patients, renovascular hypertension results from either atherosclerosis (especially in older men) or fibromuscular diseases of the renal artery wall layers (for example, medial fibroplasia and, less commonly, intimal and subadventitial fibroplasia). Other causes include arteritis, anomalies of the renal arteries, embolism, trauma, tumor, and renal artery aneurysm or dissection.

Renal artery stenosis stimulates the affected kidney to release renin, an enzyme that converts angiotensinogen (a plasma protein) to angiotensin I. As angiotensin I circulates through the lungs and liver, it converts to angiotensin II, which causes peripheral vasoconstriction, increased arterial pressure and aldosterone secretion and, eventually, hypertension.

PICTURING PATHO

What happens in renovascular hypertension

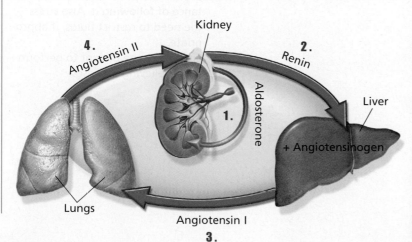

MECHANISM OF RENOVASCULAR HYPERTENSION

1. Renal artery stenosis causes reduction of blood flow to the kidneys.

2. Kidneys secrete renin in response.

3. Renin combines with angiotensinogen in the liver to form angiotensin I.

4. In the lungs, angiotensin I is converted to angiotensin II, a potent vasoconstrictor.

Signs and symptoms
▶ Elevated blood pressure
▶ Reduced urine output
▶ Heart failure
▶ Systolic bruit over the renal artery in upper abdomen
▶ Headache
▶ Nausea
▶ Anorexia
▶ Fatigue
▶ Palpitations
▶ Tachycardia
▶ Anxiety
▶ Hypertension
▶ Alterations in level of consciousness (with renal failure)
▶ Bibasilar crackles

Treatment
▶ Angioplasty with renal artery stenting to maintain adequate blood flow to the kidney (except complete occlusion)
▶ Renal artery bypass, endarterectomy, and arterioplasty
▶ Antihypertensives and ACE inhibitors
▶ Diuretics
▶ Sodium-restricted diet

Nursing considerations
▶ Accurately monitor and record intake and output and daily weight. Weigh the patient at the same time each day (before a meal) and with the same amount of clothing.
▶ Frequently assess urine specific gravity, blood urea nitrogen, serum creatinine, and protein levels.
▶ Check blood pressure in both arms regularly, with the patient lying down and standing. A decrease of 20 mm Hg or more in either systolic or diastolic pressure on arising may necessitate a dosage adjustment in antihypertensive medications.
▶ Administer drugs as ordered.
▶ Maintain fluid and sodium restrictions.
▶ If the patient is anorexic, offer appetizing, high-calorie meals to ensure adequate nutrition.
▶ Provide postoperative care. Watch for bleeding and hypotension. Monitor vital signs and report hypotension, which can precipitate acute renal failure.

LESSON PLANS

Teaching about renovascular hypertension

▶ Help the patient and his family understand the disorder, and emphasize the importance of following the prescribed treatment regimen.
▶ Describe the purpose of diagnostic tests, and explain each procedure. If the patient is scheduled for surgery, explain the procedure and postoperative care.
▶ Familiarize the patient with his medications, and encourage him to take them as ordered. Suggest taking diuretics in the morning so that sleep patterns aren't disturbed.
▶ Suggest regular blood pressure screenings.
▶ Explain the purpose of a low-sodium diet, and stress the importance of following it. Also stress the need to restrict fluids, if appropriate.
▶ Encourage the patient to perform stress-relieving exercises.

TESTS
Laboratory tests

BLOOD UREA NITROGEN

Urea, the chief end product of protein metabolism, constitutes 40% to 50% of the blood's nonprotein nitrogen. It's formed from ammonia in the liver, filtered by the glomeruli, reabsorbed (to a limited degree) in the tubules, and finally excreted. Insufficient urea excretion elevates the blood urea nitrogen (BUN) level.

For the most accurate interpretation of test results, examine BUN levels in conjunction with serum creatinine levels and in light of the patient's underlying condition.

CREATININE CLEARANCE

The creatinine clearance test, commonly used to assess the glomerular filtration rate, determines how efficiently the kidneys clear creatinine from blood. Normal values depend on the patient's age.

SERUM CREATININE

Creatinine, another nitrogenous waste, results from muscle metabolism of creatine. Diet and fluid intake don't alter serum creatinine levels.

The serum creatinine test measures renal damage more reliably than BUN level measurements because severe, persistent renal impairment is virtually the only reason that creatinine levels rise significantly. Creatinine levels greater than 1.5 mg/dl indicate 66% or greater loss of renal function; levels greater than 2 mg/dl indicate renal insufficiency.

URINALYSIS

Urinalysis evaluates the physical characteristics of urine; determines specific gravity and pH; detects and measures protein, glucose, and ketone bodies; and examines sediment for blood cells, casts, and crystals. Test types include visual examination, reagent strip screening, refractometry for specific gravity, and microscopic inspection of centrifuged sediment.

URINE CULTURE

Urine culture evaluates urinary tract infection (UTI) and bladder infection. It identifies pathogenic fungi such as *Coccidioides immitis*. A quick urine screen determines if urine contains high bacteria or white blood cell (WBC) counts and processes only urine with bacteria or WBCs. To distinguish true bacteriuria from contamination, it's necessary to know the number of organisms in a milliliter of urine, estimated by a culture technique known as a *colony count;* an additional quick centrifugation test determines where a UTI originates.

Radiologic and imaging studies

CYSTOMETRY

In cystometry, sterile water or carbon dioxide is used to evaluate intravesical pressure, sensation, and capacity in response to filling.

CYSTOSCOPY

In cystoscopy, the physician visualizes the urethral orifice, the ureters, and the inside of the bladder with a fiberoptic scope to diagnose and sometimes treat a urologic disorder.

EXCRETORY UROGRAPHY

In excretory urography, X-rays and a contrast medium are used to visualize the renal parenchyma, renal pelves, ureters, and bladder.

NEPHROTOMOGRAPHY

After I.V. injection of a contrast medium, nephrotomography is used to visualize the renal parenchyma, calices, and pelves in layers.

RENAL ANGIOGRAPHY

Renal angiography involves the injection of a contrast medium into a catheter in the femoral artery or vein, allowing the visualization of the arterial tree, capillaries, and venous drainage of the kidneys.

RENAL SCAN

A renal scan exhibits renal function by showing the appearance and disappearance of radioisotopes within the kidneys.

RENAL DUPLEX SCAN

Renal duplex scan uses high-frequency sound waves and Doppler to image the kidneys and vasculature. It can determine the speed, direction, and patterns of blood flow and identify stenoses or occlusions.

RENAL ULTRASONOGRAPHY

Renal ultrasonography is a safe, painless procedure that allows visualization of the renal parenchyma, calices,

pelves, ureters, and bladder. Because this test doesn't depend on renal function, it's useful in patients with renal failure and in detecting complications after kidney transplantation.

RENAL X-RAYS

A plain film of the abdomen discloses the size, shape, and position of the kidneys, ureters, and bladder and possible areas of calcification.

VIDEOURODYNAMIC STUDIES

A videourodynamic study is a combination of fluoroscopy and complex cystometry. It's used to document voiding dysfunction.

VOIDING CYSTOURETHROGRAPHY

In voiding cystourethrography, X-rays and a contrast medium are used to determine the size and shape of the bladder and urethra.

Other tests

PERCUTANEOUS RENAL BIOPSY

During renal biopsy, a specimen is obtained to develop a histologic diagnosis and determine therapy and the prognosis.

HANDS ON

Assisting with a percutaneous renal biopsy

To prepare a patient for a percutaneous renal biopsy, position him on his abdomen. To stabilize his kidneys, place a sandbag beneath his abdomen as shown.

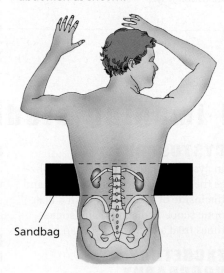

Sandbag

After administering a local anesthetic, the physician instructs the patient to hold his breath and remain immobile. Then the physician inserts a needle with the obturator between the patient's last rib and the iliac crest as shown below. After asking the patient to breathe deeply, the physician removes the obturator and inserts cutting prongs, which gather blood and tissue samples. This test is commonly performed in the radiology department so that special radiographic procedures may be used to help guide the needle.

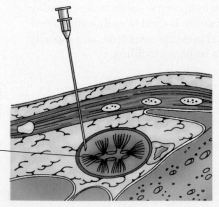

Kidney

TREATMENTS AND PROCEDURES
Drug therapy

Ideally, drug therapy should be effective and not impair renal function. However, because renal disorders alter the chemical composition of body fluids and the pharmacokinetic properties of many drugs, standard regimens of some drugs may require adjustment. For instance, dosages of drugs that are excreted by the kidneys unchanged or as active metabolites may require adjustment to avoid nephrotoxicity. In renal failure, potentially toxic drugs should be used cautiously and sparingly.

Drug therapy for renal and urologic disorders include analgesics, antibiotics, antispasmodics, and diuretics.

ANALGESICS
▶ Used to relieve pain, burning, urgency, and frequency resulting from irritation of the lower urinary tract
▶ Example: phenazopyridine (Pyridium, Urogesic)

ANTIBIOTICS
▶ Used to treat acute and chronic urinary tract infections
▶ Examples: quinolones, such as ciprofloxacin (Cipro) and ofloxacin (Floxin); penicillins, such as amoxicillin (Amoxil); cephalosporins, such as cefadroxil (Duricef) and cefixime (Suprax)

ANTISPASMODICS
▶ Decrease bladder spasm and promote complete bladder emptying
▶ Example: hyoscyamine (Anaspaz, Cystospaz-M)

DIURETICS
Loop diuretics
▶ Inhibit sodium and chloride reabsorption from the loop of Henle and the distal tubule
▶ Used to treat edema associated with renal disease and heart failure
▶ Examples: bumetanide (Bumex), ethacrynic acid (Edecrin), and furosemide (Lasix)

Osmotic diuretics
▶ Increase osmotic pressure of the glomerular filtrate, inhibiting reabsorption of water and electrolytes
▶ Used to treat cerebral edema and renal failure and to promote urinary excretion of toxic substances (mannitol [Osmitrol])
▶ Examples: mannitol, isosorbide (Ismotic), and urea (Ureaphil)

Potassium-sparing diuretics
▶ Act in the distal tubule to cause excretion of sodium, bicarbonate, and calcium, but conserve potassium excretion
▶ Used to enhance the effects of loop or thiazide diuretics or to conserve potassium
▶ Examples: amiloride (Midamor), spironolactone (Aldactone), and triamterene (Dyrenium)

Thiazide and thiazide-like diuretics
▶ Increase water excretion by either increasing the glomerular filtration rate or decreasing or inhibiting sodium reabsorption from the tubules
▶ Used to treat hypertension, edema, and heart failure
▶ Examples: chlorothiazide (Diuril), chlorthalidone (Hygroton)

Dialysis

CONTINUOUS RENAL REPLACEMENT THERAPY

Continuous renal replacement therapy (CRRT) is used to treat patients with acute renal failure. Unlike the more traditional intermittent hemodialysis (IHD), CRRT is administered around the clock, providing patients with continuous therapy and sparing them the destabilizing hemodynamic and electrolyte changes characteristic of IHD. It's used for patients, such as those who have hypotension, who can't tolerate traditional hemodialysis. For such patients, CRRT is usually the only choice of treatment; however, it can also be used in those who can tolerate IHD. CRRT methods vary in complexity and include:
▶ In continuous venovenous hemodialysis, a double-lumen catheter provides access to a vein, and a pump moves blood through the hemofilter.
▶ Continuous venovenous hemodiafiltration provides simultaneous use of dialysate and replacement fluids and removes smaller substances.

HEMODIALYSIS

Hemodialysis removes toxic wastes and other impurities from the blood of a patient with renal failure. In this technique, blood is removed through a surgically created access site, pumped through a dialyzing unit to remove toxins, and then returned to the body. The extracorporeal dialyzer works through a combination of osmosis, diffusion, and filtration. By extracting byproducts of protein metabolism—notably urea and uric acid—as well as creatinine and excess water, hemodialysis helps restore or maintain acid-base and electrolyte balance and prevent the complications associated with uremia.

CVVHD setup

During continuous venovenous hemodialysis (CVVHD), a pump pulls blood from the patient to the arterial line. A hemofilter removes water and toxic solutes (ultrafiltrate) from the blood. Filter replacement fluid is infused into a port on the arterial side; this same port can be used to infuse heparin. The venous line carries the replacement fluid, along with purified blood, to the patient. This illustration shows one of several CVVHD setups.

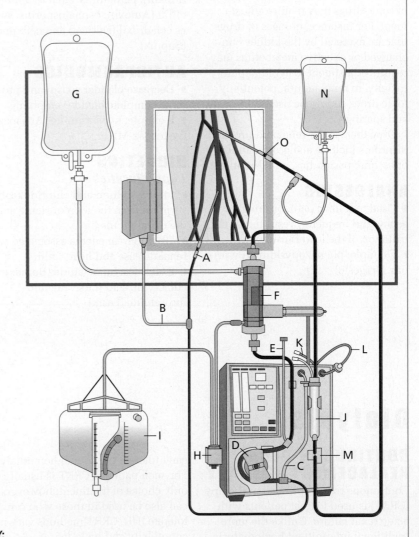

KEY:

A. Blood exiting the body
B. Heparin infusion
C. Arterial pressure monitor (prefilter pressure)
D. Blood pump
E. Saline infusion line (saline not shown here)
F. Filter
G. Dialysate

H. Blood leak detector
I. Graduated collection device
J. Air and foam detector
K. Syringe line
L. Venous pressure monitor (postfilter pressure)
M. Clamp
N. Replacement fluid
O. Blood returns to body

Hemodialysis access sites

Hemodialysis requires vascular access. The site and type of access may vary, depending on the expected duration of dialysis, the surgeon's preference, and the patient's condition.

Subclavian vein catheterization

This is a double-lumen, cuffed hemodialysis catheter used for acute hemodialysis. The blood is pumped from the patient to the dialyzer using the lumen with the red adapter and from the dialyzer to the patient using the lumen with the blue adapter.

Arteriovenous fistula

To create a fistula, the surgeon makes an incision into the patient's wrist or lower forearm, then a small incision in the side of an artery, and another in the side of a vein. He sutures the edges of the incisions together to make a common opening 3 to 7 mm long.

Arteriovenous graft

To create a graft, the surgeon makes an incision in the patient's forearm, upper arm, or thigh. He then tunnels a natural or synthetic graft under the skin and sutures the distal end to an artery and the proximal end to a vein.

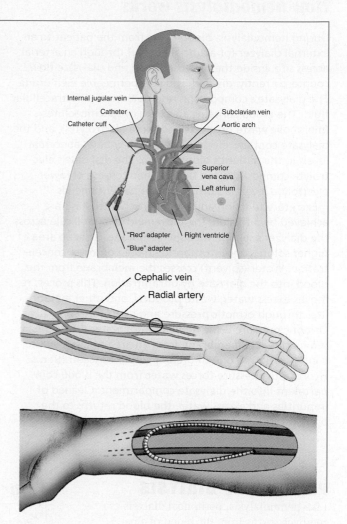

How hemodialysis works

During hemodialysis, blood flows from the patient to an external dialyzer (or artificial kidney) through an arterial access site. Inside the dialyzer, blood and dialysate flow countercurrently, divided by a semipermeable membrane. The dialysate's composition resembles normal extracellular fluid. The blood contains an excess of specific solutes (metabolic waste products and some electrolytes), and the dialysate contains electrolytes that may be at abnormal levels in the patient's bloodstream. The dialysate's electrolyte composition can be modified to raise or lower electrolyte levels, according to the patient's needs.

Excretory function and electrolyte homeostasis are achieved by diffusion, the movement of a molecule across the dialyzer's semipermeable membrane, from an area of higher solute concentration to an area of lower concentration. Water (solvent) crosses the membrane from the blood into the dialysate by ultrafiltration. This process removes excess water, waste products, and other metabolites through osmotic pressure and hydrostatic pressure. Osmotic pressure is the movement of water across the semipermeable membrane from an area of lesser solute concentration to one of greater solute concentration. Hydrostatic pressure forces water from the blood compartment into the dialysate compartment. Cleaned of impurities and excess water, the blood returns to the body through a venous site.

Types of dialyzers

There are three types of dialyzers: the hollow-fiber, the flat-plate or parallel flow-plate, and the coil.

The **hollow-fiber dialyzer**, the most commonly used dialyzer, contains fine capillaries, with a semipermeable membrane enclosed in a plastic cylinder. Blood flows through these capillaries as the system pumps dialysate in the opposite direction on the outside of the capillaries.

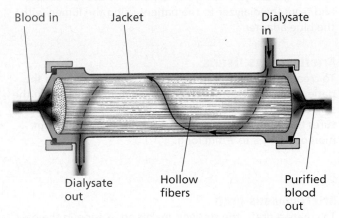

Blood in   Jacket   Dialysate in

Dialysate out   Hollow fibers   Purified blood out

PERITONEAL DIALYSIS

Like hemodialysis, peritoneal dialysis removes toxins from the blood of a patient with acute or chronic renal failure that doesn't respond to other treatments. Unlike hemodialysis, it uses the patient's peritoneal membrane as a semipermeable dialyzing membrane. With this technique, a hypertonic dialyzing solution (dialysate) is instilled through a catheter inserted into the peritoneal cavity. Then by diffusion, excess concentrations of electrolytes and uremic toxins in the blood move across the peritoneal membrane into the dialysis solution. Next, through osmosis, excess water in the blood does the same. After appropriate dwelling time, the dialysate is drained, taking toxins and wastes with it.

Principles of peritoneal dialysis

Peritoneal dialysis works through a combination of diffusion and osmosis.

Diffusion

In diffusion, particles move through a semipermeable membrane from an area of high-solute concentration to an area of low-solute concentration.

In peritoneal dialysis, the water-based dialysate being infused contains glucose, sodium chloride, calcium, magnesium, acetate or lactate, and no waste products. Therefore, the waste products and excess electrolytes in the blood cross through the semipermeable peritoneal membrane into the dialysate. Removing the waste-filled dialysate and replacing it with fresh solution keeps the waste concentration low and encourages further diffusion.

The **flat-plate or parallel flow-plate dialyzer** isn't widely used but has two or more layers of semipermeable membranes, bound by a semirigid or rigid structure. Blood ports are located at both ends, between the membranes. Blood flows between the membranes, and dialysate flows in the opposite direction along the outside of the membranes.

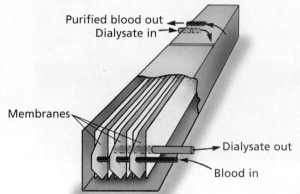

Purified blood out
Dialysate in

Membranes

Dialysate out

Blood in

The **coil dialyzer** (no longer widely used) consists of one or more semipermeable membrane tubes supported by mesh and wrapped concentrically around a central core. Blood passes through the coils as dialysate circulates at high speed around the coils and meshwork.

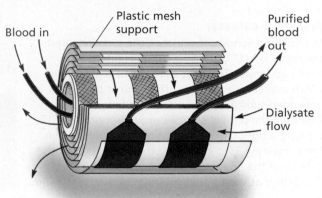

Blood in

Plastic mesh support

Purified blood out

Dialysate flow

The flat-plate and hollow-fiber dialyzers may be used several times on each patient. Heparin is given to prevent clot formation during hemodialysis. Three system types can be used to deliver dialysate. The batch system uses a reservoir for recirculating dialysate. The regenerative system uses sorbents to purify and regenerate recirculating dialysate. The proportioning system (the most common) mixes concentrate with water to form dialysate, which then circulates through the dialyzer and goes down a drain after a single pass, followed by fresh dialysate.

Osmosis

In osmosis, fluids move through a semipermeable membrane from an area of low-solute concentration to an area of high-solute concentration. In peritoneal dialysis, dextrose is added to the dialysate to give it a higher solute concentration than the blood, creating a high osmotic gradient. Water migrates from the blood through the membrane at the beginning of each infusion, when the osmotic gradient is highest.

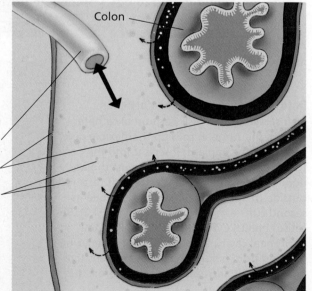

Colon

Catheter

Peritoneal membrane

Waste products

Comparing peritoneal dialysis catheters

The first step in any type of peritoneal dialysis is the insertion of a catheter to allow instillation of dialyzing solution. The surgeon may insert one of three different catheters described here.

Tenckhoff catheter

To implant a Tenckhoff catheter, the surgeon inserts the first 6¾″ (17 cm) of the catheter into the patient's abdomen. The next 2¾″ (7 cm) segment, which may have a Dacron cuff at one or both ends, is imbedded subcutaneously. Within a few days after insertion, the patient's tissues grow around the cuffs, forming a tight barrier against bacterial infiltration. The remaining 3⅞″ (10 cm) of the catheter extends outside of the abdomen and is equipped with a plastic adapter at the tip that connects to dialyzer tubing.

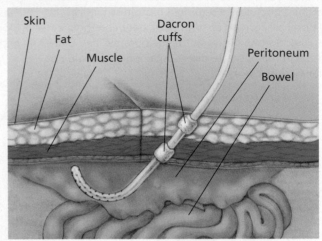

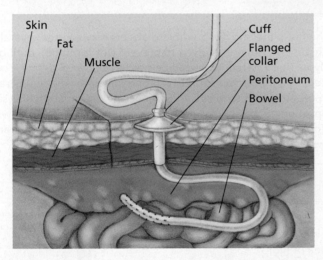

Flanged-collar catheter

To insert this type of catheter, the surgeon positions its flanged collar just below the dermis so that the device extends through the abdominal wall. He keeps the cuff's distal end from extending into the peritoneum, where it could cause adhesions.

Column-disk peritoneal catheter

To insert a column-disk peritoneal catheter (CDPC), the surgeon rolls up the flexible disk section of the implant, inserts it into the peritoneal cavity, and retracts it against the abdominal wall. The implant's first cuff rests just outside the peritoneal membrane, while its second cuff rests just underneath the skin. Because the CDPC doesn't float freely in the peritoneal cavity, it keeps inflowing dialyzing solution from being directed at the sensitive organs, which increases patient comfort during dialysis.

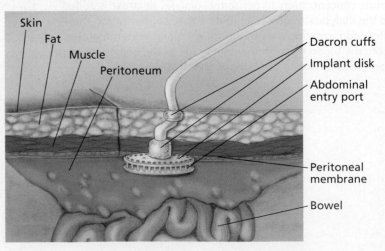

Nonsurgical procedures

Several nonsurgical procedures may be employed to treat renal or urologic disorders, including calculi basketing, catheterization, and extracorporeal shock-wave lithotripsy (ESWL).

CALCULI BASKETING

When ureteral calculi are too large for normal elimination, removal with a basketing instrument is the treatment of choice, helping to relieve pain and prevent infection and renal dysfunction. In this technique, a basketing instrument is inserted through a cystoscope into the ureter to capture the calculus and then is withdrawn to remove it.

CATHETERIZATION

The insertion of a drainage device into the bladder, catheterization may be intermittent or continuous. Intermittent catheterization drains urine remaining in the bladder after voiding. It's used for patients with urinary incontinence, urethral stricture, cystitis, prostatic obstruction, neurogenic bladder, or other disorders that interfere with bladder emptying. It may also be used postoperatively.

Catheterization helps relieve bladder distention caused by such conditions as urinary tract obstruction and neurogenic bladder. It allows continuous urine drainage in patients with a urinary meatus swollen from local trauma or childbirth as well as from surgery. Continuous catheterization can also provide accurate monitoring of urine output in critically ill patients or when normal voiding is impaired.

Teaching self-catheterization

Female patient
Instruct the female patient to hold the catheter in her dominant hand as if it were a pencil or dart, about ½" (1 cm) from its tip. Keeping the vaginal folds separated, she should slowly insert the lubricated catheter about 3" (7.5 cm) into the urethra. Tell her to press down with her abdominal muscles to empty the bladder, allowing all urine to drain through the catheter and into the toilet or drainage container.

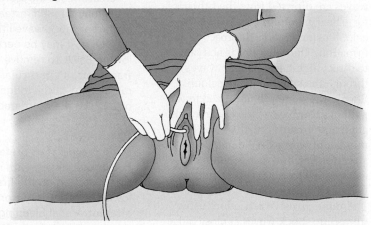

Male patient
Teach the male patient to hold his penis in his nondominant hand, at a right angle to his body. He should hold the catheter in his dominant hand as if it were a pencil or dart and slowly insert it 7" to 10" (17.5 to 25 cm) into the urethra—until urine begins flowing. Then he should gently advance the catheter about 1" (2.5 cm) farther, allowing all urine to drain into the toilet or drainage container.

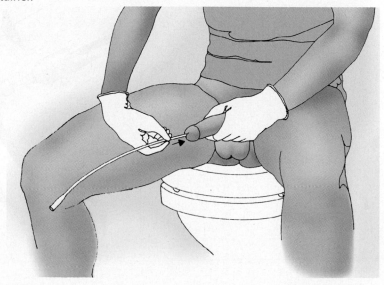

Extracorporeal shock-wave lithotripsy

A noninvasive technique for removing obstructive renal calculi, extracorporeal shock-wave lithotripsy (ESWL) uses high-energy shock waves to break up calculi and allow their normal passage.

In this procedure, the patient is placed in a semi-reclining or supine position on a hydraulic stretcher of the ESWL machine on a water-filled cushion through which the shock waves are directed from the lithotriptor. The generator is focused on the calculi using biplane fluoroscopy confirmation. The generator is activated to direct high-energy shock waves through the cushion at the calculi. Shock waves are synchronized to the patient's R waves on the electrocardiogram and fired during diastole. The number of waves fired depends on the size, number, and composition of the calculi (500 to 2,000 shocks may be delivered during a treatment).

A more invasive procedure using ultrasonic shock waves at close range is percutaneous ultrasonic lithotripsy (PUL). In PUL, the patient receives local anesthesia or oral sedation. Calculi can be broken up by several percutaneous fragmentation devices besides ultrasound, such as laser pulses and electrohydraulic electric sparks.

Understanding percutaneous ultrasonic lithotripsy

HANDS ON

In this lithotripsy technique, an ultrasonic probe inserted through a nephrostomy tube into the renal pelvis generates ultrahigh-frequency sound waves to shatter calculi, while continuous suctioning removes the fragments. (See the illustration below.)

Percutaneous ultrasonic lithotripsy (PUL) may be used instead of extracorporeal shock-wave lithotripsy (ESWL), or it may be performed following ESWL to remove residual fragments. It's particularly useful for radiolucent calculi lodged in the kidney, which aren't treatable by ESWL.

Two stages

Some practitioners prefer to perform PUL in two stages, with nephrostomy tube insertion on the first day followed by lithotripsy 1 or 2 days later, after intrarenal bleeding has subsided and the calculi can be better visualized. The day before scheduled treatment, the patient has excretory urography or lower abdominal radiographs to locate the calculi.

Potential complications

Because PUL is an invasive procedure, it has many of the risks associated with surgical methods. In addition to possibly causing hemorrhage and infection, it may lead to renal damage from nephrostomy tube insertion and ureteral obstruction from incomplete passage of calculi fragments.

Postprocedure care

After PUL, care measures include increased fluid intake, frequent nephrostomy tube irrigations, and straining of urine to capture passed calculi fragments and allow laboratory analysis of their composition. One or 2 days after treatment, the patient has a kidney, ureter, and bladder radiograph or a nephrostogram to check for retained fragments. If none are revealed, the practitioner usually removes the nephrostomy tube. Occasionally, a patient is discharged with the tube temporarily in place.

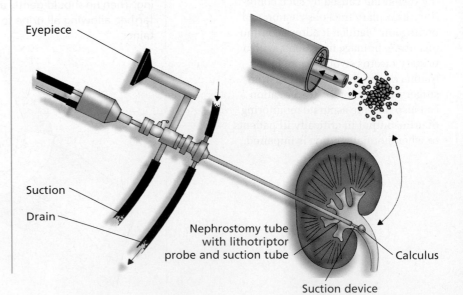

Eyepiece

Suction

Drain

Nephrostomy tube with lithotriptor probe and suction tube

Calculus

Suction device

Surgery

KIDNEY TRANSPLANTATION

In kidney transplantation, a healthy kidney is removed from a donor and implanted in a patient with nonfunctional kidneys. Two surgical teams are used in living donor transplants. One team procures the donor kidney and the other team implants it into the recipient. If the kidney is from a cadaver, only one surgical team is needed.

URINARY DIVERSION

Urinary diversion provides an alternative urine excretion route when a disease or disorder impedes normal urine flow through the bladder. The procedure may involve either a cutaneous method, such as an ileal conduit—the preferred and most common procedure for diverting urine through an ileal segment to a stoma on the abdomen—or a continent method. Continent urinary diversions include the Indiana pouch, continent ileal reservoir (Koch pouch), and modified Koch pouch. Each of these procedures begins with a cystectomy.

Kidney transplantation site and vascular connections

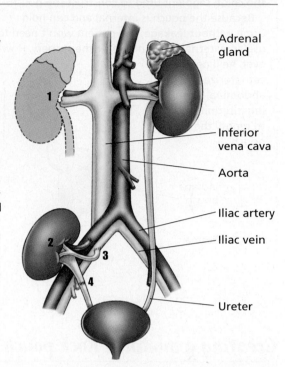

1. The diseased kidney may be removed. If it is, the renal artery and vein are ligated.

2. The donor kidney is placed in the recipient's iliac fossa.

3. Next, the renal artery of the donor kidney is sutured to the recipient's iliac artery, and the renal vein of the donor kidney is sutured to his iliac vein.

4. Then the ureter of the donor kidney is sutured to the recipient's bladder or ureter.

- Adrenal gland
- Inferior vena cava
- Aorta
- Iliac artery
- Iliac vein
- Ureter

Creating an ileal conduit

To create an ileal conduit, the surgeon excises a segment of the ileum and closes the two resulting ends. Then he dissects the ureters from the bladder and anastomoses them to the ileal segment. He closes one end of the ileal segment with sutures and brings the opposite end through the abdominal wall to form a stoma.

Because urine empties continuously, the patient must wear a collecting device or pouch after the procedure.

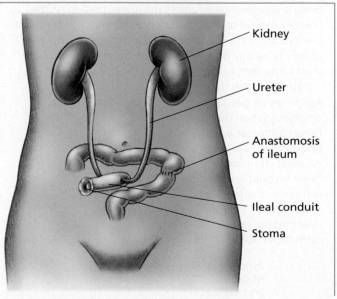

- Kidney
- Ureter
- Anastomosis of ileum
- Ileal conduit
- Stoma

Creating an Indiana pouch

To create an Indiana pouch, the surgeon uses a segment of the small bowel or colon to form an internal pouch. He tunnels the ureters through the colon segment used to construct the pouch.

Because the pouch is internal and can hold urine without leakage, the patient won't need to use an external appliance after the surgery. However, he'll need to catheterize the abdominal opening intermittently to empty the pouch.

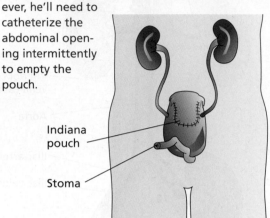

Indiana
pouch

Stoma

Creating a modified Kock pouch

To create a modified Kock pouch, the surgeon modifies a continent ileal reservoir so that both ureters and the urethra connect to it. This eliminates the need for an abdominal wall opening and helps preserve the patient's body image; however, unless the lower portion of the bladder can be spared, continence depends solely on the urethra and external sphincter. For this reason, the procedure is usually done only in men because their longer urethra permits better external sphincter control.

Internal pouch drainage relies on passive emptying when the external sphincter is relaxed as well as on abdominal straining. If these techniques aren't sufficient, the patient must learn to perform intermittent self-catheterization.

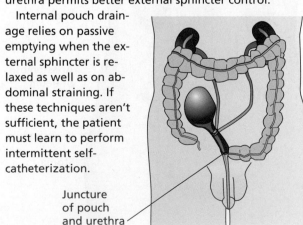

Juncture
of pouch
and urethra

Creating a continent ileal reservoir

To create a continent ileal reservoir (Kock pouch), the surgeon forms an internal pouch from a segment of the small bowel or colon. He implants the ureters into the sides of the pouch, with each ureter intussuscepted to create a nipple valve. Then he brings the efferent ureter and nipple valve to the skin surface of the anterior abdomen as a stoma and to prevent urine leakage from the pouch. The afferent ureter and nipple valve prevent urine reflux.

Because the pouch is internal and can hold urine without leakage, the patient won't need to use an external appliance. However, he'll need to catheterize the abdominal opening intermittently to empty the pouch.

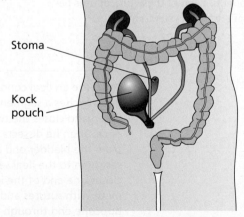

Stoma

Kock
pouch

Hematologic and immunologic care

DISEASES
Acquired immunodeficiency syndrome

Currently one of the most widely publicized diseases, acquired immunodeficiency syndrome (AIDS) is marked by progressive failure of the immune system. Although it's characterized by gradual destruction of cell-mediated (T-cell) immunity, it also affects humoral immunity and even autoimmunity because of the central role of the CD4$^+$ T lymphocyte in immune reactions. The resultant immunodeficiency makes the patient susceptible to opportunistic infections, unusual cancers, and other abnormalities that define AIDS.

A retrovirus—the human immunodeficiency virus (HIV) type I—is the primary causative agent. Transmission of HIV occurs by contact with infected blood or body fluids and is associated with identifiable high-risk behaviors. It's therefore disproportionately represented in homosexual and bisexual men, I.V. drug users, neonates of HIV-infected women, recipients of contaminated blood or blood products (dramatically decreased since mid-1985),

and heterosexual partners of people in the former groups. Because of similar routes of transmission, AIDS shares epidemiologic patterns with hepatitis B and sexually transmitted diseases.

HIV is transmitted by direct inoculation during intimate sexual contact, especially associated with the mucosal trauma of receptive rectal inter-

PICTURING PATHO

HIV life cycle

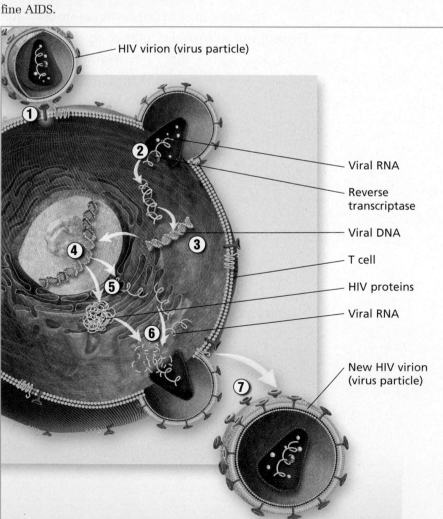

- HIV virion (virus particle)
- Viral RNA
- Reverse transcriptase
- Viral DNA
- T cell
- HIV proteins
- Viral RNA
- New HIV virion (virus particle)

1. HIV binds to the T cell.

2. Viral RNA is released into the host cell.

3. Reverse transcriptase converts viral RNA into viral DNA.

4. Viral DNA enters the T cell's nucleus and inserts itself into the T cell's DNA.

5. The T cell begins to make copies of the HIV components.

6. Protease (an enzyme) helps create new virus particles.

7. The new HIV virion (virus particle) is released from the T cell.

course; transfusion of contaminated blood or blood products (a risk diminished by routine testing of all blood products); sharing of contaminated needles; and transplacental or postpartum transmission from infected mother to fetus (by cervical or blood contact at delivery and in breast milk).

HIV isn't transmitted by casual household or social contact. The average time between exposure to the virus and diagnosis of AIDS is 8 to 10 years, but shorter and longer incuba-

tion times have been recorded. Most people develop antibodies within 6 to 8 weeks of contracting the virus.

Signs and symptoms

▶ Mononucleosis-like syndrome, which may be attributed to a flu or other virus and then may remain asymptomatic for years (after a high-risk exposure and inoculation); in the latent stage, laboratory evidence of seroconversion only sign of HIV infection

▶ When signs and symptoms appear, they may take many forms:
— Persistent generalized adenopathy
— Weight loss, fatigue, night sweats, fevers (nonspecific signs and symptoms)
— Neurologic symptoms resulting from HIV encephalopathy, such as memory loss, partial paralysis, loss of coordination
— Opportunistic infection or cancer
— Diarrhea

Stages of HIV infection

1. Primary stage
This stage occurs about 1 to 2 weeks after initial infection with human immunodeficiency virus (HIV). During this stage, the virus undergoes massive replication. Patients may be asymptomatic or have a flulike syndrome.

2. Asymptomatic HIV
During this stage, also called the clinical latency stage, chronic signs or symptoms aren't present. T-cell count may be used to monitor the progression of the disease. With the patient's own resistance and drug therapy, this stage can last 8 years or longer.

3. Symptomatic HIV
This stage has two phases: early and late. When the T-cell count in blood falls below 200 cells/mm^3, it's the late phase. This stage of HIV infection is defined mainly by the emergence of opportunistic infections and cancers to which the immune system normally helps maintain resistance.

4. AIDS
A T-cell count of 50 cells/mm^3 or less represents advanced HIV. With the onset of this stage, patients are at the highest risk for opportunistic infections and malignancies.

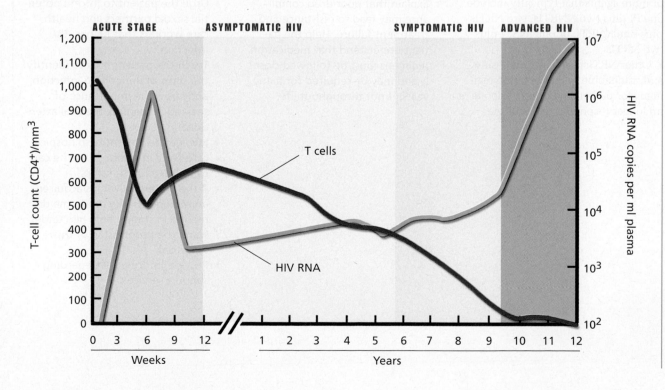

Treatment

❯ No cure; however, the World Health Organization recommends treatment for patients with CD4+ counts of 350 cells/mm³ or less, regardless of clinical stage. Primary therapy for HIV infection includes these types of antiretroviral agents:

– protease inhibitors (PIs), such as ritonavir, indinavir, nelfinavir, and atazanavir

– nucleoside reverse transcriptase inhibitors (NRTIs), such as tenofovir, emtricitabine, zidovudine, didanosine, zalcitabine, lamivudine, and stavudine

– nonnucleoside reverse transcriptase inhibitors (NNRTIs), such as efavirenz, nevirapine, and delavirdine.

❯ Integrase strand transfer inhibitors (INSTIs), such as raltegravir and elvitegravir

❯ Immunomodulators designed to boost the weakened immune system

❯ Anti-infective and antineoplastic agents to combat opportunistic infections and associated cancers

❯ Treatment protocols combining two or more agents that typically include one PI plus two NNRTIs, two NRTIs plus one NNRTI, or one INSTI plus two NRTIs

❯ Other NRTIs, such as didanosine and zalcitabine in combination regimens for patients who can't tolerate or no longer respond to zidovudine

Nursing considerations

❯ Recognize that a diagnosis of AIDS is profoundly distressing because of the disease's social impact and the discouraging prognosis. The patient may lose his job and financial security as well as the support of his family and friends. Coping with an altered body image, the emotional burden of a serious illness, and the threat of death may overwhelm the patient.

❯ Monitor the patient for fever, noting any pattern, and for signs of skin breakdown, cough, sore throat, and diarrhea. Assess him for swollen, tender lymph nodes, and check laboratory values regularly, especially CD4+ counts and viral loads.

❯ Avoid glycerine swabs for mucous membranes, and have the patient use normal saline or bicarbonate mouthwash for daily oral rinsing.

❯ Record the patient's caloric intake.

❯ Ensure adequate fluid intake during episodes of diarrhea.

❯ Provide meticulous skin care, especially if the patient is debilitated.

❯ Encourage the patient to maintain as much physical activity as he can tolerate. Make sure his schedule includes time for both exercise and rest.

❯ If the patient develops Kaposi's sarcoma, monitor the progression of lesions.

❯ Monitor opportunistic infections or signs of disease progression, and treat infections as ordered.

❯ Note that a patient who also has hepatitis or tuberculosis may have different regimens or start treatments at different points.

LESSON PLANS

Teaching about AIDS

❯ Explain that poor drug compliance may lead to resistance and treatment failure. Help the patient understand that medication regimens must be followed closely and may be required for many years, if not throughout life.

❯ Urge the patient to inform potential sexual partners and health care workers that he has HIV infection.

❯ Teach the patient how to identify the signs of impending infection, and stress the importance of seeking immediate medical attention.

❯ Involve the patient with hospice care early in treatment so he can establish a relationship.

❯ If the patient develops acquired immunodeficiency syndrome dementia in stages, help him understand the progression of this symptom.

❯ Provide information regarding support services.

Acute leukemia

Acute leukemia begins as a malignant proliferation of white blood cell (WBC) precursors, or blasts, in bone marrow or lymph tissue. It results in an accumulation of these cells in peripheral blood, bone marrow, and body tissues.

The most common forms of acute leukemia include acute lymphoblastic (lymphocytic) leukemia (ALL), characterized by abnormal growth of lymphocyte precursors (lymphoblasts); acute myeloblastic (myelogenous) leukemia (AML), which causes rapid accumulation of myeloid precursors (myeloblasts); and acute monoblastic (monocytic) leukemia, or Schilling's type, which results in a marked increase in monocyte precursors (monoblasts). Other variants include acute myelomonocytic leukemia and acute erythroleukemia.

Untreated, acute leukemia is invariably fatal, usually because of complications resulting from leukemic cell infiltration of bone marrow or vital organs. With treatment, the prognosis varies.

With ALL, treatment induces remission in 95% of children (average survival time: 5 years) and in 65% of adults (average survival time: 1 to 2 years). Children between ages 2 and 8 have the best survival rate—about 50%—with intensive therapy.

With AML, the average survival time is only 1 year after diagnosis, even with aggressive treatment. Remission lasting 2 to 10 months occurs in 50% of children; adults survive only about 1 year after diagnosis, even with treatment. Duration of remission is linked to age; younger patients have a greater chance of obtaining remission.

The exact cause of acute leukemia is unknown; however, radiation (especially prolonged exposure), certain chemicals and drugs, viruses, genetic abnormalities, and chronic exposure to benzene are likely contributing factors.

Although the pathogenesis isn't clearly understood, immature, nonfunctioning WBCs appear to accumulate first in the tissue where they originate (lymphocytes in lymph tissue, granulocytes in bone marrow). These immature WBCs then spill into the bloodstream. They then overwhelm the red blood cells (RBCs) and the platelets. From there, immature white blood cells infiltrate other tissues.

Histologic findings of acute lymphocytic leukemia

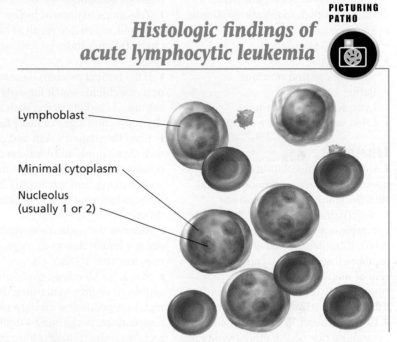

Lymphoblast

Minimal cytoplasm

Nucleolus (usually 1 or 2)

Histologic findings of acute myelogenous leukemia

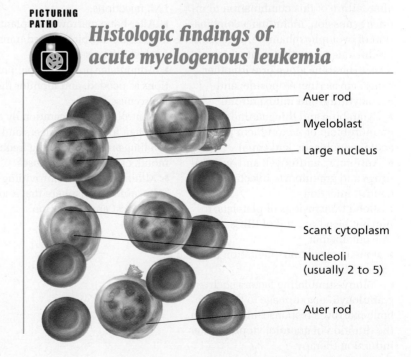

Auer rod

Myeloblast

Large nucleus

Scant cytoplasm

Nucleoli (usually 2 to 5)

Auer rod

Signs and symptoms
▶ High fever
▶ Abnormal bleeding
▶ Fatigue
▶ Night sweats
▶ Weakness and lassitude
▶ Recurrent infections
▶ Chills
▶ Abdominal or bone pain (ALL, AML, or acute monoblastic leukemia)
▶ Tachycardia
▶ Decreased ventilation
▶ Palpitations
▶ Systolic ejection murmur
▶ Pallor
▶ Lymph node enlargement
▶ Liver or spleen enlargement

Treatment
▶ Intrathecal instillation of methotrexate or cytarabine with cranial radiation (for meningeal infiltration)
▶ Vincristine, prednisone, high-dose cytarabine, and daunorubicin (for ALL); intrathecal methotrexate or cytarabine (because ALL carries a 40% risk of meningeal infiltration); radiation therapy for brain or testicular infiltration, which may occur with ALL
▶ Combination I.V. daunorubicin and cytarabine (for AML); other treatments after failure of this combination to induce remission, including a combination of cyclophosphamide, vincristine, prednisone, or methotrexate; high-dose cytarabine alone or with other drugs; amsacrine; etoposide; and 5-azacytidine and mitoxantrone
▶ Cytarabine and thioguanine with daunorubicin or doxorubicin (for acute monoblastic leukemia)
▶ Antibiotic, antifungal, and antiviral drugs and granulocyte injections to control infection
▶ Blood transfusions of platelets, to prevent bleeding, and of RBCs, to prevent anemia
▶ Bone marrow transplantation (for some patients)
▶ Colony-stimulating factors such as granulocyte-macrophage to boost the bone marrow's response and decrease the duration of granulocytopenia after induction therapy.

Nursing considerations
▶ Before treatment begins, help establish an appropriate rehabilitation program for the patient during remission.
▶ Watch for signs of meningeal infiltration (confusion, lethargy, and headache).
▶ Check the lumbar puncture site often for bleeding.
▶ Take steps to prevent hyperuricemia, a possible result of rapid, chemotherapy-induced leukemic cell lysis.
▶ If the patient receives daunorubicin or doxorubicin, watch for early indications of cardiotoxicity, such as arrhythmias and signs of heart failure.
▶ Keep the patient's skin and perianal area clean, apply mild lotions or creams to keep the skin from drying and cracking, and thoroughly clean the skin before all invasive skin procedures.
▶ Monitor the patient's temperature every 4 hours. Report a temperature rise over 101° F (38.3° C).
▶ Watch for bleeding. Avoid giving aspirin or aspirin-containing drugs or rectal suppositories, taking a rectal temperature, performing a digital rectal examination, or administering I.M. injections.
▶ After bone marrow transplantation, administer antibiotics, and transfuse packed RBCs as necessary.
▶ Administer prescribed pain medications as needed, and monitor their effectiveness.
▶ Control mouth ulceration by checking often for obvious ulcers and gum swelling and by providing frequent mouth care and saline rinses.
▶ Minimize stress by providing a calm, quiet atmosphere that's conducive to rest and relaxation.

Teaching about acute leukemia

▶ Explain the course of the disease to the patient.
▶ Teach the patient and his family how to recognize signs and symptoms of infection (fever, chills, cough, sore throat). Tell them to report an infection to the practitioner.
▶ Explain to the patient that his blood may not have enough platelets for proper clotting, and teach him the signs of abnormal bleeding (bruising, petechiae). Explain that he can apply pressure and ice to the area to stop such bleeding. Teach him steps he can take to prevent bleeding. Urge him to report excessive bleeding or bruising to the practitioner.
▶ Inform the patient that drug therapy is tailored to his type of leukemia. Explain that he'll probably need a combination of drugs; teach him about the ones he'll receive. Make sure he understands their adverse effects and the measures he can take to prevent or alleviate them.
▶ Explain that if the chemotherapy causes weight loss and anorexia, the patient will need to eat and drink high-calorie, high-protein foods and beverages.
▶ Instruct the patient to use a soft toothbrush and to avoid hot, spicy foods and commercial mouthwashes, which can irritate the mouth ulcers that result from chemotherapy.
▶ If the patient receives cranial radiation, explain what the treatment is and how it will help him. Be sure to discuss potential adverse effects and the steps he can take to minimize them.
▶ If the patient needs a bone marrow transplant, reinforce the practitioner's explanation of the treatment, its possible benefits, and the potential adverse effects.
▶ Advise the patient to limit his activities and to plan rest periods during the day.

Aplastic and hypoplastic anemias

Aplastic and hypoplastic anemias are potentially fatal and result from injury to or destruction of stem cells in bone marrow or the bone marrow matrix, causing pancytopenia (anemia, leukopenia, thrombocytopenia) and bone marrow hypoplasia.

Aplastic anemias usually develop when damaged or destroyed stem cells inhibit red blood cell (RBC) production. Less commonly, they develop when damaged bone marrow microvasculature creates an unfavorable environment for cell growth and maturation. About one-half of such anemias result from drugs (such as chloramphenicol), toxic agents (such as benzene), or radiation. The rest may result from immunologic factors (suspected but unconfirmed), severe disease (especially hepatitis), viral infection (especially in children), and preleukemic and neoplastic infiltration of bone marrow.

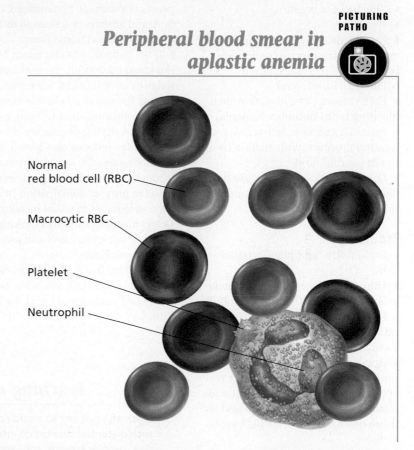

PICTURING PATHO

Peripheral blood smear in aplastic anemia

Normal red blood cell (RBC)

Macrocytic RBC

Platelet

Neutrophil

Causes of acquired aplastic anemias

Drugs, toxic agents, and radiation cause about one-half of all cases of acquired aplastic anemias. Examples and other causes are listed here.

Drugs
Antiarrhythmics (procainamide), antibiotics (chloramphenicol, cephalosporins, sulfonamides and, rarely, penicillins), anticonvulsants (especially phenytoin, ethosuximide, and carbamazepine), antidiabetics, anti-inflammatory drugs (phenylbutazone, indomethacin, gold, and penicillamine), antimalarials, antineoplastics, antithyroid drugs, diuretics (including hydrochlorothiazide), phenothiazines, zidovudine

Chemicals and toxins
Aromatic hydrocarbons (benzene), heavy metals, pesticides

Infections
Cytomegalovirus, hepatitis C, Epstein-Barr virus, miliary tuberculosis, Venezuelan equine encephalitis

Rheumatoid and autoimmune diseases
Graft-versus-host disease, systemic lupus erythematosus, rheumatoid arthritis

Other causes
Paroxysmal nocturnal hemoglobinuria, pregnancy, idiopathic causes, radiation, thymoma

Signs and symptoms

◗ Progressive weakness and fatigue
◗ Shortness of breath
◗ Headache
◗ Easy bruising and bleeding (especially from the mucous membranes [nose, gums, rectum, vagina])
◗ Pallor (with anemia)
◗ Ecchymosis, petechiae, or retinal bleeding (with thrombocytopenia)
◗ Bibasilar crackles, tachycardia, and a gallop murmur (with anemia resulting in heart failure)
◗ Opportunistic infections, such as fever, oral and rectal ulcers, and sore throat

Treatment

◗ Packed RBC and platelet transfusions
◗ Human leukocyte antigen-matched leukocytes or antithymocyte globulin used alone or with cyclosporine (improves outcomes for children and severely neutropenic patients)
◗ Bone marrow transplantation, preferably from a human leukocyte antigen–matched sibling (for anemia resulting from severe aplasia and for those needing constant RBC transfusions)
◗ Frequent hand washing and air flow filtration to prevent infection
◗ Antibiotics (for infection; however, they aren't given prophylactically because they tend to encourage resistant strains of organisms)
◗ Respiratory support with oxygen and blood transfusions (for low hemoglobin levels)
◗ An immunosuppressant (if patient isn't responding to other therapy)
◗ Colony-stimulating factors (agents that encourage the growth of specific cellular components, including granulocyte colony-stimulating factor, granulocyte-macrophage colony-stimulating factor, and erythropoietic stimulating factor

Nursing considerations

◗ Focus your efforts on helping to prevent or manage hemorrhage, infection, and adverse reactions to drug therapy or blood transfusion.
◗ If the patient's platelet count is low (less than 20,000/μl), prevent hemorrhage by avoiding I.M. injections, suggesting the use of an electric razor and a soft toothbrush, humidifying oxygen to prevent drying of mucous membranes (dry mucosa may bleed), and promoting regular bowel movements through the use of a stool softener and a diet to prevent constipation (which can cause rectal mucosal bleeding). Detect bleeding early by checking for blood in urine and stool and assessing skin for petechiae.
◗ Make sure that throat, urine, nasal, stool, and blood cultures are done regularly and correctly to check for infection.

◗ If the patient has a low hemoglobin level, which causes fatigue, schedule frequent rest periods. Administer oxygen therapy as needed.
◗ Ensure a comfortable environmental temperature for a patient experiencing hypothermia or hyperthermia.
◗ If a blood transfusion is necessary, assess the patient for a transfusion reaction by checking his temperature and watching for the development of other signs and symptoms, such as rash, urticaria, pruritus, back pain, restlessness, and shaking chills.
◗ Be sure to monitor blood studies carefully in the patient receiving an anemia-inducing drug, to prevent aplastic anemia.

LESSON PLANS

Teaching about aplastic anemia

◗ Teach the patient to avoid contact with potential sources of infection, such as crowds, soil, and standing water, which can harbor organisms.
◗ Reassure and support the patient and his family by explaining the disease and its treatment, particularly if the patient has recurring acute episodes. Explain the purpose of all prescribed drugs, and discuss possible adverse reactions, including those he should report promptly.
◗ Review signs and symptoms of bleeding and when to seek medical attention.

◗ Tell the patient who doesn't require hospitalization that he can continue his normal lifestyle with appropriate restrictions (such as regular rest periods) until remission occurs.
◗ Refer the patient to the Aplastic Anemia Foundation and MDS International Foundation for additional information and assistance.

Disseminated intravascular coagulation

Disseminated intravascular coagulation (DIC) is also known as *consumption coagulopathy* and *defibrination syndrome*. DIC occurs as a complication of diseases and conditions that accelerate clotting, causing thrombosis of small blood vessels, organ necrosis, depletion of circulating clotting factors and platelets, and activation of the fibrinolytic system. This, in turn, can provoke severe hemorrhage.

Clotting in the microcirculation usually affects the kidneys and extremities but can occur in the brain, lungs, pituitary and adrenal glands, and GI mucosa. Other conditions, such as vitamin K deficiency, hepatic disease, and anticoagulant therapy, can cause similar hemorrhage.

DIC is usually acute but can be chronic for patients with cancer. The prognosis depends on early detection and treatment, the severity of the hemorrhage, and treatment of the underlying disease or condition.

DIC may result from:
▶ infection (most common cause)—gram-negative or gram-positive septicemia; viral, fungal, or rickettsial infection; protozoal infection
▶ obstetric complications—abruptio placentae, amniotic fluid embolism, retained dead fetus, eclampsia, septic abortion, postpartum hemorrhage
▶ neoplastic disease—acute leukemia, metastatic carcinoma, lymphoma
▶ a disorder that produces necrosis—extensive burns and trauma, brain tissue destruction, transplant rejection, hepatic necrosis, anorexia

▶ another disorder or condition—heatstroke, shock, poisonous snakebite, cirrhosis, fat embolism, incompatible blood transfusion, a drug reaction, cardiac arrest, surgery necessitating cardiopulmonary bypass, giant hemangioma, extensive venous thrombosis, purpura fulminans, adrenal disease, acute respiratory distress syndrome, diabetic ketoacidosis, pulmonary embolism, or sickle cell anemia.

Why such conditions and disorders lead to DIC is unclear, as is whether they lead to DIC through a common mechanism. In many patients, the triggering mechanisms may be the entrance of foreign protein into the circulation and vascular endothelial injury.

Normal clotting process

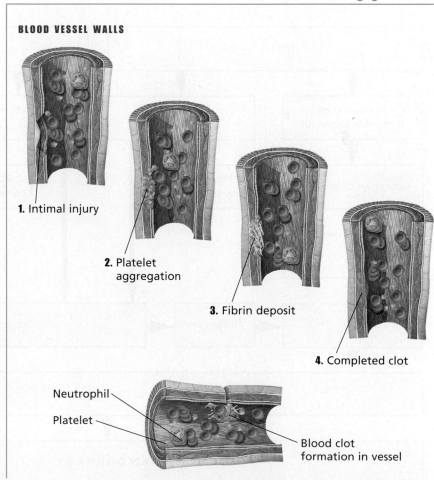

BLOOD VESSEL WALLS

1. Intimal injury

2. Platelet aggregation

3. Fibrin deposit

4. Completed clot

Neutrophil

Platelet

Blood clot formation in vessel

Regardless of how DIC begins, the typical accelerated clotting results in generalized activation of prothrombin and a consequent excess of thrombin. Excess thrombin converts fibrinogen to fibrin, producing fibrin clots in the microcirculation. This process consumes exorbitant amounts of coagulation factors (especially platelets, factor V, prothrombin, fibrinogen, and factor VIII), causing thrombocytopenia, deficiencies in factors V and VIII, hypoprothrombinemia, and hypofibrinogenemia.

Circulating thrombin activates the fibrinolytic system, which lyses fibrin clots into fibrinogen degradation products (FDPs). The hemorrhage that occurs may result largely from the anticoagulant activity of FDPs as well as from depletion of plasma coagulation factors.

Three mechanisms of DIC

However disseminated intravascular coagulation (DIC) begins, accelerated clotting (characteristic of DIC) usually results in excess thrombin, which in turn causes fibrinolysis with excess fibrin formation and fibrin degradation products (FDPs), activation of fibrin-stabilizing factor (factor XIII), consumption of platelet and clotting factors and, eventually, hemorrhage.

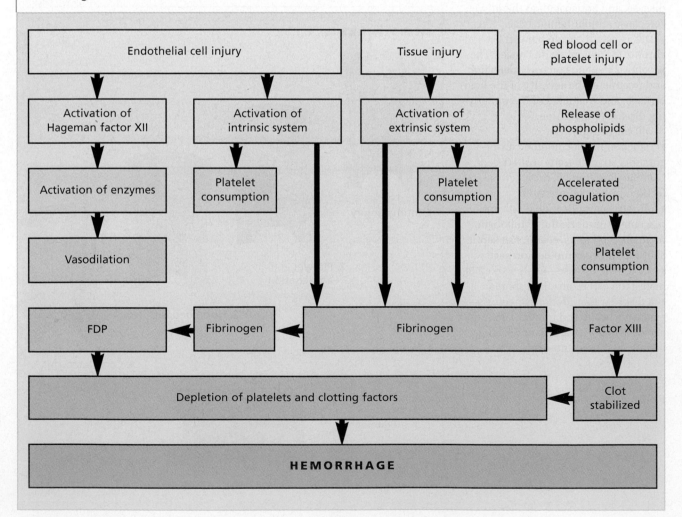

Signs and symptoms
▶ Abnormal bleeding without a history of a serious hemorrhagic disorder (usually the first sign)
▶ Signs of bleeding into the skin, such as cutaneous oozing, petechiae, ecchymoses, and hematomas
▶ Excessive bleeding from I.V. sites
▶ Nausea and vomiting
▶ Chest pain
▶ Hemoptysis
▶ Epistaxis
▶ Seizures
▶ Oliguria
▶ Severe muscle, back, and abdominal pain
▶ Acrocyanosis
▶ Dyspnea
▶ Diminished peripheral pulses
▶ Decreased blood pressure
▶ Mental status changes, including confusion

Treatment
▶ Recognition and treatment of cause of DIC
▶ Blood, fresh frozen plasma, platelets, or packed red blood cell transfusions to support hemostasis (for active bleeding)
▶ Heparin therapy (remains controversial); administered (in most cases) with transfusion therapy; in early stages to prevent microclotting; as a late resort for active bleeding; mandatory if thrombosis occurs
▶ Drugs such as antithrombin III to inhibit clotting cascade

Nursing considerations
▶ Focus on early recognition of signs of abnormal bleeding, prompt treatment of the underlying disorders, and prevention of further bleeding.
▶ Keep the family informed of the patient's progress. Prepare them for his appearance (I.V. lines, nasogastric tubes, bruises, dried blood). Give emotional support. Listen to the patient's and family's concerns. When possible, encourage the patient. As needed, enlist the aid of a social worker, a chaplain, and other health care team members in providing support.

▶ If the patient can't tolerate activities because of blood loss, provide rest periods.
▶ Administer the prescribed analgesic for pain as needed.
▶ Reposition the patient every 2 hours, and provide meticulous skin care to prevent skin breakdown.
▶ Administer oxygen therapy as ordered.
▶ Test stool and urine for occult blood.
▶ To prevent clots from dislodging and causing fresh bleeding, don't vigorously rub these areas when washing. Use a 1:1 solution of hydrogen peroxide and water to help remove crusted blood.
▶ Protect the patient from injury. Enforce complete bed rest during bleeding episodes. If the patient is agitated, pad the side rails.
▶ If bleeding occurs, use pressure and topical hemostatic agents, such as absorbable gelatin sponges (Gelfoam), microfibrillar collagen hemostat (Avitene Hemostat), or thrombin (Thrombinar), to control it.
▶ Check all venipuncture sites frequently for bleeding.
▶ Monitor intake and output hourly in patients with acute DIC, especially when administering blood products.
▶ Watch for bleeding from the GI and genitourinary (GU) tracts. If you suspect intra-abdominal bleeding, measure the patient's abdominal girth at least every 4 hours and monitor closely for signs of shock. Perform bladder irrigations, as ordered, for GU bleeding.
▶ Monitor the results of serial blood studies (particularly hematocrit, hemoglobin level, coagulation times, and fibrin split products and fibrinogen levels).

LESSON
PLANS

 Teaching about DIC

▶ Explain disseminated intravascular coagulation (DIC) to the patient and his family.
▶ Teach them about the signs and symptoms of DIC, the diagnostic tests required, and the treatment that the patient is to receive.
▶ Explain that injury can cause bleeding. Tell the patient to exercise caution when moving to avoid bumping into the bed or other objects.
▶ Advise the patient to take frequent rest periods.

Hemophilia

A hereditary bleeding disorder, hemophilia results from deficiency of specific clotting factors. Hemophilia A (classic hemophilia), which affects more than 80% of all hemophiliacs, results from deficiency of factor VIII; hemophilia B (Christmas disease), which affects 15% of hemophiliacs, results from deficiency of factor IX. Other evidence suggests that hemophilia may result from nonfunctioning factors VIII and IX, rather than from deficiency of these factors.

Hemophilia produces abnormal bleeding, which may be mild, moderate, or severe, depending on the degree of factor deficiency. After a hemophiliac forms a platelet plug at a bleeding site, the lack of clotting factors impairs formation of a stable fibrin clot. Immediate hemorrhage isn't prevalent, but delayed bleeding is common.

Signs and symptoms

▶ Pain and swelling in a weight-bearing joint, such as the hip, knee, and ankle
▶ Bleeding after circumcision (usually the first sign)
▶ Spontaneous bleeding or severe bleeding after minor trauma that may produce large subcutaneous and deep intramuscular hematomas
▶ Abdominal, chest, or flank pain, indicating internal bleeding
▶ Hematuria or hematemesis
▶ Tarry stools
▶ Hematomas on the extremities, the torso, or both
▶ Limited joint range of motion

Treatment

▶ Careful management by a hematologist (for patients undergoing surgery)
▶ Replacement of the deficient factor before and after surgery (even for minor surgery such as dental extraction)
▶ Aminocaproic acid (for oral bleeding, to inhibit the active fibrinolytic system in oral mucosa)

Normal clotting and clotting in hemophilia

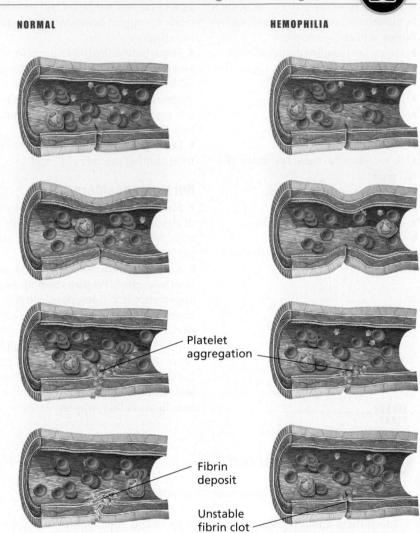

NORMAL   HEMOPHILIA

Platelet aggregation

Fibrin deposit

Unstable fibrin clot

Hemophilia A

▶ Cryoprecipitated antihemophilic factor (AHF), lyophilized AHF, or both in doses large enough to raise clotting factor levels above 25% of normal to permit normal hemostasis
▶ AHF before surgery to raise clotting factors to hemostatic levels until wound heals; fresh frozen plasma administration (has some drawbacks)
▶ Inhibitors to factor VIII develop after multiple transfusions in 10% to 20% of patients with severe hemophilia, rendering the patient resistant to factor VIII infusions
▶ Desmopressin to stimulate the release of stored factor VIII, raising the level in the blood

Hemophilia B

▶ Administration of factor IX concentrate during bleeding episodes to increase factor IX levels

Recognizing and managing bleeding

In patients with hemophilia, bleeding may occur spontaneously or stem from an injury. Inform your patient and his family about possible types of bleeding and their associated signs and symptoms. Accordingly, advise them which actions to take and when to call for medical help.

Bleeding site	Signs and symptoms	Interventions
Intracranial	Change in personality or level of consciousness, headache, nausea	Instruct the patient or his family to notify the practitioner immediately and to treat symptoms as an emergency.
Joints (hemarthroses) Usually the knees, followed by elbows, ankles, shoulders, hips, and wrists	Joint pain and swelling, joint tingling and warmth (at onset of hemorrhage)	Tell the patient to begin antihemophilic factor (AHF) infusions and then to notify the practitioner.
Kidney	Pain in the lower back near the waist, decreased urine output	Instruct the patient to notify the practitioner and to start AHF infusion if bleeding results from a known recent injury.
Muscles	Pain and reduced function of the affected muscle; tingling, numbness, or pain in a large area away from the affected site (referred pain)	Urge the patient to notify the practitioner and to start an AHF infusion if the patient is reasonably certain that bleeding results from recent injury (otherwise, call the practitioner for instructions).
Subcutaneous tissue or skin	Pain, bruising, and swelling at the site (delayed oozing may also occur after an injury)	Show the patient how to apply appropriate topical agents, such as ice packs and absorbable gelatin sponges (Gelfoam), to stop bleeding.
Heart (cardiac tamponade)	Chest tightness, shortness of breath, swelling (usually occurs in patients who are very young or who have severe disease)	Instruct the patient to contact the practitioner or to go to the nearest emergency department immediately.

Nursing considerations

▶ Provide emotional support, and listen to the patient's fears and concerns.
▶ Watch for signs and symptoms of decreased tissue perfusion.
▶ Monitor the patient's blood pressure and pulse and respiratory rates. Observe him frequently for bleeding from the skin, mucous membranes, and wounds.

During bleeding episodes

▶ If the patient has surface cuts or epistaxis, apply pressure—usually the only treatment needed.
▶ With deeper cuts, pressure may stop the bleeding temporarily. Cuts deep enough to require suturing may also require factor infusions to prevent further bleeding.

▶ Give the deficient clotting factor or plasma as ordered.
▶ Apply cold compresses or ice bags, and elevate the injured part.
▶ To prevent recurrence of bleeding, restrict activity for 48 hours after bleeding is under control.
▶ Control pain with an analgesic, such as acetaminophen, propoxyphene, codeine, or morphine as ordered. Avoid I.M. injections. Aspirin and aspirin-containing medications are contraindicated.
▶ If the patient can't tolerate activities because of blood loss, provide rest periods between activities.

Bleeding into a joint

▶ Immediately elevate the joint.
▶ To restore joint mobility, if ordered, begin range-of-motion exercises at least 48 hours after the bleeding is controlled. Tell the patient to avoid weight bearing until bleeding stops and swelling subsides.
▶ Administer an analgesic for pain. Also, apply ice packs and elastic bandages to alleviate the pain.

After bleeding episodes and surgery

▶ Watch closely for signs and symptoms of further bleeding, such as increased pain and swelling, fever, and symptoms of shock.
▶ Closely monitor partial thromboplastin time.

Teaching about hemophilia

- Teach the patient the benefits of regular exercise. Explain that isometric exercises can also help to prevent muscle weakness and recurrent joint bleeding. Refer him for physical therapy as indicated.
- Advise parents to protect their child from injury while avoiding unnecessary restrictions that impair his normal development. An older child must not participate in contact sports, such as football, but he can be encouraged to swim or play golf.
- Tell the patient to avoid such activities as lifting heavy items and using power tools because they increase the risk of injury that can result in serious bleeding problems.
- If an injury occurs, direct the parents to apply cold compresses or ice bags and elevate the injured part or to apply light pressure to the bleeding. To prevent recurrence of bleeding after treatment, instruct the parents to restrict the child's activity for 48 hours after bleeding is under control.
- Advise the parents to notify the physician immediately after even a minor injury, especially to the head, neck, or abdomen.
- Instruct parents to watch for signs of internal bleeding, such as severe pain and swelling in joints or muscles, stiffness, decreased joint movement, severe abdominal pain, blood in urine, tarry stools, and severe headache.

- Explain to the patient and, if appropriate, his parents the importance of avoiding aspirin, combination medications that contain aspirin, and over-the-counter anti-inflammatory agents such as ibuprofen compounds. Tell them to use acetaminophen instead.
- Stress the importance of good dental care, including regular, careful toothbrushing, to prevent the need for dental surgery. Have the child use a soft toothbrush to avoid gum injury. Emphasize that poor dental hygiene can lead to bleeding from inflamed gums.
- Tell the parents to check with the physician before allowing dental extractions or other surgery. Advise them to get the names of other physicians they can contact in case their regular physician isn't available.
- Teach the patient the importance of protecting his veins for lifelong therapy.
- As necessary, encourage the patient to remain independent and be self-sufficient. Refer him for counseling as necessary.
- Tell the parents to make sure that the child wears a medical identification bracelet at all times.
- Refer new patients to a hemophilia treatment center for evaluation.

For patients receiving blood components:
- Train the parents to administer blood factor components at home to avoid frequent hospitalization. Teach them proper venipuncture and infusion techniques, and urge them not to delay treatment during bleeding episodes. Tell parents to keep blood factor concentrate and infusion equipment available at all times, even on vacation.

- Review possible adverse reactions, such as blood-borne infection and factor inhibitor development, that can result from replacement factor procedures.
- If the patient develops flushing, headache, or tingling from replacement factors, inform him or his parents that these reactions are most common with freeze-dried concentrate. Slowing the infusion rate may cause signs and symptoms to abate.
- If fever and chills occur, indicating an allergy to white blood cell antigens, instruct the patient or his parents that this reaction occurs most commonly with plasma infusions. Acetaminophen may relieve the patient's discomfort.
- Tell the patient that urticaria is the most common reaction to cryoprecipitate or plasma.
- Review the signs and symptoms of anaphylaxis: rapid or difficult breathing, wheezing, hoarseness, stridor, and chest tightness. Teach the patient to administer epinephrine and then to contact the physician immediately.
- Tell the patient or the parents to watch for early signs and symptoms of hepatitis: headache, fever, decreased appetite, nausea, vomiting, abdominal tenderness, and pain over the liver. Explain that patients who receive blood components risk hepatitis, which may appear 3 weeks to 6 months after treatment with blood components.
- Inform the patient that all donated blood and plasma are screened for antibodies to human immunodeficiency virus (HIV), which causes acquired immunodeficiency syndrome. Also, all freeze-dried products are heat-treated to kill HIV.
- For more information, refer the patient's family to the National Hemophilia Foundation.

Hodgkin disease

A neoplastic disorder, Hodgkin disease is characterized by painless, progressive enlargement of the lymph nodes, spleen, and other lymphoid tissue. This enlargement results from proliferation of lymphocytes, histiocytes, eosinophils, and Reed-Sternberg cells. The latter cells are the special histologic feature of the disease.

Hodgkin disease occurs in all races but is slightly more common in whites. Its incidence peaks in two age-groups—15 to 38 and after age 50. It occurs most commonly in young adults, except in Japan, where it occurs exclusively among people older than age 50. It has a higher incidence in males than in females. A family history of Hodgkin disease increases the likelihood of acquiring the disorder.

Untreated, Hodgkin disease follows a variable but relentlessly progressive and ultimately fatal course. However, recent advances in therapy make Hodgkin disease potentially curable, even in advanced stages. Appropriate treatment in the early stage yields a 5-year survival rate of about 90%.

Although the cause of Hodgkin disease is unknown, some studies point to genetic, viral, or environmental factors.

Ann Arbor staging system for Hodgkin disease

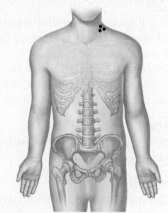

STAGE I

▶ Involvement of single lymph node region
OR
▶ Involvement of single extralymphatic site (stage I_E)

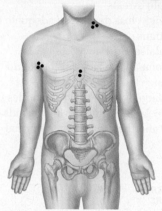

STAGE II

▶ Involvement of two or more lymph node regions on same side of diaphragm
▶ May include localized extralymphatic involvement on same side of diaphragm (stage II_E)

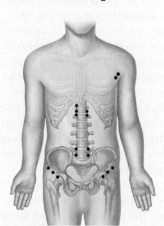

STAGE III

▶ Involvement of lymph node regions on both sides of diaphragm
▶ May include involvement of spleen (stage III_S) or localized extranodal disease (stage III_E)
▶ Hodgkin disease stage III_1: disease limited to upper abdomen—spleen, splenic hilar, celiac, or portohepatic nodes
▶ Hodgkin disease stage III_2: disease limited to lower abdomen—periaortic, pelvic, or inguinal node

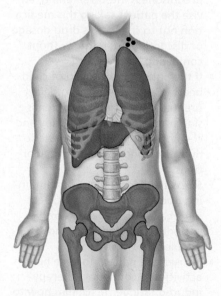

STAGE IV

▶ Diffuse extralymphatic disease (for example, in liver, bone marrow, lung, skin)

Signs and symptoms

▸ Painless swelling of one of the cervical lymph nodes or sometimes the axillary or inguinal lymph nodes
▸ A persistent fever
▸ Night sweats
▸ Weight loss despite an adequate diet
▸ Fatigue
▸ Malaise
▸ Edema of the face and neck and jaundice (advanced stages)
▸ Enlarged, rubbery lymph nodes in the neck (enlarging during periods of fever and then reverting to normal size)

Treatment

▸ Chemotherapy consisting of various drug combinations including:
– ABVD (doxorubicin [Adriamycin], bleomycin, vinblastine, and dacarbazine)
– MOPP protocol (mechlorethamine, vincristine [Oncovin], procarbazine, and prednisone)
▸ Concomitant administration of antiemetics, sedatives, and antidiarrheals to combat GI adverse effects

Stage I or II

▸ Radiation therapy alone or with chemotherapy (ABVD)

Stage III

▸ Chemotherapy with or without radiation

Stage IV

▸ Chemotherapy alone (sometimes inducing a complete remission)
▸ Chemotherapy and radiation therapy to involved sites (as an alternative)
▸ Autologous bone marrow transplantation or autologous peripheral blood sternal transfusions and immunotherapy (which by itself hasn't proved effective)

Nursing considerations

▸ Watch for complications during chemotherapy, including anorexia, nausea, vomiting, alopecia, and mouth ulcers.
▸ Provide a well-balanced, high-calorie, high-protein diet. If the patient is anorexic, provide frequent, small meals. Consult with the dietitian to incorporate foods the patient enjoys into his diet.
▸ Be alert for adverse effects of radiation therapy, such as hair loss, nausea, vomiting, and anorexia.
▸ Offer the patient ginger ale to alleviate nausea and vomiting.
▸ Perform comfort measures that promote relaxation. Provide for periods of rest if the patient tires easily. Administer pain medication as ordered, and monitor its effectiveness.
▸ Watch for the development of hypothyroidism, sterility, and a second neoplastic disease, including late-onset leukemia and non-Hodgkin lymphoma. Although these are complications of the treatments, they also indicate the success of treatment.
▸ Throughout therapy, listen to the patient's fears and concerns. Encourage him to express his feelings, and stay with him during periods of extreme stress and anxiety. Provide emotional support to the patient and his family.
▸ Involve the patient and his family in all aspects of his care.

LESSON PLANS

Teaching about Hodgkin disease

▸ Explain all procedures and treatments associated with the care plan.
▸ Because sudden withdrawal of prednisone is life-threatening, advise the patient taking this medication not to change his drug dosage or discontinue the drug without contacting his physician.
▸ If the patient is a woman of childbearing age, advise her to delay pregnancy until long-term remission occurs. Radiation therapy and chemotherapy can cause genetic mutations and spontaneous abortions.
▸ Stress the importance of maintaining good nutrition (aided by eating small, frequent meals of the patient's favorite foods) and drinking plenty of fluids.
▸ Instruct the patient to pace his activities to counteract therapy-induced fatigue. Teach him how to use relaxation techniques to promote comfort and reduce anxiety.
▸ Encourage smoking cessation or discontinuation of tobacco use, if appropriate. Provide information on available programs.

▸ Stress the importance of good oral hygiene to prevent stomatitis. To control pain and bleeding, teach the patient to use a soft toothbrush, a cotton swab, or an anesthetic mouthwash such as viscous lidocaine (as prescribed); to apply petroleum jelly to his lips; and to avoid astringent mouthwashes.
▸ Advise the patient to avoid crowds and any person with a known infection. Emphasize that he should notify the physician if he develops an infection.
▸ Because enlarged lymph nodes may indicate disease recurrence, teach the patient the importance of checking his lymph nodes.
▸ Make sure the patient understands the possible adverse effects of his treatments. Tell him to notify the physician if these signs and symptoms persist.
▸ When appropriate, refer the patient and his family members to community organizations, such as psychological counseling services, support groups, and hospices.
▸ Advise the patient to seek follow-up care after he has completed the initial treatment.

Iron deficiency anemia

Iron deficiency anemia is a common disease worldwide; it affects 10% to 30% of the adult population of the United States. It's most prevalent among premenopausal women, infants (particularly premature or low-birth-weight neonates), children (especially ages 1 to 3 whose diet primarily includes cow's milk), adolescents (especially girls), alcoholics, and elderly people (especially those who are unable to cook for themselves). The prognosis after replacement therapy is favorable.

Iron deficiency anemia stems from an inadequate supply of iron for optimal formation of red blood cells (RBCs), which produces smaller (microcytic) cells with less color on staining. Body stores of iron, including plasma iron, decrease, as does transferrin, which binds with and transports iron. Insufficient body stores of iron lead to a depleted RBC mass and, in turn, to a decreased hemoglobin level (hypochromia) and decreased oxygen-carrying capacity of the blood.

Causes of iron deficiency

▶ Inadequate dietary intake of iron (less than 2 mg/day), as in prolonged nonsupplemented breast- or bottle-feeding of infants (not eating solid foods after age 6 months); during periods of stress, such as rapid growth in children and adolescents; and in elderly patients existing on a poorly balanced diet
▶ Iron malabsorption, as in chronic diarrhea, partial or total gastrectomy, and malabsorption syndromes such as celiac disease
▶ Blood loss (a common cause in adults) secondary to drug-induced GI bleeding (from anticoagulants, aspirin, steroids) or due to heavy menses, hemorrhage from trauma, a GI ulcer, a malignant tumor, or varices
▶ Pregnancy, in which the mother's iron supply is diverted to the fetus for erythropoiesis

▶ Intravascular hemolysis-induced hemoglobinuria or paroxysmal nocturnal hemoglobinuria
▶ Mechanical erythrocyte trauma caused by a prosthetic heart valve or vena cava filter

Iron absorption and storage

Iron is essential to erythropoiesis and is abundant throughout the body. Two-thirds of total body iron is found in hemoglobin; the other third, mostly in the reticuloendothelial system (liver, spleen, and bone marrow), with small amounts in muscle, serum, and body cells.

Adequate dietary ingestion of iron and recirculation of iron released from disintegrating red cells maintain iron supplies. The duodenum and upper part of the small intestine absorb dietary iron. Such absorption depends on gastric acid content, the amount of reducing substances (ascorbic acid, for example) present in the gastrointestinal tract, and dietary iron intake. If iron intake is deficient, the body gradually depletes its iron stores, causing a decreased hemoglobin level and, eventually, signs and symptoms of iron deficiency anemia.

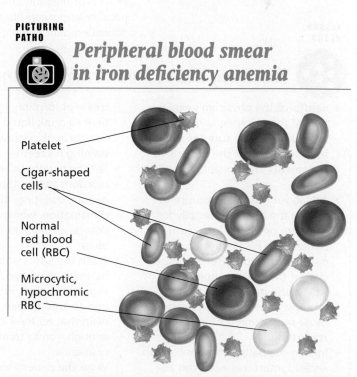

PICTURING PATHO

Peripheral blood smear in iron deficiency anemia

Platelet

Cigar-shaped cells

Normal red blood cell (RBC)

Microcytic, hypochromic RBC

Signs and symptoms

▶ Fatigue
▶ Inability to concentrate
▶ Headache
▶ Shortness of breath (especially on exertion)
▶ Increased frequency of infections
▶ Pica (an uncontrollable urge to eat strange substances, such as clay, starch, ice and, in children, lead)
▶ History of menorrhagia
▶ Dysphagia
▶ Vasomotor disturbances
▶ Numbness and tingling of the extremities
▶ Neuralgic pain
▶ Red, swollen, smooth, shiny, and tender tongue (with glossitis)
▶ Corners of the mouth may be eroded, tender, and swollen (with angular stomatitis)
▶ Spoon-shaped, brittle nails
▶ Tachycardia, increased cardiac output, and oxygen saturation level that may be below 90% (with severe iron deficiency anemia)

Treatment

▶ Iron replacement that includes an oral preparation of iron or a combination of iron and ascorbic acid (which enhances iron absorption)
▶ Parenterally administered iron (in some cases)
▶ Total-dose I.V. infusions of supplemental iron, for pregnant and elderly patients with severe iron deficiency anemia

Nursing considerations

▶ Note signs or symptoms of decreased perfusion to vital organs (dyspnea, chest pain, dizziness) and signs of neuropathy, such as tingling in the periphery. Provide oxygen therapy, as needed, to help prevent and reduce hypoxia.
▶ Assess the family's dietary habits for iron intake, noting the influence of childhood eating patterns, cultural food preferences, and family income on adequate nutrition.
▶ Because a sore mouth and tongue make eating painful, ask the dietitian to give the patient nonirritating foods. Provide diluted mouthwash or, in especially severe conditions, swab the patient's mouth with tap water or

warm saline solution. An oral anesthetic diluted in saline solution can also be used.
▶ Administer an analgesic for headache and other discomfort, as ordered, and monitor its effectiveness.
▶ Evaluate the patient's drug history. Certain drugs, such as pancreatic enzymes and vitamin E, can interfere with iron metabolism and absorption; aspirin, steroids, and other drugs can cause GI bleeding.
▶ Provide frequent rest periods to decrease physical exhaustion.
▶ The patient should receive total-dose I.V. infusions of iron dextran in normal saline solution over 8 hours. To minimize the risk of an allergic reaction to iron, an I.V. test dose of 0.5 ml should be given first.
▶ Use the Z-track injection method when administering iron I.M. to prevent skin discoloration, scarring, and irritating iron deposits in the skin.
▶ Monitor the patient for iron replacement overdose.
▶ Provide good nutrition and meticulous care of I.V. sites, such as those used for blood transfusions, to help prevent infection.
▶ Monitor the patient's compliance with the prescribed iron supplement therapy.

LESSON
PLANS

Teaching about iron deficiency anemia

▶ Reinforce the physician's explanation of the disorder, and answer any questions. Be sure the patient fully understands the prescribed treatments and possible complications.
▶ Ask about possible exposure to lead in the home (especially for children) or on the job. Teach the patient and his family about the dangers of lead poisoning, especially if the patient reports pica.
▶ Advise the patient not to stop therapy, even if he feels better, because replacement of iron stores takes time.
▶ Inform the patient that milk or an antacid interferes with iron absorption but that vitamin C can in-

crease absorption. Instruct the patient to drink liquid supplemental iron through a straw to avoid staining his teeth.
▶ Tell the patient to report adverse reactions to iron therapy, such as nausea, vomiting, diarrhea, and constipation, which may require a dosage adjustment or a stool softener.
▶ Teach the basics of a nutritionally balanced diet—red meats, green vegetables, eggs, whole wheat, iron-fortified bread, and milk. Explain that no food in itself contains enough iron to treat iron deficiency anemia.
▶ Warn the patient to guard against infections because his weakened

condition may increase his susceptibility to them. Stress the importance of meticulous wound care, periodic dental checkups, good hand-washing techniques, and other measures to prevent infection. Also tell the patient to report any signs of infection, including temperature elevation and chills.
▶ Because an iron deficiency may recur, explain the need for regular checkups and to comply with prescribed treatments.
▶ Inform the patient that his hemoglobin level should rise after taking oral iron supplements for 1 month and if it doesn't, reassessment is indicated.

Multiple myeloma

Multiple myeloma is a disseminated neoplasm of marrow plasma cells. It's also called *malignant plasmacytoma, plasma cell myeloma,* and *myelomatosis.* The disease infiltrates bone to produce osteolytic lesions throughout the skeleton (flat bones, vertebrae, skull, pelvis, and ribs). In late stages, it infiltrates the body organs as well (liver, spleen, lymph nodes, lungs, adrenal glands, kidneys, skin, and GI tract).

Multiple myeloma strikes mostly males older than age 40. It usually carries a poor prognosis because by the time it's diagnosed, it has already infiltrated the vertebrae, pelvis, skull, ribs, clavicles, and sternum. By then, skeletal destruction is widespread and, without treatment, leads to vertebral collapse. The average 5-year survival rate is 35%. If the disease is diagnosed early, treatment can often prolong life by 3 to 5 years.

Although the cause of multiple myeloma isn't known, genetic factors and occupational exposure to radiation have been linked to the disease.

Signs and symptoms
▶ Severe, constant back pain, which may increase with exercise
▶ Aches, joint swelling, and tenderness
▶ Numbness, prickling, and tingling of the extremities (with peripheral paresthesia)
▶ Pain on movement or weight bearing, especially in the thoracic and lumbar vertebrae

Treatment
▶ Chemotherapy (combinations of melphalan and prednisone thalidomide, lanalidomide, bortezomib, or cyclophosphamide and prednisone) to suppress plasma cell growth and control pain
▶ Adjuvant local radiation
▶ Bone marrow transplantation
▶ Analgesics (for pain)

Bone marrow aspirate in multiple myeloma

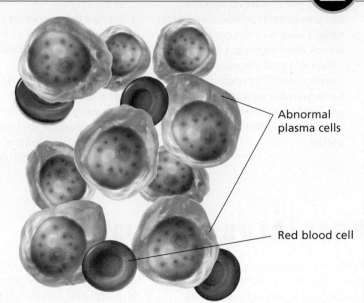

Abnormal plasma cells

Red blood cell

▶ Laminectomy (for vertebral compression)
▶ Dialysis (for renal complications)
▶ Hydration, diuretics, corticosteroids, oral phosphate, and gallium I.V. to decrease serum calcium levels to control hypercalcemia
▶ Plasmapheresis to remove the M protein from blood and return the cells to the patient (provides only temporary effect)

Nursing considerations
▶ Encourage the patient to drink 3,000 to 4,000 ml of fluids daily, particularly before excretory urography. Monitor fluid intake and output, which shouldn't fall below 1,500 ml.
▶ Administer ordered analgesics for pain as needed. Provide comfort measures, such as repositioning and relaxation techniques.
▶ During chemotherapy, watch for complications, such as fever and malaise, which may signal the onset of infection. Also watch for signs of other problems, such as severe anemia and fractures.

▶ If the patient is taking prednisone, closely watch for signs of infection, which this drug masks.
▶ After laminectomy, try to get the patient out of bed within 24 hours, if possible, and encourage him to walk; these patients are particularly vulnerable to pathologic fractures.
▶ If the patient is bedridden, change his position every 2 hours. Provide passive range-of-motion and deep-breathing exercises; promote active exercises when he can tolerate them.
▶ Check for hemorrhage, motor or sensory deficits, and loss of bowel or bladder function. Position the patient as ordered, maintain alignment, and logroll him when turning.
▶ Involve the patient and his family in decisions about his care whenever possible.

Teaching about multiple myeloma

▶ Reinforce the physician's explanation of the disease, diagnostic tests, treatment options, and prognosis. Make sure the patient understands what to expect from the treatment and diagnostic tests (including painful procedures, such as bone marrow aspiration and biopsy). Tell him to notify the physician if the adverse effects of treatment persist.

▶ Prepare the patient for the effects of surgery.
▶ Explain the procedures the patient will undergo, such as insertion of an I.V. line and an indwelling urinary catheter.
▶ Emphasize the importance of deep breathing and changing his position every 2 hours after surgery.
▶ Tell the patient to dress appropriately because multiple myeloma may make him particularly sensitive to the cold.

▶ Caution the patient to wash his hands frequently and protect himself from infections because chemotherapy diminishes the body's natural resistance to infection.
▶ If appropriate, direct the patient and family to community resources, such as the American Cancer Society or the Multiple Myeloma Research Foundation, for support.

Pernicious anemia

Pernicious anemia is a megaloblastic anemia characterized by decreased gastric production of hydrochloric acid and deficiency of intrinsic factor, a substance normally secreted by the parietal cells of the gastric mucosa that's essential for vitamin B_{12} absorption in the small bowel. The resulting deficiency of vitamin B_{12} causes serious neurologic, psychological, gastric, and intestinal abnormalities. Increasingly fragile cell membranes induce widespread destruction of red blood cells (RBCs), resulting in a low hemoglobin level.

Familial incidence of pernicious anemia suggests a genetic predisposition. This disorder is significantly more common among patients with immunologically related diseases, such as thyroiditis, myxedema, and Graves' disease.

An inherited autoimmune response may cause gastric mucosal atrophy and, consequently, decreases hydrochloric acid and intrinsic factor production. Intrinsic factor deficiency impairs vitamin B_{12} absorption. The resultant vitamin B_{12} deficiency inhibits the growth of all cells, particularly RBCs, leading to insufficient and deformed RBCs with poor oxygen-carrying capacity.

Pernicious anemia also impairs myelin formation. Initially, it affects the peripheral nerves, but gradually it extends to the spinal cord, causing neurologic dysfunction.

Secondary pernicious anemia can result from partial removal of the stomach, which limits the amount of productive mucosa.

PICTURING PATHO

Peripheral blood smear in pernicious anemia

Platelet

Hypersegmented polymorphonuclear neutrophil

Macrocytic red blood cell (RBC)

Normal RBC

Signs and symptoms

◗ Weakness
◗ A beefy red, smooth tongue
◗ Numbness and tingling in the extremities
◗ Nausea
◗ Vomiting
◗ Anorexia and weight loss
◗ Flatulence
◗ Diarrhea
◗ Constipation
◗ Slightly jaundiced sclera and pale to bright yellow skin (with hemolysis-induced hyperbilirubinemia)
◗ Rapid pulse rate
◗ Systolic murmur
◗ Enlarged liver and spleen
◗ Irritability
◗ Depression
◗ Delirium
◗ Ataxia
◗ Memory loss
◗ Positive Babinski's and Romberg's signs
◗ Optic muscle atrophy

Treatment

◗ Early I.M. vitamin B_{12} replacement to reverse disorder and help prevent permanent neurologic damage
◗ An initial high dose of parenteral vitamin B_{12} that causes rapid RBC regeneration increasing hemoglobin levels to normal within 2 weeks
◗ Concomitant iron replacement to prevent iron deficiency anemia (necessary because rapid cell regeneration increases the patient's iron requirements)
◗ Oral vitamin B_{12} therapy, especially if the patient is a strict vegetarian
◗ Bed rest (until hemoglobin levels increase)
◗ Blood transfusion and a cardiac glycoside (for severe anemia and cardiopulmonary distress)
◗ A diuretic and low-sodium diet (for heart failure)
◗ An antibiotic (for infection)
◗ A topical anesthetic (for mouth pain)

Nursing considerations

◗ If the patient has severe anemia, plan activities, rest periods, and necessary diagnostic tests to conserve his energy. Monitor pulse rate often; tachycardia indicates that his activities are too strenuous.
◗ Advise the patient to report signs and symptoms of decreased perfusion to vital organs (dyspnea, chest pain, dizziness) and symptoms of neuropathy, such as tingling in his arms or legs.
◗ To ensure accurate Schilling test results, make sure that all urine excreted over a 24-hour period is collected and that the specimens remain uncontaminated by bacteria.
◗ Provide a well-balanced diet, including foods high in vitamin B_{12} (meat, liver, fish, eggs, and milk).
◗ Because the mouth and tongue may become sore and make eating painful, ask the dietitian to avoid giving the patient irritating foods. Provide diluted mouthwash or, with severe conditions, swab the patient's mouth with tap water or warm saline solution. An oral anesthetic diluted in normal saline solution may also be used.
◗ If the patient is incontinent, establish a regular bowel and bladder routine. After the patient is discharged, a visiting nurse should follow up on this schedule and make adjustments as needed.
◗ After the patient's condition improves, decrease vitamin B_{12} doses to maintenance levels and give monthly. Because such injections must be continued for life, teach the patient about self-administration.
◗ If neurologic damage causes behavioral problems, assess mental and neurologic status often; if necessary, give a tranquilizer as ordered, and if needed, apply a soft restraint at night.
◗ Institute safety precautions to prevent falls.

LESSON PLANS

Teaching about pernicious anemia

◗ Warn the patient to guard against infections, and tell him to report signs of infection promptly, especially pulmonary and urinary tract infections, because the patient's weakened condition may increase susceptibility.
◗ Caution the patient with a sensory deficit to avoid exposure to extreme heat or cold on the extremities.
◗ If neurologic involvement is present, advise the patient to avoid clothing with small buttons and activities of daily living that require fine motor skills.
◗ Stress that vitamin B_{12} replacement isn't a permanent cure and that these supplements must be continued for life, even after symptoms subside.

◗ If needed, teach the patient or his caregiver proper injection or nasal administration techniques.
◗ Teach family members to observe for confusion and irritability and to report these findings to the physician.
◗ If the patient has had extensive gastric resection or follows a strict vegetarian diet, emphasize the importance of vitamin B_{12} supplements to prevent pernicious anemia.

Polycythemia vera

Polycythemia vera (also known as *primary polycythemia, erythema, polycythemia rubra vera, splenomegalic polycythemia,* and *Vaquez-Osler disease*) is a chronic myeloproliferative disorder. It's characterized by increased red blood cell (RBC) mass, leukocytosis, thrombocytosis, and an increased hemoglobin level, with a normal or decreased plasma volume. It usually occurs between ages 40 and 60, most commonly among men of Jewish ancestry. It seldom affects children or blacks and doesn't appear to be familial.

The onset of polycythemia is gradual, and the disease runs a chronic but slowly progressive course. The prognosis depends on age at diagnosis, treatment used, and complications. Mortality is high if polycythemia is untreated or is associated with leukemia or myeloid metaplasia.

For patients with polycythemia vera, uncontrolled and rapid cellular reproduction and maturation cause proliferation or hyperplasia of all bone marrow cells (panmyelosis). The cause of such uncontrolled cellular activity is unknown, but it's probably the result of a multipotential stem cell defect.

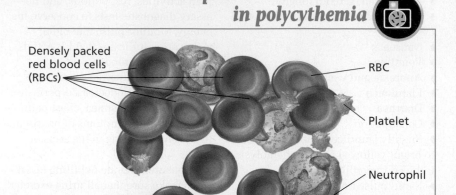

PICTURING PATHO

Peripheral blood smear in polycythemia

Densely packed red blood cells (RBCs)

RBC

Platelet

Neutrophil

Signs and symptoms

▶ In early stages, possibly no signs or symptoms
▶ Fullness in the head
▶ Rushing in the ears
▶ Tinnitus
▶ Headache
▶ Dizziness
▶ Vertigo
▶ Epistaxis
▶ Night sweats
▶ Epigastric and joint pain
▶ Scotomas, double vision, and blurred vision
▶ Decreased urine output
▶ Pruritus (which worsens after bathing and may be disabling)
▶ A sense of abdominal fullness

▶ Pleuritic chest pain or left-upper-quadrant pain

Treatment

▶ Phlebotomy therapy to promptly reduce RBC mass (Typically, 350 to 500 ml of blood can be removed every other day until the patient's hematocrit is reduced to the low-normal range. The goal is to keep the hematocrit below 45%.)
▶ Myelosuppressive therapy (for patients with severe symptoms, such as extreme thrombocytosis, a rapidly enlarging spleen, or hypermetabolism)
▶ Radioactive phosphorus (^{32}P) or a chemotherapeutic agent, such as melphalan, busulfan, or chlorambucil, to control the disease (in most cases)
▶ Pheresis technology that allows removal of RBCs, white blood cells, and platelets individually or collectively (cellular components given to blood banks)
▶ Administration of cyproheptadine and allopurinol to reduce the serum uric acid level

Nursing considerations

▶ Keep the patient active and ambulatory to prevent thrombosis. If bed rest is necessary, prescribe a daily program of both active and passive range-of-motion exercises.
▶ Watch for complications, such as hypervolemia, thrombocytosis, signs and symptoms of impending stroke (decreased sensation, numbness, transitory paralysis, fleeting blindness, headache, and epistaxis), hypertension, and heart failure (caused by prolonged hyperviscosity).
▶ Regularly examine the patient for bleeding.
▶ To compensate for increased uric acid production, give the patient additional fluids (at least 3,000 ml/day), administer allopurinol as ordered, and alkalinize the urine to prevent uric acid calculus formation.
▶ If the patient has symptomatic splenomegaly, suggest or provide small, frequent meals followed by a rest period to prevent nausea and vomiting.

Common clinical features of polycythemia vera

Signs and symptoms	Causes
Eye and ear	
▶ Vision disturbances (blurring, diplopia, scotoma, engorged veins of fundus and retina) and congestion of conjunctiva, retina, and retinal veins	▶ Hypervolemia and hyperviscosity ▶ Engorgement of capillary beds
Nose and mouth	
▶ Epistaxis or gingival bleeding ▶ Oral mucous membrane congestion	▶ Hypervolemia and hyperviscosity ▶ Engorgement of capillary beds
Central nervous system	
▶ Headache or fullness in the head, lethargy, weakness, fatigue, syncope, dizziness, vertigo, tinnitus, paresthesia of digits, and impaired mentation	▶ Hypervolemia and hyperviscosity
Cardiovascular system	
▶ Hypertension ▶ Intermittent claudication, thrombosis and emboli, angina, thrombophlebitis ▶ Hemorrhage	▶ Hypervolemia and hyperviscosity ▶ Hypervolemia, thrombocytosis, and vascular disease ▶ Engorgement of capillary beds
Skin	
▶ Pruritus (especially after hot bath) ▶ Urticaria ▶ Ruddy cyanosis ▶ Night sweats ▶ Ecchymosis	▶ Basophilia (secondary histamine release) ▶ Altered histamine metabolism ▶ Hypervolemia and hyperviscosity from congested vessels, an increased oxyhemoglobin level, and a decreased hemoglobin level ▶ Hypermetabolism ▶ Hemorrhage
GI system	
▶ Epigastric distress ▶ Early satiety and fullness ▶ Peptic ulcer pain ▶ Hepatosplenomegaly ▶ Weight loss	▶ Hypervolemia and hyperviscosity ▶ Hepatosplenomegaly ▶ Gastric thrombosis and hemorrhage ▶ Congestion, extramedullary hematopoiesis, and myeloid metaplasia ▶ Hypermetabolism
Respiratory system	
▶ Dyspnea	▶ Hypervolemia and hyperviscosity
Musculoskeletal system	
▶ Arthralgia	▶ Increased urate production secondary to nucleoprotein turnover

▶ If the patient has pruritus, give medications as ordered, and provide distractions to help him cope.

▶ Report acute abdominal pain immediately; it may signal splenic infarction, renal calculus formation, or abdominal thrombosis.

▶ Before phlebotomy, check the patient's blood pressure and pulse and respiratory rates. Stay alert for tachycardia, clamminess, and complaints of vertigo. If any of these occurs, the procedure should be stopped.

▶ Immediately after phlebotomy, check the patient's blood pressure and pulse rate. Have the patient sit up for about 5 minutes before allowing him to walk; this prevents vasovagal attack and orthostatic hypotension. Administer 24 oz (710 ml) of juice or water, or I.V. fluids if indicated, to replenish fluid volume.

Teaching about polycythemia vera

- Determine what the patient knows about the disease, especially if he has been diagnosed for some time. As necessary, reinforce the practitioner's explanation of the disease, its signs and symptoms, and prescribed treatment.
- Tell the patient to remain as active as possible to help maintain his self-esteem.
- Instruct the patient to use an electric razor to prevent accidental cuts and to keep his environment free from clutter to minimize falls and contusions.
- Advise the patient to avoid high altitudes, which may exacerbate polycythemia.

- If the patient develops thrombocytopenia, tell him the most common bleeding sites (such as the nose, gingiva, and skin) so he can check for bleeding. Advise him to promptly report any abnormal bleeding.
- If the patient requires phlebotomy, describe the procedure and explain that it will relieve distressing symptoms. Tell the patient to watch for and report any signs or symptoms of iron deficiency (pallor, weight loss, asthenia, glossitis).
- If the patient requires myelosuppressive therapy, tell him about adverse effects (nausea, vomiting, and susceptibility to infection) that may follow administration of an alkylating agent. As appropriate, mention that alopecia may follow

use of busulfan, cyclophosphamide, or uracil mustard and that sterile hemorrhagic cystitis may follow use of cyclophosphamide. (Ensuring that the patient takes in plenty of fluids can prevent this adverse effect.)
- If an outpatient develops leukopenia, reinforce instructions about preventing infection. Warn the patient that his resistance to infection is low; advise him to avoid crowds, and make sure he knows the symptoms of infection.
- If the patient requires treatment with ^{32}P, explain the procedure. Tell him that he may require repeated phlebotomies until ^{32}P takes effect.
- Refer the patient to the social service department and local home health care agencies, as appropriate.

Sickle cell anemia

Sickle cell anemia is a congenital hemolytic disease that results from a defective hemoglobin molecule (hemoglobin S) that causes red blood cells (RBCs) to become sickle shaped. Such cells impair circulation, resulting in chronic ill health (fatigue, dyspnea on exertion, swollen joints), periodic crises, long-term complications, and premature death.

Sickle cell anemia results from homozygous inheritance of the hemoglobin S–producing gene. Heterozygous inheritance of this gene results in the sickle cell trait, a condition with minimal or no symptoms. The patient with the sickle cell trait is a carrier, which can be passed to offspring.

For patients with sickle cell anemia, the abnormal hemoglobin S found in RBCs becomes insoluble whenever hypoxia occurs. As a result, these RBCs become rigid, rough, and elongated, forming a crescent or sickle shape. Such sickling can produce hemolysis (cell destruction).

PICTURING
PATHO

Comparing normal and sickled red blood cells

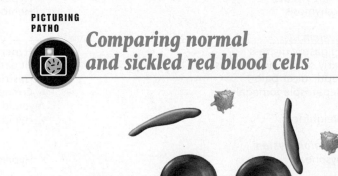

Normal red blood cell

Sickled cell

Each person with sickle cell anemia has a different hypoxic threshold and different factors that precipitate a sickle cell crisis. Illness, cold exposure, hypoxia, and stress are known to precipitate sickling crises in most people.

In addition, these altered cells accumulate in capillaries and smaller blood vessels, making the blood more viscous. Normal circulation is impaired, causing pain, tissue infarctions, and swelling. Such blockage causes anoxic changes that lead to further sickling and obstruction.

Signs and symptoms
▶ Developing after age 6 months
▶ Chronic fatigue
▶ Unexplained dyspnea with or without exertion
▶ Joint swelling
▶ Aching bones
▶ Chest pain
▶ Ischemic leg ulcers (especially around the ankles)
▶ An increased susceptibility to infection
▶ History of pulmonary infarctions and cardiomegaly
▶ Jaundice or pallor
▶ Small-for-age appearance (in a young child); growth and puberty delays (in an older child)
▶ Spiderlike body build—narrow shoulders and hips, long extremities, curved spine, and barrel chest (in an adult)
▶ Tachycardia
▶ Hepatomegaly
▶ Systolic and diastolic murmurs
▶ Avascular necrosis

Sickle cell crisis
▶ History of recent infection, stress, dehydration, or other conditions that provoke hypoxia, such as exposure to strenuous exercise, high altitude, unpressurized aircraft, cold, or vasoconstrictive drugs
▶ Sleepiness with difficulty awakening
▶ Severe pain
▶ Hematuria
▶ Pale lips, tongue, palms, and nail beds; lethargy; listlessness; and, commonly, irritability
▶ Body temperature over 104° F (40° C) or a temperature of 100° F (37.8° C) that persists for 2 days or longer

Treatment
▶ Polyvalent pneumococcal and *Haemophilus influenzae* B vaccines; an anti-infective, such as low-dose oral penicillin; and a chelating agent, such as deferoxamine, to minimize complications resulting from the disease and from transfusion therapy
▶ Analgesics (for pain of vaso-occlusive crisis)
▶ Iron supplements (for decreased folic acid levels)
▶ Hydroxyurea to increase hemoglobin level
▶ Prophylactic penicillin (beginning before age 4 months)
▶ Transfusion of packed RBCs, which is the mainstay of treatment for children to decrease stroke risk
▶ Hematopoietic cell transplantation using sibling donors (has curative potential)

Acute sequestration crisis
▶ Sedation and administration of an analgesic
▶ Blood transfusion
▶ Oxygen therapy
▶ Large amounts of oral or I.V. fluids

PICTURING PATHO

What happens in sickle cell crisis

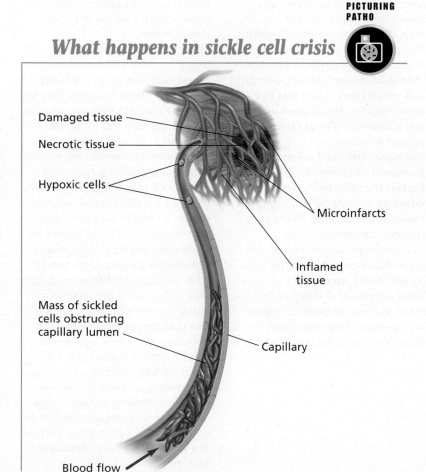

Damaged tissue

Necrotic tissue

Hypoxic cells

Microinfarcts

Inflamed tissue

Mass of sickled cells obstructing capillary lumen

Capillary

Blood flow

Nursing considerations

▶ Encourage the patient to talk about his fears and concerns. Remain with him during periods of severe crisis and anxiety.

▶ If a male patient develops sudden, painful priapism, reassure him that episodes lasting 1 to 2 hours are common and have no permanent harmful effects. However, an episode that lasts more than 3 hours is a medical emergency, and the patient should receive prompt medical treatment.

▶ Make sure that the patient receives adequate amounts of folic acid–rich foods such as leafy, green vegetables. Encourage adequate fluid intake to hydrate the patient; give parenteral fluids, if needed.

▶ Apply warm compresses, warmed thermal blankets, and warming pads or mattresses to painful areas of the patient's body.

▶ Administer an analgesic and an antipyretic as needed. Each patient's level of pain is different.

▶ When cultures demonstrate the presence of infection, administer an antibiotic as ordered.

▶ Encourage bed rest with the head of the bed elevated to decrease tissue oxygen demand. Administer oxygen only if the patient is experiencing severe dyspnea.

▶ Administer blood transfusions as ordered.

▶ If the patient requires general anesthesia for surgery, help ensure that he receives adequate ventilation to prevent hypoxic crisis. Make sure the surgeon and the anesthesiologist are aware that the patient has sickle cell anemia, and provide a preoperative transfusion of packed RBCs as needed.

LESSON PLANS

Teaching about sickle cell anemia

▶ To help prevent exacerbation of sickle cell anemia, advise the patient to avoid tight clothing that restricts circulation.

▶ Warn against strenuous exercise, vasoconstricting medications, cold temperatures (including drinking large amounts of ice water and swimming), unpressurized aircraft, high altitude, and other conditions that provoke hypoxia.

▶ Stress the importance of standard childhood immunizations, meticulous wound care, good oral hygiene, regular dental checkups, and a balanced diet as safeguards against infection.

▶ Emphasize the need for prompt treatment of infection.

▶ Explain the need to increase fluid intake to prevent dehydration that results from impaired ability to properly concentrate urine.

▶ To encourage normal mental and social development, warn parents against being overprotective.

▶ Refer parents of children with sickle cell anemia for genetic counseling to answer their questions about the risk to future offspring.

▶ Because delayed growth and late puberty are common, reassure an adolescent patient that he will grow and mature.

▶ Review the symptoms of vaso-occlusive crisis so that the patient and his family will recognize and treat it early. As appropriate, explain how to care for this condition at home.

▶ Inform the patient and his parents that if he must be hospitalized for a vaso-occlusive crisis, I.V. fluids and a parenteral analgesic may be administered. He may also receive oxygen therapy and blood transfusions.

▶ If appropriate, discuss how special conditions, such as surgery and pregnancy, may affect the patient.

▶ Stress to the patient the need to inform all health care providers that he has this disease before he undergoes any treatment, especially major surgery. Urge him to wear medical identification stating that he has sickle cell anemia.

▶ Warn women with sickle cell anemia that they are poor obstetric risks. However, their use of oral contraceptives is also risky; refer them for birth control counseling.

▶ If necessary, arrange for psychological counseling to help the patient cope. Suggest that he join an appropriate support group such as the Sickle Cell Disease Association of America.

Thalassemia

Thalassemia, a group of hereditary hemolytic anemias, is characterized by defective synthesis in one or more of the polypeptide chains necessary for hemoglobin production. Because thalassemia affects hemoglobin production, it also impairs red blood cell (RBC) synthesis.

The most severe form of alpha-thalassemia—hydrops fetalis—results in severe anemia and heart failure. The fetus is stillborn or dies shortly after birth. Genetic counseling and prenatal testing can be performed to detect the condition and to help guide pregnancy planning.

Beta-thalassemia (the most common form of this disorder) occurs in three clinical forms: thalassemia major, intermedia, and minor. The severity of the resulting anemia depends on whether the patient is homozygous or heterozygous for the thalassemic trait. The prognosis for patients with beta-thalassemia varies. Patients with thalassemia major seldom survive to adulthood, unless there's strict adherence to the therapeutic regimen throughout childhood and early adulthood; children with thalassemia intermedia develop normally into adulthood, although puberty is usually delayed; and patients with thalassemia minor can expect a normal life span.

Signs and symptoms

Thalassemia major

▶ Severe anemia, bone abnormalities, failure to thrive, and life-threatening complications (in infants)
▶ Pallor and yellow skin and scleras (first signs at ages 3 to 6 months)
▶ Abdominal enlargement (with splenomegaly or hepatomegaly)

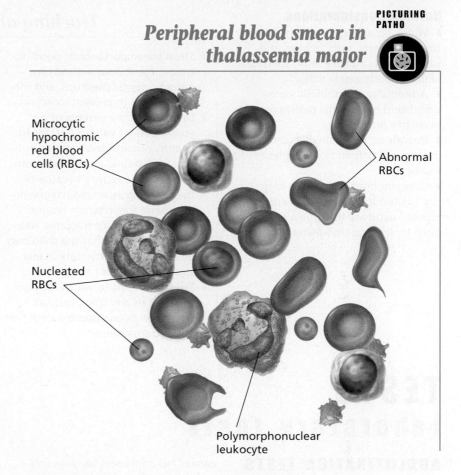

PICTURING PATHO

Peripheral blood smear in thalassemia major

Microcytic hypochromic red blood cells (RBCs)

Abnormal RBCs

Nucleated RBCs

Polymorphonuclear leukocyte

▶ Frequent infections
▶ Bleeding tendencies (especially toward epistaxis)
▶ Anorexia
▶ Small body and large head
▶ Mental disability
▶ Mongoloid features (due to bone marrow hyperactivity that thickens bone at the base of the nose)

Thalassemia intermedia

▶ Some degree of anemia
▶ Jaundice
▶ Splenomegaly

Thalassemia minor

▶ Mild anemia
▶ Usually producing no signs or symptoms; commonly overlooked

Treatment

▶ Antibiotics (for infection)
▶ Folic acid supplement to help maintain folic acid level
▶ Transfusions of packed RBCs to raise hemoglobin level
▶ Continuous subcutaneous infusions of deferoxamine, a chelating agent, to help eliminate excess iron from the body

For children

▶ Regular blood transfusions to minimize physical and mental retardation (but can cause increased risk of deadly hemosiderosis and iron overload)
▶ Continuous subcutaneous infusion of an iron-chelating agent to help produce a negative overall iron balance
▶ Splenectomy (if rapid splenic sequestration of transfused RBCs necessitates more transfusions)

Nursing considerations

▶ Watch for adverse reactions (shaking chills, fever, rash, itching, and hives) during and after RBC transfusions for thalassemia major.
▶ Administer an antibiotic, as ordered, and observe the patient for adverse reactions.
▶ Provide an adequate diet, and encourage the patient to drink plenty of fluids.
▶ Give emotional support to help the patient and his family cope with the chronic nature of the illness and the need for lifelong transfusions.

Teaching about thalassemia

▶ Stress the importance of good nutrition, meticulous wound care, periodic dental checkups, and other measures to prevent infection.
▶ Discuss with the parents of a young patient various options for healthy physical and creative outlets. Such a child must avoid strenuous athletic activity because of the resulting increased oxygen demand and the inherent tendency toward pathologic fractures. Reassure the parents that the child may be allowed to participate in less stressful activities.
▶ Tell the parents to watch for signs of hepatitis and iron overload, which are always possible with frequent transfusions.

▶ Teach the child and parents how to administer deferoxamine infusions.
▶ Refer the parents of a child with thalassemia for genetic counseling if they have concerns or questions about the vulnerability of future offspring to this disorder. Also refer adult patients with thalassemia for genetic counseling; they need to recognize the risk of transmitting thalassemia major to their children if they have a child with another person who has thalassemia. If they choose to have children, all their children should be evaluated for thalassemia by age 1.
▶ Be sure to tell patients with thalassemia minor that their condition is benign.

TESTS
Laboratory tests

AGGLUTINATION TESTS

The following tests are used to evaluate the ability of the blood's formed elements to react to foreign substances by clumping together:

▶ *ABO blood typing* helps to prevent lethal transfusion reactions. It types blood into A, B, AB, and O groups, according to the presence of major antigens A and B on red blood cell (RBC) surfaces and according to serum antibodies anti-A and anti-B.
▶ *Antibody screening test (indirect Coombs' test),* a two-step test, detects the presence of immunoglobulin (Ig) G antibodies on RBCs in recipient or donor serum before transfusion.
▶ *Crossmatching* establishes the compatibility or incompatibility of donor and recipient blood before transfusion.
▶ *Direct antiglobulin test (direct Coombs' test)* demonstrates the presence of IgG antibodies (such as antibodies to Rh factor), complement, or both on the surface of circulating RBCs. It's used to diagnose hemolytic disease of the neonate and aids in differential diagnosis of hemolytic anemias.
▶ *Leukoagglutinin test* differentiates between transfusion reactions by detecting antibodies that react with white blood cells (WBCs).
▶ *Rh typing* classifies blood by the presence or absence of the $Rh_0(D)$ antigen on the surface of RBCs to ensure compatibility of transfused blood.

BLOOD COMPOSITION TESTS

▶ *Complete blood count* is used to determine the number of blood elements in relation to volume and to quantify abnormalities (RBCs, WBCs, and platelets).

▶ *Peripheral blood smear* shows maturity and morphologic characteristics of blood elements and determines qualitative abnormalities.

COAGULATION TESTS

▶ *Activated partial thromboplastin time* is used to evaluate intrinsic pathway clotting factors. It helps in preoperative screening for bleeding tendencies and aids in monitoring heparin therapy.
▶ *Antithrombin III test* helps to determine the cause of impaired coagulation, especially hypercoagulation. Antithrombin III levels are decreased in clotting disorders, such as disseminated intravascular coagulation (DIC), and may be increased during therapy with oral anticoagulants.

▶ *Bleeding time (Ivy bleeding time)* is used to assess the platelets' capacity to stop bleeding in capillaries and small vessels by measuring the duration of bleeding after a standard skin incision. Used along with the platelet count, it can help to detect the presence of such disorders as von Willebrand's disease, DIC, severe hepatic or renal disease, and hemolytic disease of the neonate.

▶ *Capillary fragility test* is used to measure the capillaries' ability to remain intact under increasing intracapillary pressure. It can help detect thrombocytopenia, DIC, polycythemia vera, and von Willebrand's disease.

▶ *D-dimer test* measures a specific fibrin monomer fragment of fibin degradation procucts (FDPs) to determine whether FDPs are caused by normal mechanisms or by excessive fibrinolysis. The fibrin monomer fragments are present in severe clotting disorders such as DIC.

▶ *Factor VIII assay* identifies the quantity of this factor, which commonly is reduced in hemophilia.

▶ *Fibrin degradation products (fibrin split products)* show the amount of clot breakdown products in serum. Although FDPs are normally cleared rapidly, the FDP level is elevated in patients with clotting disorders such as DIC.

▶ *One-stage factor assays: Extrinsic coagulation system* helps to detect a deficiency of factor II, V, or X when prothrombin time (PT) and partial thromboplastin time (PTT) are prolonged. The *intrinsic coagulation system* helps to identify a deficiency of factor VIII, IX, or XII when PT is normal and PTT is abnormal.

▶ *Plasma fibrinogen test* is used to determine the amount of fibrinogen (factor I) available in plasma to help form fibrin clots. Fibrinogen levels are decreased in patients with hepatic failure and DIC but increased in those with hepatic cirrhosis and some lymphoproliferative disorders such as lymphoma.

▶ *Plasma thrombin time (thrombin clotting time),* which measures how quickly a clot forms, detects abnormalities in thrombin fibrinogen reaction. It helps to identify a fibrinogen deficiency or defect, diagnose DIC and hepatic disease, and monitor heparin, streptokinase, and urokinase therapy.

▶ *Platelet count* discloses the number of platelets.

▶ *Prothrombin time (PT, Quick's test, or pro time)* indirectly measures prothrombin and helps to evaluate prothrombin, fibrinogen, and extrinsic coagulation factors V, VII, and X. It's used to monitor oral anticoagulant therapy. PT is usually reported as the International Normalized Ratio (INR). INR is a standardization of PT.

PLASMA TESTS

▶ *Electrophoresis of serum proteins* determines the amount of various serum proteins, which are classified by mobility in response to an electrical field. Abnormalities are commonly seen in patients with multiple myeloma or multiple sclerosis.

▶ *Erythrocyte sedimentation rate* measures the rate of RBC settling out of plasma. It may detect infection or inflammation.

▶ *Immunoelectrophoresis of serum proteins* separates and classifies serum antibodies (immunoglobulins), using specific antisera.

RBC FUNCTION TESTS

▶ *Hematocrit,* or packed cell volume, indicates the percentage of RBCs per fluid volume of whole blood.

▶ *Hemoglobin electrophoresis* demonstrates abnormal hemoglobin, as in sickle cell anemia.

▶ *Hemoglobin level* is used to measure the amount (grams) of hemoglobin per 1 ml of whole blood to determine oxygen-carrying capacity.

▶ *Mean corpuscular hemoglobin (MCH)* indicates the average amount of hemoglobin per RBC. The MCH is decreased in iron deficiency anemia.

▶ *Mean corpuscular hemoglobin concentration* determines the average hemoglobin concentration of 100 ml of packed RBCs.

▶ *Mean corpuscular volume (MCV)* describes the RBC in terms of size. Immature or iron-deficient cells have increased MCV.

▶ *Red blood cell distribution width* reflects cell size and is increased in iron and vitamin B_{12} deficiency anemias.

▶ *Reticulocyte count* is used to assess RBC production by determining the concentration of this erythrocyte precursor (which is normally present in the peripheral circulation in small amounts).

▶ *Schilling test* is used to determine absorption of vitamin B_{12} (necessary for erythropoiesis) by measuring excretion of radioactive B_{12} in the urine.

▶ *Sideroblast test* detects stainable iron (available for hemoglobin synthesis) in normoblastic RBCs.

▶ *Sucrose hemolysis test* assesses the susceptibility of RBCs to hemolyze with complement.

WBC FUNCTION TESTS

▶ *Absolute T4 helper count* provides the CD4$^+$-cell count, which is used to monitor patients with HIV infection.

▶ *Complement fixation ratio* detects the quantity of complement and antibody complexes indicative of infection.

▶ *Immunoglobulin (Ig) test* measures the levels of IgG, IgA, and IgM to detect immune incompetence caused by low antibody levels.

▶ *Quantified T4/T8 lymphocyte test* determines helper and suppressor agents important to immune function in human immunodeficiency virus (HIV) infection; it may also be reported as a T4-T8 ratio.

▶ *WBC count and differential* establish the quantity and maturity of polymorphonuclear granulocytes or bands, basophils, eosinophils, lymphocytes, and monocytes.

Other tests

BONE MARROW ASPIRATION AND NEEDLE BIOPSY

Because most hematopoiesis occurs in bone marrow, histologic and hematologic bone marrow examination yields valuable diagnostic information about blood disorders. Bone marrow aspiration and needle biopsy provide the material for this examination.

Aspiration biopsy removes a fluid specimen containing bone marrow cells in suspension. Needle biopsy removes a marrow core containing cells but no fluid. Using both methods provides the best possible marrow specimens.

Bone marrow biopsy helps to diagnose granulomas, leukemias, lymphomas, myelofibrosis, thrombocytopenia, and aplastic, hypoplastic, and vitamin B_{12} deficiency anemias. It also helps evaluate primary and metastatic tumors, determine infection causes, stage such diseases as Hodgkin disease, evaluate chemotherapy effectiveness, and monitor myelosuppression.

Hematologic analysis, including the white blood cell differential and myeloid-erythroid ration, can suggest various disorders.

Bone marrow aspiration and biopsy sites

The most common sites for bone marrow aspiration and biopsy are the iliac crest, spinous process, and sternum. These sites are used because the involved bone structures are relatively accessible and rich in marrow cavities.

Posterior superior iliac crest
The posterior superior iliac crest is the preferred site because no vital organs or vessels are nearby. With the patient lying in a prone or lateral position with one leg flexed, the practitioner anesthetizes the bone and inserts the needle several centimeters lateral to the iliosacral junction. Directed downward, the needle enters the bone plane crest and is advanced toward the anterior interior spine. In some cases, the needle enters a few centimeters below the crest at a right angle to the bone surface.

Spinous process
The spinous process is preferred if multiple punctures are necessary or if marrow is absent at other sites. The patient sits on the edge of the bed, leaning over the bedside stand. (If he's unable, he may be placed in the prone position with restraints.) The practitioner selects the spinous process of the third or fourth lumbar vertebrae and inserts the needle at the crest or slightly to one side, advancing it in the direction of the bone plane.

Sternum
The sternum involves the greatest risk but provides the best access. The patient is placed in a supine position on a firm bed or an examination table, with a small pillow beneath his shoulders to raise his chest and lower his head. The practitioner secures the needle guard 3 to 4 mm from the tip of the needle to avoid accidentally puncturing the heart or a major vessel. Then he inserts the needle at the midline of the sternum at the second intercostal space.

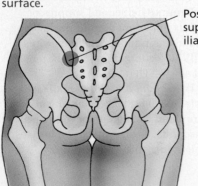

Posterior superior iliac crest

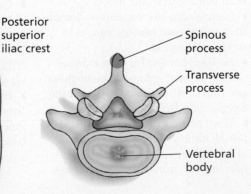

Spinous process

Transverse process

Vertebral body

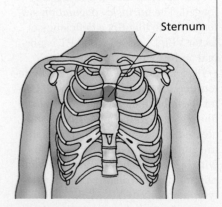

Sternum

TREATMENTS AND PROCEDURES
Drug therapy

Drug therapy includes anticoagulants, antiplatelets, biologic response modifiers, colony-stimulating factor, corticosteroids, immunosuppressants, iron products, thrombolytics, and vitamins.

ANTICOAGULANTS

▶ Prevent extension and formation of clots by inhibiting factors in the clotting cascade
▶ Used to prevent and treat thromboembolic disorders
▶ Examples: argatroban, bivalirudin (Angiomax), dalteparin sodium (Fragmin), enoxaparin sodium (Lovenox), fondaparinux sodium (Arixtra), heparin sodium, lepirudin (Refludan), tinzaparin sodium (Innohep), warfarin sodium (Coumadin)

ANTIPLATELETS

▶ Interfere with platelet aggregation in different drug-specific and dose-specific ways, preventing thromboembolic events
▶ Used as prophylaxis for thromboembolic events and intermittent claudication
▶ Examples: aspirin, cilostazol (Pletal), clopidogrel (Plavix), dipyridamole (Persantine), ticlopidine

BIOLOGIC RESPONSE MODIFIERS

▶ Stimulate red blood cell (RBC) production in the bone marrow by boosting the production of erythropoietin
▶ Used to treat anemia associated with chronic renal failure, whether or not the patient is on dialysis
▶ Examples: epoetin alfa (Epogen, Procrit) that treats anemia associated with end-stage renal disease, chemotherapy, or zidovudine therapy; darbepoetin alfa (Aranesp)

COLONY-STIMULATING FACTOR

▶ Stimulates production of granulocytes and macrophages in the bone marrow by binding to specific cell surface receptors
▶ Used to treat aplastic anemia secondary to chemotherapy, to accelerate bone marrow recovery in malignant lymphoma and Hodgkin disease, to treat delayed or failed bone marrow transplant, and to increase white blood cells in a patient taking zidovudine
▶ Examples: filgrastim (Neupogen), pegfilgrastim (Neulasta), sargramostim (Leukine)

CORTICOSTEROIDS

▶ Glucocorticoids (normally secreted by the adrenal cortex): produce metabolic effects, suppress inflammation, and alter the normal immune response; also promote sodium and water retention and potassium excretion
▶ Used to treat neoplastic diseases, septic shock, and autoimmune disease
▶ Examples: glucocorticoids: betamethasone (Celestone), cortisone (Cortone), methylprednisolone (Medrol), prednisolone (Prelone); mineralocorticoids: fludrocortisone (Florinef)

IMMUNOSUPPRESSANTS

▶ Antithymocyte globulin, antilymphocyte globulin, and antilymphocyte serum: used in organ or bone marrow transplant to reduce circulating T lymphocytes without affecting other immune cells
▶ Cyclosporine (Sandimmune, Neoral) and sirolimus: inhibit proliferation and function of the T lymphocytes
▶ Mycophenolate mofetil (CellCept): inhibits the proliferation of T lymphocytes and B lymphocytes; inhibits the recruitment of leukocytes to the sites

of inflammation; and suppresses the antibody formation by B lymphocytes
▶ Prednisone (Deltasone): inhibits macrophage formation and hinders migration of macrophages and leukocytes to inflamed areas

IRON PRODUCTS

▶ Supplement and replace depleted iron stores in the bone marrow and assist in erythropoiesis (RBC production)
▶ Used to prevent and treat iron deficiency anemia and as a dietary supplement
▶ Examples: ferrous fumarate (Femiron, Feostat), ferrous gluconate (Fergon), ferrous sulfate (Feosol, Fer-In-Sol), iron dextran (INFeD, Dex-Ferrum), iron sucrose (Venofer), sodium ferric gluconate (Ferrlecit)

THROMBOLYTICS

▶ Activate plasminogen, leading to its conversion to plasmin (a substance that degrades clots)
▶ Used to produce lysis of thrombi and to reduce mortality in patients with severe sepsis associated with acute organ dysfunction and a high risk of death
▶ Examples: alteplase (tissue plasminogen activator [Activase], drotrecogin alfa (activated) (Xigris), reteplase (Retavase), tenecteplase (TNKase), urokinase (Abbokinase)

VITAMINS

▶ Replace depleted vitamin stores
▶ Used to treat vitamin deficiencies such as B_{12} deficiency and megaloblastic anemia due to folic acid deficiency
▶ Examples: cyanocobalamin (Nascobal), hydroxocobalamin, vitamin B_{12} (Big Shot B_{12}), folic acid or vitamin B_9 (Folvite), leucovorin calcium (folinic acid citrovorum factor)

Injecting iron solutions

For deep I.M. injections of iron solutions, use the Z-track technique to avoid subcutaneous irritation and discoloration from leaking medication.

1. Choose an injection site

Rotate the injection sites in the upper outer quadrant of the buttocks.

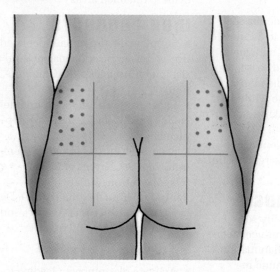

2. Displace tissues

Choose a 19G to 20G, 2″ to 3″ (5- to 7.5-cm) needle. After drawing up the solution, change to a fresh needle to avoid tracking the solution through to subcutaneous tissue. Draw 0.5 cc of air into the syringe, creating an airlock.

Displace the skin and fat at the injection site firmly to one side.

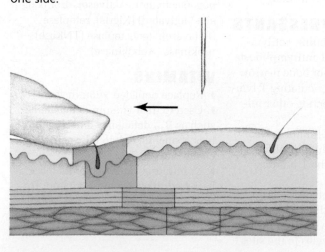

3. Inject the solution

Clean the area, and insert the needle. Aspirate to check for entry into a blood vessel. Inject the solution slowly followed by the 0.5 cc of air in the syringe.

After injecting the solution, wait 10 seconds.

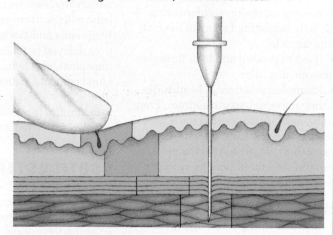

4. Release the tissues

Pull the needle straight out, and release the tissues. Apply direct pressure to the site, but don't massage it. Caution the patient not to exercise vigorously for at least 15 minutes after the injection.

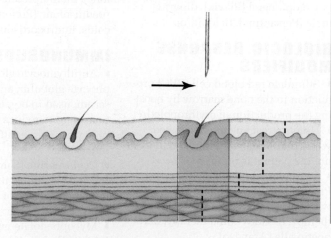

Plasmapheresis

In plasmapheresis, blood from the patient flows into a cell separator, which separates plasma from formed elements. The plasma is then filtered to remove toxins and disease mediators, such as immune complexes and autoantibodies, from the patient's blood.

The cellular components are then transferred back into the patient using fresh frozen plasma or albumin to replace the plasma that was removed.

Transfusions

Transfusion procedures allow administration of a wide range of blood products. Some examples include:
▶ red blood cell transfusions to revive oxygen-starved tissues
▶ leukocyte transfusions to combat infections beyond the reach of antibiotics
▶ transfusion of clotting factors, plasma, and platelets to help patients with hemophilia live virtually normal lives.

FACTOR REPLACEMENT

I.V. infusion of deficient clotting factors is a major part of treatment of coagulation disorders. Factor replacement typically corrects clotting factor deficiencies, thereby stopping or preventing hemorrhage. The blood product used depends on the specific disorder being treated.

Fresh frozen plasma (FFP), for instance, helps treat clotting disorders whose causes aren't known. Other uses for FFP include clotting factor deficiencies resulting from hepatic disease or blood dilution, consumed clotting factors secondary to disseminated intravascular coagulation, anticoagulant toxicity, and deficiencies of clotting factors (such as factor V) for which no specific replacement product exists.

Administration of cryoprecipitate, which forms when FFP thaws slowly, helps treat von Willebrand's disease, fibrinogen deficiencies, and factor XIII deficiencies. It's also used for hemophiliacs who are young or whose disease is mild.

Factor VIII (antihemophilia factor) concentrate is the long-term treatment of choice for hemophilia A because it contains a less viable amount of factor VIII than cryoprecipitate. It's given I.V. to hemophiliacs who have sustained injuries.

Prothrombin complex—which contains factors II, VII, IX, and X—is used to treat hemophilia B, severe liver disease, and acquired deficiencies of the factors it contains. However, it carries a high risk of transmitting hepatitis because it's collected from large pools of donors.

Transfusing blood and selected components

Blood component	Indications	Compatibility	Nursing considerations
Whole blood			
Complete (pure) blood	▶ To restore blood volume lost from hemorrhaging, trauma, or burns ▶ Exchange transfusion in sickle cell disease	▶ ABO identical: Group A receives A; group B receives B; group AB receives AB; group O receives O ▶ Rh type must match	▶ Remember that whole blood is seldom administered. ▶ Use blood administration tubing to infuse within 4 hours. ▶ Closely monitor patient volume status for volume overload. ▶ Warm blood if giving a large quantity. ▶ Use only with normal saline solution.
Packed red blood cells (RBCs)			
Same RBC mass as whole blood but with 80% of the plasma removed	▶ To restore or maintain oxygen-carrying capacity ▶ To correct anemia and surgical blood loss ▶ To increase RBC mass ▶ Red cell exchange	▶ Group A receives A or O ▶ Group B receives B or O ▶ Group AB receives AB, A, B, or O ▶ Group O receives O ▶ Rh type must match	▶ Use blood administration tubing to infuse within 4 hours. ▶ Use only with normal saline solution. ▶ Avoid administering packed RBCs for anemic conditions correctable by nutritional or drug therapy.
Leukocyte-depleted RBCs			
Same as packed RBCs with about 70% of the leukocytes removed	▶ Same as packed RBCs ▶ To prevent febrile reactions from leukocyte antibodies and decrease the possibility of cytomegalovirus transmission ▶ To treat immunocompromised patients ▶ To restore RBCs to patients who have had two or more nonhemolytic febrile reactions	▶ Same as packed RBCs ▶ Rh type must match	▶ Use blood administration tubing to infuse within 4 hours. ▶ May require a 40-micron filter suitable for hard-spun, leukocyte-depleted RBCs. ▶ Other considerations are the same as those for packed RBCs. ▶ Cells expire 24 hours after washing.
White blood cells (leukocytes)			
Whole blood with all the RBCs and about 80% of the plasma removed	▶ To treat sepsis that's unresponsive to antibiotics (especially if patient has positive blood cultures or a persistent fever exceeding 101° F [38.3° C]) and life-threatening granulocytopenia (granulocyte count less than 500/µl)	▶ Same as packed RBCs ▶ Compatibility with human leukocyte antigen (HLA) preferable but not necessary unless patient is sensitized to HLA from previous transfusions ▶ Rh type must match	▶ Use a blood administration set. Give 1 unit daily for 4 to 6 days or until the infection resolves. ▶ As prescribed, premedicate with antihistamines, acetaminophen (Tylenol), or steroids. ▶ If fever occurs, administer an antipyretic and don't discontinue the transfusion; instead, reduce the flow rate, as ordered, for patient comfort. ▶ Because reactions are common, administer slowly over 2 to 4 hours. Check the patient's vital signs, and assess him every 15 minutes throughout the transfusion. ▶ Give the transfusion with antibiotics to treat infection.

Transfusing blood and selected components (continued)

Blood component	Indications	Compatibility	Nursing considerations
Platelets			
Platelet sediment from RBCs or plasma platelets	▶ To treat bleeding caused by decreased circulating platelets or functionally abnormal platelets ▶ To improve platelet count preoperatively in a patient whose count is 50,000/µl or less	▶ ABO compatibility identical; Rh-negative recipients should receive Rh-negative platelets	▶ Use a blood filter or leukocyte-reduction filter and infuse over 30 minutes. ▶ As prescribed, premedicate with antipyretics and antihistamines if the patient's history includes a platelet transfusion reaction or to reduce chills, fever, and allergic reactions. ▶ Use single donor platelets if the patient needs repeated transfusions. ▶ Platelets aren't used to treat autoimmune thrombocytopenia or thrombocytopenic purpura unless the patient has a life-threatening hemorrhage.
Fresh frozen plasma (FFP)			
Uncoagulated plasma separated from RBCs and rich in coagulation factors V, VIII, and IX	▶ To treat postoperative hemorrhage ▶ To correct an undetermined coagulation factor deficiency ▶ To replace a specific factor when that factor isn't available ▶ Warfarin reversal	▶ ABO compatibility required ▶ Rh match not required	▶ Use a blood administration set, and administer the infusion rapidly. ▶ Keep in mind that large-volume transfusions of FFP may require correction for hypocalcemia because citric acid in FFP binds calcium. ▶ Must be infused within 24 hours of being thawed.
Albumin 5% (buffered saline); albumin 25% (salt-poor)			
A small plasma protein prepared by fractionating pooled plasma	▶ To replace volume lost because of shock from burns, trauma, surgery, hemodialysis, or infections ▶ To treat hypoproteinemia (with or without edema)	▶ Not required	▶ Use the administration set supplied by the manufacturer, and set the rate based on the patient's condition and response. ▶ Keep in mind that albumin is contraindicated in severe anemia. ▶ Administer cautiously in cardiac and pulmonary disease because heart failure may result from circulatory overload.
Factor VIII concentrate (hemophilic factor)			
Cold insoluble portion of plasma recovered from FFP	▶ To treat a patient with hemophilia A ▶ To treat a patient with von Willebrand's disease	▶ ABO compatibility not required	▶ Administer by I.V. injection using a filter needle, or use the administration set supplied by the manufacturer.
Cryoprecipitate			
Insoluble plasma portion of FFP containing fibrinogen, factor VIIIc, factor VIIvWF, factor XIII, and fibronectin	▶ To treat factor VIII deficiency and fibrinogen disorders ▶ To treat significant factor XIII deficiency	▶ ABO compatibility required ▶ Rh match not required	▶ Administer with a blood administration set. ▶ Add normal saline solution to each bag of cryoprecipitate, as necessary, to facilitate infusion. ▶ Keep in mind that cryoprecipitate must be administered within 6 hours of thawing. ▶ Before administration, check laboratory studies to confirm a deficiency of one of the specific clotting factors present in cryoprecipitate.

Surgery

Surgery for hematologic or immuno-logic disorders includes bone marrow transplant. Surgical removal of the spleen is sometimes performed to treat various hematologic disorders.

BONE MARROW TRANSPLANT

Bone marrow transplant is standard treatment for leukemia. The procedure can also be used to treat aplastic ane-mia, lymphoma, and sickle cell dis-ease. The recipient receives chemo-therapy to try to eradicate as many leukemic cells from the bone marrow as possible. The patient then receives bone marrow cells from a compatible donor. The new marrow begins ery-thropoiesis that results in healthy, properly functioning cells.

SPLENECTOMY

The spleen may be removed to reduce the rate of red blood cell and platelet destruction or to stage Hodgkin dis-ease. It's also done as an emergency procedure to stop hemorrhage after traumatic splenic rupture.

Splenectomy is the treatment of choice for such diseases as hereditary spherocytosis and chronic idiopathic thrombocytopenic purpura in patients who don't respond to steroids or dana-zol therapy. Besides bleeding and in-fection, splenectomy can cause other complications, such as pneumonia and atelectasis.

Keep in mind that the spleen's loca-tion close to the diaphragm and the need for a high abdominal incision re-strict lung expansion after surgery. Also, splenectomy patients—especial-ly children—are vulnerable to infec-tion because of the spleen's role in the immune response.

Chapter 9

Endocrine care

DISEASES
Adrenal hypofunction

Adrenal hypofunction, also called *adrenal insufficiency,* may be classified as primary or secondary. Primary adrenal hypofunction (Addison's disease) originates within the adrenal gland and is characterized by decreased mineralocorticoid, glucocorticoid, and androgen secretion. A relatively uncommon disorder, Addison's disease occurs in people of all ages and both sexes. Adrenal hypofunction may also occur secondary to a disorder outside the gland, such as with a pituitary tumor with corticotropin deficiency, but, unlike the primary form, aldosterone secretion remains unaffected.

With early diagnosis and adequate replacement therapy, the prognosis for both forms of adrenal hypofunction is promising.

Adrenal crisis—also called *addisonian crisis*—is a critical deficiency of mineralocorticoids and glucocorticoids that generally follows acute stress, sepsis, trauma, surgery, or the discontinuation of steroid therapy. Adrenal crisis is a medical emergency that necessitates immediate, vigorous treatment.

Signs and symptoms
▶ Confusion, depression, delirium, and possibly psychosis
▶ Bronze coloration of the skin that resembles a deep suntan, especially in the creases of the hands and over the metacarpophalangeal joints, elbows, and knees (Addison's disease)
▶ Cravings for salty food
▶ Decreased tolerance for even minor stress
▶ Dry skin and mucous membranes
▶ Fatigue
▶ Hypotension
▶ Light-headedness (when rising from a chair or bed)
▶ Muscle weakness, myalgia, arthralgia
▶ Nausea, vomiting, anorexia, chronic diarrhea, and weight loss
▶ Poor coordination
▶ Weak, irregular pulse
▶ Decreased pubic hair, diminished libido, and amenorrhea in women

 How adrenal crisis develops

Adrenal crisis is the most serious complication of adrenal hypofunction. It can occur gradually or with catastrophic suddenness, making prompt emergency treatment essential. It's also known as *acute adrenal insufficiency.*

This potentially lethal condition usually develops in a patient who doesn't respond to hormone replacement therapy, undergoes marked stress without adequate glucocorticoid replacement, or abruptly stops hormonal therapy. It can also result from trauma, bilateral adrenalectomy, or adrenal gland thrombosis after a severe infection (Waterhouse-Friderichsen syndrome).

Signs and symptoms
Signs and symptoms of adrenal crisis include profound weakness, fatigue, nausea, vomiting, hypotension, dehydration and, occasionally, high fever followed by hypothermia. If untreated, this condition can ultimately cause vascular collapse, renal shutdown, coma, and death.

The flowchart (shown at right) summarizes what happens in adrenal crisis and pinpoints its warning signs and symptoms.

Treatment
Primary and secondary adrenal hypofunction
▶ Lifelong corticosteroid replacement
▶ Fludrocortisone, a synthetic drug that acts as a mineralocorticoid, to

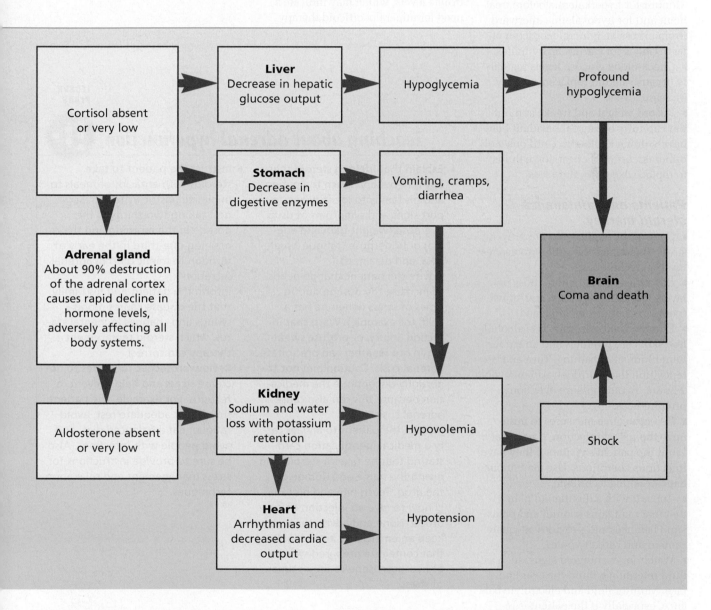

prevent dangerous dehydration and hypotension (Addison's disease)

Adrenal crisis

▶ I.V. bolus administration of dexamethasone followed by an I.V. bolus of hydrocortisone.

▶ To correct hypovolemia: infusion of 3 to 5 L of I.V. normal saline or 5% dextrose solution during the acute stage

▶ After the crisis, maintenance doses of hydrocortisone to preserve physiologic stability

Nursing considerations

◗ In adrenal crisis, monitor vital signs carefully, especially for hypotension, volume depletion, and other signs of shock. Check for decreased level of consciousness and reduced urine output, which may also signal shock. Monitor for hyperkalemia before treatment and for hypokalemia afterward (from excessive mineralocorticoid effect). Check for cardiac arrhythmias.

◗ Check blood glucose levels regularly because steroid replacement may increase levels.

◗ Record weight and intake and output carefully because the patient may have volume depletion. Until onset of mineralocorticoid effect, force fluids to replace excessive fluid loss.

Patients on maintenance steroid therapy

◗ Control the environment to prevent stress. Encourage the patient to use relaxation techniques.

◗ Encourage the patient to dress in layers to retain body heat, and adjust room temperature, as indicated.

◗ Provide good skin care. Use alcohol-free skin care products and an emollient lotion after bathing. Turn and reposition the bedridden patient every 2 hours. Avoid pressure over bony prominences.

◗ Use protective measures to minimize the risk of infection, if necessary. Limit the patient's visitors if they have infectious conditions. Use meticulous hand-washing technique.

◗ Consult with a dietitian to plan a diet that maintains sodium and potassium balances and provides adequate protein and carbohydrates.

◗ Watch for cushingoid signs, such as fluid retention around the eyes and face. Monitor fluid and electrolyte balance, especially if the patient is receiving mineralocorticoids. Monitor weight and check blood pressure to assess body fluid status. Check for petechiae because these patients bruise easily.

◗ In women receiving testosterone injections, watch for and report facial hair growth and other signs of masculinization.

◗ If the patient is receiving only glucocorticoids, observe for orthostatic hypotension or abnormal serum electrolyte levels, which may indicate a need for mineralocorticoid therapy.

Teaching about adrenal hypofunction

◗ Explain that lifelong steroid therapy is necessary. Teach the patient and his family to identify and report signs and symptoms of drug overdose (weight gain and edema) or underdose (fatigue, weakness, and dizziness).

◗ Advise the patient that he needs to increase the dosage during times of stress (when he has a cold, for example). Warn that infection, injury, or profuse sweating in hot weather can precipitate adrenal crisis. Caution him not to abruptly discontinue the medication because this can also cause adrenal crisis.

◗ Instruct the patient to always carry a medical identification card stating that he takes a steroid and giving the name and dosage of the drug. Teach him and his family how to give an injection of hydrocortisone and advise them to keep an emergency kit available that contains a prepared syringe of hydrocortisone to use in times of stress.

◗ Instruct the patient to take steroids with antacids or meals to minimize gastric irritation. Suggest taking two-thirds of the dosage in the morning and the remaining one-third in the early afternoon to mimic diurnal adrenal secretion.

◗ Inform the patient and his family that the disease causes mood swings and changes in mental status, which steroid replacement therapy can correct.

◗ Review protective measures to decrease stress and help prevent infections. For example, the patient should get adequate rest, avoid fatigue, eat a balanced diet, and avoid people with infections. Also be sure to provide instructions for stress management and relaxation techniques.

Cushing's syndrome

Cushing's syndrome is the clinical manifestation of glucocorticoid (particularly cortisol) excess. Excess secretions of mineralocorticoids and androgens may also cause Cushing's syndrome. In about 70% of patients, Cushing's syndrome results from excess production of corticotropin and consequent hyperplasia of the adrenal cortex.

The disorder is classified as primary, secondary, or iatrogenic, depending on its cause, and is most common in females.

The hallmark signs of Cushing's syndrome include adiposity of the face, neck, and trunk, and purple striae on the skin. The nature of the prognosis depends largely on early diagnosis, identification of the underlying cause, and effective treatment.

Signs and symptoms

- Fatigue
- Muscle weakness
- Sleep disturbances
- Water retention
- Amenorrhea
- Decreased libido
- Irritability
- Emotional instability
- Thin hair
- Moon-shaped face
- Hirsutism
- Acne
- Buffalo humplike back
- Thin extremities
- Petechiae, ecchymoses, and purplish striae
- Delayed wound healing
- Swollen ankles
- Hypertension

PICTURING PATHO

Manifestations of Cushing's syndrome

Increased cortisol levels
Mood changes
Depression
Psychosis
Cataracts

Increased androgen production
Acne
Increased facial and body hair
Virilization
Hyperpigmentation
Menstrual changes

Protein loss
Capillary weakness
Ecchymosis

Increased gastric acidity
Peptic ulcer

Sodium/water retention
Edema
Hypertension

Increased gluconeogenesis
Diabetes mellitus

Potassium excretion
Hypokalemic alkalosis

Body fat redistribution
Moon face
Buffalo hump
Supraclavicular fat pad
Truncal obesity
Thin extremities
Purple striae

Increased calcium loss
Bone thinning and osteoporosis
Fractures

Immunosuppression
Poor wound healing

Treatment

▶ Possibly, radiation, drug therapy, or surgery to restore hormone balance and reverse Cushing's syndrome
▶ Transsphenoidal microadenomectomy
▶ Pituitary irradiation
▶ Bilateral adrenalectomy
▶ In a patient with a nonendocrine corticotropin-producing tumor, excision of the tumor, followed by drug therapy with mitotane, metyrapone, or aminoglutethimide
▶ Lifelong steroid replacement therapy

Nursing considerations

▶ Keep accurate records of vital signs, fluid intake, urine output, and weight. Monitor serum electrolyte levels daily.
▶ Consult a dietitian to plan a diet high in protein and potassium and low in calories, carbohydrates, and sodium.
▶ Use protective measures to reduce the risk of infection, if necessary. Use meticulous hand-washing technique.
▶ Schedule activities around the patient's rest periods to avoid fatigue. Gradually increase activity, as tolerated.
▶ Institute safety precautions to minimize the risk of injury from falls.
▶ Help the bedridden patient turn every 2 hours. Use extreme caution while moving the patient to minimize skin trauma and bone stress. Provide frequent skin care, especially over bony prominences. Provide support with pillows and a convoluted foam mattress.
▶ Encourage the patient to verbalize feelings about body image changes and sexual dysfunction. Offer emotional support and a positive, realistic assessment of the patient's condition. Help the patient to develop coping strategies. Refer to a mental health professional for additional counseling, if necessary.

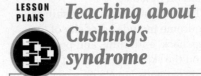

LESSON PLANS

Teaching about Cushing's syndrome

▶ Advise the patient that lifelong steroid replacement is necessary. Teach the patient and family members to identify and report signs of drug overdose (edema and weight gain) or underdose (fatigue, weakness, and dizziness). Tell the patient not to abruptly discontinue the drug because this may precipitate adrenal crisis.
▶ Instruct the patient to take steroids with antacids or meals to minimize gastric irritation. Advise taking two-thirds of a dose in the morning and the remaining third in the early afternoon to mimic diurnal adrenal secretion.
▶ Encourage the patient to wear a medical identification bracelet and carry medication at all times.
▶ Teach the patient protective measures to decrease stress and infections: for example, get adequate rest and avoid fatigue, eat a balanced diet, and avoid people with infections. Also teach relaxation and stress-reduction techniques.

Diabetes insipidus

A disorder of water metabolism, diabetes insipidus results from a deficiency of circulating vasopressin (also called *antidiuretic hormone*, or *ADH*), a resistance to vasopressin at the receptor sites in the kidneys, or an abnormal thirst mechanism. A decrease in ADH levels leads to altered intracellular and extracellular fluid control, causing renal excretion of a large amount of urine. Diabetes insipidus can strike people of all ages, from infancy to adulthood.

In uncomplicated diabetes insipidus and with adequate water replacement, the prognosis is good and patients usually can lead normal lives. However, in cases complicated by an underlying disorder, such as cancer, the prognosis is variable.

Signs and symptoms

▶ Extreme polyuria (usually 4 to 16 L/day of dilute urine, but sometimes as much as 30 L/day)
▶ Extreme thirst
▶ Weight loss
▶ Dizziness
▶ Weakness
▶ Constipation
▶ Slight to moderate nocturia
▶ Dry skin and mucous membranes
▶ Fever
▶ Dyspnea
▶ Pale and voluminous urine
▶ Poor skin turgor
▶ Tachycardia
▶ Decreased muscle strength
▶ Hypotension

PICTURING PATHO

Mechanism of ADH deficiency

```
        Decreased antidiuretic hormone (ADH) release
                      from pituitary
                            │
                            ▼
              Decreased renal tubular
              permeability to water
                            │
                            ▼
                  Decreased water
                   reabsorption
               │                    │
               ▼                    ▼
    Excessive urine output    Increased serum
         (polyuria)             osmolality

   Decreased urine osmolality    Increased thirst
     and specific gravity          (polydipsia)
```

Treatment

◗ Desmopressin acetate (DDAVP) administered nasally, orally, or by injection; affects prolonged antidiuretic activity and has no pressor effects, depending on dosage

◗ Chlorpropamide (Diabinese): a sulfonylurea used in diabetes mellitus; also sometimes used to stimulate endogenous release of antidiuretic hormone and is effective if some pituitary function is intact

◗ Carbamazepine to enhance the patient's response to ADH; clofibrate to increase the release of ADH

◗ Low-sodium, low-protein diet and thiazide diuretics to treat nephrogenic diabetes insipidus

Nursing considerations

◗ Make sure that you keep accurate records of the patient's hourly fluid intake and urine output, vital signs, and daily weight. Be sure to administer adequate replacement fluids.

◗ Closely monitor the patient's urine specific gravity. Also monitor serum electrolyte and blood urea nitrogen levels.

◗ Watch the patient for signs of hypovolemic shock. Monitor blood pressure, pulse rate, and body weight. Also watch for changes in mental or neurologic status.

◗ If the patient has any complaints of dizziness or muscle weakness, institute safety precautions to help prevent injury.

◗ Make sure that the patient has easy access to the bathroom or bedpan. Insert an indwelling urinary catheter if the patient is incontinent so output can be monitored.

◗ Provide meticulous skin and mouth care. Use a soft toothbrush and mild mouthwash to avoid trauma to the oral mucosa. If the patient has cracked or sore lips, apply petroleum jelly, as needed. Use alcohol-free skin care products, and apply emollient lotion to the patient's skin after baths.

◗ Use caution when administering vasopressin to a patient with coronary artery disease because the drug can cause coronary artery constriction. Therefore, closely monitor the patient's electrocardiogram, looking for changes and exacerbation of angina.

◗ Urge the patient to verbalize feelings. Offer encouragement, and provide a realistic assessment of the situation.

◗ Help the patient identify his strengths, and help him see how he can use these strengths to develop effective coping strategies.

◗ As necessary, refer the patient to a mental health professional for additional counseling.

◗ Advise the patient to wear a medical identification bracelet at all times. Tell him he should always keep his medication with him.

**LESSON
PLANS**

Teaching about diabetes insipidus

◗ Before the water restriction test, tell the patient to take nothing by mouth until the test is over, and explain the need for hourly urine tests, vital sign and weight checks and, if necessary, blood tests. Reassure the patient that he'll be closely monitored.

◗ Teach the patient and family about the disorder and treatment. Answer all questions as completely as possible.

◗ Instruct the patient and family members to identify and report signs of severe dehydration and impending hypovolemia.

◗ Tell the patient to record his weight daily, and teach him and family members how to monitor intake and output and how to use a hydrometer to measure urine specific gravity.

◗ Encourage the patient to maintain fluid intake during the day to prevent severe dehydration but to limit fluids in the evening to prevent nocturia.

◗ Inform the patient and family members about long-term hormone replacement therapy. Instruct the patient to take the medication as prescribed and to avoid abrupt discontinuation of the drug without the physician's order. Teach them how to give subcutaneous or I.M. injections or how to use nasal applicators. Discuss the drug's adverse effects and when to report them.

◗ Teach the parents of a child with diabetes insipidus about normal growth and development; discuss how their child may differ. Encourage the parents to identify the child's strengths and use them to develop coping strategies. Refer family members for counseling, if necessary.

◗ Explain all testing and what patient participation is required.

Diabetes mellitus

Diabetes mellitus is a chronic disease of absolute or relative insulin deficiency or resistance. It's characterized by disturbances in carbohydrate, protein, and fat metabolism. Insulin deficiency compromises the body tissues' ability to access essential nutrients for fuel and storage.

Diabetes mellitus occurs in two primary forms: type 1, characterized by absolute insufficiency; and the more prevalent type 2, characterized by insulin resistance with varying degrees of insulin secretory defects.

Onset of type 1 usually occurs before age 30, although it may occur at any age. Type 2 usually occurs in obese adults after age 40; however, it's becoming more common in North American youths.

Diabetes mellitus is thought to affect about 7% of the population of the United States (24 million people); about 6 million cases are undiagnosed. Incidence is essentially the same between males and females and increases with age.

In type 1 diabetes, pancreatic beta-cell destruction or primary defect in beta-cell function results in a failure to release insulin and ineffective glucose transport. Type 1 immune-mediated diabetes is caused by cell-mediated destruction of pancreatic beta cells. In type 2 diabetes, beta cells release insulin, but receptors resist insulin, glucose transport is variable and ineffective.

Type 1 and type 2 diabetes mellitus

TYPE 1 DIABETES
Pancreas with no insulin production

Cell

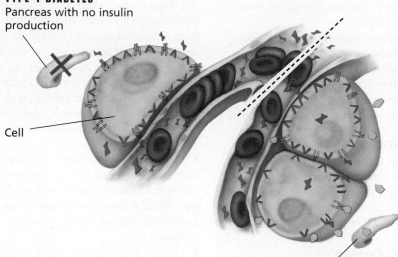

TYPE 2 DIABETES
Pancreas producing little or ineffective insulin

Closed glucose channel

Open glucose channel

Insulin

Insulin receptor

Glucose

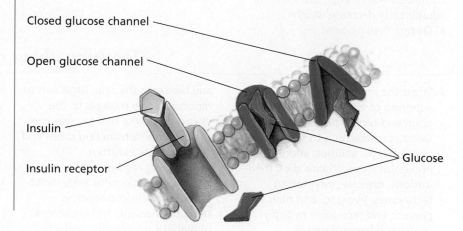

Signs and symptoms

- Polyuria
- Polydipsia
- Polyphagia
- Nausea and anorexia
- Weight loss
- Headaches, fatigue, lethargy, reduced energy levels, impaired school or work performance
- Muscle cramps, irritability, emotional lability
- Vision changes such as blurring
- Numbness and tingling
- Abdominal discomfort and pain; diarrhea or constipation
- Recurrent infections
- Delayed wound healing

Treatment

Type 1 diabetes
- Exogenous insulin
- Dietary management
- Exercise therapy
- Islet cell or pancreas transplantation

Type 2 diabetes
- Insulin therapy
- Oral antidiabetic drugs
- Exercise therapy
- Lipase inhibitor (such as orlistat) combined with a low-calorie diet to significantly decrease weight
- Dietary management

Nursing considerations

- Keep accurate records of vital signs, weight, fluid intake, urine output, and calorie intake. Monitor serum glucose and urine acetone levels.
- Monitor for acute complications of diabetic therapy, especially hypoglycemia (vagueness, slow cerebration, dizziness, weakness, pallor, tachycardia, diaphoresis, seizures, and coma); immediately give carbohydrates in the form of fruit juice, hard candy, honey or, if the patient is unconscious, glucagon or I.V. dextrose. Also be alert for signs of hyperosmolar coma (polyuria, thirst, neurologic abnormalities, and stupor). This hyperglycemic crisis requires I.V. fluids and insulin replacement.
- Monitor diabetic effects on the cardiovascular system, such as cerebrovascular, coronary artery, and peripheral vascular impairment, and on the peripheral and autonomic nervous systems.
- Provide meticulous skin care, especially to the feet and legs. Treat all injuries, cuts, and blisters. Avoid constricting clothing, slippers, or bed linens. Refer the patient to a podiatrist if indicated.

- Observe for signs of urinary tract and vaginal infections. Encourage adequate fluid intake.
- Monitor the patient for signs of diabetic neuropathy (numbness or pain in the hands and feet, footdrop, and neurogenic bladder).
- Consult a dietitian to plan a diet with the recommended allowances of calories, protein, carbohydrates, and fats, based on the patient's particular requirements.
- Encourage the patient to verbalize feelings about diabetes and its effects on lifestyle and life expectancy. Offer emotional support and a realistic assessment of his condition. Stress that with proper treatment, he can lead a relatively normal life. Help the patient to develop coping strategies. Refer him and his family for counseling, if necessary. Encourage them to join a support group.

LESSON PLANS

Teaching about diabetes mellitus

- Stress the importance of carefully adhering to the prescribed program and blood glucose control. Tailor your teaching to the patient's needs, abilities, and developmental stage. Discuss diet, medications, exercise, monitoring techniques, hygiene, and how to prevent and recognize hypoglycemia and hyperglycemia.
- To encourage compliance to lifestyle changes, emphasize how blood glucose control affects long-term health. Teach the patient how to care for his feet: He should wash them daily, carefully dry between his toes, and inspect for corns, calluses, redness, swelling, bruises,

and breaks in the skin. Urge him to report any skin changes to the physician. Advise him to wear comfortable, nonconstricting shoes and never to walk barefoot.
- Urge annual regular ophthalmologic examinations for early detection of diabetic retinopathy.
- Describe the signs and symptoms of diabetic neuropathy and emphasize the need for safety precautions because decreased sensation can mask injuries.
- Teach the patient how to manage diabetes when he has a minor illness, such as a cold, flu, or upset stomach.

- To prevent diabetes, teach people at high risk to maintain proper weight and exercise regularly. Advise genetic counseling for adult diabetic patients who are planning families.
- Teach the patient and his family how to monitor the patient's diet. Teach how to read labels in the supermarket to identify fat, carbohydrate, protein, and sugar content.
- Encourage the patient and his family to contact the Juvenile Diabetes Foundation, the American Association of Diabetes Educators, and the American Diabetes Association to obtain additional information.

Hyperthyroidism

Thyroid hormone overproduction results in the metabolic imbalance hyperthyroidism, which is also called *thyrotoxicosis*.

The most common form is Graves' disease, which increases thyroxine (T_4) production, enlarges the thyroid gland (goiter), and causes multiple systemic changes. Incidence of Graves' disease is highest between ages 30 and 40, especially in people with family histories of thyroid abnormalities; only 5% of hyperthyroid patients are younger than age 15. With treatment, most patients can lead normal lives.

However, thyrotoxic crisis (or *thyroid storm*), an acute exacerbation of hyperthyroidism, is a medical emergency that can lead to life-threatening cardiac, hepatic, or renal failure.

Signs and symptoms

▶ Enlarged thyroid
▶ Nervousness
▶ Heat intolerance
▶ Weight loss despite increased appetite
▶ Sweating
▶ Frequent bowel movements
▶ Tremor
▶ Palpitations
▶ Exophthalmos (considered most characteristic but is absent in many patients with thyrotoxicosis)

PICTURING PATHO

Histologic changes in Graves' disease

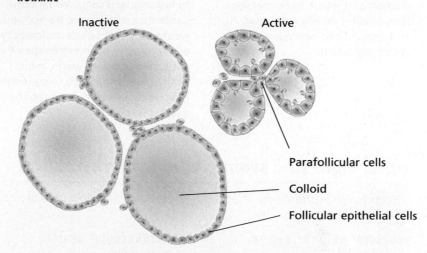

NORMAL

Inactive

Active

Parafollicular cells

Colloid

Follicular epithelial cells

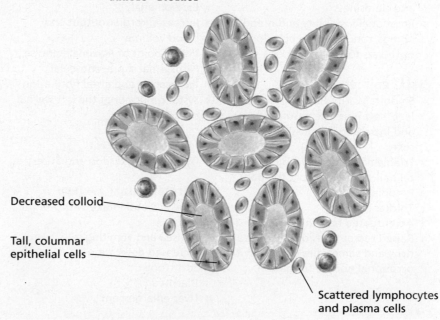

GRAVES' DISEASE

Decreased colloid

Tall, columnar epithelial cells

Scattered lymphocytes and plasma cells

Understanding thyrotoxic crisis

Thyrotoxic crisis—also known as *thyroid storm*—is an acute manifestation of hyperthyroidism. It usually occurs in patients with preexisting (though often unrecognized) thyrotoxicosis. Left untreated, it's invariably fatal.

Pathophysiology

The thyroid gland secretes the thyroid hormones triiodothyronine and thyroxine. When it overproduces them in response to any of the precipitating factors listed at right, systemic adrenergic activity increases. This results in epinephrine overproduction and severe hypermetabolism, leading rapidly to cardiac, GI, and sympathetic nervous system decompensation.

Assessment findings

Initially, the patient may have marked tachycardia, vomiting, and stupor. If left untreated, he may experience vascular collapse, hypotension, coma, and death. Other findings may include a combination of agitation and psychosis progressing to lethargy and coma; visual disturbance such as diplopia; tremor and weakness; heart failure, pulmonary edema; and swollen extremities. Palpation may disclose warm, moist flushed skin and a high fever (beginning insidiously and rising rapidly to a lethal level).

Precipitating factors

Onset is almost always abrupt, evoked by a stressful event, such as trauma, surgery, or infection. Other, less-common precipitators include:

▸ insulin-induced hypoglycemia or diabetic ketoacidosis
▸ cardiovascular accident
▸ myocardial infarction
▸ pulmonary embolism
▸ sudden discontinuation of antithyroid drug therapy
▸ initiation of radioiodine therapy
▸ preeclampsia
▸ subtotal thyroidectomy with accompanying excess intake of synthetic thyroid hormone.

Other signs and symptoms of hyperthyroidism

Thyrotoxicosis profoundly affects virtually every body system, thus producing additional signs and symptoms of hyperthyroidism.

Central nervous system

▸ Difficulty in concentrating
▸ Excitability or nervousness
▸ Fine tremor, shaky handwriting, and clumsiness
▸ Emotional instability and mood swings, ranging from occasional outbursts to overt psychosis

Skin, hair, and nails

▸ Smooth, warm, flushed skin
▸ Fine, soft hair; premature graying and increased hair loss in both sexes
▸ Friable nails and onycholysis (distal nail separated from the bed)
▸ Pretibial myxedema
▸ Thickened skin
▸ Accentuated hair follicles
▸ Raised red patches of skin that are itchy and sometimes painful, with occasional nodule formation

Cardiovascular system

▸ Tachycardia
▸ Full, bounding pulse
▸ Wide pulse pressure
▸ Cardiomegaly
▸ Increased cardiac output and blood volume
▸ Visible point of maximal impulse
▸ Paroxysmal supraventricular tachycardia and atrial fibrillation
▸ Systolic murmur at the left sternal border

Respiratory system

▸ Dyspnea on exertion and at rest

Gastrointestinal system

▸ Excessive oral intake with weight loss
▸ Nausea and vomiting
▸ Increased defecation
▸ Soft stools
▸ Diarrhea
▸ Liver enlargement

Musculoskeletal system

▸ Weakness (especially in proximal muscles)
▸ Fatigue
▸ Muscle atrophy

Reproductive system

Females
▸ Oligomenorrhea or amenorrhea
▸ Decreased fertility
▸ Higher incidence of spontaneous abortions
▸ Diminished libido

Males
▸ Gynecomastia
▸ Diminished libido

Eyes

▸ Exophthalmos
▸ Occasional inflammation of conjunctivae, corneas, or eye muscles
▸ Diplopia
▸ Increased tearing

Treatment
Graves' disease
▶ Antithyroid drug therapy to treat children, young adults, pregnant women, and patients who refuse surgery or radioiodine treatment
▶ Thyroid hormone antagonists, including propylthiouracil (PTU) and possibly methimazole, which block thyroid hormone synthesis
▶ Propranolol to manage tachycardia and other peripheral effects of excessive sympathetic activity
▶ Treatment with radioactive iodine (^{131}I)
▶ Subtotal (partial) thyroidectomy

Thyrotoxic crisis
▶ PTU
▶ I.V. propranolol to block sympathetic effects; corticosteroid to inhibit the conversion of T_3 to T_4 and to replace depleted cortisol
▶ Iodide to block release of the thyroid hormones

Nursing considerations
▶ Keep accurate records of vital signs, weight, fluid intake, and urine output. Measure neck circumference daily to check for progression of thyroid enlargement.
▶ Monitor serum electrolyte levels and check for hyperglycemia and glycosuria.
▶ Monitor the patient's electrocardiogram for arrhythmias and ST-segment changes.
▶ Monitor for signs of heart failure, such as dyspnea, jugular vein distention, pulmonary crackles, and peripheral or sacral edema.
▶ Minimize physical and emotional stress.

▶ Consult a dietitian to ensure a nutritious diet with adequate calories and fluids. Offer frequent, small meals.
▶ Monitor the frequency and characteristics of stools, and give antidiarrheals, as ordered.
▶ Reassure the patient and family members that mood swings and nervousness usually subside with treatment.
▶ If iodide is part of the treatment, mix it with milk, juice, or water to prevent GI distress and give it through a straw to prevent tooth discoloration.
▶ Monitor the patient taking propranolol for signs of hypotension (dizziness and decreased urine output).
▶ If the patient is taking PTU or methimazole, monitor complete blood count results periodically to detect leukopenia, thrombocytopenia, and agranulocytosis.
▶ If the patient has exophthalmos or other ophthalmopathy, moisten the conjunctivae often with isotonic eyedrops.
▶ Avoid excessive palpation of the thyroid, which can precipitate thyroid storm.

After thyroidectomy
▶ Check the dressings for spots of blood, which may indicate hemorrhage into the neck. Change dressings and perform wound care, as ordered. Also check the back of the dressing for drainage. Keep the patient in semi-Fowler's position and support his head and neck with sandbags to ease tension on the incision.
▶ Check for dysphagia or hoarseness from possible laryngeal nerve injury.
▶ Watch for signs of hypocalcemia (tetany and numbness), a complication that results from accidental removal of the parathyroid glands during surgery.

LESSON PLANS

Teaching about hyperthyroidism

▶ Stress the importance of regular medical follow-up visits after discharge because hypothyroidism may develop 2 to 4 weeks postoperatively and after radioisotope therapy. Advise the patient that he'll need lifelong thyroid hormone replacement. Encourage him to wear a medical identification bracelet and to carry his medication with him at all times.
▶ Tell the patient who's had radioisotope therapy not to expectorate or cough freely because his saliva remains radioactive for 24 hours. Stress the need for repeated measurement of serum thyroxine levels. Be sure he understands that he must not resume antithyroid drug therapy.
▶ Instruct the patient taking propylthiouracil (PTU) or methimazole to take these drugs with meals to minimize GI distress and to avoid over-the-counter cough preparations because many contain iodine.
▶ Tell the patient taking PTU to rise slowly after sitting or lying down to prevent feeling faint.
▶ Instruct the patient taking antithyroid drugs or radioisotope therapy to identify and report symptoms of hypothyroidism.
▶ Advise the patient with exophthalmos or other ophthalmopathy to wear sunglasses or eye patches to protect the eyes from light. If he has severe lid retraction, warn him to avoid sudden physical movements that might cause the lid to slip behind the eyeball. Instruct him to report signs of decreased visual acuity.

Hypothyroidism in adults

In hypothyroidism in adults, metabolic processes slow down because of a deficiency of the thyroid hormones triiodothyronine (T_3) or thyroxine (T_4).

Hypothyroidism is classified as primary or secondary. Primary hypothyroidism stems from a disorder of the thyroid gland itself. Hashimoto's thyroiditis (autoimmune disease in which the immune system attacks the thyroid) is the most common cause of primary hypothyroidism in the United States. Secondary hypothyroidism is caused by a failure to stimulate normal thyroid function or by a failure of target tissues to respond to normal blood levels of thyroid hormones. Either type may progress to myxedema, which is considerably more severe and a medical emergency.

Signs and symptoms

- Fatigue and loss of energy
- Forgetfulness
- Sensitivity to cold
- Unexplained weight gain
- Constipation
- Decreased mental stability (slight mental slowing to severe obtundation)
- Thick, dry tongue, causing hoarseness and slow, slurred speech
- Dry, flaky, inelastic skin
- Puffy face, hands, and feet
- Periorbital edema
- Drooping upper eyelids
- Enlarged tongue and hoarseness
- Hair that may be dry and sparse with patchy hair loss and loss of the outer third of the eyebrow
- Nails that may be thick and brittle with visible transverse and longitudinal grooves
- Ataxia
- Intention tremor
- Nystagmus
- Cool, doughy skin with decreased sweating
- Weak pulse and bradycardia
- Weak muscles
- Sacral or peripheral edema
- Delayed reflex relaxation time (especially in the Achilles tendon)
- Thyroid tissue that may not be easily palpable unless a goiter is present
- Absent or decreased bowel sounds
- Hypotension
- Gallop or distant heart sounds
- Adventitious breath sounds
- Abdominal distention or ascites

PICTURING PATHO

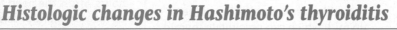

Histologic changes in Hashimoto's thyroiditis

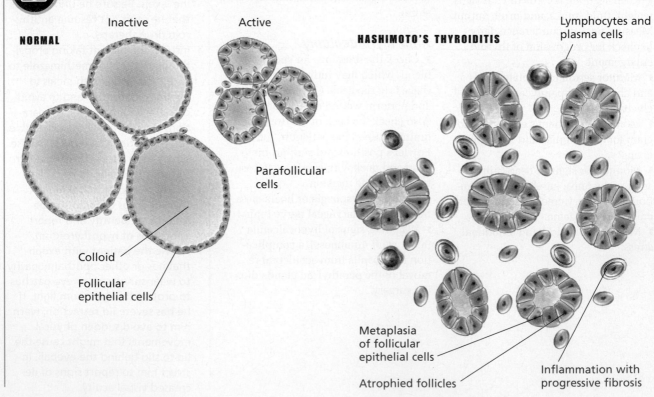

NORMAL

Inactive

Active

Parafollicular cells

Colloid

Follicular epithelial cells

HASHIMOTO'S THYROIDITIS

Lymphocytes and plasma cells

Metaplasia of follicular epithelial cells

Atrophied follicles

Inflammation with progressive fibrosis

Treatment
◗ Gradual thyroid hormone replacement with the synthetic hormone levothyroxine (T_4) and, occasionally, liothyronine (T_3)

Nursing considerations
◗ Routinely monitor and keep accurate records of the patient's vital signs, fluid intake, urine output, and daily weight.
◗ Monitor the patient's cardiovascular status. Auscultate heart and breath sounds, and watch closely for chest pain or dyspnea. Provide rest periods, and gradually increase activity to avoid fatigue and to decrease myocardial oxygen demand. Observe for dependent and sacral edema, apply antiembolism stockings, and elevate extremities to assist venous return.
◗ Encourage the patient to cough and breathe deeply to prevent pulmonary complications. Maintain fluid restrictions and a low-salt diet.
◗ Auscultate for bowel sounds, check for abdominal distention, and monitor the frequency of bowel movements. Provide the patient with a high-bulk, low-calorie diet and encourage activity to combat constipation and promote weight loss. Administer cathartics and stool softeners, as needed.
◗ Monitor mental and neurologic status. Observe the patient for disorientation, decreased level of consciousness, and hearing loss. If needed, reorient him to person, place, and time and use alternative communication techniques if he has impaired hearing. Explain all procedures slowly and carefully and avoid sedation, if possible. Provide a consistent environment to decrease confusion and frustration. Offer support and encouragement to the patient and his family.
◗ Provide meticulous skin care. Turn and reposition the patient every 2 hours if on extended bed rest. Use alcohol-free skin care products and an emollient lotion after bathing.
◗ Provide extra clothing and blankets for a patient with decreased cold toler-

ance. Dress the patient in layers and adjust room temperature, if indicated.
◗ During thyroid replacement therapy, watch for symptoms of hyperthyroidism, such as restlessness and sweating.
◗ Encourage the patient to verbalize his feelings and fears about changes in body image and possible rejection by others. Help him identify his strengths and use them to develop coping strategies, and encourage him to develop interests that foster a positive self-image. Reassure the patient that his appearance will improve with thyroid replacement therapy.

LESSON PLANS

Teaching about hypothyroidism in adults

◗ Help the patient and family members understand the patient's physical and mental changes. Teach them that hypothyroidism commonly causes mood changes and altered thought processes. Stress that these problems usually subside with proper treatment. Urge family members to encourage and accept the patient and to help him adhere to his treatment regimen. If necessary, refer the patient and his family to a mental health professional for additional counseling.
◗ Instruct the patient and his family to identify and report the signs and symptoms of life-threatening myxedema. Stress the importance of obtaining prompt medical care for respiratory problems and chest pain.
◗ Teach the patient and his family about long-term hormone replacement therapy. Emphasize that lifelong administration of this medication is necessary, that he should take it exactly as prescribed, and that he should never abruptly discontinue it. Advise the patient always to wear a medical identification bracelet and to carry his medication with him.

◗ Advise the patient and his family to keep accurate records of daily weight.
◗ Instruct the patient to eat a well-balanced diet that's high in fiber and fluids to prevent constipation, to restrict sodium to prevent fluid retention, and to limit calories to minimize weight gain.
◗ Tell the patient to schedule activities to avoid fatigue and to get adequate rest.
◗ Emphasize the importance of complying with periodic laboratory tests to assess thyroid function.
◗ Tell the patient that improvement of most symptoms occurs within 3 to 4 weeks after starting medicaton.

Metabolic syndrome

Metabolic syndrome—also called *syndrome X, insulin resistance syndrome, dysmetabolic syndrome,* and *multiple metabolic syndrome*—is a cluster of conditions characterized by abdominal obesity, high blood glucose (type 2 diabetes mellitus), insulin resistance, high blood cholesterol and triglycerides, and high blood pressure. More than 22% of people in the United States meet three or more of these criteria, raising their risk of heart disease and stroke and placing them at high risk for dying of myocardial infarction.

In the normal digestion process, the intestines break down food into its basic components, one of which is glucose. Glucose provides energy for cellular activity, while excess glucose is stored in cells for future use. Insulin, a hormone secreted in the pancreas, guides glucose into storage cells. However, in people with metabolic syndrome, glucose is insulin-resistant and doesn't respond to insulin's attempt to guide it into storage cells. Excess insulin is then required to overcome this resistance. This excess in quantity and force of insulin causes damage to the lining of the arteries, promotes fat storage deposits, and prevents fat breakdown. This series of events can lead to diabetes, blood clots, and coronary events.

PICTURING PATHO

What happens in metabolic syndrome

ORGANS AFFECTED BY UNTREATED METABOLIC SYNDROME

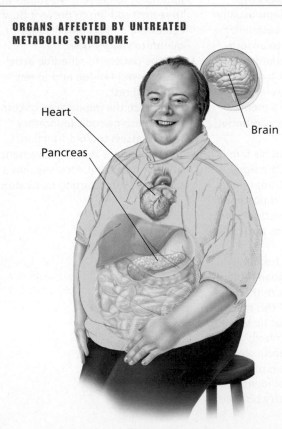

Brain

Heart

Pancreas

FIBROUS PLAQUE (ATHEROSCLEROSIS)

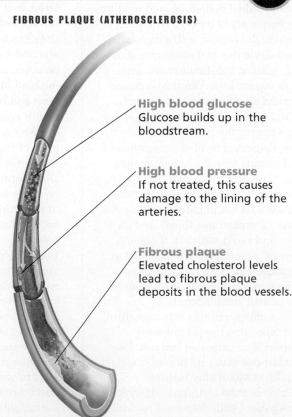

High blood glucose
Glucose builds up in the bloodstream.

High blood pressure
If not treated, this causes damage to the lining of the arteries.

Fibrous plaque
Elevated cholesterol levels lead to fibrous plaque deposits in the blood vessels.

Signs and symptoms

▶ Abdominal obesity (waist circumference of more than 40″ [101.6 cm] in men and 35″ [88.9 cm] in women)
▶ Serum triglyceride levels > 150 mg/dl
▶ Serum HDL levels < 40 mg/dl in men and < 50 mg/dl in women, or low HDL-C levels
▶ History of sedentary lifestyle
▶ Family history of metabolic syndrome
▶ Blood pressure 130/85 mm Hg or higher
▶ Fasting blood glucose level that's 100 mg/dl or higher
▶ Tiredness, especially after eating
▶ Difficulty losing weight

Treatment

▶ Lifestyle modifications that focus on dietary changes and exercise therapy to promote weight loss, improve insulin sensitivity, and reduce blood glucose levels
▶ Phentermine for short-term treatment of obesity in conjunction with diet and exercise
▶ Orlistat for long-term weight loss
▶ Gastric bypass procedures such as bariatric surgery

Nursing considerations

▶ Monitor the patient's blood pressure, blood glucose, blood cholesterol, and insulin levels.
▶ To improve compliance, schedule frequent follow-up appointments with the patient. At that time, review his food diaries and exercise logs. Be positive and promote his active participation and partnership in his treatment plan.
▶ Assist with dietary choices to comply with a low-fat, low-cholesterol diet. Refer the patient to a dietician if needed.
▶ Encourage increased activity.
▶ Monitor patients taking atypical antipsychotics such as clozapine (Clozaril) for signs and symptoms of metabolic syndrome.

LESSON PLANS

 Teaching about metabolic syndrome

▶ Teach the patient about the disorder including any diagnostic tests and the treatment regimen.
▶ Explain medication dosages, routes, and possible adverse reactions and when to call the practitioner.
▶ Teach the patient the principles of a healthy diet and the importance of regular excersise.
▶ Because research indicates that longer lifestyle modification programs are associated with improved weight loss maintenance, encourage patients with metabolic syndrome to begin an exercise and weight loss program with a friend or family member. Assist him in exploring options and support his efforts.
▶ Encourage compliance with follow-up appointments and blood tests.

Syndrome of inappropriate antidiuretic hormone

Syndrome of inappropriate antidiuretic hormone (SIADH) is a potentially life-threatening condition marked by excessive release of antidiuretic hormone (ADH), which disturbs fluid and electrolyte balance. SIADH occurs secondary to diseases that affect the osmoreceptors (supraoptic nucleus) of the hypothalamus. The prognosis depends on the underlying disorder and the patient's response to treatment.

What happens in SIADH

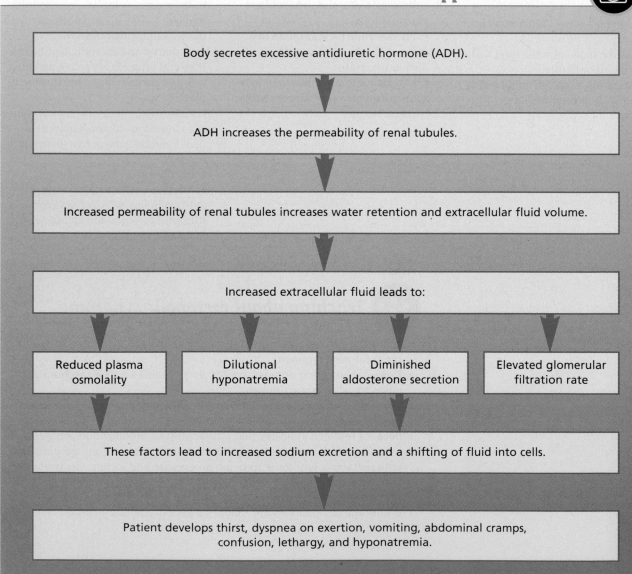

Body secretes excessive antidiuretic hormone (ADH).

ADH increases the permeability of renal tubules.

Increased permeability of renal tubules increases water retention and extracellular fluid volume.

Increased extracellular fluid leads to:

| Reduced plasma osmolality | Dilutional hyponatremia | Diminished aldosterone secretion | Elevated glomerular filtration rate |

These factors lead to increased sodium excretion and a shifting of fluid into cells.

Patient develops thirst, dyspnea on exertion, vomiting, abdominal cramps, confusion, lethargy, and hyponatremia.

Signs and symptoms

▶ History of cerebrovascular disease, cancer, pulmonary disease, or recent head injury
▶ History of drug therapy, such as chlorpropamide (Diabinese), carbamazepine (Tegrelol), cyclophosphamide (Cytoxan)
▶ Anorexia
▶ Nausea and vomiting
▶ Weight gain
▶ Lethargy
▶ Headaches
▶ Emotional and behavioral changes
▶ Tachycardia associated with increased fluid volume
▶ Disorientation, which may progress to seizures and coma
▶ Sluggish deep tendon reflexes
▶ Muscle weakness
▶ Thirst
▶ Abdominal cramping

Treatment

▶ Restricted water intake (500 to 1,000 ml/day)
▶ High-salt, high-protein diet or urea supplements
▶ Correction of the underlying cause of SIADH, such as infection or adrenal insufficiency; if due to cancer, surgery, irradiation, or chemotherapy to alleviate water retention
▶ Demeclocycline to block the renal response to ADH (if fluid restriction proves ineffective)
▶ Discontinuing drugs known to cause SIADH

Nursing considerations

▶ Closely monitor and record the patient's intake and output, vital signs, and daily weight. Watch for hyponatremia.
▶ Restrict fluids, and provide comfort measures for thirst, including ice chips, mouth care, lozenges, and staggered water intake.
▶ Perform frequent neurologic checks, depending on the patient's status. Look for and report early changes in level of consciousness (LOC). Reduce unnecessary environmental stimuli and orient the patient, as needed. Elevate the head of the bed to prevent cerebral edema.
▶ Provide a safe environment for the patient with an altered LOC. Institute seizure precautions, as needed.
▶ Observe for signs and symptoms of heart failure, which may occur due to fluid overload.

LESSON PLANS

Teaching about SIADH

▶ If SIADH doesn't resolve by the time of discharge, explain to the patient and family members why he *must* restrict fluid intake. Review ways to decrease the patient's discomfort from thirst, such as chewing sugar-free gum, sucking on sugar-free candy, and practicing relaxation techniques such as yoga.
▶ If drug therapy is prescribed, teach the patient and family about the regimen, including dosage, action, and possible adverse effects.
▶ Discuss self-monitoring techniques for fluid retention, including measurement of intake and output and daily weight. Teach the patient to recognize signs and symptoms that require immediate medical intervention.

Thyroid cancer

Although thyroid cancer occurs in all age groups, patients who have had radiation therapy in the neck area are especially susceptible. Papillary and follicular carcinomas are the most common forms of thyroid cancers and are usually associated with the longest survival times.

Papillary carcinoma

Papillary carcinoma accounts for about half of thyroid cancer in adults. It can occur at any age but is most common in young adult females. Usually multifocal and bilateral, it metastasizes slowly into regional nodes of the neck, mediastinum, lungs, and other distant organs. It's the least virulent form of thyroid cancer.

Follicular carcinoma

Less common, follicular carcinoma is more likely to recur and metastasize to the regional lymph nodes and spread through blood vessels into the bones, liver, and lungs.

Medullary (solid) carcinoma

Medullary carcinoma originates in the parafollicular cells derived from the last branchial pouch and contains amyloid and calcium deposits. This form of thyroid cancer is familial, possibly inherited as an autosomal dominant trait and usually associated with pheochromocytoma. It's most curable when detected before it causes symptoms. If left untreated, however, it grows rapidly, frequently metastasizing to bones, liver, and kidneys.

Anaplastic carcinoma

Also known as *giant* and *spindle cell cancer,* it resists radiation and is almost never curable by resection. This cancer metastasizes rapidly, causing death by invading the trachea and compressing adjacent structures.

PICTURING PATHO

Early, localized thyroid cancer

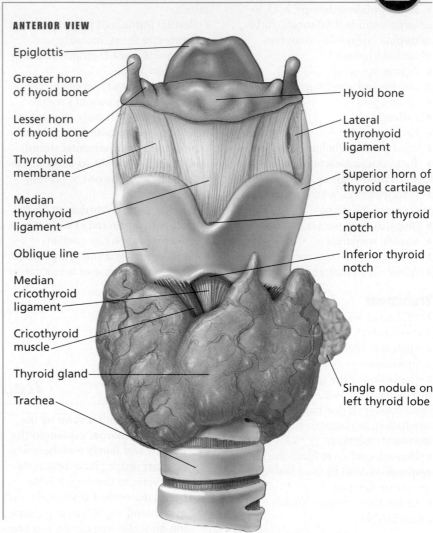

ANTERIOR VIEW

- Epiglottis
- Greater horn of hyoid bone
- Lesser horn of hyoid bone
- Thyrohyoid membrane
- Median thyrohyoid ligament
- Oblique line
- Median cricothyroid ligament
- Cricothyroid muscle
- Thyroid gland
- Trachea
- Hyoid bone
- Lateral thyrohyoid ligament
- Superior horn of thyroid cartilage
- Superior thyroid notch
- Inferior thyroid notch
- Single nodule on left thyroid lobe

Signs and symptoms

- Painless nodule
- Sensitivity to cold and mental apathy (hypothyroidism, if tumor has destroyed the thyroid)
- Sensitivity to heat
- Restlessness
- Overactivity (hyperthyroidism, if excess thyroid hormone production)
- Diarrhea
- Dysphagia
- Anorexia
- Irritability
- Ear pain
- Hoarseness
- Vocal stridor
- Disfiguring thyroid mass
- Hard nodule in an enlarged thyroid gland
- Palpable lymph nodes with thyroid enlargement
- Bruits

Treatment

▶ Total or subtotal thyroidectomy with modified node dissection (bilateral or homolateral) on the side of the primary cancer (for papillary or follicular carcinoma)
▶ Total thyroidectomy and radical neck excision (for medullary or anaplastic carcinoma); minimally invasive video-assisted thyroidectomy (for small masses)
▶ Radioisotope (^{131}I) therapy with external radiation (sometimes postoperatively in lieu of radical neck excision) or alone (for metastasis)
▶ Adjunctive thyroid suppression with exogenous thyroid hormones
▶ Chemotherapy limited to treating symptoms of widespread metastasis, as a palliative measure (doxorubicin has some antitumor activity in about 20% of cases)

Nursing considerations

▶ Prepare the patient for scheduled surgery.
▶ Encourage the patient to voice his concerns, and offer reassurance.
▶ Before surgery, establish a way for the patient to communicate postoperatively (pad and pencil, head nodding for yes and no, or other ways).
▶ Postoperatively, keep the patient in semi-Fowler's position with the head supported with sandbags and pillows.
▶ Monitor the patient's neck dressing for drainage. Assess patency of the patient's airway and notify the physician if the patient complains of difficulty swallowing or breathing.

▶ Check serum calcium levels daily because hypocalcemia may develop if the parathyroid glands were removed.
▶ Watch for and report other complications, such as hemorrhage and shock (elevated pulse rate and hypotension), tetany (carpopedal spasm, twitching, and seizures), thyroid storm (high fever, severe tachycardia, delirium, dehydration, and extreme irritability), and respiratory obstruction (dyspnea, crowing respirations, and retraction of neck tissues).
▶ Keep a tracheotomy set and oxygen equipment handy in the event respiratory obstruction occurs. Use continuous steam inhalation in the patient's room until his chest sounds clear. Administer pain medications, as ordered, and make sure that the patient feels as comfortable as possible.
▶ Provide I.V. fluids or a soft diet, as ordered. Many patients can tolerate a regular diet within 24 hours of surgery.
▶ Provide the same postoperative care after extensive tumor and node excision as you would after radical neck surgery.

PICTURING PATHO

Anaplastic thyroid cancer

The most disfiguring, destructive, and deadly form of thyroid cancer, anaplastic carcinoma has the poorest prognosis. Although this tumor rarely metastasizes to distant organs, its rapid growth and size produce severe anatomic distortion of nearby structures. Treatment usually consists of total thyroidectomy, which seldom is successful.

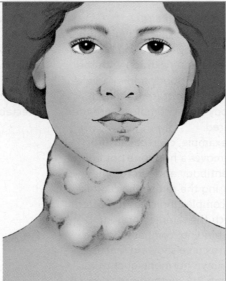

LESSON PLANS

Teaching about thyroid cancer

▶ Preoperatively, advise the patient to expect temporary voice loss or hoarseness for several days after surgery. Also, explain the operation and postoperative procedures and positioning.
▶ Before discharge, ensure that the patient knows the date and time of his next appointment. Answer his questions about his treatment and home care. Be sure he understands the purpose of his medications, dosage, administration times, and possible adverse effects.
▶ Refer the patient to resource and support services, such as the social service department, home health care agencies, hospices, and the American Cancer Society.

TESTS

Various tests are used to suggest, confirm, or rule out an endocrine disorder. Some test results also identify a dysfunction as hyperfunction or hypofunction or indicate whether a problem is primary, secondary, or functional. Endocrine function is tested by direct, indirect, provocative, and radiographic studies.

Direct testing

BLOOD TESTS

▶ Cortisol measurement to evaluate adrenocortical function
▶ Catecholamine measurement to assess adrenal medulla function
▶ Parathyroid hormone measurement to evaluate parathyroid function
▶ Growth hormone (GH) radioimmunoassay to evaluate GH oversecretion

▶ Thyroxine (T_4) radioimmunoassay to evaluate thyroid function and monitor iodine or antithyroid therapy
▶ Triiodothyronine radioimmunoassay to detect hyperthyroidism if T_4 levels are normal
▶ Follicle-stimulating hormone and luteinizing hormone measurements to distinguish a primary gonadal problem from pituitary insufficiency

URINE STUDIES

▶ 17-ketosteroid test to evaluate adrenocortical and gonadal function
▶ 17-hydroxycorticosteroid test to evaluate adrenal function
▶ Free cortisol test
▶ 24-hour urine test

Methods of direct testing

Methods of direct testing to measure hormone levels in the blood or urine include immunoradiometric assay (IRMA), radioimmunoassay (RIA), and 24-hour urine testing.

Immunoradiometric assay
IRMA measures levels of peptide and protein in hormones. These tests use a receptor antiserum labeled with radioiodine. Immunochemiluminometric assay (ICMA) uses a chemical reagent that emits a specific light waveform when activated by a particular substance. IRMA and ICMA are more specific, stable, precise, and easier to use than RIA. Tests called radioreceptor assays measure the activity of a hormone.

Radioimmunoassay
RIA determines several types of hormone levels by incubating blood or urine (or a urine extract) with the hormone's antibody and a radiolabeled hormone tracer (antigen). Antibody-tracer complexes are then measured.

For example, charcoal absorbs and removes a hormone not bound to its antibody-antigen complex. Measuring the remaining radiolabeled complex indicates the extent to which the sample hormone blocks binding, compared with a standard curve showing reactions with known hormone quantities. Although RIA method provides reliable results, it doesn't measure every hormone.

24-hour urine testing
A 24-hour urine test may be ordered to confirm adrenal, renal, and gonadal disorders. Metabolite measurement is used to evaluate hormones excreted in virtually undetectable amounts.

Indirect testing

Indirect testing is used to measure the substance controlled by a hormone—not the hormone itself. For example, glucose measurements are used to evaluate insulin levels and calcium measurements are used to assess parathyroid hormone (PTH) activity. Although radioimmunoassays measure these substances directly, indirect testing is easier and less costly.

Glucose levels obtained indirectly accurately reflect insulin's effectiveness. However, various factors that affect calcium may also alter PTH levels and, thus, the results of indirect testing. For example, abnormal protein levels can lead to abnormal calcium levels, because nearly half of calcium binds to plasma proteins. Therefore, other possibilities must be ruled out before assuming that an abnormal calcium level reflects a PTH imbalance.

Such tests include:
◗ oral glucose tolerance test to detect impaired glucose tolerance and hypoglycemia
◗ calcium measurement to detect bone and parathyroid disorders
◗ phosphorus test to detect parathyroid disorders and renal failure
◗ glycosylated hemoglobin test to monitor the degree of glucose control in diabetes mellitus over 3 months.

Provocative testing

Provocative testing is used to determine an endocrine gland's reserve function when other tests show borderline hormone levels or don't quite pinpoint the site of the abnormality. For example, an abnormally low cortisol level may indicate adrenal hypofunction or indirectly reflect pituitary hypofunction.

Provocative testing works on the principle that an underactive gland should be stimulated and an overactive gland should be suppressed (depending on the patient's underlying disorder). A hormone level that doesn't increase with stimulation confirms primary hypofunction. Hormone secretion that continues after suppression confirms hyperfunction.

Such tests include:
◗ insulin-induced hypoglycemia test to detect hypopituitarism
◗ thyroid-stimulating hormone test to detect primary hypothyroidism.

Radiographic studies

Imaging studies are done with or after other tests. Imaging studies include X-rays, computed tomography (CT) scans, ultrasound studies, magnetic resonance imaging (MRI), as well as nuclear studies.

X-RAYS

Routine X-rays are used to evaluate how an endocrine dysfunction affects body tissues, although they don't reveal endocrine glands. For example, a bone X-ray, routinely ordered for a suspected parathyroid disorder, can show the effects of a calcium imbalance.

CT SCAN AND MRI

CT scan and MRI are used to assess an endocrine gland by providing high-resolution, tomographic, three-dimensional (3-D) images of the gland's structure and may be used to identify tumors.

ULTRASOUND

An ultrasound uses high-frequency sound waves to create images of soft-tissue structures and masses. It's noninvasive and should be used to evaluate all patients with known or suspected thyroid nodules.

NUCLEAR STUDIES

Nuclear studies include radioactive iodine uptake (RAIU) test and radionuclide thyroid testing.

RAIU

The RAIU test evaluates thyroid function and helps to distinguish between primary and secondary thyroid disorders. After ingesting an oral dose of radioactive iodine, the patient's thyroid is scanned at 2 hours, 6 hours, and 24 hours using an external single counting probe.

The amount of radioactivity detected by the probe is compared with the amount of radioactivity contained in the original dose to determine the percentage of radioactive iodine retained by the thyroid.

Below-normal iodine uptake may indicate hypothyroidism and above-normal uptake may indicate hyperthyroidism or early Hashimoto's thyroiditis.

Radionuclide thyroid imaging

This test is performed to evaluate thyroid function and to assess the size, structure, and position of the thyroid gland. Such testing typically follows discovery of a palpable mass, enlarged gland, or asymmetrical goiter. After oral administration or I.V. injection of a radioisotope, such as radioactive iodine (^{131}I), ^{123}I, or technetium 99m pertechnetate, images are taken of the thyroid gland.

Hyperfunctioning nodules (areas of excessive iodine uptake) appear as black regions called hot spots. Hypofunctioning nodules (areas of little or no iodine uptake) appear as white or light-gray regions called cold spots. Biopsies may be performed to rule out malignancy.

Thyroid uptake imaging

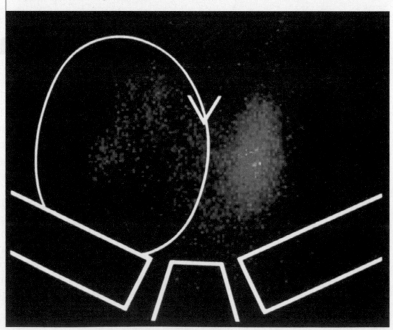

This is a nuclear image involving scanning of the thyroid gland to visualize radioactive accumulation of previously injected isotopes to detect thyroid nodules or tumors. The circled area is suggestive of hypofunctioning nodules.

TREATMENTS AND PROCEDURES
Drug therapy

Drugs commonly used to treat endocrine disorders include antidiabetics, antidiuretic hormones, thyroid hormone antagonists, and thyroid hormones.

ANTIDIABETICS

▶ Includes insulin and oral hypoglycemics
▶ Reduces the serum glucose level by increasing glucose transport into the cells and promoting glucose conversion to glycogen
▶ Lower blood glucose levels for type 1 and type 2 diabetes mellitus

▶ Examples of types of insulin: *rapid-acting*: insulin aspart (NovoLog), lispro (Humalog), regular insulin (Humulin-R); *intermediate-acting*: isophane insulin (NPH [Humulin N]), and insulin zinc suspension (lente [Humulin L]); *long-acting*: extended insulin zinc suspension (ultralente [Humulin U, Ultralente Insulin]), and glargine (Lantus)
▶ Examples of oral hypoglycemics: metformin (Glucophage) and glipizide (Glucotrol)

ANTIDIURETIC HORMONES

▶ Enhance reabsorption of water in the kidneys and smooth muscle contraction (vasoconstriction), promoting an antidiuretic effect and regulating fluid balance
▶ Treat diabetes insipidus

▶ Examples: desmopressin (DDAVP) and vasopressin (Pitressin)

THYROID HORMONE ANTAGONISTS

▶ Inhibit the synthesis of thyroid hormones
▶ Treat hyperthyroidism
▶ Examples: propylthiouracil, methimazole (Tapazole)

THYROID HORMONES

▶ Control the metabolic rate of tissues and accelerate heat production and oxygen consumption
▶ Treat primary and secondary hypothyroidism
▶ Examples: levothyroxine sodium (T_4 [Levothroid, Levoxine, Synthroid]), liothyronine sodium (T_3 [Cytomel], Triostat)

Insulin therapy

There are several routes of administration and devices for injection of insulin.

Subcutaneous route
Insulin is usually given by subcutaneous injection with a standard insulin syringe. Subcutaneous insulin can also be given with a penlike injection device that uses a disposable needle and replaceable insulin cartridges, eliminating the need to draw insulin into a syringe.

Jet-injection devices
Jet-injection devices are expensive and require special cleaning procedures, but they disperse insulin more rapidly and speed absorption. These devices draw up insulin from standard containers, which enables the patient to mix insulins, if necessary, but requires a special procedure for drawing it up. After the insulin is drawn up, it's delivered into the subcutaneous tissue with a pressure jet.

Insulin pumps
Multiple-dose regimens may use an insulin pump to deliver insulin continuously into subcutaneous tissue. The infusion rate selector automatically releases about half of the total daily insulin requirement evenly over 24 hours. The patient releases the remainder in bolus amounts before meals and snacks.

Site rotation
When administering insulin injections subcutaneously the injection sites should be rotated. Because absorption rates differ at each site, diabetic educators recommend rotating the injection site within a specific area such as the abdomen.

I.V. and I.M. routes
Regular insulin or insulin lispro may also be administered I.V. or I.M. during severe episodes of hyperglycemia. These are the only types of insulin that should ever be administered by these routes.

Investigational routes
Researchers are working on newer, more efficient ways of administering insulin. One newer method of insulin administration is the intranasal delivery method. This method is still expeimental.

Locating subcutaneous injection sites

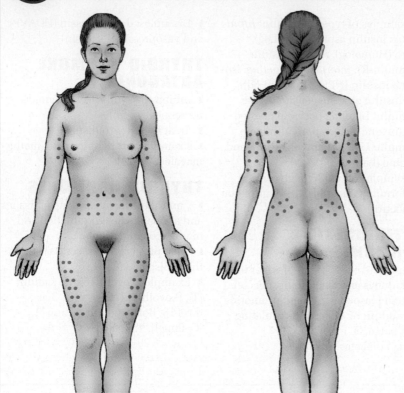

Subcutaneous injection sites (as indicated by the dotted areas in the illustration as shown at left) include the fat pads on the abdomen, upper hips, upper back, and lateral upper arms and thighs. For subcutaneous injections administered repeatedly, such as insulin, rotate sites. Choose one injection site in one area, move to a corresponding injection site in the next area, and so on.

When returning to an area, choose a new site in that area. Preferred injection sites for insulin are the arms, abdomen, thighs, and buttocks.

Using an insulin pen

When patients require multiple injections of insulin each day, an insulin pen is a convenient method that requires less equipment and may be easier to use than traditional syringes and insulin vials. The insulin pen may be prefilled with insulin (disposable type) or reusable (reloaded with disposable insulin cartridges.) Prefilled pens and insulin cartridges need to be refrigerated until used, and once in use, they may be kept at room temperature according to the type of insulin used. A disposable needle is attached to the pen and the pen is primed according to the manufacturer's directions. The patient then selects the dose to be delivered on the pen's dial and injects the insulin according to his provider's instructions. Once the insulin is injected, the needle is removed from the pen and disposed of safely. The pen is recapped for the next use.

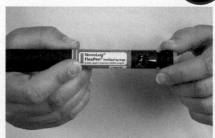

Nonsurgical treatments

Nonsurgical treatments for endocrine disorders include meal planning for diabetes mellitus and radioactive iodine (^{131}I) administration.

DIABETIC MEAL PLANNING

Diabetic specialists regard meal planning as the cornerstone of diabetes care because the patient's food intake can be carefully controlled to prevent widely fluctuating blood glucose levels. If the patient is taking insulin or sulfonylureas, he must adhere to his meal plan even more carefully to avoid hypoglycemia.

The patient's diet should be well-balanced, containing all the necessary nutrients. However, to avoid wide blood glucose variations, the patient must closely regulate his protein, fat, and carbohydrate intake. Currently, the American Dietetic Association and the American Diabetes Association recommend an individual nutritional assessment to determine appropriate medical nutrition therapy. Carbohydrate and protein composition will vary, depending on therapeutic goals, and fat should be less than 30% of total calories. The relatively low fat content may help reduce the risk of cardiovascular disease.

^{131}I ADMINISTRATION

A form of radiation therapy, the administration of ^{131}I, treats hyperthyroidism, particularly Graves' disease, and is an adjunctive treatment for thyroid cancer. It shrinks functioning thyroid tissue, decreasing circulating thyroid hormone levels and destroying malignant cells. After oral ingestion, ^{131}I is rapidly absorbed and concentrated into the thyroid as if it were normal iodine, resulting in acute radiation thyroiditis and gradual thyroid atrophy. ^{131}I causes symptoms to subside after about 3 weeks and exerts its full effect in 3 to 6 months.

Surgery

Surgical treatments for endocrine disorders include adrenalectomy, bariatric surgery for weight reduction, hypophysectomy, parathyroidectomy, and thyroidectomy.

ADRENALECTOMY

Adrenalectomy is the surgical resection or removal of one or both adrenal glands. It's the treatment of choice for adrenal hyperfunction and hyperaldosteronism. It's also used to treat adrenal tumors, such as adenomas and pheochromocytomas (with variable prognoses), and has been used to aid treatment of breast and prostate cancer.

HYPOPHYSECTOMY

Microsurgical techniques have dramatically reversed the high mortality previously associated with removal of the pituitary and sella turcica tumors. Transsphenoidal hypophysectomy is now the treatment of choice for pituitary tumors, which can cause acromegaly, giantism, and Cushing's syndrome. The surgery is also a palliative measure (for patients with metastatic breast or prostate cancer) to relieve pain and reduce the hormonal secretions that spur neoplastic growth.

Hypophysectomy may be performed subfrontally (approaching the sella turcica through the cranium) or transsphenoidally (entering from the inner aspect of the upper lip through the sphenoid sinus). The subfrontal approach carries a high risk of mortality or complications, such as loss of smell and taste and permanent, severe diabetes insipidus. As a result, this approach is only used in cases where a tumor causes marked subfrontal or subtemporal extension with optic chiasm involvement.

Adenectomy: Alternative to hypophysectomy

Both adenectomy and hypophysectomy can be used to remove pituitary tumors. In hypophysectomy, the surgeon removes the tumor and all or part of the pituitary gland. However, for a tumor confined to the sella turcica, the surgeon may be able to perform an adenectomy, in which he removes the lesion while leaving the pituitary gland intact. Both surgeries involve the transsphenoidal approach shown here.

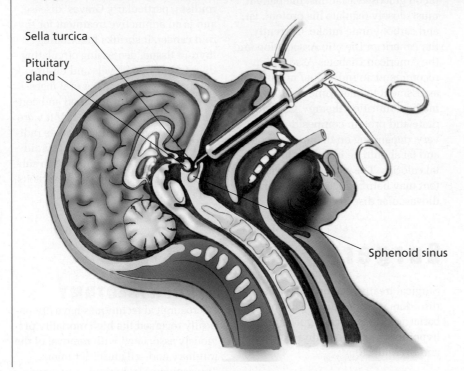

Sella turcica

Pituitary gland

Sphenoid sinus

BARIATRIC SURGERY

Bariatric or weight loss surgery is performed on the stomach, intestines, or both to promote weight loss in extremely obese patients. Bariatric procedures limit food intake by reducing the capacity of the stomach without interfering with normal digestion, thus sharply restricting food intake. These procedures include vertical banded gastroplasty and adjustable gastric banding.

Combined malabsorptive and restrictive procedures restrict food intake and the amount of calories and nutrients the body absorbs. These procedures include gastric bypass and biliopancreatic diversion.

Types of bariatric surgery

Vertical banded gastroplasty

In this common procedure, which may be performed by laparoscopy or laparotomy, the surgeon uses both a band and staples to create the reduced stomach pouch.

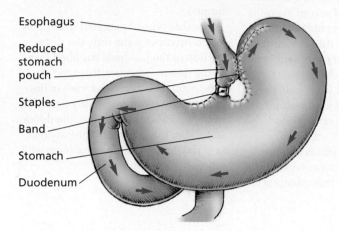

Esophagus

Reduced stomach pouch

Staples

Band

Stomach

Duodenum

Adjustable gastric banding

In this laparoscopic adjustable and reversible procedure, the surgeon places the band around the top of the stomach. The inflation and deflation tube is then inflated 4 weeks postoperatively.

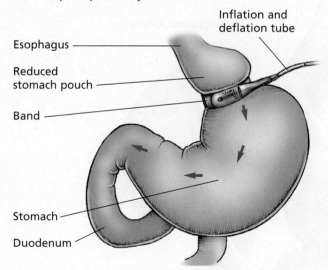

Inflation and deflation tube

Esophagus

Reduced stomach pouch

Band

Stomach

Duodenum

Gastric bypass

Also called *Roux-en Y gastric bypass,* this procedure may be performed by laparoscopy or laparotomy. The surgeon uses sutures and staples with anastomosis to the jejunum to create the reduced stomach pouch.

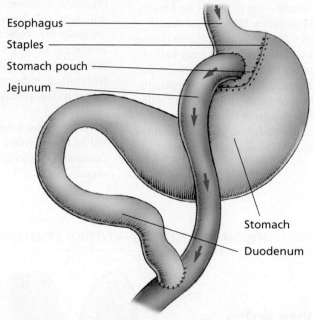

Esophagus

Staples

Stomach pouch

Jejunum

Stomach

Duodenum

Biliopancreatic diversion

In this more complex procedure, the surgeon removes the lower portion of the stomach and anastomoses the remainder of the pouch to the ileum of the small intestines.

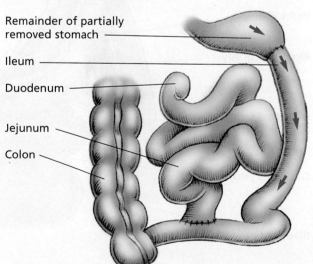

Remainder of partially removed stomach

Ileum

Duodenum

Jejunum

Colon

PANCREAS TRANSPLANTATION

Pancreas transplantation may be performed using one of two methods: whole-organ transplantation and islet beta-cell transplantation. Greater risk is involved with whole-organ transplantation, but it also offers the greatest benefit—the potential for insulin independence. However, although about 6,000 potential cadaver donors are available each year, only half of those are suitable for transplantation.

Transplantation of a pancreas, unlike a liver, lung, or heart, isn't a life-saving operation but it improves quality of life and gives the patient the potential for insulin independence.

Whole-organ pancreas transplantation

Typical candidates for pancreas transplantation are people without insulin secretion, who aren't obese, who are younger than age 50, and who have difficulty controlling blood glucose. Because of the risk of severe hypoglycemia or diabetic coma in patients with type 1 diabetes, these candidates are preferred. Typical candidates are patients with type 1 diabetes as they're at greater risk (than patients with type 2 diabetes) for developing severe hypoglycemia or diabetic coma.

Whole-organ transplantation involves identifying a tissue-compatible donor and surgically transplanting the organ.

The procedure can be done simultaneously with a kidney transplant, after a kidney transplant, or as a pancreas transplant alone. Currently, simultaneous transplantation of the pancreas and kidneys is the most common type of whole organ transplant being performed.

Another type of pancreas transplantation involves using only the distal portion of the pancreas supplied by a living donor. However, this type of transplantation is rare because of the controversy about using only a portion of the pancreas. In addition, the donor supplying the portion of the pancreas is at risk for developing problems with glucose tolerance.

Simultaneous pancreas–kidney transplantation

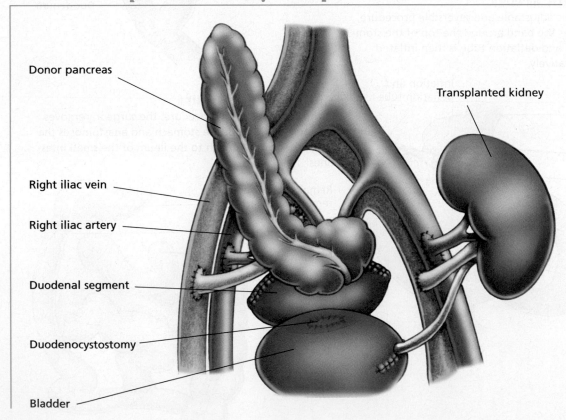

Donor pancreas

Right iliac vein

Right iliac artery

Duodenal segment

Duodenocystostomy

Bladder

Transplanted kidney

Islet cell transplantation

Islet cells (from the pancreas of a cadaver) are initially exposed to an enzyme to allow for their recovery. Once obtained, the islet cells are then injected into the patient's liver through the portal vein, using a laparoscopic or transhepatic angiographic approach. A typical transplantation requires about 1 million islet cells and usually involves the need for at least two cadaver pancreases.

The islet cells become wedged in the smaller portal vein tributaries. Here, they engraft, receiving their blood supply from the patient's vessels for growth. When implanted, the new islet cells begin to make and release insulin.

Understanding islet cell transplantation

This illustration shows the isolation of the islet cells from the donor pancreas, which are then injected into the patient's portal vein for engrafting.

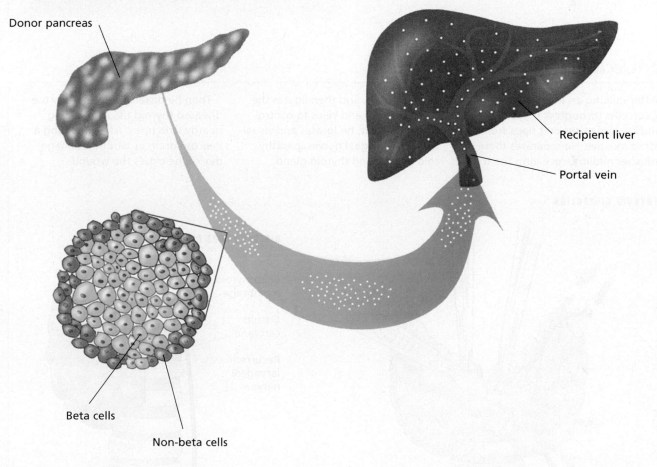

Donor pancreas

Recipient liver

Portal vein

Beta cells

Non-beta cells

THYROIDECTOMY

Thyroidectomy is the surgical removal of all or part of the thyroid gland. It's performed to treat hyperthyroidism, respiratory obstruction from goiter, and thyroid cancer. Subtotal thyroidectomy, which reduces secretion of thyroid hormone, is used to correct hyperthyroidism when drug therapy fails or radiation therapy is contraindicated. It may also effectively treat diffuse goiter. After surgery, the remaining thyroid tissue usually supplies enough thyroid hormone for normal function, although hypothyroidism may occur later.

Incision line for thyroid surgery

In thyroid surgery, the surgeon fully extends the patient's neck and determines the incision line by measuring from each clavicle.

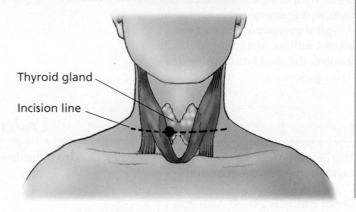

Thyroid gland

Incision line

Dissecting diseased thyroid tissue

After making an incision, the surgeon cuts through skin, fascia, and muscle and raises skin flaps from the strap muscles. He separates these muscles midline, revealing the thyroid's isthmus, and then ligates the thyroid artery and veins to control bleeding. Next, he locates and visualizes the laryngeal nerves, parathyroid glands, and thyroid gland.

Then he dissects and removes the diseased thyroid tissue, avoiding nearby structures. After inserting a Penrose drain or wound drainage device, he closes the wound.

THYROID DISSECTION

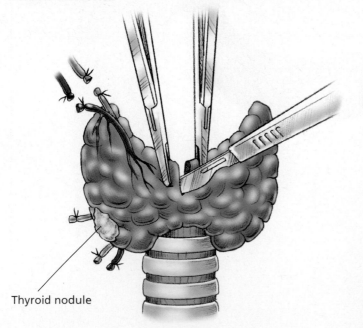

Thyroid nodule

DISEASED LOBE REMOVAL

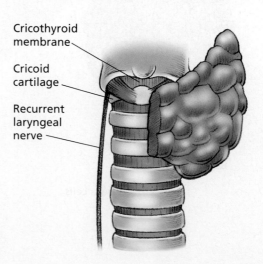

Cricothyroid membrane

Cricoid cartilage

Recurrent laryngeal nerve

Integumentary care

DISEASES
Acne vulgaris

Acne vulgaris is an inflammatory disease of the skin glands and hair follicles that appears as comedones, pustules, nodules, and nodular lesions. This disorder, which tends to run in families, affects nearly 85% of adolescents with a westernized lifestyle, although lesions can appear as early as age 8. Acne affects boys more commonly and more severely; however, it typically occurs in girls at an earlier age and tends to affect them for a longer time, sometimes into adulthood. With treatment, the prognosis is good.

PICTURING PATHO

How acne develops

EXCESSIVE SEBUM PRODUCTION

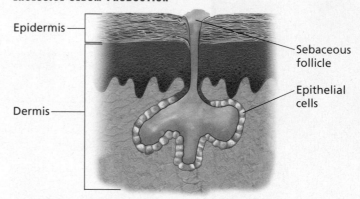

Epidermis

Sebaceous follicle

Epithelial cells

Dermis

INCREASED SHEDDING OF EPITHELIAL CELLS

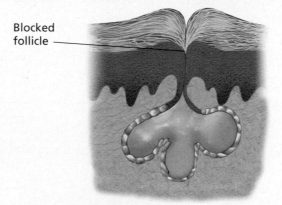

Blocked follicle

INFLAMMATORY RESPONSE IN FOLLICLE

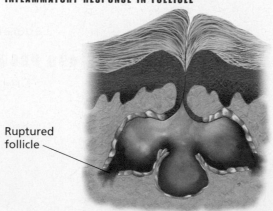

Ruptured follicle

Signs and symptoms

▶ Pain and tenderness around the area of the infected follicle

▶ Acne lesions, most commonly on the face, neck, shoulders, chest, and upper back

▶ Area around the infected follicle that appears red and swollen

▶ Acne plug that may appear as a closed comedo, or whitehead (if it doesn't protrude from the follicle and is covered by the epidermis), or as an open comedo, or blackhead (if it protrudes and isn't covered by the epidermis)

▶ Inflammation and characteristic acne pustules, papules or, in severe forms, acne cysts or abscesses

▶ Visible scars

Treatment

▶ Benzoyl peroxide (powerful antibacterial)

▶ Clindamycin (Cleocin), erythromycin (Akne-mycin), or antibacterial agents alone or in combination with tretinoin (retinoic acid [Retin-A] or topical vitamin A)

▶ Tetracycline to decrease bacterial growth

▶ Oral isotretinoin (Amnesteem)

▶ Birth control pills (such as Ortho-TriCyclen) or spironolactone to produce antiandrogenic effects (in females)

▶ Intralesional corticosteroid injections

▶ Exposure to ultraviolet light (but never when a photosensitizing agent, such as isotretinoin, is being used)

▶ Cryotherapy

▶ Acne surgery

PICTURING PATHO

Comedones of acne

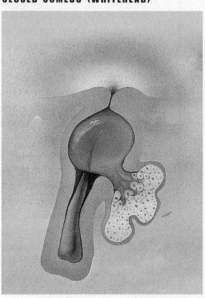

CLOSED COMEDO (WHITEHEAD)

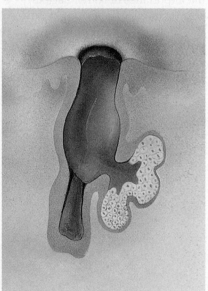

OPEN COMEDO (BLACKHEAD)

Nursing considerations

❱ Assist the patient in identifying and eliminating predisposing factors.

❱ Encourage good personal hygiene and the use of oil-free skin care products. Discourage picking, scratching, or squeezing the lesions to eliminate secondary bacterial infections and scarring.

❱ Monitor liver function studies and serum triglyceride levels when isotretinoin is used.

❱ Be alert for possible complications associated with using systemic antibiotics (such as tetracycline), including sensitivity reactions, GI disturbances, and liver dysfunction.

❱ Remember that tetracycline is contraindicated during pregnancy because it discolors the fetus's unerupted teeth.

❱ Be alert for possible adverse reactions associated with using isotretinoin, including possible skin irritation, dry skin and mucous membranes, and elevated triglyceride levels.

❱ Encourage the patient with acne to verbalize his feelings, including embarrassment, fear of rejection by others, and disturbed body image. Note the importance of body image in growth and development. Encourage him to develop interests that support a positive self-image and deemphasize appearance.

LESSON PLANS

Teaching about acne

❱ Explain the causes of acne to the patient and his family. Encourage the patient to seek medical treatment if extensive acne develops.

❱ Make sure the patient and his family understand that the prescribed treatment will improve acne more than will a strict diet or excessive scrubbing with soap and water. Advise using sunscreen whenever outdoors to prevent aggravating the skin.

❱ Instruct the patient receiving tretinoin to apply it at least 30 minutes after washing his face and at least 1 hour before bedtime. Warn against using it around the eyes or lips. Explain that after treatments, the skin should look pink and dry and that some amount of peeling is normal in the morning when tretinoin has been applied at night. Tell the patient that if the skin appears irritated, the preparation may have to be weakened or applied less often. Advise the patient to avoid exposure to sunlight while wearing the solution or to use a sunscreen.

❱ If the prescribed regimen includes tretinoin and benzoyl peroxide, advise the patient to avoid skin irritation by using one preparation in the morning and the other at night. Also advise the patient that acne typically flares up during the early course of treatment, probably because early, developing lesions are uncovered.

❱ Instruct the patient taking tetracycline to do so on an empty stomach. Advise him not to take tetracycline with antacids or milk because it interacts with their metallic ions and is then poorly absorbed. Explain that some studies suggest that a diet high in cow's milk and carbohydrates is associated with increased occurrence and severity.

❱ Tell the patient taking isotretinoin to avoid vitamin A supplements, which can worsen adverse effects. Warn the patient against giving blood during treatment with this drug and to avoid alcohol ingestion. Also, teach how to deal with the dry skin and mucous membranes that usually result during treatment. Instruct the female patient about the severe risk of teratogenicity. Encourage the patient to schedule and follow up with the necessary laboratory studies.

❱ Teach the patient and his family techniques to maintain a well-balanced diet, get adequate rest, and manage stress.

❱ Inform the patient that acne takes a long time—in some cases, years—to clear. Encourage continued local skin care even after acne clears.

Basal cell carcinoma

Basal cell carcinoma, also known as *basal cell epithelioma,* is a slow-growing, destructive skin tumor that usually occurs in people older than age 40. Forty to fifty percent of Americans age 65 or older will have either basal cell or squamous cell carcinoma at least once during their lifetime. It's most prevalent in blond, fair-skinned males, and it's the most common malignant tumor that affects whites. The two major types of basal cell carcinoma are noduloulcerative and superficial.

Prolonged sun exposure is the most common cause of basal cell carcinoma. Indeed, 90% of tumors occur on sun-exposed areas of the body. Arsenic ingestion, radiation exposure (including tanning beds), burns, immunosuppression and, rarely, vaccinations are other possible causes.

Although the pathogenesis is uncertain, some experts hypothesize that basal cell carcinoma develops when undifferentiated basal cells become carcinomatous instead of differentiating into sweat glands, sebum, and hair.

Signs and symptoms

▶ Lesions that appear as small, smooth, pinkish, and translucent papules (early-stage noduloulcerative), particularly on the forehead, eyelid margins, and nasolabial folds
▶ Telangiectatic vessels crossing the surface
▶ Lesions that may be pigmented
▶ As lesions enlarge, centers that become depressed and borders that become firm and elevated (rodent ulcers)
▶ Multiple oval or irregularly shaped, lightly pigmented plaques that may have sharply defined, slightly elevated, threadlike borders (superficial basal cell carcinomas)

Inspection of the head and neck may show waxy, sclerotic, yellow to white plaques without distinct borders. These plaques may resemble small patches of scleroderma and may suggest sclerosing basal cell carcinomas (morphea-like carcinomas).

PICTURING PATHO

Basal cell carcinoma

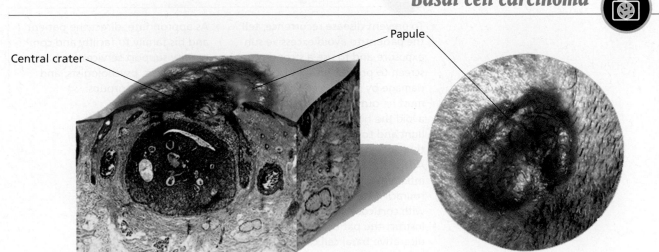

Central crater

Papule

Treatment

‣ Curettage and electrodesiccation for small lesions
‣ Topical fluorouracil for superficial lesions; produces marked local irritation or inflammation in the involved tissue but no systemic effects
‣ Microscopically controlled surgical excision to remove recurrent lesions until a tumor-free plane is achieved; possible skin grafting after removal of large lesions
‣ Irradiation, if the tumor location requires it and for elderly or debilitated patients who might not tolerate surgery
‣ Chemosurgery for persistent or recurrent lesions; consists of periodic applications of a fixative paste (such as zinc chloride) and subsequent removal of fixed pathologic tissue until the tumor is eradicated
‣ Cryotherapy, using liquid nitrogen, to freeze and, ultimately, kill cells

Nursing considerations

‣ Listen to the patient's fears and concerns. Offer reassurance, when appropriate. Remain with the patient during periods of severe stress and anxiety. Provide positive reinforcement for the patient's efforts to adapt.
‣ Arrange for the patient to interact with others who have a similar problem.
‣ Assess the patient's readiness for decision making; then involve him and family members in decisions related to his care whenever possible.
‣ Watch for complications of treatment, including local skin irritation from topically applied chemotherapeutic agents and infection.
‣ Watch for radiation's adverse effects, such as nausea, vomiting, hair loss, malaise, and diarrhea. Provide reassurance and comfort measures, when appropriate.

LESSON PLANS

 Teaching about basal cell carcinoma

‣ To prevent disease recurrence, tell the patient to avoid excessive sun exposure and to use a strong sunscreen to protect his skin from damage by ultraviolet rays. If he must be out in the sun, tell him to avoid the hours of strongest sunlight and to cover up with protective clothing.
‣ Advise the patient to relieve local inflammation from topical fluorouracil with cool compresses or with corticosteroid ointment.
‣ Instruct the patient with noduloulcerative basal cell carcinoma to wash his face gently when ulcerations and crusting occur; scrubbing too vigorously may cause bleeding.

‣ As appropriate, direct the patient and his family to facility and community support services, such as social workers, psychologists, and cancer support groups.

Burns

A major burn is a devastating injury, requiring painful treatment and a long period of rehabilitation. Burns can be fatal, permanently disfiguring, and incapacitating, both emotionally and physically.

Thermal burns, the most common type, typically result from residential fires, motor vehicle accidents, misused matches or lighters (such as a child playing with matches), improperly stored gasoline, space heater or electrical malfunctions, and arson. Other causes include improper handling of firecrackers, scalding accidents, and kitchen accidents (such as a child touching a hot stove).

Chemical burns result from the contact, ingestion, inhalation, or injection of acids, alkali, or vesicants. Electrical burns commonly occur after contact with faulty electrical wiring or high-voltage power lines, or when electric cords are chewed (by young children).

Radiation burns are caused by ionizing radiation and include sunburn and radiotherapy burns. Friction, or abrasion, burns happen when the skin is rubbed harshly against a coarse surface.

Burn severity is classified by depth of injury.

Superficial burns

Superficial burns, also referred to as *first-degree burns*, cause localized injury to the skin (epidermis only) by direct (such as a chemical spill) or indirect (such as sunlight) contact. The barrier function of the skin remains intact, and these burns aren't life-threatening.

Superficial partial-thickness burns

Superficial partial-thickness burns, also referred to as *second-degree burns*, involve destruction to the epidermis and some dermis. Thin-walled, fluid-filled blisters develop within a few minutes of the injury along with mild to moderate edema and pain. As these blisters break, the nerve endings become exposed to the air. Because pain and tactile response remains intact, subsequent treatments are very painful. The barrier function of the skin is lost.

Deep partial-thickness burns

Deep partial-thickness burns are a more severe second-degree burn that extends deeper into the dermis. The skin appears mixed red or waxy white. Blisters aren't usually present and edema usually develops. Sensation is decreased in the area of the burn.

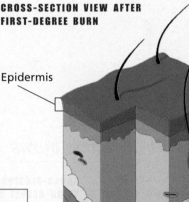

PICTURING PATHO

Superficial burns

A superficial burn causes localized injury or destruction to the epidermis only by direct (such as a chemical spill) or indirect (such as sunlight) contact. The barrier function of the skin remains intact.

CROSS-SECTION VIEW AFTER FIRST-DEGREE BURN

Epidermis

PICTURING PATHO

Superficial partial-thickness burns

Partial-thickness burns involve destruction to the epidermis and some dermis. Thin-walled, fluid-filled blisters develop within a few minutes of the injury along with mild to moderate edema and pain. As these blisters break, the nerve endings become exposed to the air. Pain and tactile responses remain intact, so subsequent treatments are painful. The barrier function of the skin is lost.

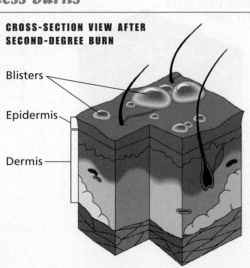

CROSS-SECTION VIEW AFTER SECOND-DEGREE BURN

Blisters

Epidermis

Dermis

Full-thickness burns

Full-thickness burns, also referred to as *third-degree burns,* affect every body system and organ. A full-thickness burn extends through the epidermis and dermis into the subcutaneous tissue. Within hours, fluid and protein shift from capillary to interstitial spaces, causing edema. The immediate immunologic response to the burn injury makes burn wound sepsis a potential threat. Last, an increased calorie demand after the burn injury increases the metabolic rate.

Fourth-degree burns

Fourth-degree burns involve muscle, bone, and interstitial tissues.

Signs and symptoms
Superficial burn

▶ Localized pain and erythema, usually without blisters in the first 24 hours, caused by injury from direct or indirect contact with a burn source
▶ Chills, headache, localized edema, and nausea and vomiting (in more severe cases)

Superficial partial-thickness burn

▶ Thin-walled, fluid-filled blisters appearing within minutes of the injury, with mild to moderate edema and pain

Deep partial-thickness burn

▶ White, waxy or mixed red appearance to the damaged area
▶ Decreased capillary refill and sensation

Full-thickness burn

▶ White, brown, or black leathery tissue and visible thrombosed vessels due to destruction of skin elasticity (dorsum of the hand is the most common site of thrombosed veins), without blisters

Fourth-degree burn

▶ Damage extends through deeply charred subcutaneous tissue to muscle and bone
▶ Usually painless because nerve fibers are burned

Treatment

▶ Immediate classification and estimation of extent or injury to guide treatment
▶ Lactated Ringer's solution through a large-bore I.V. line to expand vascular volume; volume of infusion calculated according to the extent of the area burned and the time that has elapsed since the burn injury occurred
▶ Indwelling urinary catheter to permit accurate monitoring of urine output
▶ I.V. morphine to alleviate pain and anxiety
▶ Nasogastric (NG) tube to prevent gastric distention and accompanying ileus from hypovolemic shock
▶ Booster of 0.5 ml of tetanus toxoid administered I.M.

Treatment of the burn wound

▶ Initial debriding by washing the surface of the wound area with mild soap
▶ Sharp debridement of loose tissue and blisters (blister fluid contains agents that reduce bactericidal activity and increase inflammatory response)
▶ Partial-thickness wounds: covering with hydrogel, silicone-coated nylon, or other dressing
▶ Fourth-degree wounds: covering the wound with an antimicrobial and a nonstick bulky dressing (after debridement)
▶ Escharotomy, if the patient is at risk for vascular, circulatory, or respiratory compromise

PICTURING PATHO

Full-thickness burns

A full-thickness burn extends through the epidermis and dermis and into the subcutaneous tissue layer.

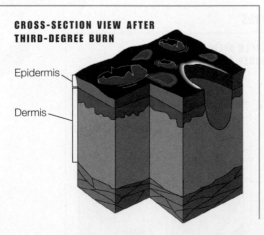

CROSS-SECTION VIEW AFTER THIRD-DEGREE BURN

Epidermis

Dermis

Nursing considerations

▶ For severe burns, provide immediate, aggressive treatment to increase the patient's chance for survival. Make sure the patient with major or moderate burns has adequate airway, breathing, and circulation. If needed, assist with endotracheal intubation. Administer 100% oxygen, as ordered, and adjust the flow to maintain adequate gas exchange.

▶ Provide sufficient I.V. fluids to maintain a urine output of 30 to 50 ml/hour; the output of a child who weighs less than 66 lb (29.9 kg) should be maintained at 1 ml/kg/hour.

▶ Remove any clothing that's still smoldering. If it continues to adhere to the patient's skin, first soak it in saline solution. Also remove jewelry and other constricting items.

▶ Cover the burns with a clean, dry, sterile bed sheet.

▶ *Never* cover large burns with saline-soaked dressings, which can drastically lower body temperature.

▶ Start I.V. therapy immediately to prevent hypovolemic shock and maintain cardiac output. Use lactated Ringer's solution or a fluid replacement formula, as ordered. Closely monitor the patient's intake and output.

▶ Assist with the insertion of a central venous pressure line and additional arterial and I.V. lines (using venous cutdown, if necessary), as needed. Insert an indwelling urinary catheter as ordered.

▶ Continue fluid therapy, as ordered, to combat fluid evaporation through the burn and the release of fluid into interstitial spaces (possibly resulting in hypovolemic shock).

▶ Check the patient's vital signs every 15 minutes. Maintain his core body temperature by covering him with a sterile blanket and exposing only small areas of his body at a time.

▶ Monitor the patient for signs and symptoms of shock—altered level of consciousness, hypotension, and respiratory distress.

▶ Insert an NG tube, as ordered, to decompress the stomach and avoid aspiration of stomach contents.

▶ Provide a diet high in potassium, protein, vitamins, fats, nitrogen, and calories to keep the patient's weight as close to his preburn weight as possible. If necessary, feed the patient through a feeding tube (as soon as bowel sounds return, if he has had paralytic ileus) until he can tolerate oral feeding. Weigh him every day at the same time.

▶ If the patient is to be transferred to a specialized burn care unit, prepare the patient for transport by wrapping him in a sterile sheet and a blanket for warmth and elevating the burned extremity to decrease edema.

▶ If the patient has only minor burns, immerse the burned area in cool saline solution (55° F [12.8° C]) or apply cool compresses, making sure he doesn't develop hypothermia. Next, soak the wound in a mild antiseptic solution to clean it, and give ordered pain medication.

▶ Debride the devitalized tissue. Cover the wound with an antibacterial agent and a nonstick bulky dressing, and administer tetanus prophylaxis, as ordered.

▶ Explain all procedures to the patient before performing them. Speak calmly and clearly to help alleviate his anxiety.

▶ Give the patient opportunities to voice his concerns, especially about altered body image. When possible, show the patient how his bodily functions are improving. If necessary, refer him for mental health counseling.

▶ Administer pain medication as ordered and evaluate its effectiveness. Provide emotional support because burns can be very painful as well as disfiguring.

LESSON PLANS

Teaching about burns

▶ If the patient has only a minor burn, stress the importance of keeping his dressing dry and clean, elevating the burned extremity for the first 24 hours, taking analgesics as ordered, and returning for a wound check in 2 days.

▶ For a patient with a moderate or major burn, discharge teaching involves the entire burn team. Teaching topics include wound management; signs and symptoms of complications; use of pressure dressings, exercises, and splints; and resocialization. Make sure the patient understands the treatment plan, including why it's necessary and how it will help his recovery.

▶ Explain to the patient that a home health nurse can assist with wound care. Provide the patient with information on available support systems.

▶ Teach the patient signs and symptoms of infection and when to seek medical attention.

▶ Give the patient written discharge instructions for later reference.

Cellulitis

An infection of the dermis or subcutaneous layer of the skin, cellulitis may follow damage to the skin, such as with a bite or a wound. If treated in a timely manner, the prognosis is usually good. If the cellulitis spreads, however, fever, erythema, and lymphangitis may occur, particularly in patients with other contributing health factors, such as diabetes, immunodeficiency, impaired circulation, or neuropathy.

Phases of acute inflammatory response

The following illustrations show the phases of acute inflammatory responses in cellulitis.

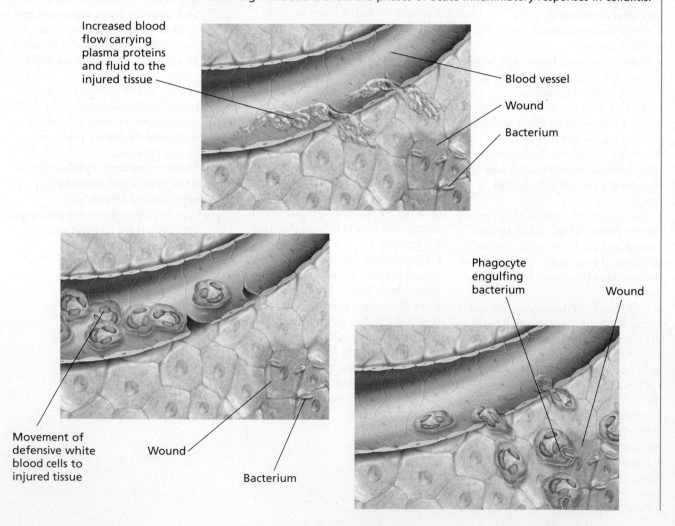

Increased blood flow carrying plasma proteins and fluid to the injured tissue

Blood vessel

Wound

Bacterium

Movement of defensive white blood cells to injured tissue

Wound

Bacterium

Phagocyte engulfing bacterium

Wound

Recognizing cellulitis

The classic signs of cellulitis are erythema and edema surrounding the initial wound. The tissue is warm to the touch.

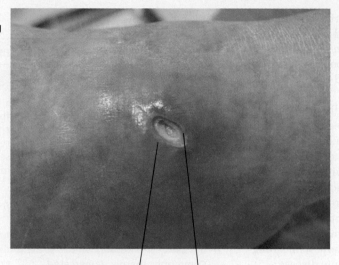

Surrounding erythema and edema   Wound

Signs and symptoms

▶ Erythema and edema
▶ Pain at the site and, possibly, the surrounding area
▶ Fever and warmth

Treatment

▶ Antibiotics, either p.o. or I.V., for the causative organism, depending on the severity
▶ Pain medication, as needed, to promote comfort
▶ Elevation of the affected extremity above heart level to promote comfort and decrease edema
▶ Modified bed rest

Nursing considerations

▶ Assess the patient for an increase in size of the affected area or worsening pain.
▶ Administer an antibiotic and an analgesic, and elevate the extremity as ordered.

LESSON PLANS

Teaching about cellulitis

▶ Emphasize the importance of complying with treatment to prevent relapse.
▶ Instruct the patient to use a properly cleaned shower instead of the bathtub until the skin problem has healed to prevent worsening of the infection.
▶ To prevent recurring cellulitis, teach the patient to maintain good general hygiene and to carefully clean abrasions and cuts. Urge early treatment to prevent the spread of infection.
▶ Describe the importance of range-of-motion exercises to prevent deep vein thrombosis.

Dermatitis

Dermatitis is characterized by inflammation of the skin and may be acute or chronic. It occurs in several forms, including contact, seborrheic, nummular, exfoliative, and stasis dermatitis.

Atopic dermatitis (discussed here), also commonly referred to as *atopic* or *infantile eczema* or *Besnier's prurigo*, is a chronic inflammatory response typically associated with other atopic diseases, such as bronchial asthma, allergic rhinitis, and chronic urticaria. It usually develops in infants and toddlers between ages 6 months and 2 years, commonly in those with strong family histories of atopic disease. These children typically acquire other atopic disorders as they grow older. In most cases, this form of dermatitis subsides spontaneously by age 3 and remains in remission until prepuberty (ages 10 to 12), when it flares up again. The disorder affects about 9 out of every 1,000 people.

Atopic dermatitis is exacerbated by certain irritants, infections (commonly *Staphylococcus aureus)*, and allergens. Common allergens include pollen, wool, silk, fur, ointment, detergent, perfume, and certain foods, particularly wheat, milk, and eggs. Flare-ups may also occur in response to temperature extremes, humidity, sweating, and stress.

Types of dermatitis

Type	Causes
Chronic dermatitis	
Characterized by inflammatory eruptions on the hands and feet	▶ Usually unknown but may result from progressive contact dermatitis ▶ Secondary factors: trauma, infections, redistribution of normal flora, photosensitivity, and food sensitivity, which may perpetuate this condition
Contact dermatitis	
Commonly, sharply demarcated skin inflammation and irritation due to contact with concentrated substances to which the skin is sensitive, such as perfumes or chemicals	▶ Mild irritants: chronic exposure to detergents or solvents ▶ Strong irritants: damage on contact with acids or alkalis ▶ Allergens: sensitization after repeated exposure
Exfoliative dermatitis	
Severe, chronic skin inflammation characterized by redness and widespread erythema and scaling	▶ Progression of preexisting skin lesions to exfoliative stage, as in contact dermatitis, drug reaction, lymphoma, or leukemia
Seborrheic dermatitis	
An acute or subacute disease that affects the scalp, face and, occasionally, other areas and is characterized by lesions covered with yellow or brownish gray scales	▶ Unknown; stress and neurologic conditions may be predisposing factors
Stasis dermatitis	
Condition usually caused by impaired circulation and characterized by eczema of the legs with edema, hyperpigmentation, and persistent inflammation	▶ Secondary to peripheral vascular diseases affecting legs, such as recurrent thrombophlebitis, postphlebitic syndrome, and resultant chronic venous insufficiency

Assessment findings	Diagnosis	Treatment and intervention
▶ Thick, lichenified, single or multiple lesions on any part of the body (commonly on the hands) ▶ Inflammation and scaling ▶ Recurrence after long remissions	▶ No characteristic pattern or course; diagnosis based on detailed history and physical findings	▶ Elimination of known allergens and decreased exposure to irritants, wearing protective clothing such as gloves, and washing immediately after contact with irritants or allergens ▶ An antibiotic for secondary infection ▶ Light therapy ▶ Avoidance of excessive washing and drying of hands and of accumulation of soaps and detergents under rings or jewelry ▶ Use of emollients with topical steroids
▶ Mild irritants and allergens: erythema and small vesicles that ooze, scale, and itch ▶ Strong irritants: blisters and ulcerations ▶ Classic allergic response: clearly defined lesions, with straight lines following points of contact ▶ Severe allergic reaction: marked edema of affected areas	▶ Patient history ▶ Patch testing to identify allergens ▶ Shape and distribution of lesions	▶ Same as for chronic dermatitis ▶ A topical anti-inflammatory (including steroids), a systemic steroid for edema and bullae, an antihistamine, and local applications of Burow's solution (for blisters)
▶ Generalized dermatitis, with acute loss of stratum corneum, and erythema and scaling ▶ Sensation of tight skin ▶ Hair loss ▶ Possibly fever, sensitivity to cold, shivering, gynecomastia, and lymphadenopathy	▶ Identification of the underlying cause	▶ Hospitalization, with protective isolation and hygienic measures to prevent secondary bacterial infection ▶ Open wet dressings, with colloidal baths ▶ Mild lotion over a topical steroid ▶ Maintenance of constant environmental temperature to prevent chilling or overheating ▶ Careful monitoring of renal and cardiac status ▶ A systemic antibiotic and a steroid
▶ Eruptions in areas with many sebaceous glands (usually scalp, face, and trunk) and in skin folds ▶ Itching, redness, and inflammation of affected areas; lesions that may appear greasy; possible fissures ▶ Indistinct, occasionally yellowish, scaly patches from excess stratum corneum (dandruff may be a mild seborrheic dermatitis)	▶ Patient history and physical findings, especially distribution of lesions in sebaceous gland areas ▶ Exclusion of psoriasis	▶ Removal of scales by frequent washing and shampooing with selenium sulfide suspension, zinc pyrithione, tar, and salicylic acid shampoo or ketoconazole shampoo ▶ Application of a topical steroid and an antifungal to nonhairy areas ▶ Immunomodulators such as tacrolimus
▶ Varicosities and edema common, but obvious vascular insufficiency not always present ▶ Usually affects the lower leg, just above internal malleolus, or sites of trauma or irritation ▶ Early signs: dusky red deposits of hemosiderin in skin, with itching and dimpling of subcutaneous tissue; later signs: edema, redness, and scaling of large area of legs ▶ Possible fissures, crusts, and ulcers	▶ Positive history of venous insufficiency and physical findings such as varicosities	▶ Treatment of the causative condition ▶ Measures to prevent venous stasis: avoidance of prolonged sitting or standing, use of compression stockings, and weight reduction for obese patients ▶ Corrective surgery for underlying cause ▶ After ulcer develops, rest periods with legs elevated; open wet dressings; Unna's boot (provides continuous pressure to areas); and an antibiotic for secondary infection after wound culture

Signs and symptoms

▶ Intense itching
▶ Erythematous patches in excessively dry areas at flexion points, such as the antecubital fossa, popliteal area, and neck; in children, may appear on the forehead, cheeks, and extensor surfaces of the arms and legs
▶ Edema, scaling, and vesiculation because of scratching
▶ Vesicles that may be pus-filled
▶ With chronic disease, multiple areas of dry, scaly skin with white dermatographism, blanching, and lichenification

What happens in contact dermatitis

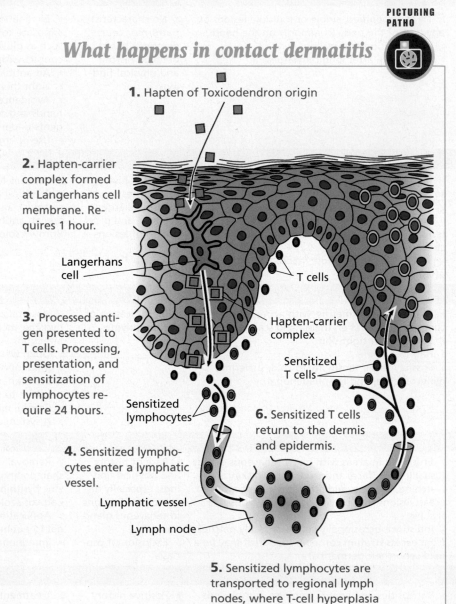

1. Hapten of Toxicodendron origin

2. Hapten-carrier complex formed at Langerhans cell membrane. Requires 1 hour.

Langerhans cell

T cells

3. Processed antigen presented to T cells. Processing, presentation, and sensitization of lymphocytes require 24 hours.

Hapten-carrier complex

Sensitized T cells

Sensitized lymphocytes

6. Sensitized T cells return to the dermis and epidermis.

4. Sensitized lymphocytes enter a lymphatic vessel.

Lymphatic vessel

Lymph node

5. Sensitized lymphocytes are transported to regional lymph nodes, where T-cell hyperplasia is induced.

Treatment

▶ Eliminating allergens and avoiding irritants, extreme temperature changes, and other precipitating factors

▶ Systemic antihistamines, such as hydroxyzine hydrochloride and diphenhydramine, to relieve pruritus

▶ Topical application of a corticosteroid cream to alleviate inflammation

▶ Systemic corticosteroid therapy only during extreme exacerbations

▶ Weak tar preparations and ultraviolet B light therapy to increase the thickness of the stratum corneum

▶ Antibiotics to fight a bacterial infection; antifungals or antivirals to fight a fungal or viral infection

Appearance of atopic dermatitis

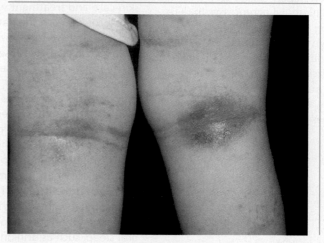

Nursing considerations

‣ Help the patient schedule daily skin care. Keep his fingernails short to limit excoriation and secondary infections caused by scratching.

‣ Be alert for possible adverse effects associated with corticosteroid use: sensitivity reactions, GI disturbances, musculoskeletal weakness, neurologic disturbances, and cushingoid symptoms.

‣ To help clear lichenified skin, apply occlusive dressings, such as a plastic film, intermittently. This treatment requires a physician's order and experience in dermatologic treatment.

‣ Apply cool, moist compresses to relieve itching and burning.

‣ Encourage the patient to verbalize feelings about his appearance, including embarrassment and fear of rejection. Offer him emotional support and reassurance and arrange for counseling, if necessary.

LESSON PLANS

Teaching about dermatitis

‣ Provide written instructions for skin care and treatment with corticosteroids. Teach the patient and his family to recognize signs of corticosteroid overdose and to notify the physician immediately if they occur.

‣ If the patient experiences an excessively dry mouth caused by antihistamine use, advise him to drink water or suck ice chips.

‣ Warn that drowsiness is possible with the use of antihistamines to relieve daytime itching. If nocturnal itching interferes with sleep, suggest methods for inducing natural sleep, such as drinking a glass of warm milk, to prevent overuse of sedatives.

‣ Advise the patient to wear loose cotton clothing to decrease itching.

‣ Stress the importance of meticulous hand washing and good personal hygiene.

‣ Caution the patient to avoid bathing in hot water because heat causes vasodilation, which induces pruritus.

‣ Instruct the patient to use plain, tepid water (96° F [35.6° C]) with a nonfatty, nonperfumed soap but to avoid using any soap when lesions are acutely inflamed. Advise him to shampoo frequently and to apply corticosteroid solution to the scalp afterward. Suggest using a lubricating lotion after a bath.

‣ With severe dermatitis, show the patient how to apply occlusive dressings. For example, severe contact dermatitis may require a topical corticosteroid and occlusion with gloves to increase drug absorption and skin hydration.

‣ Teach the patient how to apply wet-to-dry dressings to soothe inflammation, itching, and burning; to remove crusting and scales from dry lesions; and to help dry up oozing lesions.

‣ Help the patient to identify and avoid aggravating factors and allergens associated with atopic dermatitis.

Herpes zoster

Herpes zoster, also called *shingles*, is an acute, unilateral and segmental inflammation of the dorsal root ganglia and is caused by the varicella-zoster virus (herpesvirus). It produces localized vesicular skin lesions confined to a dermatome, which may produce severe neuralgic pain in the areas bordering the inflamed nerve root ganglia.

The infection is found primarily in adults ages 50 to 70, and the prognosis is usually good, with most patients re-

covering completely, unless the infection spreads to the brain.

Herpes zoster is more severe in the immunocompromised patient but seldom is fatal. Patients who have received a bone marrow transplant are especially at risk for the infection.

Although the process is unclear, the disease seems to erupt when the virus reactivates after dormancy in the cerebral ganglia (extramedullary ganglia of the cranial nerves) or the ganglia of

posterior nerve roots. The virus then may multiply as it reactivates, but antibodies remaining from the initial infection may neutralize it. Without opposition, however, the virus continues to multiply in the ganglia, destroys neurons, and spreads down the sensory nerves to the skin.

Herpes zoster is contagious until all the blisters are crusted over, but only for individuals who haven't previously had chickenpox.

Tracking herpes zoster

The blisters of herpes zoster appear along nerve distributions in the skin, called *dermatomes*.

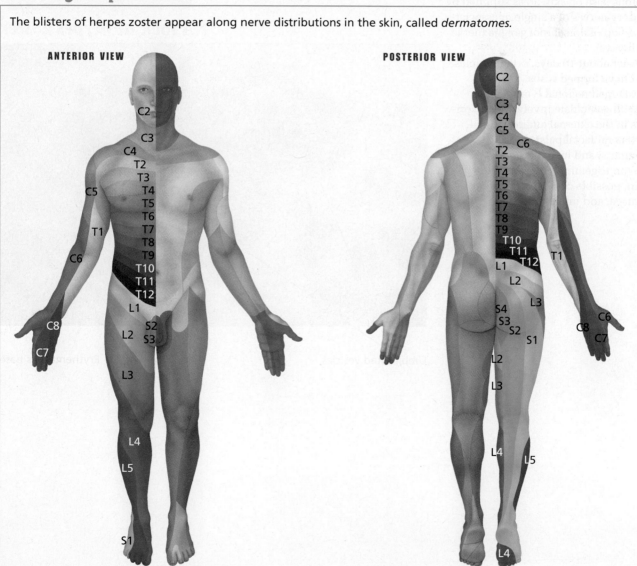

ANTERIOR VIEW

POSTERIOR VIEW

Signs and symptoms

▶ Fever
▶ Malaise
▶ Burning or sensitive skin several days before rash appears
▶ Pain that mimics appendicitis, pleurisy, musculoskeletal pain, or other conditions
▶ After 2 to 4 days, severe, deep pain; pruritus; and paresthesia or hyperesthesia (usually affecting the trunk and, occasionally, the arms and legs)
▶ Pain that may be intermittent, continuous, or debilitating, usually lasting from 1 to 4 weeks
▶ Fluid-filled vesicles with an erythematous base on skin areas supplied by sensory nerves of a single or associated group of dorsal root ganglia (nerve pathways)
▶ After about 10 days, dried vesicles that have formed scabs
▶ Enlarged regional lymph nodes
▶ With geniculate involvement, vesicles in the external auditory canal, ipsilateral facial palsy, hearing loss, dizziness, and loss of taste
▶ With trigeminal involvement, eye pain, possible corneal and scleral damage, and impaired vision

A look at herpes zoster

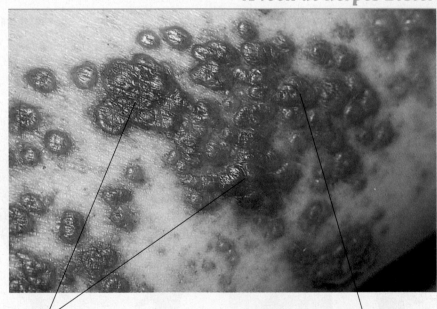

Umbilicated vesicles

Erythematous base

Treatment

▶ Oral acyclovir (Zovirax), famciclovir (Famvir), and valacyclovir (Valtrex) therapy to accelerate healing of lesions and resolution of zoster-associated pain

▶ Antipruritics (such as calamine lotion) to relieve pruritus and analgesics (such as aspirin, acetaminophen or, possibly, codeine) to relieve neuralgic pain

▶ Tricyclic antidepressants to help relieve neuritic pain

▶ Systemic corticosteroids, such as cortisone or corticotropin, to reduce inflammation and the intractable pain of postherpetic neuralgia (other possible therapies: tranquilizers, sedatives, or tricyclic antidepressants with phenothiazines)

▶ As a last resort for pain relief, transcutaneous peripheral nerve stimulation, patient-controlled analgesia, or a small dose of radiotherapy

▶ Cool compresses and use of Burow's or Domeboro solution

Nursing considerations

▶ Administer topical therapies as directed. If the physician orders calamine, apply it liberally to the patient's lesions. Avoid blotting contaminated swabs on unaffected skin areas. Be prepared to administer drying therapies, such as oxygen, if the patient has severe disseminated lesions. Use silver sulfadiazine, as ordered, to soften and debride infected lesions.

▶ Give analgesics exactly as scheduled to minimize severe neuralgic pain. For a patient with postherpetic neuralgia, consult with a pain specialist and follow his recommendations to maximize pain relief without risking tolerance to the analgesic.

▶ Maintain meticulous hygiene to prevent spreading the infection to other parts of the patient's body.

▶ If the patient has open lesions, follow contact isolation precautions to prevent the spread of infection to immunocompromised patients.

LESSON
PLANS

Teaching about herpes zoster

▶ To decrease discomfort from oral lesions, tell the patient to use a soft toothbrush, eat soft foods, and use a saline- or bicarbonate-based mouthwash and oral anesthetics.

▶ Stress the need for rest during the acute phase.

▶ Reassure the patient that herpetic pain eventually will subside. Suggest diversionary or relaxation activities to take his mind off the pain and pruritus.

▶ Advise family members who haven't had chickenpox to receive the vaccine.

▶ Advise adults age 60 and older to receive the herpes zoster vaccine (Zostavax).

Impetigo

A contagious, superficial skin infection, impetigo (*impetigo contagiosa*) occurs in nonbullous and bullous forms. This vesiculopustular eruptive disorder spreads most easily among infants, young children, and elderly people. It appears most commonly on the face and other exposed areas, usually around the nose and mouth.

Infants and young children may also develop aural impetigo, or otitis externa. These lesions usually clear without treatment in 2 to 3 weeks unless an underlying disorder, such as eczema, is present. Candidal organisms, additional bacteria, fungi, or viruses may complicate lesions in the diaper area. In addition, impetigo may complicate chickenpox or other skin disorders marked by open lesions.

Beta-hemolytic streptococci produce the nonbullous form of impetigo, which later also may harbor staphylococci, producing a mixed-organism infection. The bullous form of impetigo starts as a blister and is caused by coagulase-positive *Staphylococcus aureus*.

Signs and symptoms
▶ Painless pruritus and burning

Streptococcal (nonbullous) impetigo
▶ Small, red macule that has turned into a vesicle, becoming pustular within a few hours
▶ Characteristic thick, honey-colored crust that forms from the exudate (when the vesicle breaks)

Staphylococcal (bullous) impetigo
▶ Thin-walled vesicle that opens
▶ Thin, clear crust that forms from the exudate and a lesion that appears as a central clearing circumscribed by an outer rim—much like a ringworm lesion

Recognizing bullous impetigo

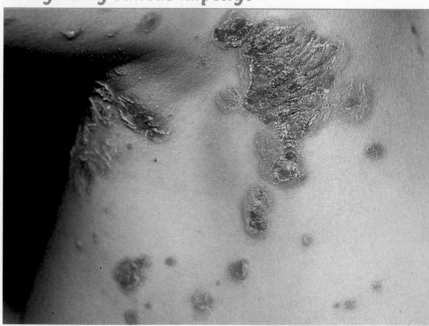

Treatment

▶ Broad-spectrum systemic antibiotics (usually a penicillinase-resistant penicillin, or erythromycin for patients who are allergic to penicillin)
▶ Removal of the exudate by washing the lesions two or three times a day with soap and water or, for stubborn crusts, using warm soaks or compresses of normal saline or diluted soap solution
▶ Topical agents, particularly mupirocin or retapamulin (Altabax) in combination with crust removal with each application
▶ Antihistamines to alleviate itching and daily bathing with bactericidal soaps as a preventive measure

Nursing considerations

▶ Use meticulous hand-washing technique and contact precautions to prevent spreading the infection.
▶ Cut the patient's fingernails short to prevent scratching, which can cause autoinoculation and new skin breaks.
▶ Remove the crusts by gently washing with bactericidal soap and water. Soften stubborn crusts with cool compresses; scrub gently to aid crust removal before applying a topical antibiotic.
▶ Give medications, as ordered, and monitor the patient's response. Remember to check for penicillin allergy.
▶ Encourage the patient to verbalize feelings about body image, and acknowledge the importance of positive self-body image.

LESSON PLANS

 ### *Teaching about impetigo*

▶ Reassure the parents that complications are rare and that residual scars are unlikely.
▶ Instruct the parents to use meticulous hand-washing and aseptic techniques when changing dressings and providing comfort measures, such as warm soaks and baths.
▶ Stress the importance of avoiding friction on the skin surface during the exfoliation stage and avoiding picking, scratching, or rubbing scales during the desquamation stage.
▶ Instruct the parents to contact the physician if adverse reactions to antibiotic therapy occur. Also, explain the importance of completing the entire regimen of antibiotic therapy, even after the lesions appear to have healed.

Malignant melanoma

Malignant melanoma is a neoplasm that arises from melanocytes. Although it's potentially the most lethal of the skin cancers, it's also relatively rare, accounting for only 1% to 2% of all malignant tumors. Melanoma is slightly more common in males than in females and is unusual in children. Peak incidence occurs between ages 50 and 70, although the incidence in younger age-groups is increasing.

Melanoma spreads through the lymphatic and vascular systems and metastasizes to the regional lymph nodes, skin, liver, lungs, and central nervous system. Its course is unpredictable, and recurrence and metastases may not appear for more than 5 years after resection of the primary lesion. The prognosis varies with the tu-

mor thickness. In most patients, superficial lesions are curable, whereas deeper lesions tend to metastasize.

Common sites for melanoma are the head and neck in males, the legs in females, and the backs of people exposed to excessive sunlight. Up to 70% of malignant melanomas arise from a preexisting nevus. It seldom appears in the conjunctiva, choroid, pharynx, mouth, vagina, or anus.

There are four types of melanoma:
▶ *Superficial spreading melanoma* is the most common type, usually developing between ages 40 and 50.
▶ *Nodular melanoma* also usually develops between ages 40 and 50. It grows vertically, invades the dermis, and metastasizes early.

▶ *Acral-lentiginous melanoma* is the most common melanoma among Hispanics, Asians, and Blacks. It occurs on the palms and soles and in sublingual locations.
▶ *Lentigo maligna melanoma* is relatively rare and is the most benign, slowest growing, and least aggressive of the four types. It most commonly occurs in areas heavily exposed to the sun, arising from a lentigo maligna, and usually occurs between ages 60 and 70.

Signs and symptoms
▶ Sore that doesn't heal
▶ Persistent lump or swelling
▶ Changes in preexisting skin markings, such as moles, birthmarks, scars, freckles, or warts

ABCDEs of malignant melanoma

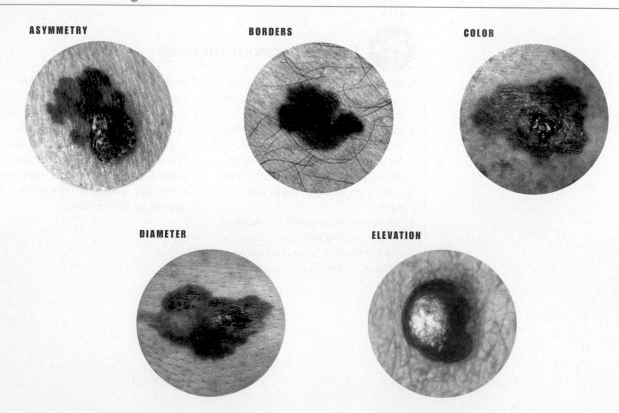

ASYMMETRY

BORDERS

COLOR

DIAMETER

ELEVATION

Superficial spreading melanoma

◗ Lesions on the ankles or the inside surfaces of the knees
◗ Lesions that may appear red, white, or blue over a brown or black background
◗ Lesions that may have an irregular, notched margin
◗ Small, elevated tumor nodules that may ulcerate and bleed

Nodular malignant melanoma

◗ Uniformly discolored nodule on the knees and ankles
◗ May appear grayish and resemble a blackberry but may also be flesh-colored with flecks of pigment around its base, which may be inflamed
◗ Polypoid nodules that resemble the surface of a blackberry

Acral lentiginous melanoma

◗ Pigmented lesions on the palms and soles and under the nails
◗ Color that may resemble a mosaic of rich browns, tans, and black
◗ Nail beds that may reveal a streak in the nail associated with an irregular tan or a brown stain that diffuses from the nail bed

Lentigo maligna melanoma

◗ Patient history of a long-standing lesion that has now ulcerated
◗ Large lesion (3 to 6 cm) that appears as a tan, brown, black, whitish, or slate-colored freckle on the face, back of the hand, or under the fingernails
◗ Irregular scattered black nodules on the surface
◗ Flat nodule with smaller nodules scattered over the surface

Looking at superficial spreading melanoma

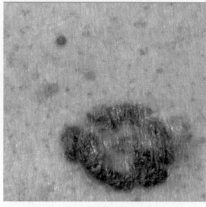

Looking at nodular malignant melanoma

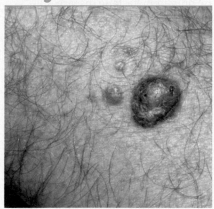

Looking at acral lentiginous melanoma

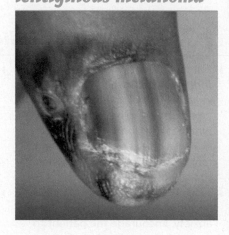

Looking at lentigo maligna melanoma

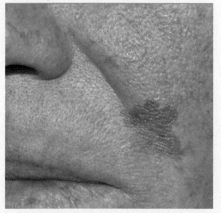

Treatment

▶ Surgical resection to remove the tumor (a 3- to 5-cm margin is desired); extent of resection dependent on the size and location of the primary lesion
▶ After surgical removal of a mass, intra-arterial isolation perfusions to prevent recurrence and metastatic spread
▶ Possible skin graft, after closure of a wide resection
▶ Regional lymphadenectomy
▶ Adjuvant chemotherapy, for deep primary lesions, including dacarbazine (DTIC-Dome) and carmustine (BiCNU)
▶ Chemotherapy and radiation therapy only in metastatic disease
▶ Immunotherapy, such as interferon alfa-2b (Intron A)

Nursing considerations

▶ Listen to the patient's fears and concerns. Stay with him during episodes of stress and anxiety. Include the patient and family members in care decisions.
▶ Provide positive reinforcement as the patient attempts to adapt to his disease.
▶ Watch for complications associated with chemotherapy, such as mouth sores, hair loss, weakness, fatigue, and anorexia. Offer orange and grapefruit juices and ginger ale to help with nausea and vomiting.
▶ Provide an adequate diet for the patient, one that's high in protein and calories. If the patient is anorectic, provide small, frequent meals. Consult with the dietitian to incorporate foods that the patient enjoys.
▶ After surgery, take precautions to prevent infection. Check dressings often for excessive drainage, foul odor, redness, and swelling. If surgery included lymphadenectomy, apply a compression stocking and instruct the patient to keep the extremity elevated to minimize lymphedema.

LESSON PLANS

Teaching about malignant melanoma

▶ Make sure the patient understands the procedures and treatments associated with his diagnosis. Review the physician's explanation of treatment alternatives. Answer all questions the patient has about surgery, chemotherapy, and radiation therapy as completely as possible.

▶ Tell the patient what to expect before and after surgery, what the wound will look like, and what type of dressing he'll have. Warn him that the donor site for a skin graft may be as painful as, if not more so than, the tumor excision site.
▶ Teach the patient and his family relaxation techniques to help relieve anxiety. Encourage the patient to continue these after he's discharged.

▶ Emphasize the need for close follow-up care to detect recurrences early. Explain that recurrences and metastases, if they occur, are commonly delayed, so follow-up must continue for years. Teach the patient how to recognize the signs of recurrence.
▶ To help prevent malignant melanoma, stress the detrimental effects of overexposure to solar radiation, especially to the fair-skinned, blue-eyed patient. Recommend that he use sunscreen at all times when outdoors.
▶ When appropriate, refer the patient and family members to community support services, such as the American Cancer Society or a hospice.

Melasma

A patchy, hypermelanotic skin disorder, melasma, also known as *chloasma* or *mask of pregnancy*, can pose a serious cosmetic problem but is never life-threatening. Although it tends to occur equally in all races, the light-brown color that's characteristic of melasma is most evident in dark-skinned whites. Melasma affects females more commonly than males and may be chronic in nature.

Melasma may be related to the increased hormonal levels associated with pregnancy, menopause, ovarian cancer, and the use of hormonal contraceptives. Progestational agents, phenytoin, and mephenytoin may also contribute to this disorder. Exposure to sunlight stimulates melasma, but it may develop without any apparent predisposing factor. Patients with acquired immunodeficiency syndrome have an increased incidence of similar hyperpigmentation.

Signs and symptoms
▶ Large, brown, irregular patches, symmetrically distributed on the forehead, cheeks, and sides of the nose
▶ Less commonly, may occur on the neck, upper lip, and temples and, occasionally, on the dorsa of the forearms

Treatment
▶ Application of bleaching agents containing 2% to 4% hydroquinone in combination with tretinoin or glycolic acid to inhibit melanin synthesis
▶ Adjunctive measures: avoidance of exposure to sunlight, use of opaque sunscreens, and discontinuation of hormonal contraceptives

Looking at melasma

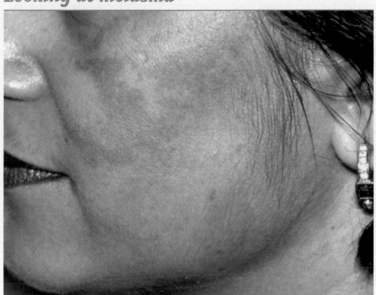

Nursing considerations
▶ Tell the patient that melasma with pregnancy usually clears within a few months after delivery and may not return with subsequent pregnancies.
▶ Advise the patient to avoid exposure by using sunscreens and wearing protective clothing. Bleaching agents may help but may require repeated treatments to maintain the desired effect. Cosmetics may help mask deep pigmentation.
▶ Reassure the patient that melasma is treatable. It may fade spontaneously with protection from sunlight, at postpartum, and after discontinuing hormonal contraceptives. Serial photographs may help show the patient that patches are improving.

LESSON PLANS

Teaching about melasma

▶ Teach the patient the importance of using sunscreen with a sun protection factor of at least 30.
▶ Suggest to the patient that she wear an additional cover-up (along with the sunscreen), such as a hat or scarf.
▶ Advise the patient to try to limit her exposure to sunlight.

Pressure ulcers

Pressure ulcers are localized areas of cellular necrosis that occur most commonly in the skin and subcutaneous tissue over bony prominences, especially the sacrum, ischial tuberosities, greater trochanter, heels, malleoli, and elbows. These ulcers—also called *decubitus ulcers, pressure sores,* or *bedsores*—may be superficial, caused by local skin irritation with subsequent surface maceration; or deep, originating in underlying tissue. Deep lesions typically go undetected until they penetrate the skin, at which time they've usually caused subcutaneous damage.

**PICTURING
PATHO**

Pressure ulcer staging

The National Pressure Ulcer Advisory Panel has updated the staging of pressure ulcers to include the original four stages plus two other stages called *suspected deep tissue injury* and *unstageable.*

Suspected deep tissue injury

Suspected deep tissue injury involves maroon or purple intact skin or a blood-filled blister due to damage from shearing or pressure on the underlying soft tissue. Before the discoloration occurs, the area may be painful, mushy or firm or boggy, and warmer or cooler than other tissue.

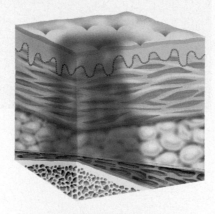

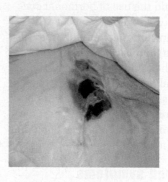

Stage I

A stage I pressure ulcer is an area of intact skin that doesn't blanch and is usually over a bony prominence. Skin that's darkly pigmented may not show blanching, but its color may differ from the surrounding area. The area may be painful, firm or soft, and warmer or cooler than the surrounding tissue.

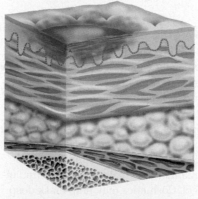

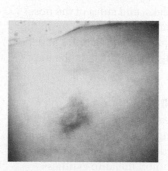

Stage II

A stage II pressure ulcer is a superficial partial-thickness wound that presents clinically as a shallow and open ulcer without slough and with a red and pink wound bed. This term shouldn't be used to describe perineal dermatitis, maceration, tape burns, skin tears, or excoriation. Examples include an abrasion, a blister, or a shallow crater involving the epidermis and dermis.

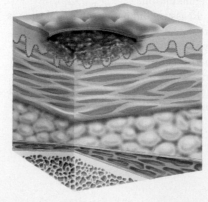

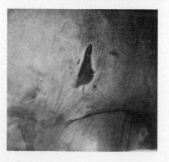

Signs and symptoms

The signs and symptoms of pressure ulcers depend on the extent of damage and are classified as suspected deep tissue injury, stage I, stage II, stage III, stage IV, or unstageable.

Stage III

A stage III pressure ulcer is a full-thickness wound with tissue loss. The subcutaneous tissue may be visible but muscle, tendon, or bone isn't exposed. Slough may be present, but it doesn't hide the depth of the tissue loss. Undermining and tunneling may be present.

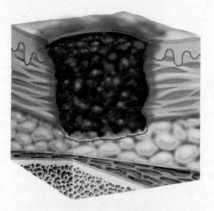
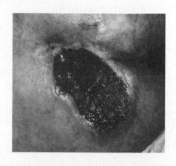

Stage IV

A stage IV pressure ulcer involves full-thickness skin loss with exposed muscle, bone, and tendon. Eschar and sloughing may be present as well as undermining and tunneling.

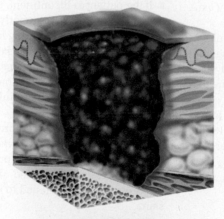
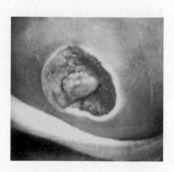

Unstageable

An unstageable pressure ulcer involves full-thickness tissue loss. The base of the ulcer is covered by yellow, tan, gray, green, or brown slough or tan, brown, or black eschar. Some may have both slough and eschar. The pressure ulcer can't be staged until enough eschar or slough is removed to expose the base of the wound.

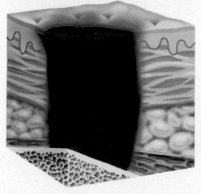
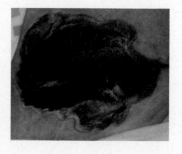

Treatment

‣ Devices, such as pads, mattresses, and special beds to redistribute pressure
‣ Turning and repositioning the patient frequently
‣ Diet high in protein, iron, and vitamin C to promote healing

Stage I

‣ Lubricants (Lubriderm), clear plastic dressings (Op-Site), gelatin-type wafers (DuoDERM), vasodilator sprays (Proderm), and whirlpool baths to increase tissue pliability, stimulate local circulation, promote healing, and prevent skin breakdown

Stage II

‣ Cleaning the ulcer with normal saline solution to remove ulcer debris and help prevent further skin damage and infection

Stage III or IV

‣ Cleaning the ulcer with normal saline solution and applying granular and absorbent dressings to promote wound drainage and absorb any exudate
‣ Enzymatic ointment (collagenase) to break down dead tissue; healing ointments to clean deep or infected ulcers
‣ Debridement of necrotic tissue to allow healing
‣ Debridement using surgical, mechanical, or chemical techniques (on occasion); skin grafting (in severe cases)

Nursing considerations

‣ During each shift, check the immobile patient's skin for changes in color, turgor, temperature, and sensation. Examine an existing ulcer for any change in size or degree of damage.
‣ Reposition the immobile patient at least every 2 hours around the clock with his heels elevated off the bed at all times. Minimize the effects of shearing force by using a footboard and not raising the head of the bed to an angle that exceeds 60 degrees. Keep the patient's knees slightly flexed for short periods.
‣ Perform passive range-of-motion exercises, or encourage the patient to do active exercises, if possible.
‣ To prevent pressure ulcers in an immobilized patient, use pressure redistribution aids on the bed.
‣ Give the patient meticulous skin care. Keep the skin clean and dry without using harsh soaps. Apply moisturizing lotions to the skin to reduce maceration of the skin surface. Change bed linens frequently for a diaphoretic or incontinent patient.
‣ If the patient is incontinent, offer a bedpan or commode frequently. Use only a single layer of padding for urine and fecal incontinence because excessive padding increases perspiration, which leads to maceration. Excessive padding may also wrinkle, irritating the skin.
‣ Clean open lesions with normal saline solution. If possible, expose the lesions to air and sunlight to promote healing. Dressings, if needed, should be porous and lightly taped to healthy skin.

‣ Encourage adequate nutrition and fluid intake to maintain body weight and promote healing. Consult the dietitian to provide a diet that promotes granulation of new tissue. Encourage the debilitated patient to eat frequent, small meals that include protein- and calorie-rich supplements. Assist the weakened patient with meals.
‣ Because anemia and elevated blood glucose levels may lead to skin breakdown, monitor hemoglobin and blood glucose levels and hematocrit.

 LESSON PLANS

Teaching about pressure ulcers

‣ Explain the function of pressure redistribution aids and topical agents, and demonstrate their proper use.
‣ Teach the patient and his family position-changing techniques and active and passive range-of-motion exercises.
‣ Stress good hygiene. Teach the patient to avoid skin-damaging agents, such as harsh or antibacterial soaps, alcohol-based products, tincture of benzoin, and hexachlorophene.
‣ As indicated, explain debridement procedures and prepare the patient for skin graft surgery.
‣ Teach the patient and his family to recognize and record signs of healing. Explain that treatment typically varies according to the stage of healing.
‣ Encourage the patient to eat a well-balanced diet and consume an adequate amount of fluids, explaining their importance for skin health. Point out dietary sources rich in vitamin C, which aids wound healing, promotes iron absorption, and helps in collagen formation.

Psoriasis

Psoriasis is a chronic skin disease marked by epidermal proliferation and characterized by recurring remissions and exacerbations. Lesions appear as erythematous papules and plaques covered with silvery scales and vary widely in severity and distribution.

The tendency to develop psoriasis is based strongly on genetic and environmental factors. Trauma can trigger the isomorphic effect, or Koebner phenomenon, in which lesions develop at injury sites. Infections, especially those resulting from beta-hemolytic streptococci, may cause a flare of guttate (drop-shaped) lesions. Other contributing factors include pregnancy, endocrine changes, climatic conditions (cold weather tends to exacerbate psoriasis), and emotional stress.

A skin cell normally takes 14 days to move from the basal layer to the stratum corneum, where, after an additional 14 days of normal wear and tear, it's sloughed off. In contrast to this 28-day cycle, the life cycle of a psoriatic cell is only 4 days, which doesn't allow time for the cell to mature. Consequently, the stratum corneum becomes thick and flaky, producing the cardinal signs and symptoms of psoriasis.

Signs and symptoms

▶ Skin lesions that itch and burn and may be painful, erythematous, well-defined plaques covered with characteristic silver scales; usually appear on the scalp, chest, elbows, knees, back, and buttocks
▶ In mild psoriasis, plaques scattered over a small skin area
▶ Scales that flake off easily (on palpation); scales that have thickened and have covered the lesion
▶ Fine bleeding points, or Auspitz sign, when attempting to remove scales
▶ Small guttate lesions, either alone or with plaques; typically thin and erythematous, with few scales

Looking at a psoriatic lesion

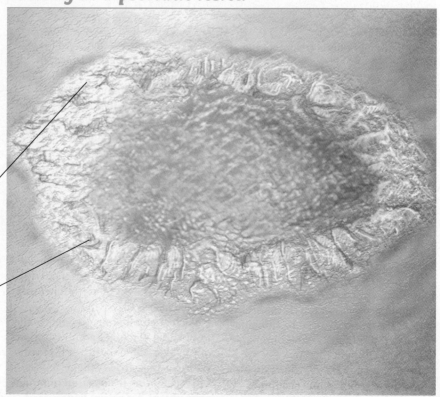

Clear margins

Plaque with thick, silver scales

Identifying types of psoriasis

Psoriasis occurs in various forms, ranging from one or two localized plaques that seldom require long-term medical attention to widespread lesions and crippling arthritis.

Erythrodermic psoriasis

Erythrodermic psoriasis is marked by extensive flushing, pain, and itching all over the body, which may or may not result in scaling. The rash may begin rapidly, signaling new psoriasis; it may develop gradually as chronic psoriasis; or it may occur as an adverse reaction to a drug.

Guttate psoriasis

Guttate psoriasis typically affects children and young adults. Erupting in drop-sized plaques over the trunk, arms, legs and, sometimes, scalp, this rash of plaques generalizes in several days. It's commonly associated with upper respiratory tract streptococcal infections.

Inverse psoriasis

Smooth, dry, bright red plaques characterize inverse psoriasis. Located in skin folds—for example, the armpits and groin—the plaques fissure easily.

Plaque psoriasis

Plaque psoriasis is the most common type of psoriasis. It begins with red, dotlike lesions that gradually enlarge and produce dry, silvery scales. The plaques usually appear symmetrically on the knees, elbows, extremities, genitalia, scalp, and nails.

Pustular psoriasis

Pustular psoriasis features an eruption of local or extensive small, raised, pus-filled plaques on the soles or palms or diffusely over the body. Precursors include emotional stress, sweat, infections, and adverse drug reactions.

Psoriatic arthritis

Psoriatic arthritis affects the feet and hands of up to 30% of patients with skin symptoms. Pain, stiffness, and joint damage may occur.

Treatment

▶ No permanent cure; treatment palliative
▶ Lukewarm baths and application of occlusive ointment bases, such as petroleum jelly, or preparations that contain urea or salicylic acid that may soften and help remove psoriatic scales
▶ Steroid creams
▶ Methods to retard rapid cell production, such as exposure to ultraviolet B (UVB) light or natural sunlight to the point of minimal erythema
▶ Coal tar preparations to retard skin cell growth and relieve inflammation, itching, and scaling
▶ Topical corticosteroids for mild to moderate psoriasis of the trunk, arms, and legs; commonly used in combination with emollients, coal tar preparations, and UV light therapy
▶ Topical vitamin D
▶ 0.025% triamcinolone acetonide (Kenalog) ointment for mild psoriasis involving the extremities
▶ 1% desonide cream or alclometasone dipropionate (Aclovate) for facial, groin, or axillary plaques
▶ 0.1% betamethasone valerate (Valisone) or 0.1% triamcinolone acetonide for moderate psoriasis
▶ Anthralin for large plaques that don't respond to coal tar or topical corticosteroid preparations
▶ Methotrexate (Rheumatrex), a drug that inhibits cell replication, for severe, unresponsive psoriasis
▶ Acitretin, a potent retinoic acid derivative, for psoriasis that's resistant to other drugs or treatments
▶ Goeckerman treatment, which combines topical coal tar treatment with UVA or UVB light therapy, for severe chronic psoriasis
▶ Photochemotherapy program, called *PUVA*, that combines administration of psoralen, either orally or topically, with exposure to UVA light
▶ Cyclosporine (Neoral), an immunosuppressant, for severe widespread psoriasis that results in dramatic clearing
▶ Ustekinumab (Stelara) to inhibit the production of proteins involved in inflammatory and immune responses
▶ Low-dose antihistamine therapy, oatmeal baths, emollients (perhaps with phenol and menthol), and open wet dressings to help relieve pruritus; aspirin and local heat to help alleviate the pain of psoriatic arthritis; nonsteroidal anti-inflammatory drugs for severe cases
▶ For psoriasis of the scalp, coal tar shampoo, followed by the application of a steroid lotion while the hair is still wet; no effective treatment for psoriasis of the nails—usually improves as skin lesions improve
▶ Tumor necrosis factor inhibitors, such as infliximab (Remicade) or etanercept (Enbrel); may decrease the inflammatory process in plaque psoriasis

Nursing considerations

▶ Ensure proper patient teaching, and offer emotional support.

▶ Apply all topical medications, especially those that contain anthralin and coal tar, with a downward motion to avoid rubbing them into the follicles. Wear gloves because anthralin stains and injures the skin. After application, allow the patient to dust himself with powder to help prevent anthralin from rubbing off on his clothes.

▶ Watch for adverse reactions to therapeutic agents, which may include allergic reactions to anthralin; atrophy and acne from steroids; and burning, itching, nausea, and squamous cell epitheliomas from PUVA.

▶ Initially, evaluate the patient on methotrexate weekly and then monthly for red blood cell, white blood cell, and platelet counts because cytotoxins may cause hepatic or bone marrow toxicity. Liver biopsy may be done to assess the effects of methotrexate.

▶ Monitor triglycerides, cholesterol, and liver function tests for acitretin. Patients on cyclosporine need renal function and blood pressure monitoring.

▶ Encourage the patient to verbalize feelings about his appearance; feelings of embarrassment, frustration, or powerlessness; or fear of rejection. Involve his family in the treatment regimen to reduce the patient's feelings of social isolation. Help the patient build a positive self-image by encouraging his participation in activities that deemphasize appearance.

Teaching about psoriasis

LESSON PLANS

▶ Explain the causes, predisposing factors, and course of psoriasis to the patient and his family. Stress that psoriasis isn't communicable. Advise them that exacerbations and remissions commonly occur but that they can usually control the disorder by adhering to the treatment regimen.

▶ Make sure the patient understands his prescribed therapy; provide written instructions to avoid confusion. Teach correct application of prescribed ointments, creams, and lotions.

▶ Instruct the patient to avoid scratching the plaques. Suggest that he wear gloves to help protect the skin from unconscious scratching. Tell him that pressing ice cubes against the lesions or applying a mentholated shaving cream may provide relief. Recommend using a humidifier in the winter to avoid dry skin, which may increase itching.

▶ Caution the patient to avoid scrubbing his skin vigorously. If a medication has been applied to the scales to soften them, suggest that the patient use a soft brush to remove them.

▶ Warn the patient never to put an occlusive dressing over anthralin. Suggest the use of mineral oil and then soap and water to remove anthralin.

▶ Caution the patient receiving PUVA therapy to stay out of the sun on the treatment day and to protect his eyes with sunglasses that screen UVA for 24 hours after treatment. Tell him to wear goggles during exposure to this light.

▶ If the patient is using acitretin, inform him that the drug may remain in his body for up to 3 years after the treatment ends. For this reason, discourage female patients who may want to become pregnant from using this drug.

▶ Caution the patient using methotrexate not to drink alcoholic beverages; explain that alcohol ingestion increases the risk of hepatotoxicity.

▶ Warn the patient and his family about possible adverse effects associated with the therapeutic agents; tell them to notify the physician if any occur.

▶ Teach the patient stress-reduction techniques and injury prevention strategies to prevent exacerbations.

▶ Explain the relation between psoriasis and arthritis, but point out that psoriasis causes no other systemic disturbances.

▶ Refer the patient to the National Psoriasis Foundation.

Rosacea

A chronic skin eruption, rosacea produces flushing and dilation of the small blood vessels in the face, especially around the nose and cheeks. Papules and pustules may also occur but without the characteristic comedones of acne vulgaris. Rosacea is most common in white women age 30 to 50. When it occurs in men, however, it's usually more severe and commonly associated with rhinophyma, which is characterized by dilated follicles and thickened, bulbous skin on the nose. Ocular involvement may result in blepharitis, conjunctivitis, uveitis, or keratitis. Rosacea usually spreads slowly and rarely subsides spontaneously.

Although the exact cause of rosacea is unknown, stress, infection, vitamin deficiency, menopause, and endocrine abnormalities can aggravate the condition. Spicy foods; physical activity; sunlight; hot beverages, such as tea or coffee; tobacco; alcohol; and extreme heat or cold can also aggravate rosacea, producing the characteristic flushing.

Signs and symptoms

▶ Periodic flushing across the central oval of the face
▶ Telangiectasia
▶ Papules
▶ Pustules
▶ Nodules

Rhinophyma is commonly associated with severe untreated rosacea but may also occur alone. Initially, rhinophyma appears on the lower half of the nose and produces red, thickened skin and follicular enlargement. It's found almost exclusively in men older than age 40.

Looking at rosacea

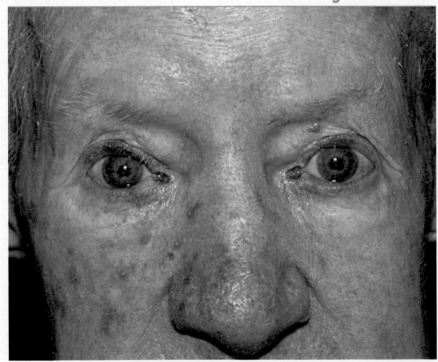

Treatment

▶ Prevention through avoidance of aggravating factors
▶ Oral tetracycline or erythromycin in gradually decreasing doses over 1 to 2 months for the acneiform component of rosacea
▶ Oral minocycline or doxycycline isotretinoin for resistant cases and in those with severe disease
▶ Topical metronidazole gel to help decrease papules, pustules, and erythema
▶ Sulfacet-R lotion, available in flesh tones, to control pustules and hide redness; can be used alone or with oral antibiotics
▶ Electrolysis to destroy large, dilated blood vessels and remove excess tissue (in patients with rhinophyma)

Nursing considerations

▶ Instruct the patient to avoid hot beverages, spicy foods, alcohol, extended sun exposure, and other possible causes of flushing.
▶ Assess the effect of rosacea on body image. Because it's always apparent on the face, your support is essential.
▶ Tell the patient to avoid topical hydrocortisone preparations because they worsen rosacea.

LESSON PLANS

Teaching about rosacea

▶ Assist the patient in identifying and eliminating aggravating factors. If stress and anxiety seem to trigger the disease, teach relaxation techniques and encourage him to use them often.
▶ Instruct the patient to use meticulous hand washing and personal hygiene to avoid irritating and aggravating the condition. To prevent infection, stress the importance of not picking or squeezing the lesions.
▶ Provide directions for antibiotic therapy, and tell the patient to report any adverse effects.
▶ Instruct the patient to wear sunscreen with a sun protection factor of 15 or higher to protect his face from the sun.
▶ Tell the patient to protect his face in the winter with a scarf or ski mask.
▶ Have the patient avoid irritating his facial skin by not rubbing or touching it too much.
▶ Advise the patient to avoid facial products that contain alcohol or other skin irritants.
▶ When using moisturizer with a topical medication, instruct the patient to apply the moisturizer after the medication has dried.

▶ Caution the patient to use products that are labeled noncomedogenic. These won't clog oil and sweat gland openings (pores) as much.
▶ Advise the patient to avoid overheating.
▶ Instruct the patient to avoid alcohol.

Squamous cell carcinoma

Squamous cell carcinoma of the skin is an invasive tumor arising from keratinizing epidermal cells and has the potential for metastasis. It occurs most commonly in fair-skinned white males older than age 60 and is the second most common form of skin cancer. Outdoor employment and residence in a sunny, warm climate (southern United States and Australia, for example) greatly increase the risk of squamous cell carcinoma.

Lesions on sun-damaged skin tend to be less invasive with less tendency to metastasize than lesions on unexposed skin. Notable exceptions are squamous cell lesions on the lower lip and the ears; almost invariably, these are markedly invasive metastatic lesions with a poor prognosis.

A premalignant lesion may progress with induration and inflammation of the preexisting lesion. When arising from normal skin, the nodule grows slowly on a firm, indurated base. If untreated, this nodule eventually ulcerates and invades underlying tissues.

PICTURING PATHO

Looking at squamous cell carcinoma

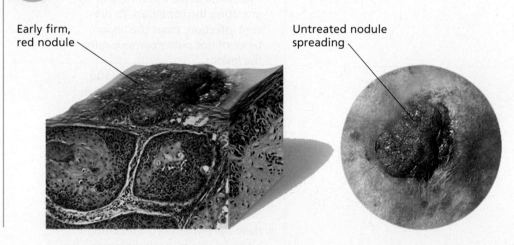

Early firm, red nodule

Untreated nodule spreading

Comparing premalignant skin lesions

Review this chart to help you differentiate among diseases associated with premalignant skin lesions, including their causes, the people at risk, lesion descriptions, and treatment.

Disease	Cause	People at risk	Lesion description	Treatment
Actinic keratosis	Solar radiation	White males with fair skin (middle-age to elderly)	Reddish brown lesions 1 mm to 1 cm in size (may enlarge if untreated) on face, ears, lower lip, bald scalp, and dorsa of hands and forearms	Topical fluorouracil, cryosurgery using liquid nitrogen, or curettage and electrodesiccation
Bowen's disease	Unknown	White males with fair skin (middle-age to elderly)	Brown to reddish brown lesions, with scaly surface on exposed and unexposed areas	Surgical excision, topical fluorouracil
Erythroplasia of Queyrat	Bowen's disease of the mucous membranes	Males (middle-age to elderly)	Red lesions with a glistening or granular appearance on mucous membranes, particularly the glans penis in uncircumcised males	Surgical excision
Leukoplakia	Smoking, alcohol, chronic cheek-biting, ill-fitting dentures, mis-aligned teeth	Males (middle-age to elderly)	Lesions on oral, anal, and genital mucous membranes, varying in appearance from smooth and white to rough and gray	Elimination of irritating factors, surgical excision, or curettage and electrodesiccation (if lesion is still premalignant)

Signs and symptoms

▶ Areas of chronic ulceration, especially on sun-damaged skin
▶ Lesions on the face, ears, and dorsa of the hands and forearms and on other sun-damaged skin areas
▶ Lesions that may appear scaly and keratotic with raised, irregular borders
▶ In late disease, lesions that grow outward (exophytic), are friable, and tend toward chronic crusting
▶ Pain, malaise, and anorexia and resulting fatigue and weakness (as the disease progresses and metastasizes to the regional lymph nodes)

Treatment

▶ Mohs surgery if lesions are 2 cm or larger, or have recurred on the face, mucosal, membranes, or genitals
▶ Wide surgical excision or curettage and electrodesiccation, for smaller lesions; radiation therapy, for older or debilitated patients; chemotherapy; and chemosurgery, for resistant or recurrent lesions
▶ Chemotherapeutic agent fluorouracil (Efudex) in various strengths (1%, 2%, and 5%) as a cream or solution
▶ Fluorouracil continued only until lesions reach the ulcerative and necrotic stages (usually 2 to 4 weeks); then, application of corticosteroid preparation such as an anti-inflammatory agent; complete healing within 1 to 2 months

Nursing considerations

▶ Disfiguring lesions are distressing. Accept the patient as he is to increase his self-esteem and to strengthen a caring relationship.

▶ Listen to the patient's fears and concerns. Offer reassurance, when appropriate. Remain with the patient during periods of severe stress and anxiety.

▶ Help the patient and his family set realistic goals and expectations.

▶ Assess the patient's readiness for decision making, and then involve him in making choices and decisions related to his care. Provide positive reinforcement for the patient's efforts to adapt.

▶ Coordinate a consistent care plan for changing the patient's dressings. A standard routine helps the patient and his family learn how to care for the wound.

▶ To promote healing and prevent infection, keep the wound dry and clean.

▶ Try to control odor with balsam of Peru, yogurt flakes, oil of cloves, or other odor-masking substances, even though they may be ineffective for long-term use. Topical or systemic antibiotics also temporarily control odor and eventually alter the lesion's bacterial flora.

▶ Provide periods of rest between procedures if the patient fatigues easily.

▶ Be prepared for the adverse effects of radiation therapy, such as nausea, vomiting, hair loss, malaise, and diarrhea.

▶ Provide small, frequent meals that are high in protein and calories if the patient is anorexic. Consult with the dietitian to incorporate foods that the patient enjoys.

LESSON PLANS

Teaching about squamous cell carcinoma

▶ Explain all procedures and treatments to the patient and his family. Encourage the patient to ask questions, and answer them as completely as possible.

▶ Instruct the patient to avoid excessive sun exposure to prevent recurrence. Direct him to wear protective clothing (hats, long sleeves) when he's outdoors.

▶ Urge the use of a strong sunscreen to protect the skin from ultraviolet rays. Agents containing para-aminobenzoic acid, benzophenone, and zinc oxide are most effective. Instruct the patient to apply these agents 30 to 60 minutes before sun exposure as well as to use lip screens to protect the lips from sun damage.

▶ Advise the patient to relieve local inflammation from topical fluorouracil with cool compresses or with corticosteroid ointment.

▶ Teach the patient to regularly examine the skin for precancerous lesions and to have these removed promptly.

▶ If appropriate, direct the patient and his family to support services, such as social workers, psychologists, and cancer support groups.

▶ Tell the patient to be careful to keep fluorouracil away from the eyes, scrotum, or mucous membranes. Warn the patient to avoid excessive exposure to the sun during the course of treatment because it intensifies the inflammatory reaction. Possible adverse effects of treatment include post-inflammatory hyperpigmentation.

Vitiligo

Marked by stark-white skin patches that may cause a serious cosmetic problem, vitiligo results from the destruction and loss of pigment cells (melanocytes). This condition affects about 1% of the population in the United States, usually people ages 10 to 30, with peak incidence around age 20. It shows no racial preference, but the distinctive patches are most noticeable in blacks.

Although the cause of vitiligo is unknown, inheritance seems to be a definite etiologic factor because about 30% of patients with vitiligo have family members with the same condition. Other theories implicate enzymatic self-destructing mechanisms, autoimmune mechanisms, and abnormal neurogenic stimuli.

Some link exists between vitiligo and many other disorders that it commonly accompanies, including thyroid dysfunction, pernicious anemia, Addison's disease, aseptic meningitis, diabetes mellitus, photophobia, hearing defects, alopecia areata, uveitis, chronic mucocutaneous candidiasis, and halo nevi.

The most frequently reported precipitating factor is a stressful physical or psychological event—severe sunburn, surgery, pregnancy, loss of a job, bereavement, or some other source of distress. Chemical agents, such as phenols and catechols, may also cause this condition.

Types of vitiligo include:
▶ generalized: most common type, with more than one general area of involvement. It commonly presents with rapid loss of color on the hands, fingertips, face, neck, and scalp.
▶ segmental: starts at an early age, progresses for 1 to 2 years, then stops. Color loss is in one segment of the body.
▶ trichrome: brown, tan, and white shades on the skin.

Signs and symptoms
▶ Depigmented or stark-white patches on the skin
▶ Lesions that are usually bilaterally symmetrical with sharp borders, which occasionally are hyperpigmented
▶ Lesions that are small initially but that can enlarge and even progress to total depigmentation (universal vitiligo)
▶ Patches that generally appear over bony prominences on the back of the hands; on the face, the axillae, genitalia, nipples, or umbilicus; around orifices (such as the eyes, mouth, and anus); within body folds; and at sites of trauma

▶ Hair within these lesions that may also turn white
▶ Vitiligo that may be associated with premature gray hair and ocular pigmentary changes because hair follicles and certain parts of the eyes also contain pigment cells

Vitiligo on the hands

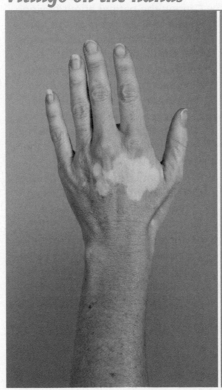 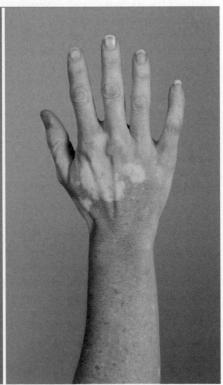

Treatment

‣ Repigmentation therapy that combines systemic or topical psoralen compounds (trimethyl psoralen or 8-methoxypsoralen) with exposure to sunlight or artificial ultraviolet A light to enhance the contrast between normal skin, which turns darker than usual, and white, vitiliginous skin.

‣ Topical class I glucosteroid ointments for single or small macules; depigmentation therapy for patients with vitiligo affecting more than 50% of the body surface; cream containing 20% monobenzone to permanently destroy pigment cells in unaffected areas of the skin and produce a uniform skin tone

‣ Commercial cosmetics to help deemphasize vitiliginous skin

Nursing considerations

‣ During application of topical class I glucosteroid ointments, monitor for skin atrophy or telangiectasia.

‣ With depigmentation therapy, the medication is applied initially to a small area of normal skin once daily to test for unfavorable reactions (contact dermatitis, for example).

‣ Provide emotional support to the patient and caregivers.

LESSON
PLANS

Teaching about vitiligo

‣ Instruct the patient to use psoralen medications three or four times weekly. (*Note:* Systemic psoralens should be taken 2 hours before exposure to sun; topical solutions should be applied 30 to 60 minutes before exposure.) Warn him to use a sunscreen (sun protection factor [SPF] of 15) to protect both affected and normal skin during exposure and to wear sunglasses after taking the medication. If periorbital areas require exposure, tell the patient to keep his eyes closed during treatment.

‣ Suggest that the patient receiving depigmentation therapy wear protective clothing and to use a sunscreen (SPF 15). Explain the therapy thoroughly, and allow the patient plenty of time to decide whether to undergo this treatment. Make sure he understands that the results of depigmentation are permanent and that he must, thereafter, protect his skin from the adverse effects of sunlight.

‣ Caution the patient about buying commercial cosmetics or dyes without trying them first because some may not be suitable.

‣ For the child with vitiligo, modify repigmentation therapy to avoid unnecessary restrictions. Tell the parents the child should wear clothing that permits maximum exposure of vitiliginous areas to the sun.

‣ Remind patients undergoing repigmentation therapy that exposure to sunlight also darkens normal skin. After being exposed to UVA for the prescribed amount of time, the patient should apply a sunscreen if he plans to be exposed to sunlight also. If sunburn occurs, advise the patient to discontinue therapy temporarily and to apply open wet dressings (using thin sheeting) to affected areas for 15 to 20 minutes, four or five times daily or as necessary for comfort. After application of wet dressings, allow the skin to air-dry. Suggest

application of a soothing lubricating cream or lotion while the skin is still slightly moist.

‣ Reinforce patient teaching with written instructions.

‣ Be sensitive to the patient's emotional needs, but avoid promoting unrealistic hope for a total cure.

Warts

Warts, also called *verrucae*, are common, benign infections of the skin and adjacent mucous membranes. Although warts may occur at any age, common warts (*verrucae vulgaris*) are most prevalent in children and young adults. Flat warts usually occur in children but can also affect adults. Genital warts may be transmitted through sexual contact. About 8% to 10% of the population has warts.

The prognosis varies: some warts disappear with treatment; others necessitate vigorous, prolonged treatment.

Warts are caused by infection with a virus from the human papillomavirus family. The mode of transmission is probably through direct contact, but autoinoculation is possible.

Signs and symptoms
Common wart
❯ Usually found on the extremities, particularly the hands and fingers; rough, elevated, rounded surfaces

Filiform wart
❯ Single, thin, threadlike projection, commonly around the face and neck

Looking at a cross-section of a wart

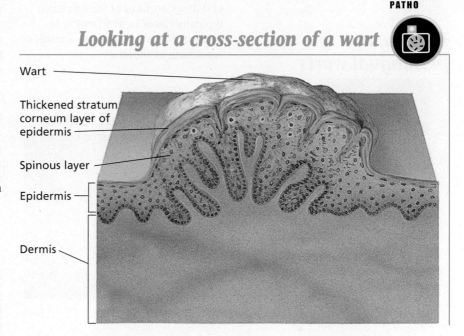

- Wart
- Thickened stratum corneum layer of epidermis
- Spinous layer
- Epidermis
- Dermis

Looking at common and filiform warts

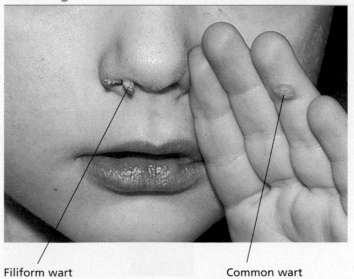

Filiform wart   Common wart

Periungual wart

▶ Rough, irregularly shaped, elevated surfaces around the nail edges; pain accompanying a wart that has extended under the nail and lifted it off the nail bed

Looking at periungual warts

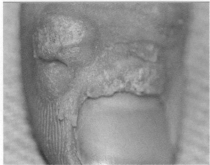

Flat wart

▶ Multiple groupings of up to several hundred slightly raised lesions with smooth, flat, or slightly rounded tops, usually found on the face, neck, chest, knees, legs, dorsa of the hands, wrists, and flexor surfaces of the forearms; typically linear in distribution because of potential spread as a result of scratching or shaving

Looking at flat warts

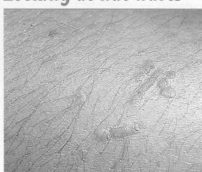

Plantar wart

▶ Possible pain in feet with pressure; inspection of pressure points that reveals slightly elevated or flat lesions appearing singly or in large clusters (mosaic warts); warts possibly obliterating natural skin lines

Digitate wart

▶ Fingerlike, horny projection, arising from a pea-shaped base

Genital wart

▶ Small pink to red warts, also known as *condyloma acuminatum,* found on the penis, scrotum, vulva, or anus; may appear singly or in large cauliflower-like clusters

Looking at plantar warts

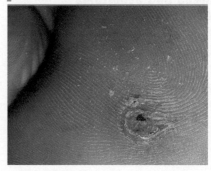

Looking at a digitate wart

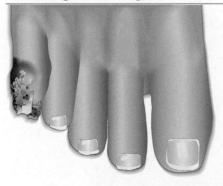

Looking at genital warts of the penis

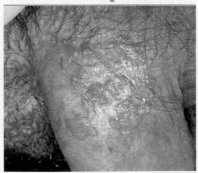

Treatment

Effective treatment varies with the location, size, and number of warts. It also depends on the patient's age, pain level (current and projected), history of therapy, and compliance with treatment. Most people develop an immune response that causes warts to disappear spontaneously, thus requiring no treatment.

Electrodesiccation and curettage

▶ High-frequency electric current that destroys the wart and is followed by surgical removal of dead tissue at the base; after application of an antibiotic ointment, area covered with a bandage for 48 hours

Cryotherapy

▶ Liquid nitrogen that kills the wart, resulting in a dried blister that's peeled off several days later; if initial treatment unsuccessful, may be repeated at 2- to 4-week intervals; method useful for periungual warts or for common warts on the face, extremities, penis, vagina, or anus

Acid therapy

▶ Used as primary or adjunctive therapy; involves application (by patient) of acid-impregnated plaster patches (such as 40% salicylic acid plasters) or acid drops (such as 5% to 20% salicylic and lactic acid in flexible collodion [DuoFilm]) every 12 to 24 hours for 2 to 4 weeks; method contraindicated for areas in which perspiration is heavy or that are likely to get wet or for exposed body parts on which patches are cosmetically undesirable

Podophyllum

▶ Application of 25% podophyllum resin in compound with tincture of benzoin solution for moist warts, such as venereal warts; after allowing to dry, left on for 4 hours and then washed off with soap and water; may be repeated every 3 to 4 days and, in some cases, must be left on a maximum of 24 hours, depending on the patient's tolerance; contraindicated in pregnant patients

Nursing considerations

▶ To protect adjacent unaffected skin during acid or podophyllum treatment, cover it with petroleum jelly or sodium bicarbonate.
▶ Encourage the patient to verbalize feelings about his appearance. Discuss any embarrassment or fear of reaction he may have. Offer emotional support, and assure him that warts respond to treatment.
▶ Be alert for possible adverse effects of acid therapy, such as burning and irritation of surrounding tissues.

LESSON PLANS

Teaching about warts

▶ Teach the patient and his family that warts are contagious and can be spread by shaving, sharing personal articles, scratching, and sexual contact. Help the patient identify all contacts, and tell him that he should encourage them to seek medical treatment. Advise him that warts commonly recur.

▶ If the patient is receiving acid therapy, make sure he knows how to apply the plaster patches. Instruct him to leave the patches on for 12 to 24 hours. Stress the importance of protecting healthy tissue and avoiding picking, rubbing, or scratching lesions. Emphasize that compliance with the treatment regimen is essential for successful wart removal and to prevent scarring.
▶ If the patient is receiving electrosurgery to remove warts, explain the procedure and give preoperative and postoperative instructions.

TESTS

A good portion of diagnosing skin disorders is in what you see on inspection. When evaluating a lesion, you need to classify it as primary (new) or secondary (a change in a primary lesion). Then determine whether it's solid or fluid-filled and describe its characteristics, pattern, location, and distribution.

Lesion shapes

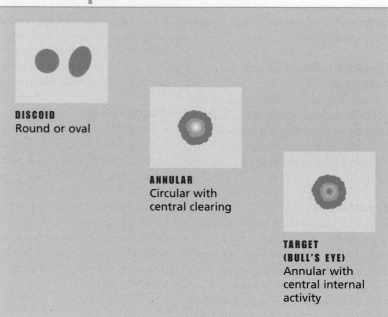

DISCOID
Round or oval

ANNULAR
Circular with central clearing

TARGET (BULL'S EYE)
Annular with central internal activity

Lesion configurations

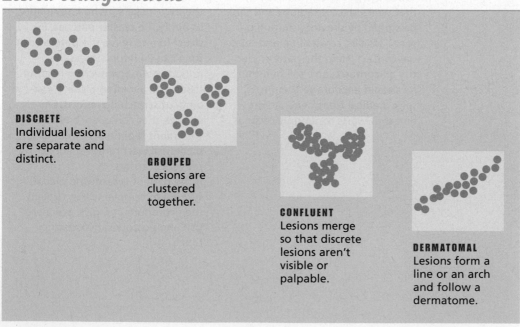

DISCRETE
Individual lesions are separate and distinct.

GROUPED
Lesions are clustered together.

CONFLUENT
Lesions merge so that discrete lesions aren't visible or palpable.

DERMATOMAL
Lesions form a line or an arch and follow a dermatome.

Types of skin lesions

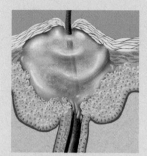

PUSTULE
A small, pus-filled lesion (called a *follicular pustule* if it contains a hair)

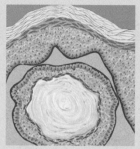

CYST
A closed sac in or under the skin that contains fluid or semisolid material

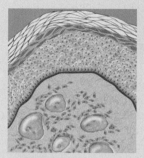

NODULE
A raised lesion detectable by touch that's usually 1 cm or more in diameter

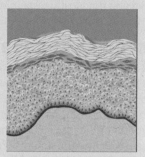

WHEAL
A raised, reddish area that's commonly itchy and lasts 24 hours or less

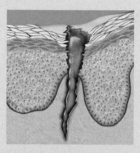

FISSURE
A painful, cracked lesion of the skin that extends at least into the dermis

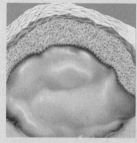

BULLA
A large, fluid-filled blister that's usually 1 cm or more in diameter

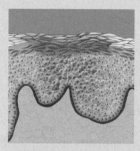

MACULE
A small, discolored spot or patch on the skin

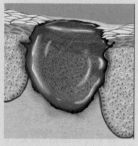

ULCER
A craterlike lesion of the skin that usually extends at least into the dermis

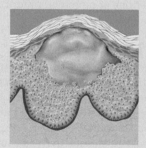

VESICLE
A small, fluid-filled blister that's usually 1 cm or less in diameter

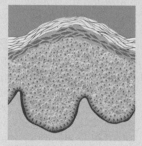

PAPULE
A solid, raised lesion that's usually less than 1 cm in diameter

Laboratory tests

Several diagnostic tests may help to identify skin disorders.

RADIOALLERGOSORBENT TEST

The radioallergosorbent test (RAST) measures immunoglobulin (Ig) E antibodies in serum by radioimmunoassay and identifies specific allergens that cause rash, asthma, hay fever, drug reactions, and other atopic complaints. The RAST is easier to perform, more specific, less painful, and less dangerous than skin testing. Careful selection of specific allergens, based on the patient's history, is crucial for effective results.

Although skin testing is still the preferred means of diagnosing IgE-mediated hypersensitivities, the RAST may be more useful when a skin disorder makes accurate reading of skin tests difficult, when a patient requires continual antihistamine therapy, or when skin tests are negative but the patient's history supports IgE-mediated hypersensitivity.

In the RAST, a sample of the patient's serum is exposed to a panel of allergen particle complexes (APCs) on cellulose disks. The patient's IgE reacts with APCs to which it's sensitive. Radiolabeled anti-IgE antibody is then added, and this binds to the IgE-APC complexes. After centrifugation, the amount of radioactivity in the particulate material is directly proportional to the amount of IgE antibodies present.

DIASCOPY

In diascopy, a lesion is covered with a microscopic slide or piece of clear plastic, which helps determine whether dilated capillaries or extravasated blood is causing a lesion's redness. Microscopic immunofluorescence identifies immunoglobulins and elastic tissue in manifestations of immune disorders.

PATCH TEST

The patch test identifies the cause of allergic contact sensitization. Indicated in patients with suspected allergies or allergies from an unknown cause, this test uses a sample of common allergies, or antigens, to determine whether one or more will produce a positive reaction.

PHOTOTESTING

Phototesting exposes small areas of the patient's skin to ultraviolet A or ultraviolet B light to detect photosensitivity. Phototesting in combination with patch testing is used to evaluate a patient's photosensitivity to compounds placed on the skin (photopatch testing).

POTASSIUM HYDROXIDE TEST

Potassium hydroxide (KOH) test helps to identify fungal skin infections. It requires scraping scales from the skin and then mixing the scales with a few drops of 10% to 25% KOH on a glass slide. After heating the slide, skin cells dissolve, leaving fungal elements visible on microscopic examination.

Performing a patch test

A patch test confirms allergic contact sensitivity and can help identify its cause. In this test, a sample series of common allergens (antigens) is applied to the skin in the hope that one or more will produce a positive reaction. A positive patch test result proves that the patient has a contact sensitivity, but it doesn't necessarily confirm that the test substance caused the clinical eruption.

If the patient has an acute inflammation, the patch test should be postponed until the inflammation subsides to avoid exacerbating the inflammation.

Keep the following points in mind when performing a patch test:

▸ Use only potentially irritating substances for a patch test. Testing with primary irritants isn't possible.
▸ To avoid skin irritation, dilute substances that may be irritating to 1% to 2% in petroleum jelly, mineral oil or, as a last choice, water. When there are no clues to a likely allergen in a person with possible contact dermatitis, use a series of common allergens available in standard patch tests.
▸ Apply the allergens to normal, hairless skin on the back or on the ventral surface of the forearm. First, apply them to a small disk of filter paper attached to aluminum and coated with plastic. Tape the paper to the skin, or use a small square of soft cotton and cover it with occlusive tape. Apply liquids and ointments to the disk or cotton. Apply volatile liquids to the skin, and allow the areas to dry before covering. Before application, powder solids and moisten powders and fabrics.
▸ Make sure that patches remain in place for 48 hours. However, remove the patch immediately if pain, pruritus, or irritation develops. Positive reactions may take time to develop, so check findings 20 to 30 minutes after removing the patch and again 96 hours (4 days) after the application.
▸ To relieve the effects of a positive reaction, tell the patient to apply topical corticosteroids as ordered.

Administering test antigens

The illustration here shows the arm of a patient undergoing a recall antigen test, which determines whether he has previously been exposed to certain antigens. A sample panel of four test antigens has been injected into his forearm, and the test site has been marked and labeled for each antigen.

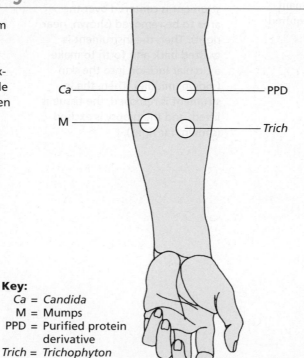

Ca — — — PPD

M — — — Trich

Key:
Ca = *Candida*
M = *Mumps*
PPD = *Purified protein derivative*
Trich = *Trichophyton*

SKIN BIOPSY

Skin biopsy determines the histology of cells and may be diagnostic, confirmatory, or inconclusive, depending on the disease. It's frequently used to help diagnose nonhealing or atypical wounds.

During a skin biopsy, a small piece of tissue from a suspected malignancy or other skin lesion is excised, using any of the following techniques.

Excision biopsy

▶ Removes a small lesion in its entirety; indicated for rapidly expanding lesions; for sclerotic, bullous, or atrophic lesions; and for examination of the border of a lesion and surrounding normal skin

Punch biopsy

▶ Removes a small cylindrical specimen by a special instrument that pierces the center of a lesion

Shave biopsy

▶ Cuts the lesion above the skin line, leaving the lower dermal layers intact (not recommended for any lesion that's suspected of being malignant where margin assessment is required)

Looking at excision biopsy

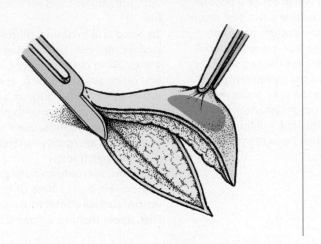

Looking at punch biopsy

In a punch biopsy, the biopsy instrument is centered over the area to be removed (shown, near right). Then the instrument is twisted back and forth to make a circular incision into the skin (shown, middle). Then, the instrument is removed, the tissue is lifted, and the biopsy is excised (shown, far right).

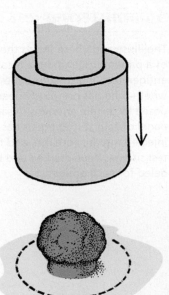

Looking at shave biopsy

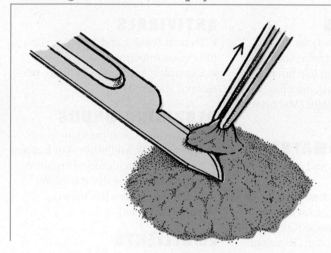

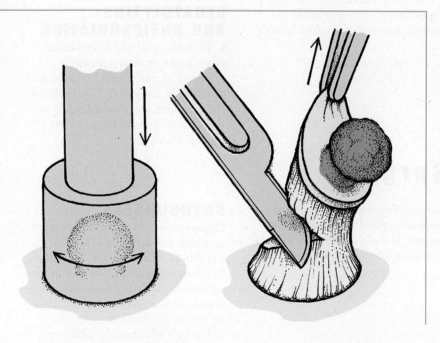

STAINS AND CULTURES

Gram stains and exudate cultures help to identify the organism responsible for an underlying infection by separating bacteria into two classifications: gram-negative and gram-positive. Although staining provides rapid, valuable diagnostic leads, firm identification must be made by culturing the organisms.

TZANCK TEST

In the Tzanck test, vesicular fluid or exudate from an ulcer is smeared on a glass slide and stained with Papanicolaou's, Wright's, Giemsa, or methylene blue stain. Herpesvirus is confirmed if microscopic examination of the slide reveals the presence of multinucleated giant cells, intranuclear inclusion bodies, and ballooning degeneration.

TREATMENTS AND PROCEDURES

Drug therapy

Categories of drugs used to treat skin disorders include acne products, antibacterials, antifungals, anti-inflammatories, antipruritics, antivirals, debriding drugs, emollients, and keratolytics and antipsoriatics.

ACNE PRODUCTS

▶ To treat acne vulgaris
▶ Examples: antibiotics (clindamycin [Cleocin T], erythromycin [Eryderm], tetracycline [Sumycin], cleaners/antiseptic drugs), azelaic acid [Azelex], benzoyl peroxide, isotretinoin [Amnesteem], tretinoin [Retin-A])

ANTIBACTERIALS

▶ To fight bacterial skin infections; some also used to treat burn wounds
▶ Examples: bacitracin, gentamicin sulfate, mafenide acetate (Sulfamylon), neomycin sulfate (Cortisporin), silver sulfadiazine (Silvadene), polymyxin B and bacitracin combination (Neosporin), and polymyxin B combination

ANTIFUNGALS

▶ To treat fungal infections
▶ Examples: clotrimazole (Lotrimin, Mycelex), griseofulvin (Grifulvin), ketoconazole (Nizoral), miconazole nitrate (Vusion), nystatin (Mycostatin), terbinafen (Lamisil)

ANTI-INFLAMMATORIES

▶ To treat dermatitis and allergic skin reactions
▶ Examples: betamethasone valerate (Beta-Val), coal tar (Fototar), dexamethasone, hydrocortisone (Cortef), triamcinolone (Aristocort, Kenalog)

ANTIPRURITICS

▶ To treat pruritus
▶ Examples: calamine lotion, cyproheptadine, diphenhydramine (Benadryl), oatmeal (Aveeno Colloidal)

ANTIVIRALS

▶ To treat types 1 and 2 herpes simplex virus infections
▶ Examples: acyclovir (Zovirax), penciclovir (Denavir)

DEBRIDING DRUGS

▶ To treat and clean pressure ulcers, burns, wounds, and other skin injuries
▶ Examples: becaplermin (Regranex), chlorophyllin derivatives (Chloresium), dextranomer (Debrisan), trypsin (Granulex)

EMOLLIENTS

▶ To lubricate and moisturize the skin to treat dryness and itching
▶ Examples: lanolin, mineral oil

KERATOLYTICS AND ANTIPSORIATICS

▶ To treat superficial fungal infections, psoriasis, and dermatitis
▶ Examples: resorcinol, salicylic acid (PROPApH Astringent, Clearasil, Sal-Acid, Stridex Pads), coal tar preparations (Estar, Fototar, Oxipor VHC, Polytar, PsoriGel)

Surgery

Surgical techniques used to treat skin disorders include cryosurgery, laser surgery, Mohs' micrographic surgery, skin grafting, and debridement.

CRYOSURGERY

Cryosurgery is a common procedure in which extreme cold is applied to the skin to induce tissue destruction. Cryosurgery causes epidermal-dermal separation above the basement membranes, helping to prevent scarring after reepithelialization.

The procedure can be performed using nothing more than a cotton-tipped applicator dipped in liquid nitrogen and applied to the skin; or, it may involve a complex cryosurgical unit.

Positioning thermocouple needles

During cryosurgery, you may be responsible for positioning thermocouple needles and then operating them according to the surgeon's direction. These needles measure the temperature of the tissue at its tip and help the surgeon gauge the depth of freezing—a vitally important factor when destroying cancerous lesions. The needle may be placed in any of several positions.

Precise temperature measurement can be difficult because a variation of only 1 mm in the needle's position can translate into a difference of 50° to 59° F (10° to 15° C). For that reason, you'll usually place two or more needles in different areas to increase the accuracy of the reading.

In this illustration, the needle is shown inserted at an angle so that its tip rests about 5 mm below the base of the tumor to give a direct reading of tissue temperature. In this position, the temperature reading may be affected by chilling of the shaft within the frozen tissue, but the error isn't likely to be significant.

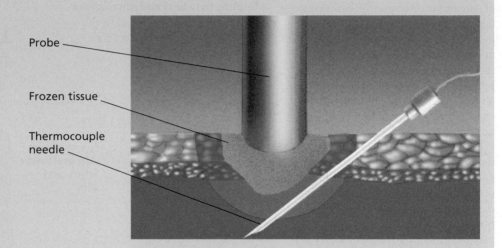

Probe

Frozen tissue

Thermocouple needle

Here the probe is placed about 5 mm to one side of the frozen tissue at a depth of about 3 mm. In this position, it registers the same temperature as the probe above because both probe tips are about the same distance from the frozen tissue.

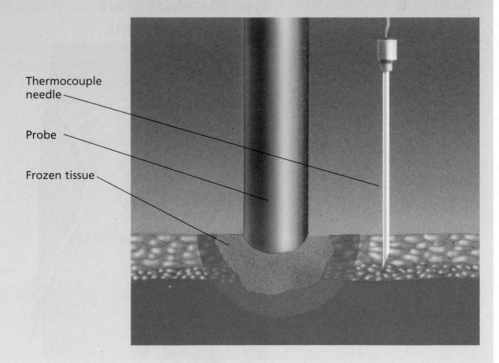

Thermocouple needle

Probe

Frozen tissue

LASER SURGERY

Laser surgery uses the intense, highly focused light of a laser beam to treat dermatologic lesions. Performed on an outpatient basis, it spares normal tissue, promotes faster healing, and helps prevent postsurgical infection.

MOHS' MICROGRAPHIC SURGERY

Mohs' micrographic surgery involves serial excision and histologic analysis of cancerous or suspected cancerous tissues. By allowing step-by-step tumor excision, Mohs' surgery minimizes the size of the scar (important if the treatment is done on the face) and helps prevent recurrence by removing all malignant tissue. This surgery is especially effective in basal cell carcinomas.

Mohs' surgery has two complications, however: bleeding and nerve damage. Bleeding is easily controlled with direct pressure and usually occurs with large flaps and repairs of previous procedures. Nerve damage may occur as small sensory fibers are severed during the procedure, but the deficits usually last only until the body regenerates the nerve fibers.

SKIN GRAFTING

Skin grafting corrects defects caused by burns, trauma, and surgery. This procedure is indicated when:
▶ primary closure isn't possible or cosmetically acceptable
▶ primary closure would interfere with functioning
▶ the defect is on a weight-bearing surface
▶ a skin tumor is excised and the site needs to be monitored for recurrence.

Grafting may be done using a general or local anesthetic and can be performed on an outpatient basis for small facial or neck defects.

Types of skin grafts include:
▶ split-thickness grafts, which consist of the epidermis and a small portion of dermis
▶ full-thickness grafts, which include all of the dermis as well as the epidermis
▶ composite grafts, which also include underlying tissues, such as muscle, cartilage, or bone.

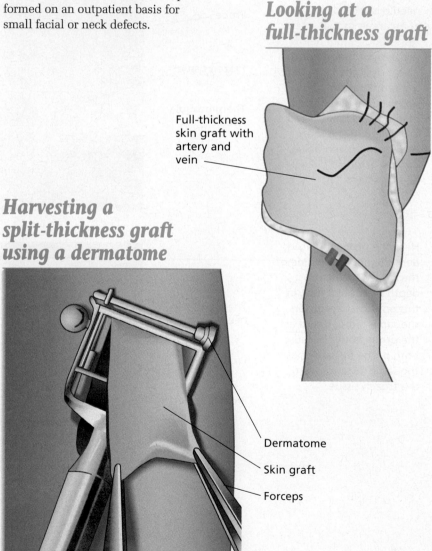

Looking at a full-thickness graft

Full-thickness skin graft with artery and vein

Harvesting a split-thickness graft using a dermatome

Dermatome

Skin graft

Forceps

Evacuating fluid from a sheet graft

When small pockets of fluid (called *blebs*) accumulate beneath a sheet graft, evacuate the fluid using a sterile scalpel and sterile cotton-tipped applicators.

First, carefully perforate the center of the bleb with the scalpel.

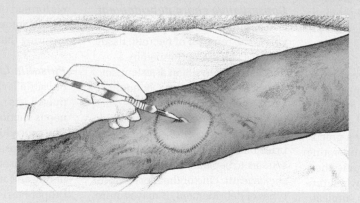

Gently express the fluid with the cotton-tipped applicators. Never express fluid by rolling the bleb to the edge of the graft. This disturbs healing in other areas.

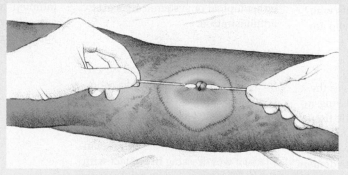

HANDS ON

Caring for the donor graft site

Autografts are usually taken from another area of the patient's body with a dermatome, an instrument that cuts uniform, split-thickness skin portions (typically 0.013-cm to 0.05-cm thick). Autografting makes the donor site a partial-thickness wound, which may bleed, drain, and cause pain.

This site needs scrupulous care to prevent infection, which could change the site to a full-thickness wound. Depending on the graft's thickness, tissue may be obtained from the donor site again in as few as 10 days.

Usually, Xeroflo gauze is applied postoperatively. The outer gauze dressing can be taken off on the 1st postoperative day; the Xeroflo will protect the new epithelial proliferation.

Care for the donor site as you care for the autograft, using dressing changes at the initial stages to prevent infection and promote healing. Follow the guidelines at right.

Dressing the wound
- Wash your hands and put on sterile gloves.
- Remove the outer gauze dressings within 24 hours. Inspect the Xeroflo for signs of infection, and then leave the wound open to the air to speed drying and healing.
- Leave small amounts of fluid accumulation alone. Using aseptic technique, aspirate larger amounts through the dressing with a small-gauge needle and syringe.
- Apply a lanolin-based cream daily to completely healed donor sites to keep skin tissue pliable and to remove crusts.

DEBRIDEMENT

Debridement may involve surgical, autolytic, chemical, or mechanical techniques to remove necrotic tissue from a wound. Although debridement can be extremely painful, it's necessary to prevent infection and promote healing of burns and skin ulcers.

Surgical debridement

Surgical debridement involves removing necrotic and healthy tissue, thus converting a chronic wound to a clean, acute wound. Surgical sharp debridement is performed by a practitioner or by a surgeon in the operating room with the patient under anesthesia. Caution should be used when providing either conservative or surgical sharp debridement on patients who have low platelet counts or who are taking anticoagulants.

Autolytic debridement

Autolytic debridement involves the use of moisture-retentive dressings to cover the wound bed. Necrotic tissue is then dissolved through self-digestion of enzymes in the wound fluid. Although autolytic debridement takes longer than other debridement methods, it isn't painful, it's easy to perform, and it's appropriate for patients who can't tolerate other methods. It shouldn't be performed if the wound is infected, however.

Chemical debridement

Chemical debridement with enzymatic agents is a selective method of debridement. Enzymes are applied topically to areas of necrotic tissue only, breaking down necrotic tissue elements. Enzymes digest only the necrotic tissue, sparing healthy tissue and ultimately producing a wound that's clean with red granulation tissue. These agents require specific conditions that vary from product to product. Indeed, effectiveness is achieved by carefully following each manufacturer's guidelines.

Mechanical debridement

Mechanical debridement includes conservative sharp debridement, wet-to-dry dressings, hydrotherapy, and pulsatile lavage.

Conservative sharp debridement

Conservative sharp debridement involves the removal of necrotic tissue only. It's usually performed by a physician, a physician assistant, an advanced practice nurse, or another certified wound specialist.

During conservative sharp debridement, loosened eschar is carefully pried out and cut with forceps and scissors to separate it from viable tissue beneath. One of the most painful types of debridement, it may require either topical or systemic analgesic administration.

Wet-to-dry dressings

Wet-to-dry dressings, typically used for wounds with extensive necrotic tissue and minimal drainage, require an appropriate technique, and the dressing materials used are critical to the outcome. The nurse or physician places a wet dressing in contact with the lesion and covers it with an outer layer of bandaging. As the dressing dries, it sticks to the wound. When the dried dressing is removed, the necrotic tissue comes off with it.

Irrigation of a wound with a pressurized antiseptic solution cleans tissue and removes wound debris and excess drainage.

Hydrotherapy

Hydrotherapy—commonly referred to as *tubbing, tanking,* or *whirlpool*—involves immersing the patient in a tank of warm water, with intermittent agitation of the water. It's usually performed on large wounds with a significant amount of nonviable tissue covering the wound surface.

Pulsatile lavage

Pulsatile lavage uses intermittent or pulsed jets of an irrigant and simultaneous suctioning to debride a wound. The procedure can loosen wound debris, thus reducing bacteria. It's especially useful in wounds where tunneling and undermining are present. Proper barrier precautions and containment are necessary to decrease aerosolized pathogens and prevent the spread of infection.

Chapter 11
Female
reproductive care

DISEASES
Breast cancer

Along with lung cancer, breast cancer is a leading killer of women ages 35 to 54.

With early detection and treatment, however, the prognosis is influenced considerably. The American Cancer Society believes the combination of mammography, clinical breast examination, and finding and reporting breast changes early offers females the best opportunity for reducing breast cancer mortalities.

About half of all breast cancers develop in the upper outer quadrant, and growth rates vary. Theoretically, slow-growing breast cancer may take up to 8 years to become palpable at 1 cm. It spreads by way of the lymphatic system and the bloodstream through the right side of the heart to the lungs and to the other breast, chest wall, liver, bone, and brain.

Risk factors for breast cancer include:
- female gender
- increasing age (risk greater after age 60)
- family history of breast cancer
- genetic mutations BRCA 1 and BRCA 2
- radiation exposure
- obesity
- menarche before age 12
- menopause after age 55
- women with their first child after age 35
- postmenopausal hormone therapy.

Classified by histologic appearance and the lesion's location, breast cancer may be described as:
- *adenocarcinoma* (ductal)—arising from the epithelium
- *intraductal*—developing within the ducts (includes Paget's disease)
- *infiltrating*—occurring in the breast's parenchymal tissue
- *inflammatory* (rare)—growing rapidly and causing overlying skin to become edematous, inflamed, and indurated
- *lobular carcinoma in situ*—involving the lobes of glandular tissue
- *medullary* or *circumscribed*—enlarging tumor with rapid growth rate.

Coupled with a staging system, these classifications provide a clearer picture of the cancer's extent. The most common system for staging, both before and after surgery, is the TNM (tumor, node, metastasis) system.

Breast tumor sources and sites

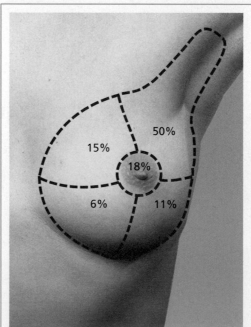

About 90% of all breast tumors arise from the epithelial cells lining the ducts. About half of all breast cancers develop in the breast's upper outer quadrant—the section containing the most glandular tissue.

The second most common cancer site is the nipple, where all of the breast ducts converge.

The next most common site is the upper inner quadrant, followed by the lower outer quadrant and, finally, the lower inner quadrant.

Staging breast cancer

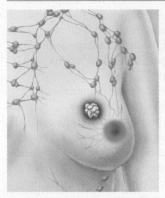

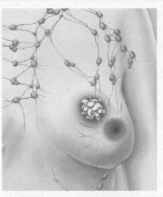

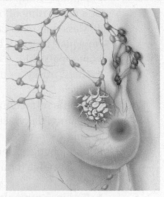

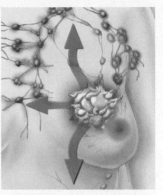

Stage I

In stage I, the tumor is less than 2 cm in size.

Stage II

In stage II, the tumor is greater than 2 cm in size.

Stage III

In stage III, the tumor is greater than 5 cm in size.

Stage IV

In stage IV, the tumor can be any size, with direct extension to the chest wall.

PICTURING PATHO

Ductal carcinoma in situ

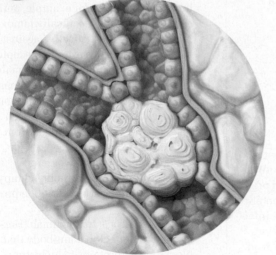

PICTURING PATHO

Infiltrating (invasive) ductal carcinoma

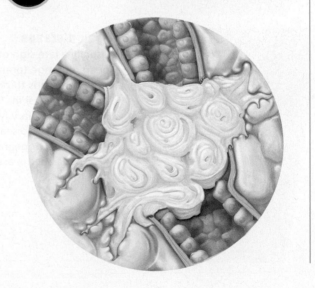

Signs and symptoms

▶ Painless lump or mass in the breast or a thickening of breast tissue
▶ Mass that most commonly appears on a mammogram before a lesion becomes palpable
▶ Clear, milky, or bloody nipple discharge
▶ Nipple retraction
▶ Peeling, flaky, scaly skin around the nipple
▶ Skin changes, such as dimpling, peau d'orange (orange peel), or inflammation
▶ Cervical supraclavicular and axillary nodes that may show lumps or enlargement

Treatment

▶ Surgery that includes lumpectomy, partial mastectomy, simple or total mastectomy, modified radical mastectomy, radical mastectomy, sentinel node biopsy, and axillary node dissection
▶ Lumpectomy, for patients with small, well-defined lesions
▶ A cell-destroying technique, called *cryolumpectomy,* for small, early, primary tumors; radiation therapy possibly following cryolumpectomy, which has few complications and may prevent local recurrence
▶ Before or after tumor removal, primary radiation therapy for a patient who has a small tumor in the early stages without distant metastasis; radiation therapy possibly also preventing or treating local recurrence
▶ Chemotherapy, such as cyclophosphamide (Cytoxan), fluorouracil, methotrexate, doxorubicin, vincristine, paclitaxel (Abraxane), and prednisone
▶ Hormonal blocking therapy that lowers levels of estrogen and other hormones suspected of nourishing breast cancer cells; for example, antiestrogen therapy (specifically tamoxifen, which is most effective against tumors identified as estrogen receptor-positive), for postmenopausal females
▶ Aromatase inhibitors such as anastrazole (Arimidex): given to postmenopausal women to decrease estrogen levels by preventing androgen from converting to estrogen
▶ For premenopausal women: oophorectomy and hormone therapy to discontinue ovarian hormone production
▶ Targeted drugs: trastuzumab (Herceptin), a monoclonal antibody that blocks HER2 proteins, which stimulate cancer cell growth; kapatinib (Tykerb), which also blocks the effects of HER2 proteins and others with tumor cells

Looking at breast dimpling and peau d'orange

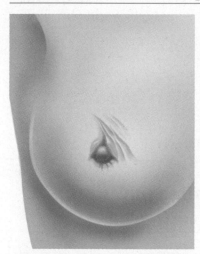

Breast dimpling

Breast dimpling—the puckering or retraction of skin on the breast—results from abnormal attachment of the skin to underlying tissue. It suggests an inflammation or malignant mass beneath the skin surface and usually represents a late sign of breast cancer.

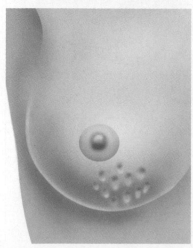

Peau d'orange

Usually a late sign of breast cancer, peau d'orange (orange peel skin) is the edematous thickening and pitting of breast skin. This sign can also occur with axillary lymph node infection or Graves' disease. Its striking orange peel appearance stems from lymphatic edema around deepened hair follicles.

Nursing considerations

▶ Evaluate the patient's feelings about her illness, and determine her level of knowledge. Listen to her concerns, and stay with her during periods of severe anxiety.

▶ Administer ordered analgesics, as required. Monitor and record their effectiveness.

▶ Perform comfort measures, such as repositioning, to promote relaxation and relieve anxiety.

▶ If immobility develops late in the disease, prevent complications by frequently repositioning the patient, using a convoluted foam mattress, and providing skin care (particularly over bony prominences).

▶ Watch for treatment complications, such as nausea, vomiting, anorexia, leukopenia, thrombocytopenia, GI ulceration, and bleeding. Provide comfort measures and prescribed treatments to relieve these complications.

After surgery

▶ Inspect the dressing anteriorly and posteriorly. Report excessive bleeding promptly.

▶ Record the amount and color of drainage. Drainage appears bloody during the first 4 hours; then it becomes serous.

▶ Monitor vital signs. If a general anesthetic was given during surgery, monitor intake and output for at least 48 hours.

▶ Prevent lymphedema of the arm, which may be an early complication of lymph node dissection. Such prevention is crucial because lymphedema can't be treated effectively.

▶ Use strict sterile technique when changing dressings or I.V. tubing or performing an invasive procedure. Monitor temperature and white blood cell count closely.

▶ Inspect the incision. Encourage the patient and her partner to look at her incision.

▶ Provide emotional support and references to available support systems.

Teaching about breast cancer surgery

LESSON PLANS

▶ Clearly explain all procedures and treatments.

▶ Besides the usual preoperative teaching, show the mastectomy patient how to ease postoperative pain by lying on the affected side or by placing a hand or pillow on the incision. Point out where the incision will be. Inform the patient that after the operation, she'll receive analgesics because pain relief encourages coughing and turning and promotes well-being. Explain that a small pillow placed under the arm anteriorly may provide comfort.

▶ Tell her that she may move about and get out of bed as soon as possible, usually as soon as the effects of the anesthetic subside or the first evening after surgery.

▶ Explain that she may have an incisional drain or some type of suction to remove accumulated fluid, relieve tension on the suture line, and promote healing.

▶ Urge the patient to avoid activities that could injure her arm and hand on the side of her surgery. Caution her not to let blood be drawn from or allow injections into that arm. She should also refuse to have blood pressure taken or I.V. therapy administered on the affected arm.

▶ To help prevent lymphedema, instruct the patient to exercise her hand and arm on the affected side regularly and to avoid activities that might allow infection of this hand or arm. Tell her that infection increases the risk of lymphedema.

▶ Inform the patient that she may experience "phantom breast syndrome," a tingling or pins-and-needles sensation in the area where the breast was removed.

▶ Females who have had breast cancer in one breast are at higher risk for cancer in the other breast or for recurrent cancer in the chest wall. For this reason, urge the patient to continue examining the other breast and to comply with recommended follow-up treatment.

▶ Teach relaxation techniques and gentle exercises to improve well-being.

▶ Provide reassurance regarding follow-up support for reconstructive surgery and rehabilitation, as appropriate.

Cervical cancer

Cervical cancer is the third most common cancer of the female reproductive system. It's classified as either preinvasive or invasive.

Preinvasive cancer ranges from minimal cervical dysplasia, in which the lower third of the epithelium contains abnormal cells, to carcinoma in situ, in which the full thickness of epithelium contains abnormally proliferating cells (also known as *cervical intraepithelial neoplasia*). Preinvasive cancer is curable in 75% to 90% of patients with early detection and proper treatment. If untreated, it may progress to invasive cervical cancer, depending on the form.

Signs and symptoms

▶ Preinvasive cancer produces no symptoms or other clinical changes.

Early invasive cancer

▶ Vaginal bleeding, such as a persistent vaginal discharge that may be yellowish, blood-tinged, and foul-smelling; postcoital pain and bleeding
▶ Bleeding between menstrual periods
▶ Unusually heavy menstrual periods

Advanced invasive cancer (into the pelvic wall)

▶ Gradually increasing flank pain (sciatic nerve involvement)
▶ Leakage of urine (metastasis into the bladder with formation of a fistula)
▶ Leakage of stool (metastasis to the rectum with a fistula)

PICTURING PATHO

Looking at cervical cancer

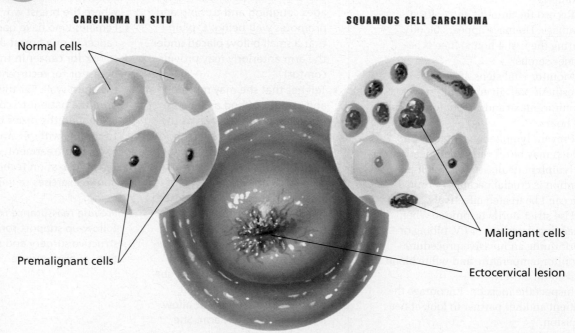

CARCINOMA IN SITU

Normal cells

Premalignant cells

SQUAMOUS CELL CARCINOMA

Malignant cells

Ectocervical lesion

Staging cervical cancer

Treatment decisions depend on accurate staging. The International Federation of Gynecology and Obstetrics defines the following cervical cancer stages.

Stage 0
Carcinoma in situ, intraepithelial carcinoma.

Stage I
Cancer is confined to the cervix (extension to the corpus should be disregarded).

Stage IA
Preclinical malignant lesions of the cervix are diagnosed only microscopically.

Stage IA1
Minimal microscopically evident stromal invasion measures less than 3 mm deep and 7 mm wide.

Stage IA2
Lesions are detected microscopically, measuring 3 to 5 mm from the base of the epithelium, either surface or glandular, from which it originates; lesion width shouldn't exceed 7 mm.

Stage IB
Lesions measure more than 5 mm deep and 7 mm wide, whether seen clinically or not (preformed space involvement shouldn't alter the staging but should be recorded for future treatment decisions).

Stage IB1
Visible lesions measure less than 4 cm.

Stage IB2
Visible lesions measure more than 4 cm.

Stage II
Extension goes beyond the cervix but not to the pelvic wall.

Stage IIA
Cancer involves the vagina but hasn't spread to the lower third.

Stage IIB
Parametrial involvement is obvious.

Stage III
Cancer extends to the pelvic wall; on rectal examination, no cancer-free space between the tumor and the pelvic wall; involves the lower third of the vagina; may block the ureters.

Stage IIIA
No extension to the pelvic wall exists.

Stage IIIB
Extension is to the pelvic wall and ureters are blocked.

Stage IV
Extension is beyond the true pelvis or involvement of the bladder or the rectal mucosa.

Stage IVA
Cancer has spread to adjacent organs.

Stage IVB
Cancer has spread to distant organs.

PICTURING PATHO

Pap smear findings in cervical cancer

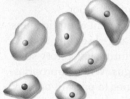

Normal
▸ Large, surface-type squamous cells
▸ Small, pyknotic nuclei

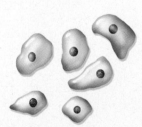

Mild dysplasia
▸ Mild increase in nuclear-to-cytoplasmic ratio
▸ Hyperchromatism
▸ Abnormal chromatin pattern

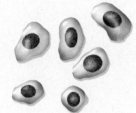

Severe dysplasia, carcinoma in situ
▸ Basal type cells
▸ Very high nuclear-to-cytoplasmic ratio
▸ Marked hyperchromatism
▸ Abnormal chromatin

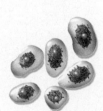

Invasive carcinoma
▸ Marked pleomorphism
▸ Irregular nuclei
▸ Clumped chromatin
▸ Prominent nucleoli

Treatment

▶ Based on accurate clinical staging
▶ Excisional biopsy, cryosurgery, laser destruction, conization (followed by frequent Papanicolaou [Pap] test follow-ups) or, rarely, hysterectomy, for preinvasive lesions
▶ Radical hysterectomy and radiation therapy (internal, external, or both), for invasive squamous cell carcinoma
▶ Rarely, pelvic exenteration (resection of the uterus, cervix, vagina, bladder, and rectum), for recurrent cervical cancer

Nursing considerations

▶ Find out whether the patient will have internal or external therapy or both. Usually, internal radiation therapy is the first procedure.
▶ Listen to the patient's fears and concerns, and offer reassurance when appropriate. Encourage her to use relaxation techniques to promote comfort during diagnostic procedures.
▶ If you assist with a biopsy, drape and prepare the patient as for a routine Pap test and pelvic examination. Have a container of formaldehyde ready to preserve the specimen during transfer to the pathology laboratory. Assist the physician, as needed, and provide support for the patient throughout the procedure.
▶ If you assist with cryosurgery or laser therapy, drape and prepare the patient as for a routine Pap test and pelvic examination. Assist the physician, as needed, and provide support for the patient throughout the procedure.
▶ Watch for and immediately report signs of complications, such as bleeding, abdominal distention, severe pain, and wheezing or other breathing difficulties. Encourage deep breathing and coughing. Administer analgesics and prophylactic antibiotics, as ordered.

For internal radiation therapy

▶ Check to see whether the radioactive source will be inserted while the patient is in the operating room (preloaded) or at the bedside (afterloaded). If the source is preloaded, the patient returns to her room "hot," and safety precautions begin immediately.
▶ Remember that safety precautions—time, distance, and shielding—begin as soon as the radioactive source is in place. Inform the patient that she'll require a private room.
▶ Encourage the patient to lie flat and to limit movement while the source is in place. If she prefers, elevate the head of the bed slightly.
▶ Avoid leg exercises and other body movements that could dislodge the source. If ordered, administer sedatives to help the patient relax and remain still. Organize your time with the patient to minimize your exposure to radiation.
▶ Check the patient's vital signs every 4 hours; watch for skin reactions, vaginal bleeding, abdominal discomfort, and evidence of dehydration. Make sure the patient can reach everything she needs without stretching or straining.
▶ Assist the patient with range-of-motion arm exercises.
▶ Provide diversional activities that require minimal movement.
▶ Inform visitors of safety precautions and post a sign listing these precautions on the patient's door.
▶ Watch for treatment complications by listening to and observing the patient and monitoring laboratory studies and vital signs. When appropriate, perform measures to prevent or alleviate complications.

Teaching about cervical cancer treatment

For biopsy

▶ Explain to the patient that she may feel pressure, minor abdominal cramps, or a pinch from the punch forceps. Reassure her that the pain will be minimal because the cervix has few nerve endings.

For cryosurgery

▶ Explain to the patient that the procedure takes about 15 minutes, during which time the physician uses refrigerant to freeze the cervix. Caution her that she may experience abdominal cramps, headache, and sweating, but reassure her that she'll feel little, if any, pain.

For laser surgery

▶ Explain that the procedure takes about 30 minutes and may cause abdominal cramps.

General

▶ After excisional biopsy, cryosurgery, or laser therapy, tell the patient to expect a discharge or spotting for about 1 week. Advise her not to douche, use tampons, or engage in sexual intercourse during this time. Caution her to report signs of infection.

For preloaded internal radiation therapy

▶ Explain to the patient that the procedure requires a 2- to 3-day hospital stay, bowel preparation, a povidone-iodine vaginal douche, a clear liquid diet, and nothing by mouth the night before the implantation. It also requires an indwelling urinary catheter.
▶ Inform the patient that the procedure is performed in the operating room under general anesthesia.

For afterloaded internal radiation therapy

▶ Explain to the patient that a member of the radiation team implants the source after the patient returns to her room from surgery.
▶ If the patient will undergo outpatient external radiation therapy, explain that it will continue for about 4 to 6 weeks. Describe the procedure and measures she can take at home to prevent complications such as providing care around the radiation site to prevent skin breakdown.
▶ Review the possible complications of radiation therapy. Remind the patient to watch for and report uncomfortable adverse effects. Because radiation therapy may increase susceptibility to infection by lowering the white blood cell count, warn the patient to avoid people with obvious infections during therapy.
▶ Inform the patient that vaginal narrowing caused by scar tissue can occur after internal radiation and may be treated with dilation.
▶ Describe the complications that can occur even years after high-dose radiation therapy.

Endometrial cancer

Cancer of the endometrium (uterine cancer) is the most common gynecologic cancer. It typically afflicts postmenopausal women between ages 50 and 60. It's uncommon between ages 30 and 40 and rare before age 30. However, in premenopausal women who develop endometrial cancer, there's usually a history of anovulatory menstrual cycles or other hormonal imbalance such as polycystic ovarian syndrome.

In most patients, endometrial cancer is an adenocarcinoma that metastasizes late, usually from the endometrium to the cervix, ovaries, fallopian tubes, and other peritoneal structures. It may spread to distant organs, such as the lungs and the brain, by way of the blood or the lymphatic system. Less common uterine tumors include adenoacanthoma, endometrial stromal sarcoma, lymphosarcoma, mixed mesodermal tumors (including carcinosarcoma), and leiomyosarcoma.

Signs and symptoms

▶ Spotting and protracted menstrual periods (in premenopausal patients)
▶ Bleeding that began 12 or more months after menses had stopped (in postmenopausal patients)
▶ Discharge that's initially watery, then blood-streaked, and gradually becoming bloodier (in both age-groups)
▶ Enlarged uterus (in more advanced stages)
▶ Lower abdominal or pelvic cramping

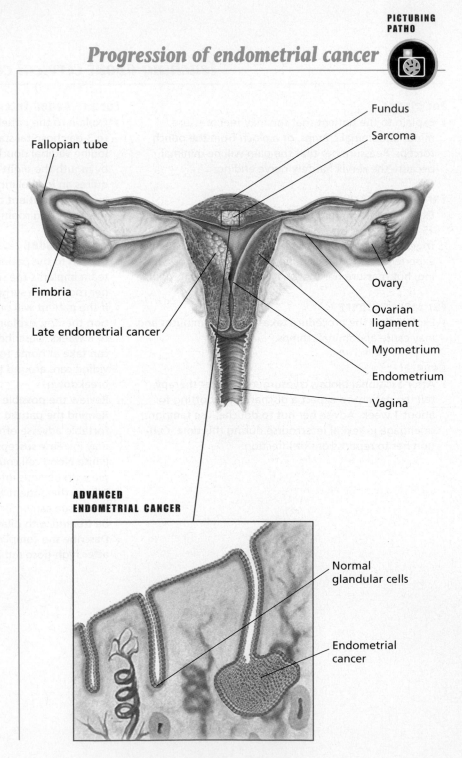

PICTURING PATHO

Progression of endometrial cancer

Fallopian tube
Fimbria
Late endometrial cancer

Fundus
Sarcoma
Ovary
Ovarian ligament
Myometrium
Endometrium
Vagina

ADVANCED ENDOMETRIAL CANCER

Normal glandular cells
Endometrial cancer

Staging endometrial cancer

Treatment decisions depend on accurate staging. The International Federation of Gynecology and Obstetrics defines the following endometrial cancer stages.

Stage 0
Carcinoma in situ.

Stage I
Cancer is confined to the corpus.

Stage IA
Cancer is limited to the endometrium.

Stage IB
Cancer has spread less than halfway through the myometrium.

Stage IC
Cancer has spread more than halfway through the myometrium, but is contained in the body of the uterus.

Stage II
Cancer has involved the corpus and the cervix but hasn't extended outside the uterus.

Stage IIA
Cancer is in the corpus and the endocervical glands.

Stage IIB
Cancer is in the corpus and the cervical stroma.

Stage III
Cancer has extended outside the uterus but not outside the true pelvis.

Stage IIIA
Cancer is in the serosa of the uterus and in the adnexa; cancer cells are present in peritoneal fluid, but not in lymph nodes or distant sites.

Stage IIIB
Cancer has spread to the vagina but not to lymph nodes or distant sites.

Stage IIIC
Cancer is in lymph nodes close to the uterus but not at distant sites.

Stage IV
Cancer has extended outside the true pelvis or has obviously involved the mucosa of the bladder or rectum.

Stage IVA
Cancer has spread to adjacent organs.

Stage IVB
Cancer has spread to distant organs.

Treatment
▶ Surgery: usually involves total abdominal hysterectomy, bilateral salpingo-oophorectomy or, possibly, omentectomy with or without pelvic or para-aortic lymphadenectomy; in rare cases in which there is an isolated central pelvic recurrence, total pelvic exenteration: removes all pelvic organs, including the rectum, bladder, and vagina, and is only performed when the disease is sufficiently contained to allow surgical removal of diseased parts (seldom curative, especially in nodal involvement)

▶ Radiation therapy: used when the tumor isn't well differentiated; intracavitary radiation, external radiation, or both possibly given 6 weeks before surgery to inhibit recurrence and lengthen survival time
▶ Hormonal therapy (using tamoxifen): shows a response rate of 20% to 40%

▶ Chemotherapy (including both cisplatin [Platinol] and doxorubicin): usually attempted when other treatments have failed

Nursing considerations

▶ Listen to the patient because she may fear for her survival and be concerned that treatment will alter her lifestyle or prevent sexual intimacy.

▶ Administer ordered pain medications, as necessary.

After surgery

▶ Measure fluid contents of the blood drainage system every shift. Notify the physician immediately if drainage exceeds 400 ml.

▶ If the patient has received prophylactic heparin, continue administration, as ordered, until she's fully ambulatory. Give prophylactic antibiotics, as ordered, and provide good indwelling urinary catheter care.

▶ Check the patient's vital signs every 4 hours. Watch for and immediately report signs of complications. Provide analgesics, as ordered.

▶ Regularly encourage the patient to breathe deeply and cough. Promote the use of an incentive spirometer once every waking hour to help keep the lungs expanded.

For internal radiation therapy

▶ Check to see whether the radioactive source will be inserted while the patient is in the operating room (preloaded) or at the bedside (afterloaded). If the source is preloaded, the patient returns to her room "hot," and safety precautions begin immediately.

▶ Remember that safety precautions—time, distance, and shielding—must be imposed as soon as the radioactive source is in place. Inform the patient that she'll require a private room.

▶ Encourage the patient to limit movement while the source is in place. Assist her in range-of-motion arm exercises; leg exercises and other body movements could dislodge the source.

▶ If ordered, administer a tranquilizer to help the patient relax and remain still.

▶ Provide diversional activities that require minimal movement.

▶ Check the patient's vital signs every 4 hours; watch for skin reaction, vaginal bleeding, abdominal discomfort, and evidence of dehydration.

▶ Inform visitors of safety precautions, and post a sign listing these precautions on the patient's door.

For internal and external radiation therapy

▶ Be alert for the possible adverse effects of radiation. Perform measures that help prevent them.

▶ Organize the time you spend with the patient to minimize your exposure to radiation.

▶ Emphasize that prompt treatment significantly improves a patient's likelihood of survival. Discuss tests used to diagnose and stage the disease, and explain treatments, which may include surgery, radiation therapy, hormonal therapy, or chemotherapy, or a combination of these.

For surgery

▶ Reinforce what the physician told the patient about the surgery, and explain routine tests (such as repeated blood tests the morning after surgery) and postoperative care. If the patient will have a lymphadenectomy and a total hysterectomy, explain that she'll probably have a blood drainage system for about 5 days after surgery. Also explain indwelling catheter care. Fit the patient with compression stockings for use during and after surgery. Make sure the patient's blood has been typed and crossmatched. If the patient is premenopausal, inform her that removal of her ovaries will induce menopause.

▶ As appropriate, explain that except in total pelvic exenteration, the vagina remains intact and that when she recovers, sexual intercourse is possible.

Teaching about endometrial cancer treatment

For internal radiation therapy

▶ Describe the procedure to the patient. Answer the patient's questions and counsel her about radiation's adverse effects. Advise her to rest frequently and to maintain a well-balanced diet.

▶ Explain that the preloaded internal radiation procedure requires a 2- to 3-day hospital stay, bowel preparation, a povidone-iodine vaginal douche, a clear liquid diet, and nothing by mouth the night before the implantation as well as an indwelling catheter. Inform the patient that the procedure is performed in the operating room under general anesthesia. She will be placed in a dorsal position, with knees and hips flexed and heels resting in footrests. The physician implants the radiation source into the vagina.

▶ Explain that in afterloaded internal radiation therapy, a member of the radiation team implants the source while the patient is in her room.

For external radiation therapy

▶ Teach the patient and her family about the therapy before it begins. Tell the patient that treatment is usually given 5 days per week for 6 weeks. Warn her not to scrub body areas marked with indelible ink because these markings direct treatment to exactly the same area each time.

▶ Instruct the patient to maintain a high-protein, high-carbohydrate, low-residue diet to reduce bulk yet maintain calories. Administer diphenoxylate with atropine, as ordered, to minimize diarrhea, a possible adverse effect of pelvic radiation.

▶ To minimize skin breakdown and reduce the risk of skin infection, tell the patient to keep the treatment area dry, avoid wearing clothes that rub against the area, and avoid using heating pads, alcohol rubs, or irritating skin creams. Because radiation therapy increases susceptibility to infection (possibly by lowering the white blood cell [WBC] count), instruct the patient to avoid people with colds or other infections.

For chemotherapy or immunotherapy

▶ Explain the therapy and make sure the patient understands what adverse effects to expect and how to alleviate them. If the patient is receiving a synthetic form of progesterone, such as hydroxyprogesterone, medroxyprogesterone (Provera), or megestrol (Megace), tell her to watch for depression, dizziness, backache, swelling, breast tenderness, irritability, and abdominal cramps. Instruct her to report signs of thrombophlebitis, such as pain in the calves, numbness, tingling, or loss of leg function.

▶ Advise the patient receiving chemotherapy that WBC counts must be checked weekly, and reinforce the importance of preventing infection. Assure her that hair loss is temporary, and teach her about side effects specific to her treatment.

▶ If the patient works and is undergoing chemotherapy, point out that continuing to work during this period may offer an important diversion. Advise her to talk with her employer about a flexible work schedule.

▶ Refer the patient to the social service department and to community services that offer psychological support and information such as the American Cancer Society.

Endometriosis

Endometriosis is the appearance of endometrial tissue outside the lining of the uterine cavity. Such ectopic tissue is generally confined to the pelvic area, most commonly around the ovaries, uterovesical peritoneum, uterosacral ligaments, and the cul-de-sac, but it can appear anywhere in the body.

This ectopic endometrial tissue responds to normal stimulation in the same way that the endometrium does. During menstruation, the ectopic tissue bleeds, which causes inflammation of the surrounding tissues, resulting in fibrosis, adhesions, pain, and sometimes infertility.

Active endometriosis usually occurs between ages 30 and 40, especially in women who postpone childbearing; it's uncommon before age 20. Severe symptoms of endometriosis may have an abrupt onset or may develop over many years. The disorder usually becomes progressively severe during the menstrual years but tends to subside after menopause.

Signs and symptoms

▶ Pain in the lower abdomen, vagina, posterior pelvis, and back that usually begins from 5 to 7 days before menses, reaches a peak, and lasts for 2 to 3 days
▶ Multiple tender nodules on uterosacral ligaments or in the rectovaginal septum
▶ Nodules that enlarge and become more tender during menses
▶ Ovarian enlargement in the presence of endometrial cysts on the ovaries or thickened, nodular adnexa

Oviducts and ovaries
▶ History of infertility and profuse menses

Ovaries and cul-de-sac
▶ Deep-thrust dyspareunia

Bladder
▶ Suprapubic pain, dysuria, and hematuria

Rectovaginal septum and colon
▶ Painful defecation, rectal bleeding with menses, and pain in the coccyx or sacrum

Small bowel and appendix
▶ Nausea and vomiting that worsen before menses and abdominal cramps

Looking at pelvic endometriosis

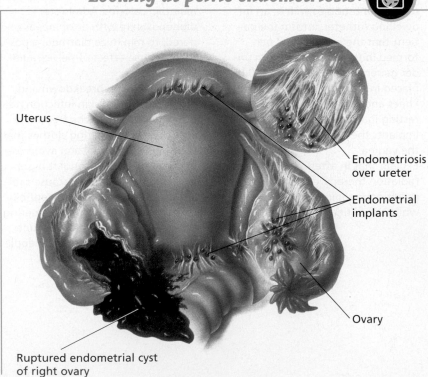

Uterus

Endometriosis over ureter

Endometrial implants

Ovary

Ruptured endometrial cyst of right ovary

Treatment

▶ In determining the course of treatment, stage of the disease and patient's age and desire to have children considered

▶ Conservative therapy (for young women who want to have children): androgens, such as danazol, which produce a temporary remission in stages I and II; over-the-counter pain medication

▶ Progestins and hormonal contraceptives, medroxy progesterone, aromatase inhibitors: relieve symptoms; gonadotropin-releasing analogues, such as leuprolide (Lupron): suppress estrogen production, which causes atrophic changes in the ectopic endometrial tissue, thus allowing healing

▶ Laparoscopy: lyse adhesions, remove small implants, and cauterize implants; also permits laser vaporization of implants; usually followed with hormonal therapy to suppress the return of endometrial implants

▶ Surgery to rule out cancer, for the patient with ovarian masses

▶ Total abdominal hysterectomy with bilateral salpingo-oophorectomy for women who don't want to bear children or for extensive disease (stages III and IV)

Nursing considerations

▶ Encourage the patient and her partner to verbalize their feelings about the disorder and its effect on their sexual relationship. Offer emotional support. Stress the need for open communication before and during intercourse to minimize discomfort and frustration.

▶ Help the patient to develop effective coping strategies. Refer her and her partner to a mental health professional for additional counseling, if necessary. Encourage her to contact a support group such as the Endometriosis Association.

PICTURING PATHO

Common sites of endometriosis

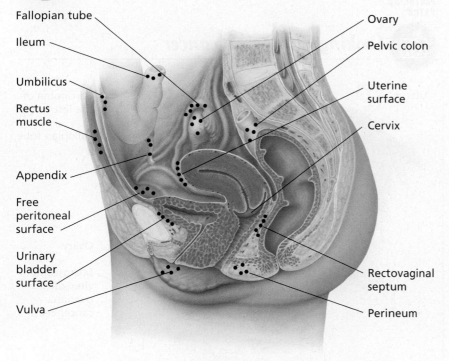

Fallopian tube

Ileum

Umbilicus

Rectus muscle

Appendix

Free peritoneal surface

Urinary bladder surface

Vulva

Ovary

Pelvic colon

Uterine surface

Cervix

Rectovaginal septum

Perineum

LESSON PLANS

Teaching about endometriosis

▶ Explain all procedures and treatment options. Clarify misconceptions about the disorder, associated complications, and fertility.

▶ Advise adolescents to use sanitary napkins instead of tampons. This can help prevent retrograde flow in girls with a narrow vagina or small vaginal meatus.

▶ Because infertility is a possible complication, counsel the patient who wants children not to postpone childbearing.

▶ Advise the patient to have an annual pelvic examination and a Papanicolaou test.

Ovarian cancer

After cancers of the lung, breast, and colon, primary ovarian cancer ranks as the most common cause of cancer death among women in the United States. In women with previously treated breast cancer, metastatic ovarian cancer is more common than cancer of another organ.

There are three main types of ovarian cancer:

▶ *Primary epithelial tumors* account for 90% of all ovarian cancers and include serous cystadenocarcinoma, mucinous cystadenocarcinoma, and endometrioid and mesonephric malignant tumors.

▶ *Germ cell tumors* include endodermal sinus malignant tumors, embryonal carcinoma (a rare ovarian cancer that appears in children), immature teratomas, and dysgerminoma.

▶ *Sex cord (stromal) tumors* include granulosa, cell tumors (which produce estrogen and may have feminizing effects), thecomas, and the rare androblastomas (which produce androgen and have virilizing effects).

Signs and symptoms

▶ Cancer usually metastasized before a diagnosis is made

▶ Signs and symptoms dependent on tumor's size and extent of metastasis, but may include the following:

– Urinary frequency

– Constipation

– Pelvic discomfort

– Distention

– Weight loss

– Pain, possibly associated with tumor rupture, torsion, or infection

– Ovarian tumors that may vary from a rocky hardness to a rubbery or cyst-like quality (on palpation)

PICTURING PATHO

 Looking at ovarian cancer

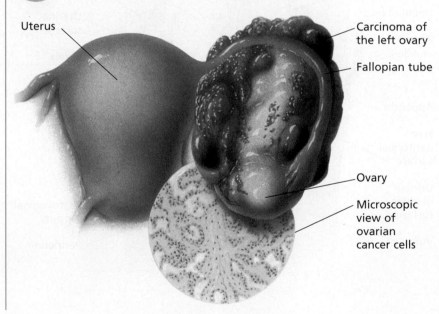

Uterus

Carcinoma of the left ovary

Fallopian tube

Ovary

Microscopic view of ovarian cancer cells

Staging ovarian cancer

The International Federation of Gynecology and Obstetrics has established this staging system, which is based on findings at clinical examination, surgical exploration, or both. Histology is taken into consideration, as is cytology in effusions. Ideally, biopsies should be obtained from any suspicious areas outside of the pelvis.

To evaluate the impact on the prognosis of the different criteria for allotting cases to stage IC or IIC, consider (1) if rupture of the capsule was (a) spontaneous or (b) caused by the surgeon, or (2) if the source of malignant cells detected was (a) peritoneal washings or (b) ascites.

Stage I
Growth is limited to the ovaries.

Stage IA
Growth is limited to one ovary, with no ascites; no tumor on the external surface; capsule is intact.

Stage IB
Growth is limited to both ovaries, with no ascites; no tumor on the external surfaces; capsules are intact.

Stage IC
Tumor is either stage IA or IB but with tumor on surface of one or both ovaries; or with capsule ruptured; or with ascites present, containing malignant cells or with positive peritoneal washings.

Stage II
Growth involves one or both ovaries with pelvic extension.

Stage IIA
There is extension, metastasis, or both to the uterus, fallopian tubes, or both.

Stage IIB
There is extension to other pelvic tissues.

Stage IIC
Tumor is either stage IIA or IIB, but with tumor on surface of one or both ovaries; or with capsule (or capsules) ruptured; or with ascites present, containing malignant cells or with positive peritoneal washings.

Stage III
Tumor involves one or both ovaries with peritoneal implants outside the pelvis or positive retroperitoneal or inguinal nodes; superficial liver metastasis equals stage III; tumor is limited to the true pelvis but with histologically proved malignant extension to small bowel or omentum.

Stage IIIA
Tumor is grossly limited to the true pelvis with negative nodes, but with histologically confirmed microscopic seeding of abdominal peritoneal surfaces.

Stage IIIB
Tumor of one or both ovaries has histologically confirmed implants of abdominal peritoneal surfaces, but none exceeding 2 cm in greatest dimension; nodes are negative.

Stage IIIC
Abdominal implants are greater than 2 cm in greatest dimension or retroperitoneal or inguinal nodes or both are positive.

Stage IV
Growth involves one or both ovaries with distant metastasis; if pleural effusion is present, positive cytology suggests stage IV; parenchymal liver metastasis equals stage IV.

Treatment
Conservative treatment (to preserve fertility)
▶ Resection of the involved ovary
▶ Biopsies of the omentum and the uninvolved ovary
▶ Careful follow-up, including periodic X-rays, to rule out metastasis

Aggressive treatment
▶ Total abdominal hysterectomy and bilateral salpingo-oophorectomy with tumor resection, omentectomy, appendectomy (upon lymph node palpation), probable lymphadenectomy, tissue biopsies, and peritoneal washings
▶ Chemotherapy after surgery to lengthen survival time, but largely palliative in advanced disease, although occasional, prolonged remissions in some patients; drugs that are usually given in combination—intraperitoneal or I.V. administration of cisplatin (Platinol) or paclitaxel (Abraxane) or carboplastin and paclitaxel (given after initial surgery)—slowing disease progression and increasing survival
▶ I.V. administration of biological response modifiers—interleukin-2, interferon, and possibly monoclonal antibodies such as bevacizumab (Avastin), which disrupts tumor blood supply
▶ External beam radiation: may be used to treat advanced cancer

Nursing considerations

▶ Listen to the patient's concerns and fears and provide emotional support.

▶ After surgery, frequently monitor the patient's vital signs and check I.V. fluids. Monitor intake and output while maintaining good catheter care. Check the dressing regularly for excessive drainage or bleeding, and watch for signs of infection.

▶ Provide abdominal support and be alert for abdominal distention. Measure abdominal girth daily or as ordered. Encourage coughing and deep breathing. Reposition the patient often, and encourage her to walk shortly after surgery.

▶ If the patient has pain, make her as comfortable as possible. Give analgesics, as needed, provide distractions, and have the patient perform relaxation techniques.

▶ Monitor and treat adverse effects of therapy. If the patient is undergoing intraperitoneal chemotherapy, help alleviate her discomfort by infusing the fluid at a slower rate and repositioning her in an attempt to distribute the fluid evenly.

▶ If the patient is receiving immunotherapy, watch for flulike symptoms that may last 12 to 24 hours after drug administration. Give aspirin or acetaminophen (Tylenol) for fever.

▶ For the malnourished patient, administer supplementary enteral or parenteral nutrition, as ordered. If the GI tract is intact, offer the patient small, frequent meals.

LESSON PLANS

Teaching about ovarian cancer treatment

▶ Teach the patient relaxation techniques and other measures that may help ease her discomfort.

▶ Stress the importance of preventing infection, emphasizing good hand-washing technique.

▶ Explain measures that may help maintain adequate nutrition, such as eating small, frequent meals and foods high in protein and calories.

▶ If the patient will undergo drug therapy or radiation therapy, explain the adverse effects that she can expect and suggest ways to alleviate and prevent them.

▶ Before surgery, thoroughly explain all preoperative tests, the expected course of treatment, and surgical and postoperative procedures.

▶ In premenopausal females, explain that bilateral oophorectomy artificially induces early menopause. Such patients may experience hot flashes, headaches, palpitations, insomnia, depression, and excessive perspiration.

▶ Encourage the patient to be as active as possible; the use of repetitive motion, such as swimming, may be helpful.

▶ As appropriate, refer the patient and her family to the social service department, home health care agencies, hospices, and support groups such as the American Cancer Society.

Ovarian cysts

Usually nonneoplastic, ovarian cysts are sacs on an ovary, which contain fluid or semisolid material. They're usually small and produce no symptoms, but they require thorough investigation as possible sites of malignant change. Common ovarian cysts include lutein cysts (granulose-lutein, corpus luteum, and theca-lutein cysts), follicular cysts, and polycystic (or sclerocystic) ovary disease. Ovarian cysts can develop anytime between puberty and menopause, including during pregnancy. Granulosa-lutein cysts occur infrequently, usually during early pregnancy. The prognosis for nonneoplastic cysts is excellent.

Follicular cysts are usually small and arise from follicles that overdistend instead of going through the atretic stage of the menstrual cycle. They appear semitransparent and are filled with a watery fluid visible through their thin walls. When such cysts persist into menopause, they secrete excessive amounts of estrogen in response to the hypersecretion of follicle-stimulating hormone and luteinizing hormone that normally occurs during menopause.

A dermoid cyst (or cystic teratoma) begins in the ovarian cell that forms into different tissue as the egg is fertilized and develops. This type of cyst can become large and can contain teeth, hair, bone, and cartilage. It's most common in young women and during pregnancy.

Looking at a follicular cyst

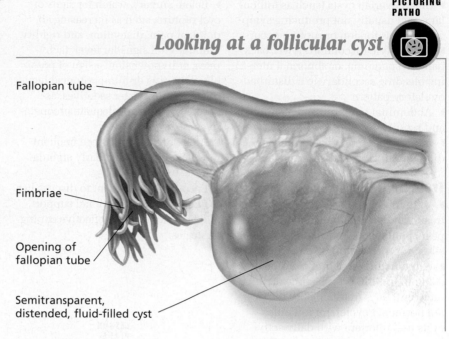

Fallopian tube

Fimbriae

Opening of fallopian tube

Semitransparent, distended, fluid-filled cyst

Looking at a dermoid cyst

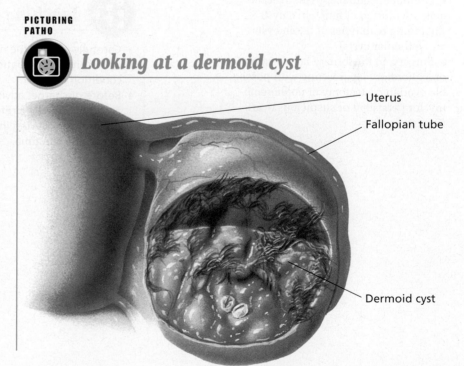

Uterus

Fallopian tube

Dermoid cyst

Signs and symptoms

▶ Small ovarian cysts (such as follicular cysts) usually not producing symptoms unless torsion or rupture occurs
▶ Mild pelvic discomfort, lower back pain, dyspareunia, or abnormal uterine bleeding secondary to a disturbed ovulatory pattern
▶ Abdominal tenderness, distention, and rigidity
▶ Indigestion, urge to defecate, or difficulty having a bowel movement

Treatment

▶ With follicular cysts, usually no treatment because they tend to disappear spontaneously by reabsorption or silent rupture within 60 days
▶ Administration of oral clomiphene (Clomid) or I.M. progesterone (Crinone) for 5 days (reestablishes the ovarian hormonal cycle), for follicular cysts that interfere with daily activities
▶ Hormonal contraceptives, to accelerate involution of functional cysts (including both types of lutein cysts and follicular cysts)
▶ Surgery, in the form of laparoscopy or exploratory laparoscopy with possible ovarian cystectomy or oophorectomy, for persistent or suspicious ovarian cyst

Nursing considerations

▶ Before surgery, watch for signs of cyst rupture, such as increasing abdominal pain, distention, and rigidity. Monitor vital signs for fever, tachypnea, or hypotension, a sign of possible peritonitis or intraperitoneal hemorrhage. Administer sedatives, as ordered, to ensure adequate preoperative rest.
▶ After surgery, encourage frequent movement in bed and early ambulation.
▶ Encourage the patient to discuss her feelings, provide emotional support, and help her develop effective coping strategies.

LESSON PLANS

Teaching about ovarian cysts

▶ Carefully explain the nature of the particular cyst, the type of discomfort the patient experiences, and how long the condition may last.
▶ Before discharge, advise the patient to increase her at-home activity gradually, preferably over 4 to 6 weeks. Tell her to abstain from having intercourse, using tampons, and douching during this time.

Pelvic inflammatory disease

Pelvic inflammatory disease (PID) is an umbrella term that refers to any acute, subacute, recurrent, or chronic infection of the oviducts and ovaries, with adjacent tissue involvement. It includes inflammation of the cervix (cervicitis), uterus (endometritis), fal-lopian tubes (salpingitis), and ovaries (oophoritis), which can extend to the connective tissue lying between the broad ligaments (parametritis).

About 60% of cases result from overgrowth of one or more of the common bacterial species found in the cervical mucus. Early diagnosis and effective treatment help prevent damage to the reproductive system; however, untreated PID may be fatal.

Forms of pelvic inflammatory disease: Features and test findings

Clinical features	Diagnostic findings
Cervicitis	
▸ *Acute:* purulent, foul-smelling vaginal discharge; vulvovaginitis, with itching or burning; red, edematous cervix; pelvic discomfort; sexual dysfunction; menorrhagia; infertility; spontaneous abortion ▸ *Chronic:* cervical dystocia, laceration or eversion of the cervix, ulcerative vesicular lesion (when cervicitis results from herpes simplex virus [HSV] 2)	▸ *Chlamydia trachomatis* is the most common organism infecting the cervix, followed by *Neisseria gonorrhoeae,* which occurs with *C. trachomatis* about 40% of the time. HSV and human papillomavirus are other common causes. ▸ Cytologic smears may reveal severe inflammation. ▸ If cervicitis isn't complicated by salpingitis, white blood cell (WBC) count is normal or slightly elevated; erythrocyte sedimentation rate (ESR) is elevated. ▸ With *acute cervicitis,* cervical palpation reveals tenderness. ▸ With *chronic cervicitis,* causative organisms are usually staphylococcus or streptococcus.
Endometritis (generally postpartum or postabortion)	
▸ *Acute:* mucopurulent or purulent vaginal discharge oozing from the cervix; edematous, hyperemic endometrium, possibly leading to ulceration and necrosis (with virulent organisms); lower abdominal pain and tenderness; fever; rebound pain; abdominal muscle spasm; thrombophlebitis of uterine and pelvic vessels (in severe forms) ▸ *Chronic:* recurring acute episodes (increasingly common because of widespread use of intrauterine devices)	▸ With severe infection, palpation may reveal a boggy uterus. ▸ Uterine and blood samples are positive for a causative organism, usually staphylococcus. ▸ WBC count and ESR are elevated.
Salpingo-oophoritis	
▸ *Acute:* sudden onset of lower abdominal and pelvic pain, usually following menses; increased vaginal discharge; fever; malaise; lower abdominal pressure and tenderness; tachycardia; pelvic peritonitis ▸ *Chronic:* recurring acute episodes	▸ Blood studies show leukocytosis—or a normal WBC count. ▸ X-rays may show ileus. ▸ Pelvic examination reveals extreme tenderness. ▸ Smear of cervical or periurethral gland exudate shows gram-negative intracellular diplococci.

Signs and symptoms

▶ Profuse, purulent vaginal discharge
▶ Low-grade fever and malaise (particularly if gonorrhea is the cause)
▶ Lower abdominal pelvic pain
▶ Vaginal bleeding
▶ Pain during movement of the cervix or palpation of the adnexa
▶ Dyspareunia

Treatment

▶ To prevent progression of PID, antibiotic therapy beginning immediately after culture specimens are obtained; therapy reevaluation needed as soon as laboratory results are available (usually after 24 to 48 hours)
▶ The Centers for Disease Control and Prevention recommendations (for inpatient treatment): doxycycline (Vibramycin) alone or a combination of clindamycin (Cleocin) and gentamicin (Garamycin); for outpatient therapy: single dose of cefoxitin (Metoxin) given concurrently with probenecid (Benemid) or a single dose of ceftriaxone (Rocephin); each regimen given with doxycycline
▶ Supplemental treatment that may include bed rest, analgesics, and I.V. fluids, as needed
▶ Inadequate treatment possibly leading to chronic infection
▶ Drainage and possible total abdominal hysterectomy with bilateral salpingo-oophorectomy, for pelvic abscess (rupture may be life-threatening)

Nursing considerations

▶ After establishing that the patient has no drug allergies, administer antibiotics and analgesics, as ordered.
▶ Monitor vital signs for fever and fluid intake and output for signs of dehydration. Watch for abdominal rigidity and distention, possible signs of developing peritonitis.
▶ Provide frequent perineal care if vaginal drainage occurs.
▶ Use meticulous hand-washing technique; institute contact precautions, if necessary.
▶ Encourage the patient to discuss her feelings, offer emotional support, and help her develop effective coping strategies.

PICTURING PATHO

Distribution of adhesions in pelvic inflammatory disease

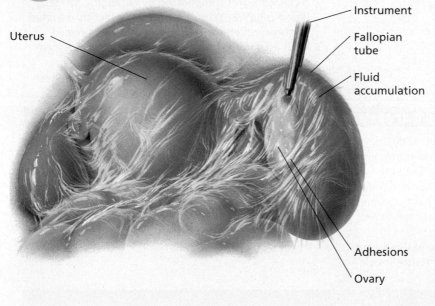

Uterus

Instrument

Fallopian tube

Fluid accumulation

Adhesions

Ovary

LESSON PLANS

Teaching about PID

▶ To prevent recurrence, encourage compliance with treatment and explain pelvic inflammatory disease (PID) and its severity.
▶ Stress the need for the patient's sexual partner to be examined and, if necessary, treated for infection.
▶ Discuss the use of safe sexual practices to reduce the risk of sexually transmitted diseases.
▶ Because PID may cause dyspareunia, advise the patient to check with her physician about sexual activity.
▶ To prevent infection after minor gynecologic procedures, such as dilatation and curettage, tell the patient to immediately report fever, increased vaginal discharge, or pain. After such procedures, instruct her to avoid douching or intercourse for at least 7 days.

Uterine leiomyomas

Uterine leiomyomas are the most common benign tumors in women. These smooth-muscle tumors are usually multiple and generally occur in the uterine corpus, although they may appear on the cervix or on the round or broad ligament. Also known as *myomas* or *fibromyomas,* uterine leiomyomas are commonly called *fibroids,* but this term is misleading because leiomyomas consist of muscle cells and not fibrous tissue.

Uterine leiomyomas occur in about 25% of all women of reproductive age and affect Blacks two to three times more commonly than Whites and at a younger age (4 to 6 years younger) than Whites. Malignant tumors (leiomyosarcomas) develop from benign tumors in only about 0.1% of patients.

Although the exact cause of uterine leiomyomas is unknown, excessive levels of estrogen and growth hormone (GH) are thought to influence tumor formation by stimulating susceptible fibromuscular elements. Large doses of estrogen and the later stages of pregnancy increase both tumor size and GH levels. Conversely, uterine leiomyomas usually shrink or disappear after menopause, when estrogen production decreases.

Signs and symptoms

‣ Usually producing no symptoms
‣ Hypermenorrhea (cardinal sign of uterine leiomyomas)
‣ Other forms of abnormal endometrial bleeding as well as dysmenorrhea
‣ Pain, if the tumors twist or degenerate after circulatory occlusion; or infection, if the uterus contracts in an attempt to expel a pedunculated submucous leiomyoma
‣ Increasing abdominal girth without weight gain
‣ Feeling of heaviness in the abdomen or pelvic pressure
‣ Constipation
‣ Urinary frequency or urgency, if the tumors press on surrounding organs, or difficulty with bladder emptying
‣ Irregular uterine enlargement
‣ Backache or leg pain

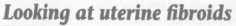

Looking at uterine fibroids

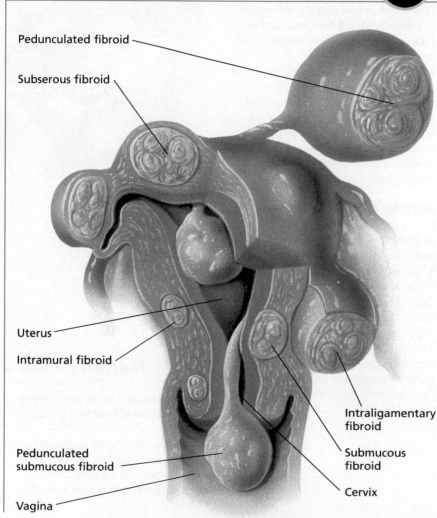

Pedunculated fibroid

Subserous fibroid

Uterus

Intramural fibroid

Pedunculated submucous fibroid

Vagina

Intraligamentary fibroid

Submucous fibroid

Cervix

Treatment

Medical management of uterine leiomyomas depends on severity of symptoms, size and location of the tumors, and patient's age, parity, pregnancy status, desire to have children, and general health.

▶ Pelvic examination every 4 to 6 months to monitor the growth of small leiomyomas that produce no symptoms

▶ Abdominal, laparoscopic, or hysteroscopic myomectomy and administration of gonadotropin-releasing hormone analogues, for patients who want to preserve fertility (reduction in tumor size before surgery, reduction in intraoperative blood loss, and an increase in prospective hematocrit all beneficial)

▶ Hysterectomy (with preservation of the ovaries, if possible), for symptomatic women who have completed childbearing; other surgical options, which may include myolysis (a laparoscopic procedure to treat fibroids), uterine artery embolization, cryomylosis, and other variants

Nursing considerations

▶ In a patient with severe anemia due to excessive bleeding, administer iron and blood transfusions, as ordered.

▶ Encourage the patient and her partner to verbalize their feelings about the disorder and its effect on their sexual relationship. Offer emotional support.

▶ Help the patient develop effective coping strategies. Refer her and her partner to a mental health professional for additional counseling, if necessary.

Fibroids compressing the bladder and rectum

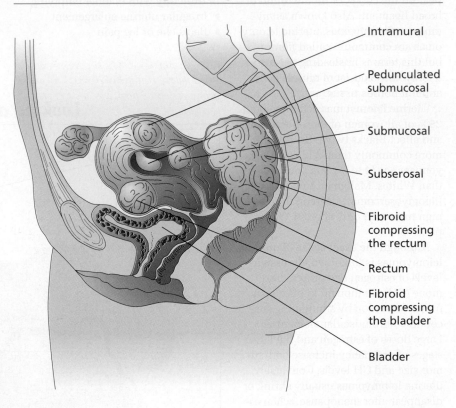

- Intramural
- Pedunculated submucosal
- Submucosal
- Subserosal
- Fibroid compressing the rectum
- Rectum
- Fibroid compressing the bladder
- Bladder

LESSON PLANS

Teaching about uterine leiomyomas

▶ Tell the patient to immediately report abnormal bleeding or pelvic pain.
▶ If a hysterectomy or oophorectomy is indicated, explain the effects of the surgery on menstruation, menopause, and sexual activity.

▶ Reassure the patient that she won't experience premature menopause if her ovaries are left intact.
▶ If the patient must have a multiple myomectomy, make sure she understands that pregnancy is still possible. However, if a hysterotomy is performed, explain that a cesarean delivery may be necessary.

TESTS
Laboratory tests

HER2/NEU TESTING

HER2/neu is a growth-promoting hormone. About 15% to 25% of women with breast cancer have too much of this protein. Tumors with increased levels of HER2/neu are referred to as *HER2 positive.* These cancers tend to grow and spread more aggressively than other breast cancers with only a normal amount of the HER2/neu gene.

HORMONE RECEPTOR ASSAY

During a biopsy of the breast tissue, the tissue is analyzed for estrogen and progesterone receptors. Breast cancers that contain these receptors are commonly referred to as *ER-positive* and *PR-positive tumors* or, simply, *hormone receptor positive.*

Tissue analysis

COLPOSCOPY

In colposcopy, the cervix and vagina are visually examined using an instrument that contains a magnifying lens and a light (colposcope). This test is primarily used to evaluate abnormal cytology or grossly suspicious lesions and to examine the cervix and vagina after a positive Papanicolaou (Pap) test.

During colposcopy, a biopsy may be performed and photographs taken of suspicious lesions with the colposcope and its attachments. Risks of biopsy include bleeding (especially during pregnancy) and infection.

CORE NEEDLE BIOPSY

In core needle biopsy, the surgeon obtains a tissue sample by inserting a cutting-type needle into a breast mass, securing the tissue sample, and withdrawing the needle.

DUCTAL LAVAGE OF BREAST TISSUE

Ductal lavage of breast tissue is a minimally invasive method for assessing a woman's risk of developing breast cancer and may be considered experimental by some. This test permits the collection of cells from inside the milk ducts of the breast that are microscopically examined to determine normal, atypical, suspicious, or malignant type. Research has demonstrated that most breast cancers begin in the cells that line the breast ducts. These cells may take 8 to 10 years to develop into a tumor that's visible with a mammogram or palpated with a breast examination. This test helps to determine if the woman has atypical cells in her milk ducts that have the potential for becoming malignant. The belief is that the earlier the abnormal cells are found, the more treatment options are available.

This test may be referred to as the *Pap smear for the breasts.* It's indicated only in those women who are considered to be at high risk for developing breast cancer based on personal and family factors. It's commonly performed in a physician's office.

Understanding breast ductal lavage

1. A syringelike aspirator is placed over the breast at the nipple area. Suction is applied to the aspirator to draw small amounts of fluid from the ducts to the nipple surface. Usually only 1 or 2 ducts produce fluid.

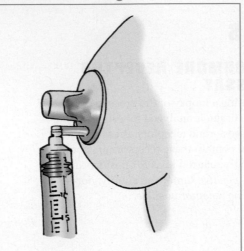

2. A microcatheter is then inserted into the ducts from which fluid was obtained.

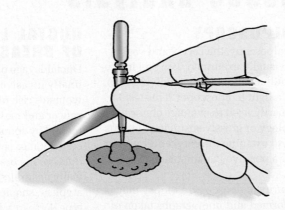

3. A small of amount of anesthetic may be instilled followed by a small amount of saline. The breast is massaged and then fluid is withdrawn into the catheter, which is attached to a syringe. The sample is then placed in a preservative and sent to the laboratory for analysis.

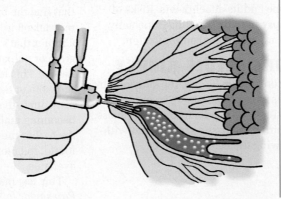

ENDOMETRIAL BIOPSY

An endometrial biopsy is used to assess hormonal secretions of the corpus luteum, determine whether normal ovulation is occurring, and check for neoplasia.

LOOP ELECTROSURGICAL EXCISION

Loop electrosurgical excision procedure (LEEP) is a method for obtaining tissue specimens of the cervix for biopsy and removing abnormal tissue from the cervix and high in the endocervical canal. This procedure is usually done after a Pap test and colposcopy as follow-up to ensure the accuracy of results and for further investigation of abnormal tissue as a means to exclude the diagnosis of invasive cancer and to determine the extent of noninvasive lesions. Complications associated with LEEP include heavy bleeding, severe cramping, infection, and accidental cutting or burning of normal tissue. Cervical stenosis is also a possible risk.

OPEN BREAST BIOPSY

In open breast biopsy, the surgeon makes an incision over the breast mass and then removes the mass. Open breast biopsy may also be performed with wire localization, in which a wire is inserted into the suspicious area before the procedure using the mammogram as a guide.

PAPANICOLAOU TEST

The Pap test is a widely known cytologic test for early detection of cervical cancer. Secretions are scraped from the patient's cervix and spread on a slide, which is sent to the laboratory for cytologic analysis. The test relies on the ready exfoliation of malignant cells from the cervix and shows cell maturity, metabolic activity, and morphology variations.

Although cervical scrapings are the most common test specimen, the test method may be used in cytologic evaluation of the vaginal pool, prostatic secretions, urine, gastric secretions, cavity fluids, bronchial aspirations, sputum, or solid tumor cells obtained by fine needle aspiration. If a cervical Pap test is positive or suggests malignancy, cervical biopsy can confirm the diagnosis.

Sentinel node biopsy

In sentinel node biopsy, the surgeon injects dye or radioactive material into the breast mass area in order to identify the sentinel node—the first lymph node along the lymphatic chair of the breast mass. He then removes the node, which is microscopically examined for the presence of cancer cells.

ThinPrep test

Cervical cells for ThinPrep test analysis may be collected in the same manner as those of a Pap test, using a cytobrush and plastic spatula. The specimens are deposited in a bottle containing a fixative and sent to the laboratory. A filter is then inserted into the bottle and excess mucus, blood, and inflammatory cells are filtered out by centrifuge. Remaining cells are then placed on a slide in a uniform, thin layer and read as a Pap test. This procedure causes fewer slides to be classified as unreadable, significantly reducing the incidence of false negatives and the need for repeat tests.

Understanding how a Pap test is performed

During a Papanicolaou (Pap) test, a speculum is inserted into the vagina. Then a special spatula is inserted into the vagina through the open speculum and placed at the cervical os.

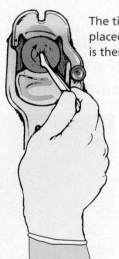

The tip of the spatula is placed in the cervical os and is then rotated 360 degrees.

Cellular material from the cervix clinging to the spatula is placed on a glass slide and sprayed with a fixative and sent to the laboratory.

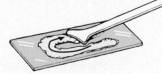

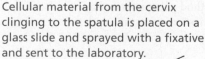

A cytobrush is rotated in the cervical os the same way as the spatula, but is then rolled onto the glass slide.

Endoscopy

HYSTEROSCOPY

Hysteroscopy involves the use of a small-diameter endoscope to visualize the interior of the uterus, usually used as an adjunct to endometrial biopsy. Usually performed as an office procedure using a local anesthetic or mild sedation, this procedure has become widely used to investigate abnormal uterine bleeding. It also aids in the removal of polyps and the diagnosis and treatment of other uterine abnormalities, such as uterine fibroid tumors and adhesions.

LAPAROSCOPY

Laparoscopy is used to evaluate infertility, dysmenorrhea, and pelvic pain and as a means of sterilization, which can be performed only in a facility while the patient is under anesthesia.

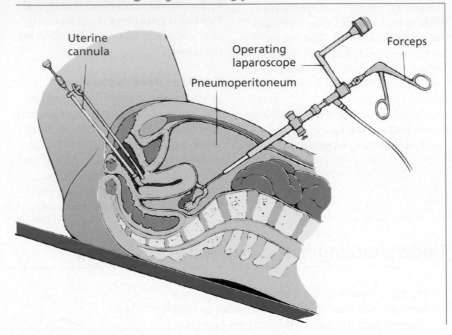

Understanding laparoscopy

Uterine cannula

Operating laparoscope

Forceps

Pneumoperitoneum

Radiography

MAMMOGRAPHY

Mammography is used as a screening test to detect breast cysts or tumors, especially those not palpable on physical examination. Biopsy of suspicious areas may be required to confirm malignancy. Mammography may follow such screening procedures as ultrasonography or thermography.

Film-screen mammograms use X-rays, which are converted to light- and gray-scale images on film.

Although mammography can detect 90% to 95% of breast cancers, the test produces many false-positive results. The American College of Radiologists and the American Cancer Society have established separate guidelines for the use and potential risks of mammography. Both groups agree that despite low radiation levels, the test is contraindicated during pregnancy. Magnetic resonance imaging, which is highly sensitive, is becoming a more popular method of breast imaging; however, it isn't very specific and leads to biopsies of many benign lesions.

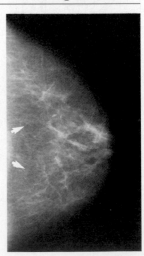

Looking at a normal mammogram

Shown here is a normal view of the left breast; the nipple is in profile and the pectoralis muscle (arrows) is seen posteriorly.

Digital mammography

Digital mammography, which also aids in screening and diagnosis, produces pictures of the breast using X-rays. Instead of film, this process uses detectors that change the X-rays into electrical signals, which are then converted to gray-scale images. For the patient, the procedure is the same as with ordinary mammography.

Digital mammography may offer the following advantages over conventional mammography:

▶ The images can be stored and retrieved electronically, which makes long-distance consultations with other mammography specialists easier.

▶ The resolution is greater and because the images can be adjusted by the radiologist, subtle differences between tissues may be noted.

▶ The number of follow-up procedures that are necessary may be reduced.

▶ The need for fewer exposures with digital mammography can reduce the already low levels of radiation.

Ultrasonography

BREAST ULTRASONOGRAPHY

Ultrasonography is especially useful for diagnosing tumors less than 0.6 cm in diameter and in distinguishing cysts from solid tumors in dense breast tissue. As in other ultrasound techniques, a transducer sends a beam of high-frequency sound waves through the patient's skin and into the breast. The sound waves are then processed and displayed for interpretation.

A benefit to ultrasonography is that it can show all areas of the breast, including the area close to the chest wall, which is difficult to study with X-rays. When used as an adjunct to mammography, ultrasound increases diagnostic accuracy; when used alone, it's more accurate than mammography in examining the denser breast tissue of a young patient.

PELVIC ULTRASONOGRAPHY

In pelvic ultrasonography, high-frequency sound waves are reflected to a transducer to provide images of the interior pelvic area on a monitor. Techniques of sound imaging include A-mode (amplitude modulation, recorded as spikes), B-mode (brightness modulation), gray scale (a representation of organ texture in shades of gray), and real-time imaging (instantaneous images of the tissues in motion, similar to fluoroscopic examination). Selected views may be photographed for later examination and a permanent record of the test.

VAGINAL ULTRASONOGRAPHY

In vaginal ultrasonography, a probe inserted into the vagina reflects high-frequency sound waves to a transducer, forming an image of the pelvic structures. This study allows better evaluation of pelvic anatomy and earlier diagnosis of pregnancy. It also circumvents poor visualization encountered with obese patients.

TREATMENTS AND PROCEDURES
Drug therapy

ANDROGENS

▶ Stimulate the action of endogenous hormones to replace deficient hormones or treat hormone-sensitive disorders
▶ Stimulate the production of red blood cells by enhancing the production of the erythropoietic stimulating factor
▶ Example: danazol

ANTI-ESTROGEN DRUGS

▶ Bind to estrogen receptors and block estrogen action
▶ Used to inhibit estrogen-mediating tumor growth in breast tissue
▶ Examples: tamoxifen, toremifene (Fareston), and fulvestrant (Faslodex)

ESTROGENS AND PROGESTINS

▶ Stimulate the endogenous hormones to restore hormonal balance and treat hormone sensitive tumors
▶ Estrogens: used to provide contraception and to treat hormonal deficiencies, breast cancer, endometriosis, and atrophic vaginitis
▶ Progestins: used to provide contraception, to regulate or restore the menstrual cycle, and to treat endometrial or renal cancer, endometriosis, and premenstrual syndrome
▶ Examples: conjugated estrogens (Premarin), estradiol (Estrace, Estraderm, Delestrogen, Depo-Estradiol), medroxyprogesterone (Provera), megestrol (Megace), progesterone (Crinone)

GONADOTROPIN-RELEASING HORMONE ANALOGUES

▶ Used to treat endometriosis
▶ Examples: leuprolide (Lupron) and nafarelin (Synarel)

Surgery

BREAST CANCER SURGERY

Types of surgery for breast cancer include lumpectomy, partial mastectomy, simple (total) mastectomy, modified radical mastectomy, radical mastectomy and, perhaps, breast reconstruction.

Lumpectomy

Lumpectomy is used to remove small, well-defined lesions. Through a small incision near the nipple, the surgeon removes the breast mass, surrounding tissue and, possibly, nearby axillary lymph nodes. Lumpectomy preserves the breast mound.

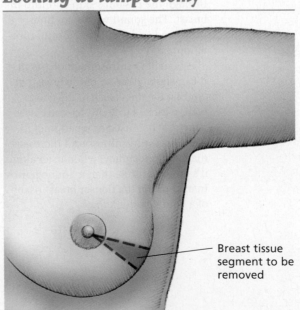

Looking at lumpectomy

Breast tissue segment to be removed

Partial mastectomy

With a partial mastectomy, the surgeon makes an incision over the breast mass. Then he removes the breast mass along with enough additional breast tissue to leave tumor-free margins. In some cases, he also removes the axillary lymph nodes.

Simple (total) mastectomy

With a simple mastectomy, the surgeon makes an elliptical incision around the breast and then removes the entire breast, leaving axillary lymph nodes and pectoral muscles intact.

Modified radical mastectomy

Through a transverse or longitudinal incision, the surgeon removes the entire breast, along with some axillary lymph nodes.

Radical mastectomy

With a radical mastectomy, the surgeon removes the entire breast, pectoralis major and minor, and axillary lymph nodes. Usually reserved for tumors that have invaded deeper tissues, use of radical mastectomy has been declining in recent years.

Looking at partial mastectomy

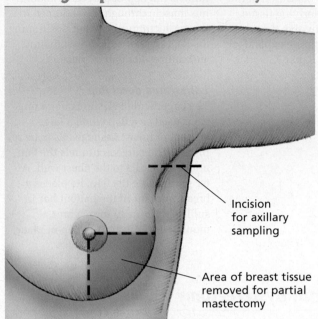

Incision for axillary sampling

Area of breast tissue removed for partial mastectomy

Looking at simple mastectomy

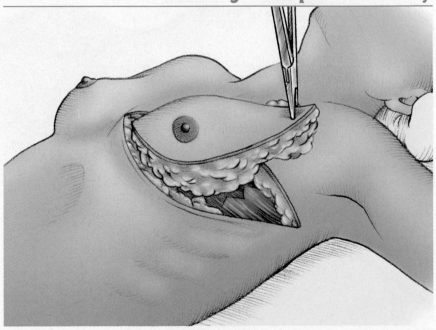

Breast reconstruction

Breast reconstruction may be performed either at the time of mastectomy or after a delay. The choice of technique depends on the condition of the patient's skin and underlying tissue. Reconstruction may involve the use of permanent implants, tissue expanders, or myocutaneous flaps.

Transverse rectus abdominis myocutaneous

In this most commonly used breast reconstruction procedure, the surgeon tunnels the flap of the rectus abdominus muscle through the abdomen to the mastectomy site. After positioning the flap, he forms the breast mound and sutures the flap in place.

Latissimus dorsi flap

The large, wide latissimus dorsi muscle is used as a flap when a large amount of breast tissue needs to be replaced. The surgeon tunnels the flap under the axilla to the chest wall. After positioning the flap, he places a breast implant (if the patient has insufficient tissue to form a breast mound) and sutures the flap in place.

HYSTERECTOMY, ABDOMINAL

Hysterectomy (removal of the uterus) may be performed using the abdominal, vaginal, or laparoscopic-assisted approach. Hysterectomies fall into the following four classifications.

Subtotal hysterectomy

With a subtotal hysterectomy, the surgeon removes the entire uterus except the cervix; however, this procedure is rarely done today.

Total abdominal hysterectomy

With a total abdominal hysterectomy, the surgeon removes the entire uterus and cervix. He makes a transverse or midline incision and dissects through the abdominal layers until the uterus is exposed. Then he removes the uterus and accompanying structures (as necessary) and closes the incision.

Total abdominal hysterectomy

Note: The dark lines below show the incision lines for uterus and cervix removal.

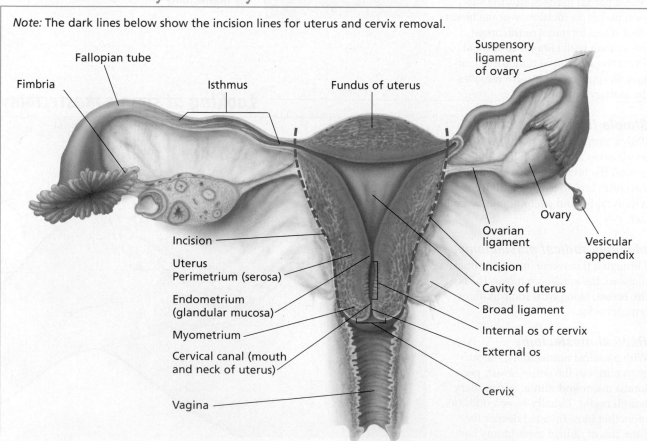

Panhysterectomy

With a panhysterectomy, the surgeon removes the entire uterus along with the ovaries and fallopian tubes (salpingo-oophorectomy).

Radical hysterectomy

With a radical hysterectomy, the surgeon removes the entire uterus, ovaries, fallopian tubes, adjoining ligaments and lymph nodes, and the upper third of the vagina and surrounding tissues. This procedure requires an abdominal approach.

HYSTERECTOMY, VAGINAL

For a hysterectomy with a vaginal approach, the surgeon makes an incision inside the vagina, above but near the cervix. He excises the uterus and removes it through the vaginal canal.

Vaginal hysterectomy

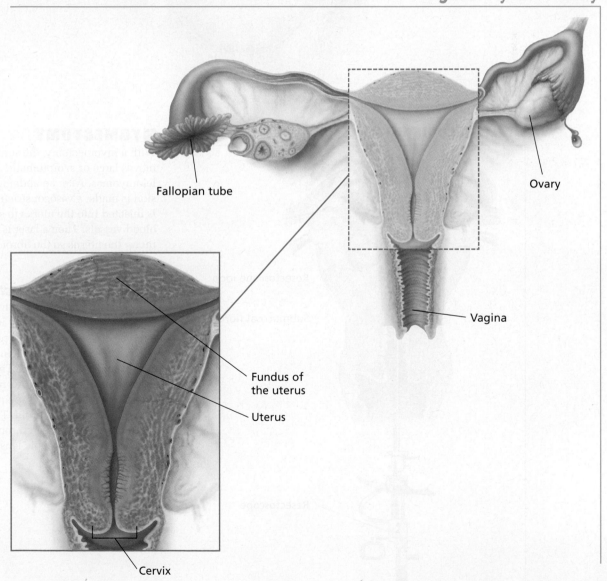

Fallopian tube

Ovary

Vagina

Fundus of the uterus

Uterus

Cervix

Laparoscopic-assisted vaginal hysterectomy

With a laparoscopic-assisted vaginal hysterectomy, the surgeon makes a small incision in the umbilicus for insertion of the laparoscope (with attached camera). He insufflates the abdomen with carbon dioxide, which allows him to view the structures. Then he inserts the laparoscope and may make additional incisions to pass the instruments and excise the uterus. After excising the uterus and accompanying structures, he removes them vaginally and closes the incision.

Viewing a laparoscopic-assisted vaginal hysterectomy

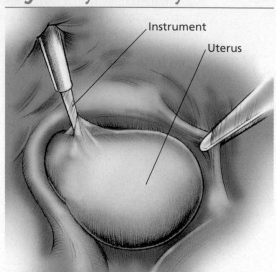

Instrument

Uterus

Understanding hysteroscopic myomectomy

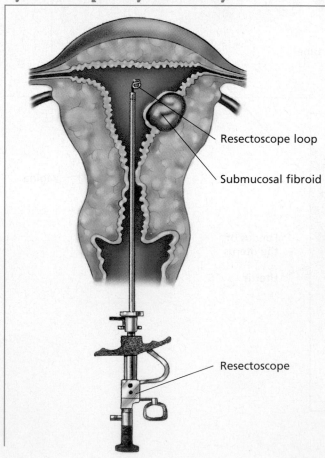

Resectoscope loop

Submucosal fibroid

Resectoscope

MYOMECTOMY

With a myomectomy, the surgeon removes large or symptomatic uterine leiomyomas. After an abdominal incision is made, a vasoconstrictive drug is injected into the uterus to shrink the blood vessels. Then a laser is used to incise the uterus so the fibroids can be removed.

Hysteroscopic myomectomy

Submucosal (and some intramural) myomas can be removed by inserting a resectoscope—a special type of hysteroscope—through the vagina and cervix and into the uterus. The resectoscope has a wire loop or a roller-type tip that directs high-frequency energy to ablate the fibroid. The fibroid tissue can be seen through the resectoscope's telescopic lens.

Other treatments and procedures

RADIATION THERAPY

Radiation therapy, also called *brachytherapy*, involves delivery of high levels of radiation (internally) to a specific body area. It may be administered locally or systemically, using various approaches.

The specially prepared applicators are inserted into the endometrial cavity and vagina under anesthesia. However, the devices aren't loaded with the radioactive material until after the patient leaves the operating room and returns to her room. Then under X-ray guidance to verify placement, the oncologist inserts the radioactive material. This procedure, called *afterloading,* limits the patient's and health care workers' exposure to the radioactive material.

Internal radiation

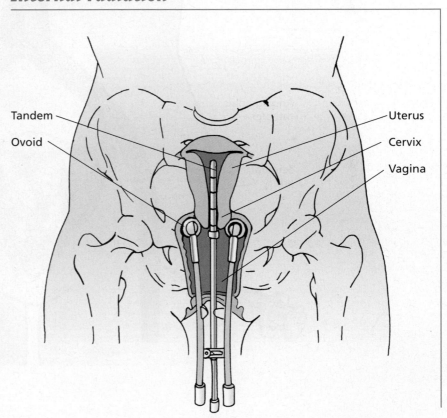

Tandem

Ovoid

Uterus

Cervix

Vagina

UTERINE FIBROID EMBOLIZATION

Under angiogram guidance, a catheter is inserted into the femoral artery and guided to the uterine artery. Tiny balls made of plastic or gelatin sponge (the size of grains of sand) are pumped through the catheter into the uterine artery on one side of the body. The procedure is then repeated on the other side of the body. The substance blocks the blood supply in both the right and left uterine arteries. Without a blood supply, the fibroids shrink and die.

Looking at fibroid embolization

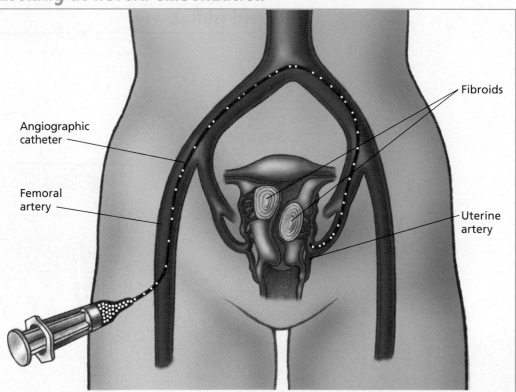

Angiographic catheter

Femoral artery

Fibroids

Uterine artery

Chapter 12

Male reproductive care

DISEASES
Benign prostatic hyperplasia

In benign prostatic hyperplasia (BPH) the prostate gland enlarges sufficiently to compress the urethra and cause some overt urinary obstruction. BPH begins with changes in periurethral glandular tissue. As the prostate enlarges, it may extend into the bladder and obstruct urine outflow by compressing or distorting the prostatic urethra. BPH may also cause a diverticulum musculature that retains urine when the rest of the bladder empties.

Recent evidence suggests a link between BPH and hormonal activity. As men age, production of androgenic hormones decreases, causing an imbalance in androgen and estrogen levels and high levels of dihydrotestosterone, the main prostatic intracellular androgen. Other theoretical causes include neoplasm, arteriosclerosis, inflammation, and metabolic or nutritional disturbances.

Signs and symptoms

Clinical features of BPH depend on the extent of prostatic enlargement and on the lobes affected:
▶ Prostatism (decreased urine stream caliber and force)
▶ Interrupted stream
▶ Urinary hesitancy
▶ Difficulty starting urination
▶ Feeling of incomplete voiding
▶ Frequent urination
▶ Nocturia
▶ Dribbling
▶ Urine retention
▶ Incontinence
▶ Possibly hematuria
▶ Visible midline mass above the symphysis pubis (incompletely emptied bladder)

PICTURING PATHO

Looking at
prostatic enlargement in BPH

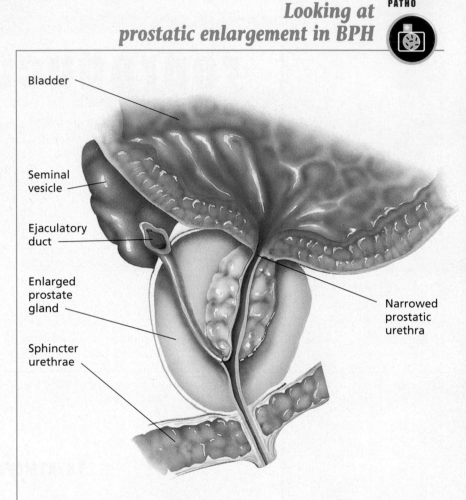

Bladder

Seminal vesicle

Ejaculatory duct

Enlarged prostate gland

Sphincter urethrae

Narrowed prostatic urethra

Treatment

▶ Prostatic massages, sitz baths, short-term fluid restriction (to prevent bladder distention), and antimicrobials (for infection)
▶ Regular sexual activity (for relief of prostatic congestion)
▶ Terazosin (Hytrin), finasteride (Propecia), and tamsulosin (Flomax)
▶ Transurethral resection (for a prostate weighing less than 2 oz [57 g]), vaporization of the prostate, or a prostate incision with a scalpel or laser
▶ Suprapubic (transvesical) prostatectomy (when prostatic enlargement remains within the bladder area)
▶ Perineal prostatectomy (for a large gland in an older patient), commonly resulting in impotence and incontinence
▶ Retropubic (extravesical) prostatectomy (allows direct visualization); potency and continence usually maintained
▶ Transurethral microwaves (heat therapy); their efficacy lies between that of an alpha-adrenergic blocker and surgery

Nursing considerations

▶ Prepare the patient for diagnostic tests and surgery as appropriate.
▶ Monitor and record the patient's vital signs, intake and output, and daily weight. Watch closely for signs of postobstructive diuresis (such as increased urine output and hypotension), which may lead to dehydration, lowered blood volume, shock, electrolyte losses, and anuria.
▶ Administer antibiotics as ordered for urinary tract infection, urethral procedures that involve instruments, and cystoscopy.
▶ If urine retention occurs, try to insert an indwelling urinary catheter. If the catheter can't be passed transurethrally, assist with suprapubic cystostomy. Watch for rapid bladder decompression.
▶ Avoid giving a patient with BPH decongestants, tranquilizers, alcohol, antidepressants, or anticholinergics because these drugs can worsen the obstruction.

After prostatic surgery

▶ Maintain the patient's comfort, and watch for and prevent postoperative complications. Observe for signs of shock and hemorrhage. Check the catheter frequently (every 15 minutes for the first 2 to 3 hours) for patency and urine color; check the dressings for bleeding.
▶ Postoperatively, many urologists insert a three-way catheter and establish continuous bladder irrigation. Keep the solution flowing at a rate sufficient to maintain patency and ensure that returns are clear. If a regular catheter is used, observe it closely. If drainage stops because of clots, irrigate the catheter as ordered, usually with 80 to 100 ml of normal saline solution, while maintaining sterile technique. Be sure to monitor intake and output closely.
▶ Watch for septic shock, the most serious complication of prostatic surgery. Immediately report severe chills, sudden fever, tachycardia, hypotension, or other signs of shock. Start rapid infusion of I.V. antibiotics as ordered.
▶ Watch for pulmonary embolism, heart failure, and acute renal failure. Monitor vital signs, central venous pressure, and arterial pressure.
▶ Make the patient comfortable after an open procedure: Administer suppositories (except after perineal prostatectomy), and give analgesics to control incisional pain. Change dressings frequently.
▶ Continue infusing I.V. fluids until the patient can drink enough on his own (2 to 3 qt [2 to 3 L]/day) to maintain adequate hydration.
▶ Administer stool softeners and laxatives, as ordered, to prevent straining. Don't check for fecal impaction because a rectal examination can cause bleeding.

LESSON PLANS

Teaching about BPH

▶ After surgery, when the catheter has been removed, the patient may experience urinary frequency, dribbling and, occasionally, hematuria. Reassure the patient and family members that he'll gradually regain urinary control.
▶ Reinforce prescribed limits on activity. Warn the patient against lifting, performing strenuous exercises, and taking long car rides for at least 1 month after surgery because these activities increase bleeding tendency. Also caution him not to have sexual intercourse for at least several weeks after discharge.
▶ Teach the patient to recognize the signs of urinary tract infection. Urge him to immediately report these signs to the physician because infection can worsen the inflammation and lead to further obstruction.
▶ Instruct the patient to follow the prescribed oral antibiotic regimen, and tell him the indications for using gentle laxatives.
▶ Urge the patient to seek medical care immediately if he can't void at all, passes bloody urine, or develops a fever.

Epididymitis

Epididymitis, infection of the epididymis (the cordlike excretory duct of the testis), is one of the most common infections of the male reproductive tract. It usually affects adults and is rare before puberty.

Epididymitis usually results from pyogenic organisms, such as staphylococci, *Escherichia coli*, streptococci, chlamydia, *Neisseria gonorrhoeae*, and *Treponema pallidum*. Infection usually results from established urinary tract infection and sexually transmitted disease (STD) or prostatitis extending to the epididymis through the lumen of the vas deferens. Rarely, epididymitis is secondary to a distant infection, such as pharyngitis or tuberculosis that spreads through the lymphatic system or, less commonly, the bloodstream.

Trauma may reactivate a dormant infection or initiate a new one. In addition, epididymitis is a complication of prostatectomy and may result from chemical irritation by extravasation of urine through the vas deferens.

Signs and symptoms

▶ Unilateral, dull, aching pain radiating to the spermatic cord, lower abdomen, and flank
▶ Extremely heavy feeling in the scrotum
▶ Erythema
▶ High fever
▶ Malaise
▶ Characteristic waddle in an attempt to protect the groin and scrotum while walking

PICTURING
PATHO

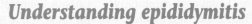

Understanding epididymitis

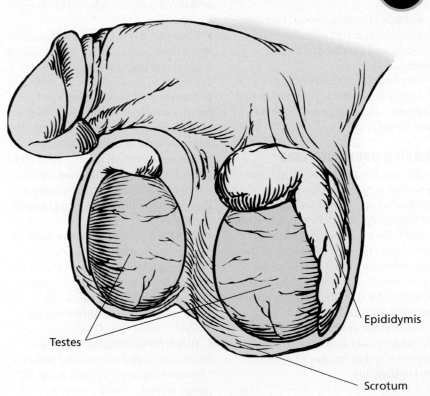

Testes

Epididymis

Scrotum

Understanding orchitis

Orchitis, an infection of the testes, is a serious complication of epididymitis. It also may result from mumps, which can lead to sterility, or less commonly, another systemic infection.

Signs and symptoms
Typical effects of orchitis include unilateral or bilateral tenderness and redness, sudden onset of pain, and swelling of the scrotum and testes. Nausea and vomiting also occur. Sudden cessation of pain indicates testicular ischemia, which can cause permanent damage to one or both testes. Hydrocele also may be present.

Treatment
Appropriate treatment consists of immediate antibiotic therapy or, in mumps orchitis, injection of 20 ml of lidocaine near the spermatic cord of the affected testis, which may relieve swelling and pain. Although corticosteroid use is experimental, such drugs may be used to treat nonspecific granulomatous orchitis. Severe orchitis may require surgery to incise and drain the hydrocele and to improve testicular circulation. Other treatments are similar to those for epididymitis.

To prevent mumps orchitis, ensure that prepubertal males receive the mumps vaccine (or gamma globulin injection after contracting mumps).

Treatment
▶ Bed rest, scrotal elevation with towel rolls or adhesive strapping, broad-spectrum antibiotics, and analgesics (acute phase)
▶ Ice bag applied to the groin area to reduce swelling and relieve pain (Heat is contraindicated because it may damage germinal cells, which are viable only at or below normal body temperature.)
▶ Athletic supporter once pain and swelling subside to prevent pain
▶ Corticosteroids to help counteract inflammation (use is controversial)
▶ Epididymectomy under local anesthesia (if refractory to antibiotics)
▶ Bilateral vasectomy in an older patient undergoing prostatectomy to prevent epididymitis as a postoperative complication (antibiotics alone may prevent it)

Nursing considerations
▶ Watch closely for signs of abscess formation (a localized, hot, red, tender area) or extension of the infection into the testes. Closely monitor temperature, and ensure adequate fluid intake.
▶ Because the patient is usually uncomfortable, administer analgesics as necessary. Allow him to rest in bed, legs slightly apart, with testes elevated on a towel roll. Suggest that he wear nonconstricting, lightweight clothing until the swelling subsides. Apply ice packs as needed for comfort.
▶ Administer antibiotics and antipyretics as ordered. If epididymitis is secondary to an STD, treat the patient and his sexual partner(s) with appropriate antibiotics.
▶ If the patient faces the possibility of sterility, suggest supportive counseling as necessary.

LESSON PLANS

Teaching about epididymitis

▶ If the patient will take antibiotics after discharge, emphasize the importance of completing the prescribed regimen even after symptoms subside.
▶ Suggest that the patient wear a scrotal support while sitting, standing, or walking.
▶ If epididymitis is secondary to an STD, encourage the patient to use a condom during intercourse and to notify sex partners so that they can be adequately treated for infection.

Erectile dysfunction

Erectile dysfunction (ED) refers to the inability to attain or maintain penile erection long enough to complete intercourse. ED is characterized as primary or secondary. The patient with primary ED has never achieved sufficient erection. Secondary ED, which is more common and less serious than the primary form, implies that, despite the current inability, the patient has succeeded in completing intercourse in the past. Transient periods of ED aren't considered dysfunctional and probably occur in 50% of males.

Three types of secondary ED occur:
▶ Partial—The patient can't achieve a full erection or keep his erection long enough to penetrate his partner.
▶ Intermittent—The patient sometimes is potent with the same partner.
▶ Selective—The patient is potent only with certain partners.

ED affects all age-groups but becomes more common with age. The prognosis depends on the severity and duration of ED and on the underlying cause.

Signs and symptoms
▶ Long-standing inability to achieve erection
▶ Sudden loss of erectile function
▶ Gradual decline in function
▶ History of medical disorders, drug therapy, or psychological trauma
▶ Ability to achieve erection through masturbation but not with a partner (psychogenic rather than organic cause)
▶ Depression (either a cause or a result of the impotence)

PICTURING
PATHO

 Understanding erectile dysfunction

Neurologic dysfunction results in a lack of signal to the autonomic nerves.

Arteriolar dilation is reduced.

Perfusion of corpus cavernosum is compromised.

Corpus spongiosum

Treatment

▶ Sex therapy that includes sensate focus therapy, improving verbal communication skills, eliminating stress, and reevaluating attitudes toward sex and sexual roles
▶ Eliminating the cause (for organic impotence); psychological counseling to help the couple deal realistically with their situation and explore alternatives for sexual expression (if cause can't be eliminated)
▶ Surgically inserted inflatable or semirigid penile prosthesis (for organic impotence)
▶ Sildenafil (Viagra), vardenafil (Levitra), or tadalafil (Cialis) as an alternative to surgery

Nursing considerations

▶ Help the patient feel comfortable about discussing his sexuality.
▶ As needed, refer the patient to a physician, nurse, psychologist, social worker, or counselor trained in sex therapy.
▶ Explore areas of stress with the patient. Help him develop relaxation techniques to reduce the stress.
▶ If there are coexisting conditions, such as diabetes mellitus or hypertension, encourage the patient to comply with prescribed treatment.

After penile prosthesis surgery

▶ Apply ice packs to the penis for 24 hours.
▶ Empty the drainage device when it's full.
▶ If the patient has an inflatable prosthesis, instruct him to pull the scrotal pump downward to ensure proper alignment.
▶ When ordered, have the patient practice inflating and deflating the device.

LESSON PLANS

Teaching about erectile dysfunction

▶ Provide instruction about the anatomy and physiology of the reproductive system and the human sexual response cycle as needed.
▶ After penile implant surgery, instruct the patient to avoid intercourse until the incision heals, usually in 6 weeks. Advise him to report signs of infection to the physician.
▶ If the patient is using medication to treat ED, be sure to explain potential side effects or interactions with other medications the patient may be taking.

▶ As a helpful guideline, inform the patient that the therapist's certification by the American Association of Sex Educators, Counselors, and Therapists or by the American Society for Sex Therapy and Research usually ensures quality treatment. If the therapist isn't certified by one of these organizations, advise the patient to ask about the therapist's training in sex counseling and therapy.

Hydrocele

A hydrocele is a collection of fluid between the visceral and parietal layer of the tunica vaginalis of the testicle or along the spermatic cord. It's the most common cause of scrotal swelling. It may be caused by an infection or trauma to the testes or epididymis or a testicular tumor.

Congenital hydrocele occurs when an opening between the scrotal sac and the peritoneal cavity allows peritoneal fluid to collect in the scrotum. The exact mechanism is unknown.

Signs and symptoms
▶ Scrotal swelling and feeling of heaviness
▶ Inguinal hernia (commonly accompanies congenital hydrocele)
▶ Fluid collection, presenting as a flaccid or tense mass
▶ Pain with acute epididymal infection or testicular torsion
▶ Scrotal tenderness due to severe swelling

Treatment
▶ Possibly no treatment, especially in newborns
▶ Surgical herniography (for inguinal hernia with bowel in the sac)
▶ Aspiration of fluid and injection of a sclerosing agent (for a tense hydrocele that impedes blood circulation)
▶ Excision of the tunica vaginalis (for recurrent hydroceles)
▶ Suprainguinal excision for a testicular tumor (detected by ultrasound)

Nursing considerations
▶ Place a rolled towel between the patient's legs and elevate the scrotum to help reduce swelling.
▶ Apply heat or ice packs to the scrotum.
▶ Monitor scrotal swelling.
▶ Provide postoperative wound care, if appropriate.

PICTURING PATHO

Looking at a hydrocele

Epididymis

Testis

Fluid accumulation in the tunica vaginalis

Tunica vaginalis:
–visceral layer
–parietal layer

Hydrocele

LESSON PLANS

Teaching about hydrocele

▶ Educate the patient about wearing a loose-fitting athletic supporter lined with soft cotton dressings.
▶ Instruct the patient on how to take a sitz bath.
▶ Advise the patient about the need to avoid tub baths (only using the sitz bath) postoperatively for 5 to 7 days.
▶ Caution the patient that the hydrocele possibly may reaccumulate during the first month after surgery because of edema.

Prostate cancer

Prostate cancer is the most common neoplasm in males older than age 50; it's a leading cause of male cancer death. Adenocarcinoma is the most common form; only seldom does prostate cancer occur as a sarcoma. Most prostate cancers originate in the posterior prostate gland, with the rest growing near the urethra. Malignant prostatic tumors seldom result from the benign hyperplastic enlargement that commonly develops around the prostatic urethra in older males.

Slow-growing prostate cancer seldom produces signs and symptoms until it's well advanced. Typically, when primary prostatic lesions spread beyond the prostate gland, they invade the prostatic capsule and then spread along the ejaculatory ducts in the space between the seminal vesicles or perivesicular fascia. When prostate cancer is fatal, there is usually widespread bone metastasis.

Risk factors for prostate cancer include age (the cancer seldom develops in males younger than age 40), race (higher incidence in Blacks), and genetic factors. Men who have a first-degree relative with prostate cancer have twice the risk of developing it. Endocrine factors may also have a role, leading researchers to suspect that androgens speed tumor growth.

PICTURING PATHO

Looking at prostate cancer

Bladder

Seminal vesicle

Ejaculatory duct

Prostatic carcinoma

Prostate gland

Sphincter urethrae

Membranous urethra

PICTURING PATHO

Pathway for metastasis of prostate cancer

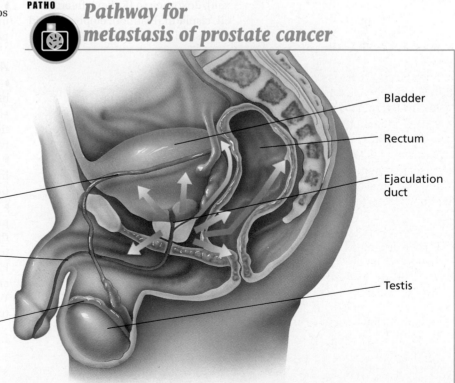

Bladder

Rectum

Ejaculation duct

Ductus deferens

Urethra

Testis

Epididymis

Signs and symptoms
▶ Dysuria
▶ Urinary frequency
▶ Urine retention
▶ Back or hip pain (signaling bone metastasis)
▶ Hematuria (uncommon)
▶ Edema of the scrotum (or leg in advanced disease)
▶ Nonraised, firm, nodular mass with a sharp edge (in early disease) or a hard lump (in advanced disease)
▶ Erectile dysfunction

Treatment
▶ Radiation, prostatectomy, orchiectomy (removal of the testes) to reduce androgen production, and hormonal therapy with leuprolide (Lupron Depot) or goserelin (Zoladex)
▶ Radical prostatectomy (for localized lesions without metastasis)
▶ Suprapubic prostatectomy
▶ Transurethral resection of the prostate to relieve an obstruction
▶ Perineal prostatectomy
▶ Radiation therapy to cure locally invasive lesions in early disease and to relieve bone pain from metastatic skeletal involvement; also used prophylactically for patients with tumors in regional lymph nodes
▶ Internal beam radiation that permits increased radiation to reach the prostate but minimizes the surrounding tissues' exposure to radiation (alternative therapy)
▶ Chemotherapy (if hormonal therapy, surgery, and radiation therapy aren't feasible or successful), including combinations of cyclophosphamide (Cytoxan), doxorubicin (Rubex), fluorouracil, cisplatin (Platinol), etoposide, and vindesine; limited benefits

Nursing considerations
▶ At all times, encourage the patient to express his fears and concerns, including those about changes in his sexual identity, because of surgery. Offer reassurance when possible.
▶ Administer ordered analgesics as necessary. Provide comfort measures to reduce pain. Encourage the patient to identify care measures that promote his comfort and relaxation.
▶ Monitor intake and output closely.

After prostatectomy
▶ Regularly check the dressing, incision, and drainage systems for excessive blood. Also watch for signs of bleeding (pallor, restlessness, decreasing blood pressure, and increasing pulse rate).
▶ Be alert for signs of infection (fever, chills, inflamed incisional area). Maintain adequate fluid intake (at least 2,000 ml daily).
▶ Give antispasmodics, as ordered, to control postoperative bladder spasms. Also provide analgesics as needed.
▶ Because urinary incontinence commonly follows prostatectomy, keep the patient's skin clean and dry.

After suprapubic prostatectomy
▶ Keep the skin around the suprapubic drain dry and free from drainage and urine leakage. Encourage the patient to begin perineal exercises between 24 and 48 hours after surgery.
▶ Allow the patient's family to assist in his care, and encourage them to provide psychological support.
▶ Give meticulous catheter care. After prostatectomy, a patient usually has a three-way catheter with a continuous irrigation system. Check the tubing for kinks, mucus plugs, and clots, especially if the patient complains of pain. Warn the patient not to pull on the tubes or the catheter.

After transurethral resection
▶ Watch for signs of urethral stricture (dysuria, decreased force and caliber of urine stream, and straining to urinate). Also observe for abdominal distention (a result of urethral stricture or catheter blockage by a blood clot). Irrigate the catheter as ordered.

After perineal or retropubic prostatectomy
▶ Avoid taking the patient's temperature rectally or inserting an enema or other rectal tubes. Provide pads to absorb draining urine. Assist the patient with frequent sitz baths to relieve pain and inflammation.
▶ Give reassurance that urine leakage after catheter removal is normal and subsides in time.

After radiation therapy
▶ Watch for the common adverse effects of radiation to the prostate. These include proctitis, diarrhea, bladder spasms, and urinary frequency. Internal radiation of the prostate almost always results in cystitis in the first 2 to 3 weeks of therapy. Encourage the patient to drink at least 2 qt (2 L) of fluid daily. Administer analgesics and antispasmodics to increase comfort.

After hormonal therapy
▶ When a patient receives hormonal therapy, watch for adverse effects (gynecomastia, fluid retention, nausea, and vomiting). Be alert for thrombophlebitis (pain, tenderness, swelling, warmth, and redness in calf).

LESSON PLANS

Teaching about prostate cancer

▶ Before surgery, discuss the expected results. Explain that radical surgery always produces impotence. Up to 7% of patients experience urinary incontinence.
▶ To help minimize incontinence, teach the patient how to do perineal exercises while he sits or stands. To develop his perineal muscles, tell him to squeeze his buttocks together and hold this position for a few seconds, then relax. He should repeat this exercise as frequently as ordered by the physician.

▶ If appropriate, discuss the adverse effects of radiation therapy. All patients who receive pelvic radiation therapy will develop such symptoms as diarrhea, urinary frequency, nocturia, bladder spasms, rectal irritation, and tenesmus.
▶ Encourage the patient to maintain a lifestyle that's as nearly normal as possible during recovery.
▶ When appropriate, refer the patient to the social service department, local home health care agencies, hospices, and other support organizations.

Prostatitis

Prostatitis is an inflammation of the prostate gland. It occurs in several forms. Acute prostatitis most commonly results from gram-negative bacteria and is easily recognized and treated. Chronic prostatitis, which affects up to 35% of men older than age 50 and is the most common cause of recurrent urinary tract infection in men, is harder to recognize.

Infection probably spreads to the prostate gland by the hematogenous route or from an ascending urethral infection, invasion of rectal bacteria by way of the lymphatic vessels, or reflux of infected bladder urine into the prostate ducts. Less commonly, infection may result from urethral procedures performed with instruments, such as cystoscopy and catheterization, or from infrequent or excessive sexual intercourse.

Chronic prostatitis usually results from bacterial invasion from the urethra. Granulomatous prostatitis occurs secondary to a miliary spread of *Mycobacterium tuberculosis*. Nonbacterial prostatitis is probably caused by the protozoa *Mycoplasma, Ureaplasma, Chlamydia,* or *Trichomonas vaginalis,* or some viruses.

Signs and symptoms
Acute prostatitis
▶ Sudden fever
▶ Chills
▶ Lower back pain
▶ Myalgia
▶ Perineal fullness
▶ Perineal pain
▶ Arthralgia
▶ Frequent urination
▶ Urinary urgency
▶ Dysuria
▶ Nocturia
▶ Transient erectile dysfunction
▶ Cloudy urine
▶ Bladder distention

Chronic bacterial prostatitis
▶ Possibly asymptomatic
▶ Urinary symptoms same as acute form (but to a lesser degree)
▶ Hemospermia
▶ Persistent urethral discharge
▶ Painful ejaculation
▶ Sexual dysfunction

Granulomatous prostatitis
▶ Stony, hard induration of the prostate (mimicking carcinoma or a calculus)

Nonbacterial prostatitis
▶ Dysuria
▶ Mild perineal or lower back pain
▶ Frequent nocturia

PICTURING PATHO

Looking at prostatic inflammation

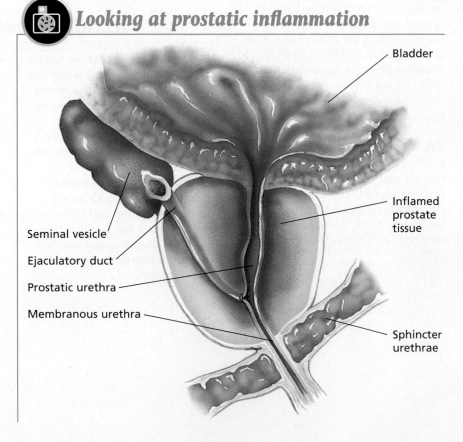

- Bladder
- Inflamed prostate tissue
- Sphincter urethrae
- Seminal vesicle
- Ejaculatory duct
- Prostatic urethra
- Membranous urethra

Treatment

▶ Bed rest, adequate hydration, analgesics, antipyretics, sitz baths, and stool softeners as necessary

Acute and chronic prostatitis

▶ Aminoglycosides, in combination with penicillins or cephalosporins (for severe cases)
▶ Trimethoprim-sulfamethoxazole (Bactrim) to prevent chronic prostatitis and to combat infections with *Escherichia coli;* other drugs used for *E. coli* infections including amoxicillin, nitrofurantoin (Macrobid), erythromycin (E-Mycin), fluoroquinolones (ciprofloxacin), and tetracycline (Sumycin)
▶ Sitz baths and regular sexual intercourse (the patient should use condoms during the treatment phase) or ejaculation to promote drainage of prostatic secretions (for chronic prostatitis)
▶ Transurethral resection of the prostate (for unsuccessful drug therapy)
▶ Total prostatectomy (possibly causing impotence and incontinence)

Granulomatous prostatitis

▶ Antitubercular drug combinations, such as minocycline (Dynacin), doxycycline (Vibramycin), or erythromycin (for nonbacterial prostatitis for 4 weeks; antibiotic therapy not repeated if symptoms don't subside)
▶ Bed rest, adequate hydration, and administration of analgesics (nonsteroidal anti-inflammatory drugs), antipyretics, and stool softeners as necessary

Nonbacterial prostatitis

▶ Anticholinergics and analgesics (for symptom relief)

Nursing considerations

▶ Administer analgesics for pain as ordered and evaluate response.
▶ Ensure bed rest and adequate hydration.
▶ Provide stool softeners and administer sitz baths as ordered. Avoid rectal examination because it can precipitate bleeding.
▶ As necessary, prepare to assist with suprapubic needle aspiration of the bladder or a suprapubic cystostomy.
▶ If transurethral resection of the prostate is performed, monitor the patient postoperatively for signs of hypovolemia (decreased blood pressure, increased pulse rate, and pale, clammy skin).
▶ Check the catheter every 15 minutes for the first 2 to 3 hours after surgery for patency, urine color and consistency, and excessive urethral meatus bleeding.
▶ If a three-way continuous bladder irrigation is being performed, keep the solution flow rate sufficient to maintain patency and keep the return light pink. Palpate for bladder distention. If the solution stops or the patient complains of pain, irrigate the catheter with normal saline solution using a 50-ml syringe. Monitor intake and output closely.
▶ Watch for septic shock, the most serious complication of prostatic surgery. Immediately report severe chills, sudden fever, tachycardia, hypotension, or other signs of shock. Start rapid infusion of I.V. antibiotics as ordered. Watch for pulmonary embolism, heart failure, and acute renal failure. Continuously monitor vital signs and central venous pressure.
▶ Administer anticholinergics as ordered to relieve painful bladder spasms that commonly occur after transurethral resection.

Teaching about prostatitis

LESSON PLANS

▶ Familiarize the patient with prescribed drugs and their possible adverse effects. Tell him to take the drugs exactly as ordered and to complete the prescribed drug regimens.
▶ Tell the patient to immediately report adverse drug reactions, such as rash, nausea, vomiting, fever, chills, and GI irritation.
▶ Instruct him to drink at least eight 8-oz glasses of fluid per day (about 2 qt [2 L]).
▶ If the patient has chronic prostatitis, recommend that he stay sexually active and ejaculate regularly to promote drainage of prostatic secretions. Tell him to use a condom during intercourse when he's having a bout of prostatitis.

For transurethral resection of the prostate

▶ Tell him that after catheter removal he may have urinary frequency, dribbling, and occasional hematuria. Reassure him that he'll gradually regain urinary control. Explain this to his family so that they can offer reassurance as well.
▶ Reinforce prescribed limits on activity. Warn the patient not to lift, exercise strenuously, or take long automobile rides because these increase bleeding tendency. Caution him to abstain from sexual activity for several weeks after discharge.
▶ Instruct the patient to take oral antibiotics exactly as prescribed and for as long as prescribed. Also review the indications for using gentle laxatives.
▶ Urge the patient to seek medical care immediately if he can't void, passes bloody urine, or develops a fever.

Testicular cancer

Malignant testicular tumors are the most prevalent solid tumors in males ages 15 to 35. Testicular cancer is rare in nonwhite males and accounts for less than 1% of all male cancer deaths. Testicular cancer rarely occurs in children.

With few exceptions, testicular tumors originate from germinal cells. About 40% become seminomas. These tumors, which are characterized by uniform, undifferentiated cells, resemble primitive gonadal cells. Other tumors—nonseminomas—show various degrees of differentiation.

Typically, when testicular cancer extends beyond the testes, it spreads through the lymphatic system to the iliac, para-aortic, and mediastinal nodes. Metastasis affects the lungs, liver, viscera, and bone.

Although researchers don't know the immediate cause of testicular cancer, they suspect that cryptorchidism (even when surgically corrected) plays a role in the developing disease. A history of mumps orchitis, inguinal hernia in childhood, or maternal use of diethylstilbestrol (DES) or other estrogen-progestin combinations during pregnancy also increases the risk of this disease.

Signs and symptoms

◗ History of previous injuries to the scrotum, viral infections (such as mumps), or the use of DES or other estrogen-progestin drugs by the patient's mother during pregnancy
◗ Feeling of heaviness or dragging sensation in the scrotum
◗ Swollen testes
◗ Painless lump found while performing testicular self-examination
◗ Gynecomastia (tumor produces chorionic gonadotropins or estrogen)
◗ Enlarged lymph nodes in surrounding areas

Late stages

◗ Weight loss
◗ Cough
◗ Hemoptysis
◗ Shortness of breath
◗ Lethargy
◗ Fatigue
◗ Decreased breath sounds
◗ Lumbar back pain
◗ Bone pain
◗ Unilateral or bilateral leg edema secondary to iliac or vena caval compression or thrombosis

PICTURING PATHO

Looking at testicular cancer

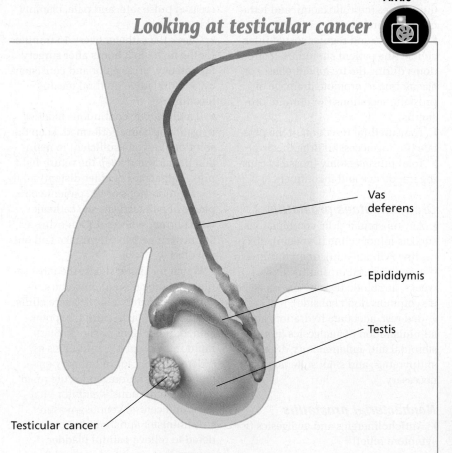

Vas deferens

Epididymis

Testis

Testicular cancer

Staging testicular cancer

Stage III
Disseminated to distant organs, such as bones, lungs, or other viscera

Stage II
Regional nodes involved

Stage I
Tumor in testis only

Cryptorchidism and testicular cancer

In men with cryptorchidism (the failure of a testicle to descend into the scrotum), testicular tumors are about 50 times more common than in men with normal anatomic structure. A simple surgical procedure called orchiopexy can bring the testicle to its normal position in the scrotum and reduce the testicular cancer risk. Nevertheless, testicular tumors occur more commonly in a surgically descended testicle than in a naturally descended one.

What happens in orchiopexy
In this procedure, the surgeon incises the groin area and separates the testicle and its blood supply from surrounding abdominal structures. Then he creates a "tunnel" into the scrotum to accommodate the descent of the testicle.

Reducing further risk
After orchiopexy, urge the patient to examine himself monthly to detect a tumor at its earliest stage.

Treatment
▶ Varying in intensity based on the tumor cell type and stage
▶ Orchiectomy and retroperitoneal node dissection to prevent disease extension and assess its stage; involves removal of the testis, not the scrotum
▶ Hormonal replacement therapy (after bilateral orchiectomy)
▶ Postoperative radiation to the retroperitoneal and homolateral iliac nodes (for seminomas)
▶ Prophylactic radiation to the mediastinal and supraclavicular nodes (for patients whose disease extends to retroperitoneal structures)

▶ Radiation directed to all cancerous lymph nodes (for nonseminoma)
▶ Chemotherapy (for late-stage seminomas and most nonseminomas when used for recurrent cancer after orchiectomy and removal of the retroperitoneal lymph nodes)
▶ High-dose chemotherapy with autologous bone marrow transplantation: involves, removing and treating the patient's bone marrow to kill remaining cancer cells, and returning the processed bone marrow to the patient (for those who don't respond to standard therapy)

Nursing considerations

▶ Focus on responding to the psychological impact of the disease, preventing postoperative complications, and minimizing and controlling the complications of radiation therapy and chemotherapy.

▶ Listen to the patient's fears and concerns. Remember that the patient with testicular cancer typically fears sexual impairment and disfigurement. When possible, provide reassurance. Stay with the patient during periods of severe anxiety and stress.

▶ Encourage the patient to ask questions. Base your relationship on trust so that he feels comfortable expressing his concerns.

After orchiectomy

▶ For the first day after surgery, apply an ice pack to the scrotum and provide analgesics, as ordered.

▶ Check for excessive bleeding, swelling, and signs of infection, such as drainage from the incision, fever, pain, and redness.

▶ Supply an athletic supporter to minimize scrotal pain during ambulation.

During chemotherapy

▶ Know what problems to expect and how to prevent or ease them.

▶ Give antiemetics as ordered to prevent severe nausea and vomiting.

▶ Offer the patient small, frequent meals to maintain oral intake despite anorexia. Devise a mouth care regimen, being sure to check regularly for stomatitis.

▶ Be alert for signs of myelosuppression. If the patient receives vinblastine, monitor for signs and symptoms of neurotoxicity (peripheral paresthesia, jaw pain, muscle cramps). If he receives cisplatin (Platinol), check for ototoxicity. To prevent renal damage, encourage increased fluid intake.

▶ To maximize hydration, give I.V. fluids as ordered with a potassium supplement for low serum potassium level.

During radiation therapy

▶ Watch for and report adverse effects.

▶ Implement appropriate comfort and safety measures. For example, avoid rubbing the skin near radiation target sites, which helps to prevent or alleviate pain, skin breakdown, and infection.

LESSON PLANS

Teaching about testicular cancer

▶ Provide reassurance that sterility and impotence usually don't follow unilateral orchiectomy. Explain that synthetic hormones can supplement depleted hormone levels. Inform the patient that most surgeons don't remove the scrotum. Also explain that a testicular prosthetic implant can correct disfigurement.

▶ As suitable, review sperm-banking procedures before the patient begins treatment, especially if infertility and erectile dysfunction may result from surgery.

▶ Explain tests and treatments that the patient is to undergo. Make sure he understands each treatment, its purpose, possible complications, and the care required during and after the treatment.

▶ Teach the patient how to perform testicular self-examination. Tell him that this is the best way to detect a new or recurrent tumor.

▶ Refer the patient to organizations such as the American Cancer Society that offer information and support during and after treatment.

Testicular torsion

With testicular torsion, the spermatic cord twists with the rotation of a testis or the mesorchium (the mesentery between the testis and epididymis), strangulating the testis. It occurs unilaterally about 90% of the time. Testicular torsion is most common in males ages 12 to 18 (although it can occur at any age). With early detection and prompt treatment, the prognosis is good.

The tunica vaginalis normally envelops the testis and attaches to the epididymis and spermatic cord. In intravaginal torsion (the most common type of testicular torsion in adolescents), testicular twisting may result from abnormal positioning of the testis in the tunica or from a narrowing of the mesentery support. In extravaginal torsion (most common in neonates), loose attachment of the tunica vaginalis to the scrotal lining causes spermatic cord rotation above the testis. A sudden, forceful contraction of the cremaster muscle may precipitate this condition.

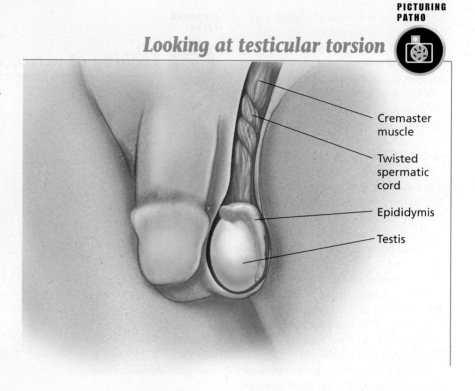

PICTURING PATHO

Looking at testicular torsion

- Cremaster muscle
- Twisted spermatic cord
- Epididymis
- Testis

Signs and symptoms
▶ Sudden excruciating pain in the affected testis or iliac fossa frequently after physical exertion or mild testicular trauma
▶ Elevated testis, which lies transversely instead of longitudinally
▶ Tense, tender swelling in the scrotum or inguinal canal
▶ Hyperemia of the overlying skin of the scrotum
▶ Nausea and vomiting

Treatment
▶ Vascular emergency that requires treatment within 4 hours of initial pain
▶ Possible manual detorsion by a urologist
▶ Immediate surgical repair by orchiopexy (fixation of a viable testis to the scrotum) or orchiectomy (excision of a nonviable testis)
▶ Analgesics for pain postoperatively

Nursing considerations
▶ Offer reassurance, and keep the patient comfortable before and after surgery. Administer pain medication as ordered.
▶ Monitor voiding, and apply a covered ice bag to the surgical site to reduce edema.
▶ Protect the wound from contamination. Otherwise, allow as many normal daily activities as possible.

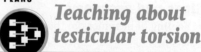

LESSON PLANS

Teaching about testicular torsion

▶ Explain the surgical procedure and postoperative care. Even if the testis must be removed, reassure the patient that sexual function and fertility should be unaffected.
▶ Recommend that the patient routinely wear a scrotal support when exercising.

Varicocele

A varicocele is a mass of dilated and torturous varicose veins in the spermatic cord. It's commonly described as a "bag of worms" and generally appears in the left scrotum.

Because of a valvular disorder in the spermatic vein, blood pools in the pampiniform venous plexus. One of the functions of the pampiniform plexus is to keep the testes slightly cooler than body temperature, which is the optimal temperature for sperm production. Incomplete blood flow through the testes then interferes with spermatogenesis. Testicular atrophy may also occur because of the reduced blood flow.

The cause of a varicocele is thought to be from incomplete or congenitally absent valves in the spermatic veins. Tumors or thrombus may also obstruct the inferior vena cava causing a unilateral left-sided varicocele.

This condition is present in 30% of all men diagnosed with infertility and occurs in 15% to 20% of all males, usually between ages 13 and 18.

Signs and symptoms

▶ Feeling of heaviness in the affected side
▶ "Bag of worms" feeling with patient in upright position
▶ Testicular tenderness or atrophy
▶ Possible infertility

Treatment

▶ Scrotal support to relieve discomfort
▶ Surgical repair or removal involving ligation of the gonadal vein

PICTURING PATHO

Looking at varicocele

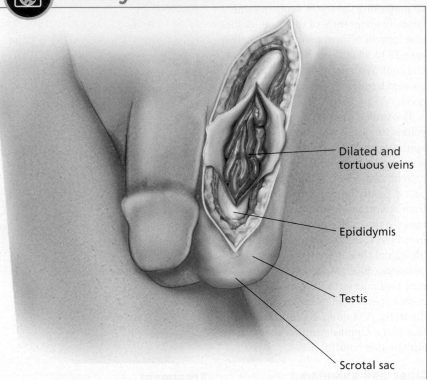

— Dilated and tortuous veins

— Epididymis

— Testis

— Scrotal sac

Nursing considerations

▶ Promote the patient's comfort before and after surgery.
▶ After surgery, administer drug therapy as prescribed.
▶ Apply an ice bag with a cover to the scrotal area to reduce edema.
▶ Protect the wound from contamination during toileting.
▶ Allow the patient to perform as many normal daily activities as possible.
▶ Monitor the patient's intake and output, comfort level, and wound healing.

LESSON PLANS

Teaching about varicocele

▶ Reinforce the practitioner's explanation of the disorder.
▶ Explain preoperative and postoperative care if the patient is scheduled for surgery.
▶ Explain the treatment procedure and reinforce the practitioner's explanation.
▶ Provide wound care to the surgical site as necessary.
▶ Provide analgesia as needed and monitor the patient's response.

TESTS
Laboratory tests

ALPHA-FETOPROTEIN

Many testicular cancers secrete high levels of certain proteins, such as alpha-fetoprotein. Testing for these proteins is important because their presence in the blood suggests that a testicular tumor is present. However, they can also be found in conditions other than cancer.

HUMAN CHORIONIC GONADOTROPIN

Human chorionic gonadotropin (hCG) is another protein secreted by many testicular tumors. The presence of hCG in the blood may suggest a testicular tumor but may also indicate other conditions besides cancer.

PROSTATE-SPECIFIC ANTIGEN

This test measures levels of prostate-specific antigen (PSA), which appears in normal, benign hyperplastic and malignant prostatic tissue, as well as in metastatic prostate cancer. Levels are used to monitor the spread or recurrence of stage B3 to D1 prostate cancer and evaluate the patient's response to treatment. PSA level measurement and a digital rectal examination are recommended to screen men over age 50 for prostate cancer.

SEMEN ANALYSIS

A semen analysis evaluates male fertility (semen count and motility analysis), validates the effectiveness of a vasectomy, and detects the presence of semen for medicolegal investigations.

TESTOSTERONE

This competitive protein-binding test measures plasma or serum testosterone levels. When combined with measurement of plasma gonadotropin levels (follicle-stimulating hormone and luteinizing hormone), it's a reliable aid in the evaluation of gonadal dysfunction in men and women. It facilitates differential diagnosis of male sexual precocity in boys younger than age 10. (True precocious puberty must be distinguished from pseudoprecocious puberty.) It's used to aid differential diagnosis of hypogonadism. (Primary hypogonadism must be distinguished from secondary hypogonadism.) It's also used to evaluate male infertility or other sexual dysfunction.

Imaging studies

Imaging studies allow examination of internal reproductive structures and can include ultrasonography and magnetic resonance imaging (MRI). X-ray imaging may be performed, but MRI has been found to be more accurate.

MAGNETIC RESONANCE IMAGING

MRI can be used to evaluate and stage prostate cancer. It can also detect prostate calculi and cysts, and cancer invasion into seminal vesicles and pelvic lymph nodes.

ULTRASONOGRAPHY

Ultrasound can be used to aid in the diagnosis of several male reproductive disorders. Duplex Doppler ultrasound can be used to evaluate arterial and venous blood flow to the penis to determine an organic cause for erectile dysfunction. It can determine if there's a twisting of the spermatic cord (testicular torsion) or a mass as in a testicular tumor or scrotal swelling. It can also support the diagnosis of epididymitis if it reveals increased blood flow to the testicle.

Other tests

PROSTATE GLAND BIOPSY

Prostate gland biopsy is the needle excision of a prostate tissue specimen for histologic examination. Indications include potentially malignant prostatic hyperplasia and prostatic nodules. A perineal, transrectal, or transurethral approach may be used—the transrectal approach is used for high prostatic lesions.

URINARY FLOW TEST

A urine flow test measures the strength and amount of urine flow by charting urine flow patterns and rate over time. Restricted urine flow can also be a sign of a weakened bladder muscle, or it may indicate prostate enlargement and urethral constriction.

URODYNAMIC STUDIES

Urodynamic studies measure internal bladder pressure by injecting water into the bladder. They also measure how effectively the bladder contracts and may be used if the practitioner suspects a bladder problem rather than prostate gland enlargement.

TREATMENTS AND PROCEDURES
Drug therapy

ALPHA-ADRENERGIC BLOCKERS
▶ Release the prostate and bladder muscles, reducing straining with urination and improving urine flow
▶ Used to treat benign prostatic hyperplasia
▶ Examples: terazosin (Hytrin), doxazosin (Cardura), and tamsulosin (Flomax), prazosin (Minipress)

ANDROGEN HORMONE INHIBITORS
▶ Inhibit steroid 5-alpha-reductase, which is an enzyme that converts testosterone into 5-alpha-dihydrotesterone (DHT)

▶ Lead to a decrease in the high levels of DHT found in men with an enlarged prostate
▶ Used to treat benign prostatic hyperplasia
▶ Examples: finasteride (Propecia, Proscar)

ERECTILE DYSFUNCTION DRUGS
▶ Inhibit the breakdown of cyclic guanosine monophosphate (cGMP) by phosphodiesterase, which leads to increased cGMP levels and prolonged smooth muscle relaxation, thereby promoting blood flow into the corpus cavernosum
▶ Examples: alprostadil (Caverject, Caverject Impulse), sildenafil (Viagra), tadalafil (Cialis), vardenafil (Levitra)

GONADOTROPIN-RELEASING HORMONE AGONISTS ANALOGUES
▶ Suppress LH by the pituitary gland, reducing testosterone levels
▶ Inhibit tumor progression by blocking the uptake of testicular and adrenal androgens at the prostate tumor site (flutamide)
▶ Examples: leuprolide (Lupron Depot), goserelin acetate (Zoladex)

Nonsurgical procedures

VACUUM CONSTRICTION DEVICE
A vacuum constriction device is an external pump with a band on it that a patient with erectile dysfunction can use to get and maintain an erection.

The device consists of an acrylic cylinder with a pump that may be attached directly to the end of the penis. A constriction ring or band is placed on the cylinder at the other end, which is applied to the body. The cylinder and pump are used to create a vacuum to help the penis become erect; the band or constriction ring is used to help maintain the erection.

Surgery

Surgical procedures include cryosurgical ablation, penile implants, prostatectomy, and orchidectomy.

CRYOSURGICAL ABLATION

Cryosurgical ablation or cryoablation is a minimally invasive procedure that's used to treat prostate cancer. It's reserved for patients whose cancer is confined to the prostate. In this procedure, an ultrasound probe is inserted into the rectum to view the prostate. Cryoprobes are then inserted into the perineum and directly into the prostate. Liquid nitrogen is injected into the prostate, freezing the prostate tissue and destroying tumor cells.

Understanding cryoablation

In cryoablation, cryoprobes are placed through the skin into the perineal area and directly into the prostate. Transrectal ultrasound guides the placement of the probes into the prostate. Liquid nitrogen is injected into the prostate.

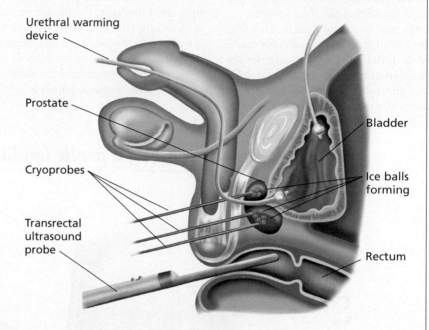

In this illustration, the liquid nitrogen has formed an "ice ball" around the prostate.

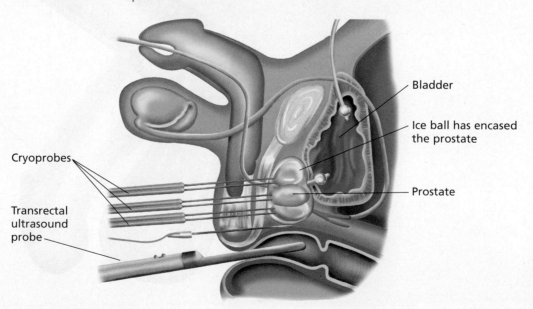

PENILE IMPLANT

Penile implants or prostheses are used when all other methods to resolve erectile dysfunction fail. Penile prostheses (rigid, semi-rigid, and malleable rods) produce varying degrees of rigidity. Inflatable prostheses include the multicomponent and self-contained inflatable prostheses. Semi-rigid prostheses allow an erection sufficient for penetration and are better suited for patients with less manual dexterity. Most rigid prostheses are associated with a low mechanical failure rate, but may produce a noticeably unsightly erection and interfere with urination. One-piece inflatable penile prostheses don't become as erect as rigid ones and don't deflate as much as multicomponent inflatable devices; these types are limited to an "average-sized penis." Multicomponent inflatable prostheses give the best appearance when erect and are the softest when deflated.

A reservoir is placed into the scrotum, and tubes carry the fluid from the reservoir into the inflatable pieces that are placed in the penis. The implants are inflated when the pump, located in the scrotum, is squeezed. To deflate the prosthesis, a release button is activated.

Understanding a penile implant

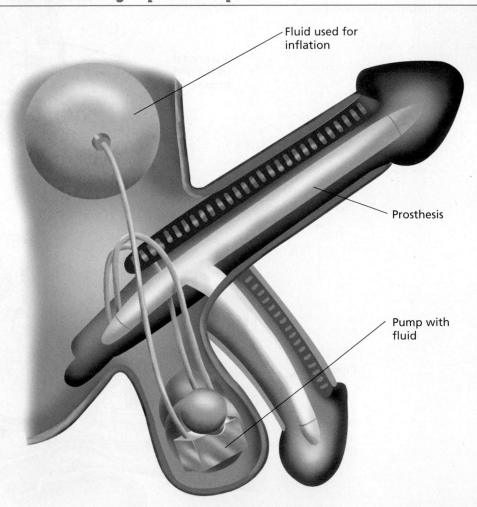

Fluid used for inflation

Prosthesis

Pump with fluid

PROSTATECTOMY

Prostatectomy removes all or part of the prostate gland. Radical prostatectomy is a treatment option for patients with early-stage prostate cancer. Total or partial prostatectomy may be used in patients with significant obstructive benign prostatic hyperplasia. The procedure removes diseased or obstructive tissue and restores urine flow through the urethra.

Transurethral resection of the prostate

With the patient in the lithotomy position, the surgeon introduces a resectoscope into the urethra and advances it to the prostate. He instills a clear, isotonic nonelectrolytic irrigating solution (such as 1.5% glycine), visualizes the obstruction, and uses the resectoscope's cutting loop to resect prostatic tissue and restore the urethral opening.

A look at transurethral resection of the prostate

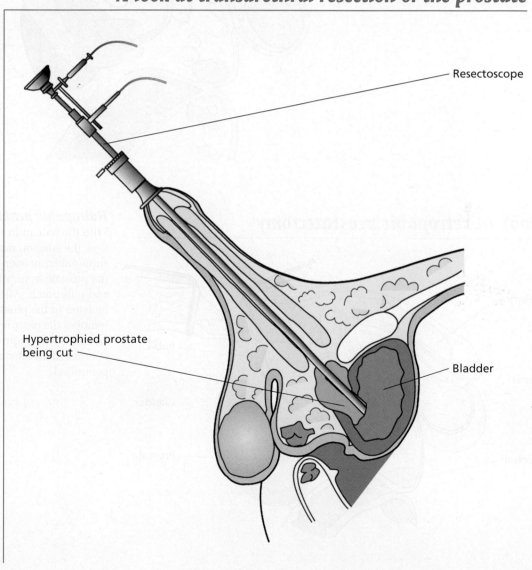

Resectoscope

Hypertrophied prostate being cut

Bladder

Suprapubic prostatectomy

With the patient in the supine position, the surgeon makes a horizontal incision above the pubic symphysis. He instills fluid into the bladder to distend it, makes a small incision in the bladder wall to expose the prostate, and shells out the obstructive prostatic tissue from the bed using his finger. Then he ligates bleeding points and usually inserts a suprapubic drainage tube and Penrose drain.

A look at suprapubic prostatectomy

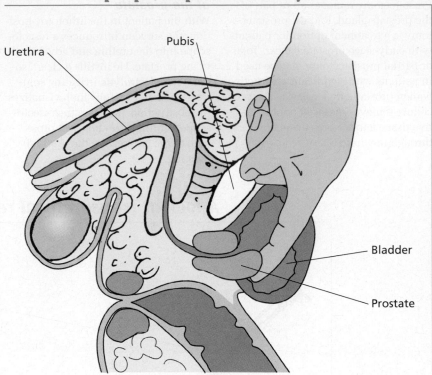

Urethra

Pubis

Bladder

Prostate

A look at retropubic prostatectomy

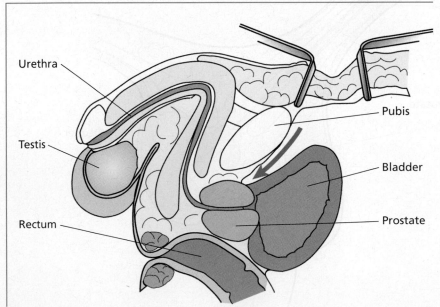

Urethra

Testis

Rectum

Pubis

Bladder

Prostate

Retropubic prostatectomy

With the patient in the supine position, the surgeon makes a horizontal suprapubic incision and approaches the prostate from between the bladder and pubic arch. After making another incision in the prostatic capsule, he removes the obstructive tissue. Usually, he inserts a suprapubic tube and Penrose drain after any bleeding is controlled.

Perineal prostatectomy

The patient is placed in an exaggerated lithotomy position with knees drawn up against the chest. The surgeon makes an inverted U-shaped incision in the perineum and removes the entire prostate and seminal vesicles. Then he anastomoses the urethra to the bladder and closes the incision, leaving a Penrose drain in place.

A look at perineal prostatectomy

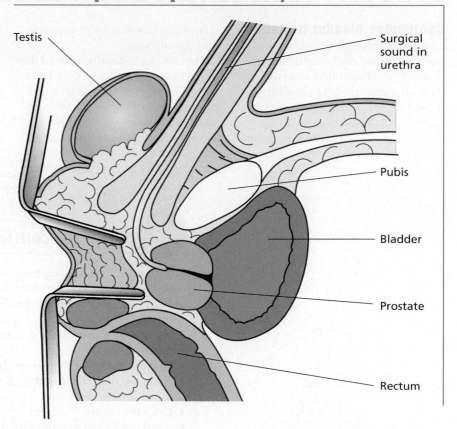

Testis

Surgical sound in urethra

Pubis

Bladder

Prostate

Rectum

ORCHIDECTOMY

A bilateral orchidectomy or removal of both testes is performed as palliative surgery and isn't meant to cure prostate cancer. The intent of the procedure is to stop cancer spread by decreasing testosterone.

Other treatments and procedures

Continuous bladder irrigation

Continuous bladder irrigation helps prevent urinary tract obstruction by flushing out small blood clots that form after prostate or bladder surgery. It can be used to treat an irritated, inflamed, or infected bladder lining. Continuous flow of irrigating solution through the bladder creates a mild tamponade that may help prevent venous hemorrhage.

The catheter is usually inserted during prostate or bladder surgery, but may be inserted at bedside for a nonsurgical patient. Use Y-type tubing to allow immediate irrigation with reserve solution. Large volumes of irrigating solution are usually required during the first 24 to 48 hours after surgery. Before starting, double-check the irrigating solution against the physician's order. If the solution contains an antibiotic, check the patient's chart to make sure he isn't allergic to the drug. The patient should remain on bed rest throughout continuous bladder irrigation, unless specified otherwise.

HANDS ON

 ## Setup for continuous bladder irrigation

After properly identifying the patient and gathering the equipment, follow these steps to perform continuous bladder irrigation.
▸ Insert the spike of the Y-type tubing into the container of irrigating solution.
▸ If you have a two-container system, insert one spike into each container.
▸ Squeeze the drip chamber on the spike of the tubing.
▸ Open the flow clamp and flush the tubing to remove air that could cause bladder distention.
▸ Close the clamp.
▸ Hang the bag of irrigating solution on the I.V. pole.
▸ Clean the opening to the inflow lumen of the catheter with the alcohol or povidone-iodine pad.
▸ Insert the distal end of the Y-type tubing securely into the inflow lumen (third port) of the catheter using sterile technique.
▸ Make sure the catheter's outflow lumen is securely attached to the drainage bag tubing.
▸ Open the flow clamp under the container of irrigating solution, and set the drip rate as ordered.
▸ To prevent air from entering the system, don't allow the primary container to empty completely before replacing it.
▸ If you have a two-container system, simultaneously close the flow clamp under the nearly empty container and open the flow clamp under the reserve container. This prevents reflux of irrigating solution from the reserve container into the nearly empty one.
▸ Hang a new reserve container on the I.V. pole, and insert the tubing, maintaining sterile technique.
▸ Empty the drainage bag about every 4 hours or as often as needed.
▸ Use sterile technique to avoid risk of contamination.
▸ Monitor vital signs at least every 4 hours during irrigation, increasing the frequency if the patient becomes unstable.

(continued)

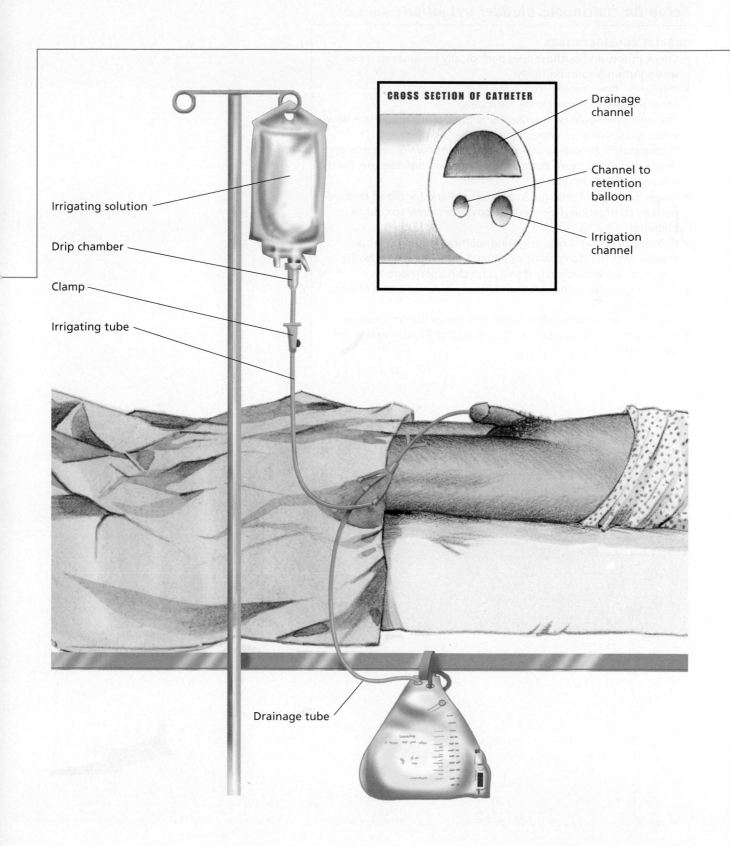

Irrigating solution

Drip chamber

Clamp

Irrigating tube

CROSS SECTION OF CATHETER

Drainage channel

Channel to retention balloon

Irrigation channel

Drainage tube

Setup for continuous bladder irrigation (continued)

Special considerations

▸ Check inflow and outflow lines periodically for kinks to make sure solution is running freely.

▸ If solution flows rapidly, check the lines frequently.

▸ Measure the outflow volume accurately.

▸ The outflow should be the same or slightly more than the inflow volume, allowing for urine production.

▸ Postoperative inflow volume exceeding outflow volume may indicate bladder rupture at the suture lines or renal damage; notify the physician immediately.

▸ Assess outflow for changes in appearance and for blood clots, especially if irrigation is being done postoperatively to control bleeding.

▸ If drainage is bright red, irrigating solution should be infused rapidly with the clamp wide open until drainage clears. Notify the physician immediately if you suspect hemorrhage.

▸ If drainage is clear, the solution is usually given at a rate of 40 to 60 drops/minute.

▸ The physician usually specifies the rate for antibiotic solutions.

▸ Encourage oral fluid intake of 2 to 3 qt (2 to 3 L)/day unless contraindicated.

Credits

Selected references

Index

Page 384: "Recognizing bullous impetigo." From Goodheart, H.P. (2003). *Goodheart's photoguide of common skin disorders* (2nd ed.). Philadelphia, PA: Lippincott Williams & Wilkins.

Page 387: "Looking at superficial spreading melanoma," "Looking at nodular malignant melanoma," "Looking at acral lentiginous melanoma," and "Looking at lentigo maligna melanoma." From Goodheart, H.P. (2003). *Goodheart's photoguide of common skin disorders* (2nd ed.) Philadelphia, PA: Lippincott Williams & Wilkins.

Page 389: "Looking at melasma." From Goodheart, H.P. (2003). *Goodheart's photoguide of common skin disorders* (2nd ed.). Philadelphia, PA: Lippincott Williams & Wilkins.

Pages 390 and 391: Photos from Nettina, S.M. (2001). *The Lippincott manual of nursing practice* (7th ed.). Philadelphia, PA: Lippincott Williams & Wilkins.

Page 396: "Looking at rosacea." From Goodheart, H.P. (2003). *Goodheart's photoguide of common skin disorders* (2nd ed.). Philadelphia, PA: Lippincott Williams & Wilkins.

Pages 403 and 404: "Looking at common and filiform warts," "Looking at periungual warts," "Looking at flat warts," "Looking at plantar warts," and "Looking at genital warts of the penis." From Goodheart, H.P. (2003). *Goodheart's photoguide of common skin disorders* (2nd ed.). Philadelphia, PA: Lippincott Williams & Wilkins.

Pages 410 and 411: "Looking at excision biopsy," "Looking at punch biopsy," and "Looking at shave biopsy." From Dircky, J.H. (Ed.). (2007). *Stedman's concise medical dictionary. Illustrated 4th edition*. Baltimore, MD: Lippincott Williams & Wilkins.

Chapter 11
Page 440: "Fibroids compressing the bladder and rectum." From Rubin, E., et al. (2005). *Rubin's pathology: Clinicopathologic foundations of medicine* (4th ed.). Philadelphia, PA: Lippincott Williams & Wilkins.

Chapter 12
Page 456: "Understanding epididymitis." From Weber, J., & Kelley, J. (2003). *Health assessment in nursing* (2nd ed.). Philadelphia, PA: Lippincott Williams & Wilkins.

Selected references

Anatomy & physiology made incredibly easy (3rd ed.). (2008). Philadelphia, PA: Lippincott Williams & Wilkins.

Asher, K., & Sachar, D. (2010). Ulcerative colitis practice guidelines in adults: American College of Gastroenterology, Practice Parameters Committee. *American Journal of Gastroenterology, 105,* 500.

Assessment made incredibly easy (6th ed.). (2008). Philadelphia, PA: Lippincott Williams & Wilkins.

Bass, N.M., et al. (2010). Rifaximin treatment in hepatic encephalopathy. *New England Journal of Medicine, 362*(12), 1071–1081.

Bingham, M., et al. (2010). Implementing a unit-level intervention to reduce the probability of ventilator-associated pneumonia. *Nursing Research, 59*(1, suppl.), S40–47.

Bornstein, S.R. (2009). Predisposing factors for adrenal insufficiency current concepts. *New England Journal of Medicine, 360*(22), 2328–2339.

Boyer, T., & Haskal, Z.J. (2010). AASLD practice guidelines: The role of transjugular intrahepatic portosystemic shunt (TIPS) in the management of portal hypertension. *Hepatology, 51*(1), 1–16.

Craven, R., & Hirnie, J. (2008). *Fundamentals of nursing* (6th ed.). Philadelphia, PA: Lippincott Williams & Wilkins.

Eron, L.J., & Steven, D.L. (2009). Cellulitis and soft tissue infections. *Annals of Internal Medicine, 150*(1), ITC1–1.

Funnell, M.M., et al. (2009). National standards for diabetes self-management education. *Diabetes Care, 32*(1), S87–96.

Ghany, M., et al. (2009). Diagnosis, management, and treatment of hepatitis C: An update. *Hepatology, 49,* 1335–1374.

Gibb, R.S., et al. (2008). *Danforth's obstetrics and gynecology* (10th ed.). Philadelphia, PA: Lippincott Williams & Wilkins.

Harris, H., et al. (2010). Understanding acute pancreatitis. *Nursing 2010 Critical Care, 5*(6), 29–33.

Hickey, J.V. (2008). *The clinical practice of neurological and neurosurgical nursing* (6th ed.). New York, NY: Lippincott Williams & Wilkins.

ICU/ER facts made incredibly quick. (2010). Philadelphia, PA: Lippincott Williams & Wilkins.

Jarvis, C. (2008). *Physical examination and health assessment* (5th ed.). Philadelphia, PA: Lippincott Williams & Wilkins.

Klippel, J.H., et al. (2008). *Primer on rheumatic diseases* (13th ed.). New York, NY: Springer.

Lee, K.S., et al. (2010). Symptom clusters in men and women with heart failure and their impact on cardiac event-free survival. *Journal of Cardiovascular Nursing, 25*(4), 263–272.

Littlejohn, L.R., & Bade, M.K. (2009). *AACN-AANN protocols for practice: Monitoring technologies in critically ill neuroscience patients.* Boston, MA: Jones & Bartlett.

McCance, K.L., et al. (Eds.). (2010). *Pathophysiology: The biologic basis for disease in adults and children* (6th ed.). St. Louis, MO: Mosby Elsevier.

Moss, L.E. (2010). Treatment of the burn patient in primary care. *Advances in Skin & Wound Care: The Journal for Prevention and Healing, 23*(11), 517–524.

Newell-Price, J. (2008). Cushing's syndrome. *Clinical Medicine, 8*(2), 204–209.

Nursing 2011 drug handbook (31st ed.). (2011). Philadelphia, PA: Lippincott Williams & Wilkins.

Oostema, J.A., & Ray, D.J. (2010). No clear winner among dressings for partial-thickness burns. *Annals of Emergency Medicine, 56*(3), 298–299.

Schorge, J.O., et al. (2008). *Williams gynecology.* New York, NY: McGraw-Hill Medical.

Smeltzer, S.C., Bare, B.G., & Hinkle, J.L. (2010). *Brunner & Suddarth's textbook of medical-surgical nursing* (12th ed., Vol. 1–2). Philadelphia, PA: Lippincott Williams & Wilkins.

Tofthagen, C., & McMillan, S. (2010). Pain, neuropathic symptoms, and physical and mental well-being in persons with cancer. *Cancer Nursing, 33*(6), 437–444.

Trigg, B.G., et al. (2008). Sexually transmitted infections and pelvic inflammatory disease in women. *Medical Clinics of North America, 92,* 1083.

Wecker, L. (Ed.). (2010). *Brody's human pharmacology* (5th ed.). Philadelphia, PA: Mosby Elsevier.

Wiegand, D.J. (2011). *AACN procedure manual for critical care* (6th ed.). St. Louis, MO: Elsevier/Saunders.

Index